As we have become accustomed to from Bob Flaws's publications, this book once again offers excellent help for daily practice. Bob's books make Chinese medicine digestible for Western readers. The biggest problem a Western physician faces when starting the practice of Chinese medicine is the need to accept the 'facts' of Chinese medicine and to be willing to integrate these into their Western medical practice. On the one hand, this book enables readers to interpret Western medical terms and diseases from a Chinese medical point of view. On the other, it forces Chinese medical aficionados to link their purely Chinese thoughts to the realities of Western biomedicine. The joining of Chinese and Western approaches offered in this book is to be called nothing less than excellent. . . . As a Western MD, I can say the Western medical information on diabetes contained in this book is reliable, comprehensive, and up-to-date. As a clinician practicing Chinese medicine on a day-to-day basis, I can also say it is an outstanding text on the Chinese medical view of diabetes. . . . In a nutshell, this book is a valuable contribution to the world's medical literature. Congratulations!"

—**Dieter Klein**, MD, acupuncturist, Germany

With diabetes being one of the leading causes of death and morbidity in the U.S., this book provides a long overdue addition to the library of the modern TCM practitioner. I was particularly pleased to read the section on the pathomechanisms of diabetes. Unlike basic sources that merely attribute DM to yin vacuity, this book lays out the clear relationship between spleen vacuity and damp heat as central factors in the pathogenesis of insulin resistance. In addition to extensive presentations of pattern discrimination for DM and all its complications, this book shines in its use of case studies and abstracts of numerous clinical audits. The section on diet is well researched and forms a critical subsection of this text that is often glossed over in other TCM presentations. The authors clearly recognize that only a combination of Eastern and Western medicines can truly be effective in treating this disorder. To that end, they have also included the latest research correlating a variety of physiological and biochemical parameters with the TCM patterns of DM. With doctoral studies about to be launched at TCM schools in the U.S., this book sets a new standard for an integrative approach to holistic medicine. I hope others will follow the lead of Blue Poppy in the development of TCM for the 21st century in America."

—**Todd Luger**, L.Ac.
Director, Chinese Herb Academy

This book is an excellent review of the approach to the treatment of diabetes mellitus from both a Chinese and Western medicine perspective. The review of current conventional integrative nutritional and lifestyle approaches is of value both to the conventional and alternative practitioner. The acupuncturist will find this an indispensable guide to the treatment of diabetes mellitus itself and its complications using acupuncture and Chinese herbal formulations. The information is also delivered along with numerous clinical cases which will enable the practitioner to correctly apply treatments in clinical situations. I highly recommend this book for every acupuncturist who deals with this metabolic disorder as well as other practitioners who are interested in the Chinese medicine approach to diabetes mellitus."

—**Leonard A. Wisneski**, M.D., F.A.C.P.
Endocrinology, Metabolism, and Medical Acupuncture
Clinical Professor of Medicine
The George Washington University Medical Center

This is an outstanding text! It contains clinical information on the Chinese medicine treatment of diabetes never before available in English combined with up-to-date biomedical information. Chinese language material is meticulously translated, and basic patterns are supplemented by formula analysis and clinical case studies. The book is well written and should prove invaluable to any practitioner of Chinese medicine. I applaud the efforts of all of the authors in completing such a text."

—**Marnae Ergil**, Ph.D.
Instructor, New York College for Wholistic Education & Research
Cotranslator, *Practical Diagnosis in Traditional Chinese Medicine*

The Treatment of Diabetes Mellitus with Chinese Medicine is impressive not only in the scope of its inquiry but in the depth of its detail. The heart of the text is a thorough discussion of diabetes and its associated conditions that is constructed in a unique and practical fashion. After a brief analysis of each condition in terms of Western medicine, the authors then provide the Chinese medical pattern differentiation and treatment. What sets this book apart, however, is the inclusion of a great deal of modern research and aptly chosen cases which illustrate the basic principles. This book is a valuable addition to the libraries of students, researchers, and clinicians alike."

—**Craig Mitchell**, M.S., Lic. Ac.
Cotranslator, *Shang Han Lun: On Cold Damage*

This book is an excellent representation of the latest evolution of TCM texts. It provides essential material for pattern differentiation and treatment strategy for patients with diabetes. All too often, we need to reference our TCM texts and then open our Western medicine texts to review allopathic approaches. In this book, diabetes is discussed from both medical paradigms, giving the practitioner a detailed understanding of the complex nature of this disease. Treatment protocols, strategies, and outcomes are outlined in a manner that enables the reader to manage this disease confidently and responsibly with Chinese medicine. The authors were meticulous in providing references to all formulas and research listed in this book, thereby, making it an invaluable resource book for all TCM practitioners."

—**John Stan**, DTCM, Reg. Ac., (Canada)
CEO, *Eastern Currents*

In 2001, Lynn Kuchinski's mother, June Kuchinski, passed away due to complications of diabetes. Therefore, Lynn would like to dedicate her portion of this book to her mother's memory.

For my mother, June
Love. Courage. Honor. Perseverance.

THE TREATMENT OF
DIABETES MELLITUS
WITH CHINESE MEDICINE

THE TREATMENT OF
DIABETES MELLITUS
WITH CHINESE MEDICINE

A TEXTBOOK
&
CLINICAL MANUAL

BY
BOB FLAWS
LYNN KUCHINSKI
& ROBERT J. CASAÑAS, MD

Published by:
BLUE POPPY PRESS
A Division of Blue Poppy Enterprises, Inc.
5441 Western Ave., Suite 2
Boulder, CO 80301
www.bluepoppy.com

First Edition, April 2002

ISBN 1-891845-21-7

Page design: Eric J. Brearton
Cover design: Frank Crawford

COMP Designation: Original work

10 9 8 7 6 5 4 3 2 1

Printed at Thomson-Shore, Inc., Dexter, MI

Library of Congress Cataloging-in-Publication Data

Flaws, Bob, 1946-
   The treatment of diabetes mellitus with Chinese medicine / by Bob Flaws, Lynn
Kuchinski & Robert Casañas.
     p. ; cm.
   Includes bibliographal references and index.
   ISBN 1-891845-21-7
   1. Diabetes–Alternative treatment. 2. Medicine, Chinese. I. Kuchinski, Lynn M. II.
Casañas, Robert, 1949- III. Title.
   [DNLM: 1. Diabetes Mellitus–therapy. 2. Medicine, Chinese Traditional. WK 815
F591t 2001]
   RC661. A47 F56 2001
   616.4'6206–dc21
                                                      2001056706

PREFACE

This book is a clinical manual on the Chinese medical treatment of diabetes mellitus (DM) and its many complications. The Chinese medical materials have been compiled by myself and Lynn Kuchinski. The Western medicine materials have been written, checked, and/or edited by Robert Casañas, MD. This book has been patterned after Blue Poppy Press's critically acclaimed *Chinese Medical Psychiatry*. Each Western medical condition contained herein is discussed in terms of its Western medical definition, epidemiology, etiology, pathophysiology, diagnosis, current standards of care, and prognosis. These Western medical sections are then followed by Chinese medical sections describing disease categorization, disease causes and mechanisms, treatment based on pattern discrimination (both acupuncture and Chinese medicinal), abstracts of representative Chinese research, representative Chinese case histories, and a concluding "Remarks" section discussing clinical tips and concerns. Other sections in this book describe the history of diabetes in both Western and Chinese medicines, Chinese materia medica and DM, Chinese formulas and DM, acupuncture, tuina, and Chinese foot relexology and DM, exercise and qigong and DM, and Western and Chinese dietary therapies and DM as well as discussions on the integration of Chinese and Western medicines, syndrome X, and dealing with such issues as patient adherence and denial. At the back of this book, the reader will find a glossary of Western medical terms pertaining to diabetes and its Western medical diagnosis and treatment. The reader will also find the most extensive Chinese medical bibliography on DM of which we are aware. However, even this extensive bibliography is only a fraction of what exists on the Chinese medical treatment of DM within the Chinese language literature. The books and articles in this bibliography only represent those which reside in my and Lynn Kuchinski's personal libraries and, as such, are random in their representation. By this I mean that they are only those articles which happened to appear in the handful of Chinese medical journals to which we individually subscribe. Nevertheless, as the reader hopefully will see through the copious reports of Chinese research and case histories included herein, Chinese medicine can be an effective complement and alternative to modern Western medicine in the prevention and treatment of this increasingly prevalent disease.

As with other Blue Poppy Press publications, the Chinese medical terminology used in this book is based on Nigel Wiseman and Feng Ye's *A Practical Dictionary of Chinese Medicine*, Paradigm Publications, Brookline, MA, 1998. Deviations from that norm are noted in the text or by endnotes the first time such deviations occur. Chinese medicinals are identified first by Latin pharmacological nomenclature followed by Pinyin romanization of their standard Chinese name in parentheses the first time they are introduced in a given section. In subsequent discussions in the same section, those medicinals are only identified by their Chinese names. Chinese formulas are identified by their Chinese names in Pinyin romanization followed by our denotative translation of those names in parentheses. Acupuncture points are identified first by their standard Chinese names in Pinyin romanization followed by standard channel abbreviation and number notation. In terms of acupuncture channel abbreviations, Blue Poppy Press uses Lu for lung, LI for large intestine, St for stomach, Sp for spleen, Ht for heart, SI for small intestine, Bl for bladder, Ki for kidney, Per for pericardium, TB for triple burner, GB for gallbladder, Liv for liver, CV for conception vessel, and GV for governing vessel, and we use O'Connor and Bensky's numbering system as it appears in *Acupuncture: A Comprehensive Text*, Eastland Press,

Seattle, 1995, for the alpha-numerical identification of extra-channel points.

We hope this book will be of great benefit to English-speaking practitioners of Chinese medicine and all of their patients suffering from diabetes and its myriad of complications. In order to continually expand, refine, and advance the materials included herein, Blue Poppy Press has created a companion web site located at www.chinesemedicaldiabetes.com. Laypersons suffering from dia-

betes who wish to learn more about Chinese medicine and what it may offer them should see Lynn Kuchinski's *Controlling Diabetes Naturally with Chinese Medicine* also available from Blue Poppy Press. The authors would sincerely appreciate any feedback on or amendments and corrections to this work.

Bob Flaws
Dec. 6, 2001

TABLE OF CONTENTS

1

DIABETES MELLITUS & WESTERN MEDICINE

DEFINITION

Diabetes mellitus (DM) is a group of metabolic diseases characterized by high levels of blood glucose resulting from defects in insulin secretion, insulin action, or both. It is by far the most commonly occurring disorder of the endocrine system in all populations and in all age groups.[1]

HISTORY

The earliest surviving description of diabetes mellitus comes from the *Ebers Papyrus* which is believed to have been written by the Egyptian physician Hesi Ra around 1550 BCE. This papyrus contains descriptions of a number of diseases and their treatments. One of the descriptions so closely resembles diabetes that it is highly unlikely the author could have been referring to anything else. Hesi Ra recommended a liquid decoction made from animal, mineral, and vegetable medicinals.

One thousand years later, physicians in India developed the first recorded clinical test for diabetes. They observed that flies and ants were attracted to the sweet tasting urine of people afflicted with certain diseases. Susruta, the father of Ayurvedic medicine, accurately described these diseases, including diabetes, around 500-600 BCE. In the second century CE, Charaka, another famous Ayurvedic practitioner, was the first to discern a difference between two groups of diabetics. He noted the difference between thin people who develop this disease at a young age and obese people who develop diabetes at an older age. He also noted that the older, heavier group seemed to live longer. This method of classifying patients with diabetes remains with us today. We now refer to the first group as type 1 and the second group as type 2 diabetes.

Around 230 BCE, Paul of Aegina described *dypsacus* (a term referring to the tremendous thirst experienced by those with diabetes) as a weakness of the kidneys combined with excessive dampness produced by the body. Paul recommended that the early stages of this condition be treated with a liquid decoction of potherbs, endive, lettuce, rock-fish, the juice of knotgrass, and elecampane in dark wine with dates and myrtle. For those with more advanced disease, he suggested the application of compresses to the hypochondrium over the kidneys made of vinegar, rose oil, and navelwort. In addition, Paul also suggested the use of bleeding. The name "diabetes" was coined by the Greco-Roman physician, Aretaeus of Cappadoccia between 30-90 CE. Diabetes means a "siphon" or "to run through." This refers to the chronic polyuria which is characteristic of this disease. Although many authors from the 15th century BCE to the second century CE described conditions characterized by polyuria, few recognized the difference between those with diabetes and people afflicted with other causes of polyuria. Demetris of Apamea was one of the first to discern a difference between diabetes and other causes of polyuria, and it was Aretaeus, mentioned above, who first distinguished between diabetes mellitus and diabetes insipidus. The Roman physician, Galen (131-201 CE), wrote that, at least in his time, diabetes was a rare affliction. It would appear that Galen encountered only two cases during his entire career. Twentieth century researchers would later use these observations as evidence that the incidence of diabetes has steadily risen since ancient times. Galen, unlike Aretaeus, labeled the condition *diarrhea urinosa* and *dipsakos*, referring to the excessive urine production and thirst experienced by diabetics.

During the 9-11th centuries CE, Greco-Roman medicine

was carried on by the Arabs as Unani medicine. However, Unani medicine is not just Greco-Roman medicine but contains a large admixture of Ayurvedic and Chinese medicines. For instance, the Arab writer Rhazea (865-925 CE) translated the Sanskrit writings on diabetes into Arabic. One of the greatest of these Arab doctors, Abu Ali al-Hussain ibn Abdallah ibn Sina (Avicenna, 960-1037 CE), published a monumental medical encyclopedia titled *Qaanun fi al-Tibb* (*The Canons of Medicine*) that accurately described the clinical features of diabetes as well as several of its complications, including gangrene and loss of sexual function. His recommended treatment included lupin, fenugreek, and zedoary seeds.

During the 10-15th centuries, despite occasional insightful observations, little progress was made in the Western diagnosis or treatment of diabetes. It was not until European medical science began to progress in the 16th century that real progress in the recognition, understanding, and treatment of diabetes was made. European medical scientists rediscovered what Eastern medical science had observed during the previous thousand years and carried their observations further. During the 16th century, European physicians advanced uroscopy or inspection of the urine to a high art. Bombastus von Hohenheim, a Swiss physician better known to history as Paracelsus, observed that a white powder was left when the urine of a person with diabetes was allowed to evaporate. He concluded, incorrectly, that this residue was salt. According to Paracelsus, this salt caused the kidneys to develop excessive thirst and produce excessive urine. In Italy, Cardona (1501-1576 CE) observed that those with diabetes seemed to put out more fluid than they took in. However, he was unable to explain this observation.

In 1684, Thomas Willis in London stressed that the urine in patients with this condition is "wonderfully sweet as if imbued with honey or sugar."[2] In addition, he surmised, quite correctly, that the incidence of diabetes had risen since ancient times because of excessive consumption of food and wine. Thomas Sydenham (1624-1689), a contemporary of Thomas Willis, came close to the modern explanation of diabetes when he hypothesized that diabetes is a systemic disease caused by the incomplete digestion of chyle. He further speculated that the increased urine production associated with diabetes is related to the excretion of the incompletely digested and non-absorbable chyle. In 1776, Matthew Dobson was the first to show conclusively that the urine of those with diabetes does, in fact, contain sugar. Thus the association between this disease and a disturbance of carbohydrate metabolism became apparent. Several years later, another British physician, John Rollo, was the first to add the adjective

mellitus to diabetes when he published a paper titled, "An Account of Two Cases of Diabetes Mellitus." Rollo applied the name mellitus, derived from the Greek and Latin for honey, to distinguish diabetes mellitus from other causes of polyuria in which the urine has no sweet taste. He termed the other causes of polyuria "diabetes insipidus" (from the Latin for tasteless), a term still used today. Rollo treated patients with diabetes mellitus with a high protein, low carbohydrate diet and compounds that would suppress the appetite, such as antimony, digitalis, and opium. In 1788, Thomas Cawley published a paper relating this disease to a disorder of the pancreas. Cawley observed the development of diabetes in people who had sustained injury to the pancreas.

In 1869, a German medical student, Paul Langerhans, published a paper identifying two types of cells in the pancreas, one which secreted normal pancreatic juices and the other whose functions were unknown. Several years later, these cells came to be known as the islets of Langerhans. In 1889, Joseph von Mering and Oskar Minkowski showed that removal of the pancreas from dogs led to a condition resembling diabetes with its characteristic rise in blood glucose and the appearance of glucose and ketones in the urine. At the turn of the century, Eugene L. Opie of the Johns Hopkins University School of Medicine and others were convinced that the islets of Langerhans functioned as an endocrine gland. However, after years of searching, they failed to isolate the active principle. In 1908, the German scientist, Georg Zuelzer created the first injectible insulin extract to suppress glycosuria. However, it caused far too many side effects. Thus, up until 1910, opium was the only widely used medicine in the Western medical treatment of diabetes. However, this only dulled the patients' despair. It did nothing to cure or treat.[3]

From 1910-1920, Frederick Madison Allen and Elliot P. Joslin were the two leading diabetes specialists in the United States. Joslin believed diabetes was "the best of the chronic diseases" because it was "clean, seldom unsightly, not contagious, often painless and susceptible to treatment."[4] In 1913, Allen published *Studies Concerning Glycosuria and Diabetes*, a book which is significant for the revolution in diabetes therapy that developed from it. In 1919, Frederick Allen published *Total Dietary Regulation in the Treatment of Diabetes*, citing exhaustive case records of 76 of the 100 diabetes patients he observed, and became the director of diabetes research at the Rockefeller Institute. Also in 1919, Allen established the first clinic in the U.S. to treat patients with diabetes, hypertension, and Bright's disease, and wealthy and desperate patients flocked to it.

On Oct. 31, 1920, Dr. Frederick Banting conceived of the idea of insulin after reading Moses Barron's "The Relation of the Islets of Langerhans to Diabetes with Special Reference to Cases of Pancreatic Lithiasis" in the November issue of *Surgery, Gynecology and Obstetrics*. For the next year, with the assistance of Charles Best, James Collip, and J.J.R. Macleod, Dr. Banting continued his research using a variety of different extracts on depancreatized dogs. In 1921, Banting and Best showed that a substance extracted from the pancreas could lower blood glucose in dogs. This substance was the protein insulin, and soon therafter insulin was being used to treat diabetes mellitus in humans. The first human to receive a dose of insulin was the 14 year-old, Leonard Thompson, on Jan. 11, 1922.[5] On May 30, 1922, Eli Lilly and Company and the University of Torontoagreed to a contract for the mass production of insulin in North America. On Oct. 23, 1923, Dr. Banting and his colleague, Prof. Macleod, were awarded the Nobel Prize in Physiology of Medicine. Dr. Banting shared his award with Best, and Prof. Macleod shared his award with Dr. Collip.

Protamine zinc insulin was introduced in the 1930s. During the 1940s, the link was made between diabetes and such long-term complications as nephropathy and retinopathy. In 1944, the standard insulin syringe was developed, helping to make diabetes management more uniform. The lente series of insulins were introduced during the 1950s, and oral drugs were introduced to help lower glycemic levels in 1955. Also in 1955, Dr. Frederick Sanger determined the complete amino acid sequence of this polypeptide, for which he was awarded the Nobel Prize in 1958. In 1960, home testing of blood glucose was developed to improve glycemic control. In 1966, the first pancreas transplant in humans was performed. Since then, 11,000 pancreas transplants have been performed worldwide, with 1,000 new transplants per year.[6] In 1969, Donald F. Steiner showed that insulin is actually synthesized as a larger precursor molecule, proinsulin.[7] Insulin meters and the insulin pump were developed in 1970, and laser surgery was introduced to treat diabetic retinopathy. Advances in chromotography in the 1960s and 70s led to even more highly purified insulins. In 1983, due to recombinant DNA technology, biosynthetic insulin was introduced. In fact, biosynthetic insulin was the first medication created through such recombinant DNA technology. More recently, DNA technology has led to the ability to synthesize insulin analogs. To date, more than 300 insulin analogs have been produced.

While the purity of insulin has increased and the needle size for injections has decreased, thus reducing the discomfort associated with subcutaneous insulin injections, no method of insulin delivery other than injection is currently available. Therefore, research, including clinical trials, is currently underway to develop nasal inhalant insulin. Research is also underway to develop orally administered insulin. Preclinical studies conducted by Unigene Laboratories, Inc. of Fairfield, NJ, have shown successful oral delivery of insulin.[8] Other recent developments include the use of combination therapy wherein two or more antidiabetic drugs are used in tandem to achieve a better, more complete therapeutic effect,[9] islet cell transplantation, noninvasive glucose meters and blood analyzers, and humanized, engineered monoclonal antibodies to suppress the immune system in those with type 1 diabetes.

EPIDEMIOLOGY

According to the U.S. Center for Disease Control (CDC), currently 15.7 million Americans have diabetes. This is 5.9% of the total U.S. population, and 10.3 million of these people have actually been diagnosed with this disease.[10] This means that 5.4 million other Americans suffer from insulin resistance or glucose intolerance but do not know they have this condition. Seven hundred ninety-eight thousand new cases of diabetes are diagnosed each year in the U.S. The majority of these individuals (90%) have type 2 or non-insulin dependent diabetes mellitus) (NIDDM), while 10% (1,600,000) have type 1 or insulin dependent diabetes mellitus) (IDDM).[11] Six point three million of these cases are 65 years old or older. In fact, 18.4% of all people in this age group in the U.S. have diabetes. Only 123,000 Americans under the age of 20 have diabetes or 0.16% of all people in this age group. In terms of sex, in those with diabetes over 20 years of age, 7.5 million are men and 8.1 million are women. In terms of ethnicity, there are 11.2 million non-Hispanic white Americans with diabetes, 2.3 million non-Hispanic blacks, and 1.2 million Mexican Americans with diabetes. Other Hispanic/Latino Americans on average are almost twice as likely to have diabetes than non-Hispanic whites of the same age. Nine percent of Native Americans have been diagnosed with diabetes. On average, Native Americans are 2.8 times as likely to have been diagnosed with diabetes as non-Hispanic whites of similar age. Although prevalence data for Asian Americans and Pacific Islanders are limited, some groups within this segment of the population are at increased risk for diabetes. For instance, data suggests that Native Hawaiians are twice as likely to have been diagnosed with diabetes as white residents of Hawaii.[12] Fifty percent of males and 70% of females with type 2 DM are obese,[13] 90% are overweight,[14] and there is a strong familial susceptibility to this condition.[15] One third of all those with diabetes smoke, one half have elevated cholesterol, half have a sedentary lifestyle, and one quarter are hypertensive.[16] The number of individuals with diabetes is currently doubling every 15 years.[17] At current rates, diabetes mellitus will affect 239 million patients worldwide in 2010.[18]

MORTALITY

Based on death certificate data, diabetes contributed to 193,140 deaths in the U.S. in 1996.[19] This made it the seventh leading cause of death listed on death certificates in America that year. However, diabetes is believed to be under-reported on death certificates both as a condition and a cause of death. The death rate in middle-aged adults for those with diabetes is twice as high as that among those without diabetes.[20] Life expectancy is eight years less than average for those diagnosed with type 2 DM before 40 years of age,[21] and mortality increases in persons with type 2 diabetes with age.[22] The younger the age of development, the greater the risk of excess mortality. Excess mortality is also greater in those using insulin and for women with DM.[23] The three leading causes of mortality for those with diabetes are:

1. Cardiovascular disease
2. Malignant neoplasms
3. Cerebrovascular disease

Ischemic heart disease accounts for 40% of deaths in those with diabetes.[24]

COSTS

The total direct and indirect costs of diabetes mellitus in the U.S. in 1997 were calculated to be $100 billion. Of this, direct medical costs were $44 billion, and indirect costs, such as disability, work loss, and premature mortality, were $54 billion.[25] In a recent study, it was found that the typical oral antidiabetic medication costs patients in the U.S. $1,700 per year. In addition, 90% of U.S. endocrinologists prescribe three or more such medications in combination for patients with type 2 DM.[26]

NOSOLOGY

There are three main types of diabetes mellitus: type 1, type 2, and gestational.

TYPE 1 DIABETES

In type 1 or insulin dependent diabetes (IDDM), the pancreas produces little or no insulin. This type of diabetes is considered an autoimmune disease. It has formerly been called juvenile diabetes, juvenile onset diabetes (JOD), ketosis-prone diabetes, and brittle diabetes. Insulin therapy is required with this form of diabetes. Although type 1 DM may occur at any age, it most commonly develops in childhood or adolescence and is the predominant type of diabetes diagnosed before age 30. Classic symptoms of type 1 diabetes include:

> increased thirst
> increased urination
> hunger
> rapid weight loss
> vision changes
> fatigue

If type 1 diabetes is left untreated, individuals can succumb to diabetic ketoacidosis which can lead to coma or even death.

TYPE 2 DIABETES

In type 2 diabetes or non-insulin dependent diabetes (NIDDM), the pancreas still produces insulin. The problem is that the insulin receptor cells do not respond to this insulin, thus causing improper hepatic glucose metabolism. This is referred to as insulin resistance. In this condition, the pancreas actually produces more insulin in an attempt to decrease elevated blood glucose. However, the cells are unable to respond, and so the blood glucose remains high. Over time, this elevated blood glucose damages the body through the accumulation of sorbitol and glycation proteins, producing symptoms including:

> fatigue
> general malaise
> nocturia
> constant thirst
> slow, unintentional weight loss
> vision changes, such as blurring or poor focusing
> decreased immunity
> slow healing ability from cuts or wounds

Left untreated, the damage from type 2 diabetes can be irreversible, leading to chronic health problems, such as renal failure, blindness, and vascular compromise. Other names for type 2 diabetes are adult or maturity onset diabetes (MOD) and ketosis-resistant diabetes. This is the most common type of diabetes diagnosed in those over 30 years of age. However, it may occur in children and adolescents, in which case it is referred to as maturity onset diabetes in the young (MODY). Although most patients are treated with diet, exercise, and oral drugs, some patients may intermittently or persistently require insulin to control symptomatic hyperglycemia and prevent non-ketotic hyperglycemic-hyperosmolar coma (NKHHC).

GESTATIONAL DIABETES

Gestational diabetes (GDM) refers to diabetes diagnosed during pregnancy. Gestational diabetes occurs in 2-5% of all pregnant women. Although this type of diabetes may spontaneously remit after delivery, if left untreated during pregnancy, it may lead to fetal death or miscarriage. It may also predispose both the mother and child to develop type 2 diabetes later on in life. A separate chapter on gestational diabetes is included below.

OTHER TYPES OF DIABETES MELLITUS

Secondary diabetes refers to the development of diabetes as a consequence of some other disease process, such as pancreatic disease, other endocrine disorders, drug or chemical-induced diabetes, insulin or its receptor abnormalities, and certain genetic syndromes, such as Bloom syndrome. There is also malnutrition-related diabetes (also called tropical diabetes), pancreatic diabetes, and ketosis-resistant diabetes of the young. Secondary and other specific types of diabetes account for only 1-2% of all DM.[27]

ETIOLOGY & PATHOPHYSIOLOGY

TYPE 1 DIABETES

In people with type 1 diabetes, the immune system mistakenly destroys more than 90% of the insulin-secreting beta cells in the pancreas, treating them as if they were a foreign invader. Cell-mediated immune mechanisms are believed to play the major role in this beta cell destruction. Other factors which may trigger or are associated with this autoimmune response are genetics, viruses, cow's milk, and oxygen free radicals. Researchers have identified several different genes that might make a person more likely to develop type 1 DM. However, they have not found one single gene which makes all people who inherit it develop this disease. Hence, one can only speak of a type 1 genetic susceptibility. In white populations, a strong association exists between type 1 DM diagnosed before age 30 and specific HLA-D phenotypes HLA-DR3, HLA-DR4, and HLA-DR3/DR4.[28] Of people newly diagnosed with type 1 diabetes, 70-80% have antibodies to their islet cells, 30-50% have antibodies to insulin, and 80-95% have antibodies to glutamic acid decarboxylase (GAD), a protein made by the beta cells in the pancreas.[29] Infection by the Coxsackie B4 virus may play a

role in the development of type 1 diabetes by provoking the production of autoantibodies to GAD, since a small region of the GAD molecule is almost identical to a region of a protein found in that virus. As for cow's milk, one group of researchers found a connection between ingestion of cow's milk before 3-4 months of age and development of type 1 DM. However, cow's milk is only one kind of food that may play a role in the development of type 1 DM. Studies in diabetes-prone rats show that withholding wheat and soy helps delay or prevent diabetes.[30] Oxygen free radicals are formed as a by-product of many chemical reactions in the body. These free radicals destroy the body's own cells, and islet cells have very low levels of the enzymes that break down such free radicals. Therefore, agents which increase free radical production, such as smoke, air pollution, and diet may result in destruction of pancreatic cells. In addition, several chemicals have been shown to trigger type 1 diabetes, such as pyriminil, a rat poison, and two prescription drugs, pentamidine and L-asparaginase. Other chemicals have been shown to induce diabetes in animals, but current data does not support extrapolation to humans. Geography may also play a role in the development of type 1 diabetes since the incidence of this condition is especially high in Finland and Sardinia.[31]

RISK FACTORS FOR TYPE 1 DIABETES

- Family history of diabetes, thyroid disease, or other endocrinopathies

- Family history of autoimmune disease, such as Hashimoto's thyroiditis, Grave's disease, myasthenia gravis, or pernicious anemia

- Cow's milk consumption in infancy

TYPE 2 DIABETES

The link to a genetic etiology is even stronger in type 2 diabetes than in type 1. The concordance rate for type 2 DM in monozygotic twins (*i.e.*, "identical" twins) is more than 90%. As described above, it is also a fact that, compared to white Americans, African Americans, Asian Americans, Hispanic Americans (excluding Cuban Americans), and Native Americans (especially Pima Indians) are all afflicted with type 2 diabetes more often. Similar to the situation in type 1 DM, rather than being a single "diabetes gene," there seems to be an even greater genetic susceptibility that includes errors on several genes. In this case, genetically determined post-insulin receptor intracellular defects lead to insulin resistance and hyperinsulinemia. In other words, in type 2 DM, there is an impaired insulin secretory response to glucose and decreased insulin effectiveness in stimulating glucose uptake by skeletal muscles and in restraining hepatic glucose production. The resulting hyperinsulinemia then leads to other common conditions, such as obesity (especially abdominal obesity), hypertension, dyslipidemia, and coronary artery disease. This constellation of five abnormalities is referred to as insulin resistance syndrome, Kaplan's syndrome, or syndrome X.

However, most persons with insulin resistance do not develop type 2 diabetes. In those people with insulin resistance who do not develop diabetes, the body compensates by adequately increasing insulin secretion in order to "push" the glucose into the cells. Since not all patients with insulin resistance develop diabetes, there must be other factors which account for this difference. These other factors in the development of type 2 diabetes are obesity, age, and lifestyle. Although some researchers believe insulin resistance leads to obesity, it also appears that obesity is the single most important trigger of type 2 DM. People with central body obesity (which means carrying too much fat above the hips) have a higher risk of developing type 2 DM than those with excess fat on the hips and thighs. It is also possible that the links between age and a sedentary lifestyle and type 2 diabetes actually have to do with obesity. People typically gain weight as they age, and a sedentary lifestyle leads to reduced burning of calories and subsequent obesity. However, there may also be other age-related changes in body composition which trigger or aggravate diabetes. Likewise, eating a high fat, high calorie diet leads to obesity which may then lead to type 2 diabetes.

Some researchers think that chronic viral infection may also play a part in initiating type 2 diabetes. Implicated viruses, include the almost ubiquitous herpes-type viruses such as cytomegalovirus (CMV) and human herpes viruses six (HHV6) and seven (HHV7). These viruses may remain dormant within the body for years or even decades but then become active due to aging, illness, stress, or poor diet.[32] Recent research into two markers of systemic inflammation, C-reactive protein and interleukin 6, suggest that the development of type 2 diabetes may be associated with systemic inflammation.[33]

In addition, researchers have shown that adults who get less than 6.5 hours of sleep per night have a 40% lower insulin sensitivity than those who get closer to a full eight hours of sleep per night. These researchers found that sleep curtailment in otherwise healthy young adults

---

RISK FACTORS FOR TYPE 2 DIABETES

- **Obesity and age over 40 years**

- **Family history of diabetes, thyroid disease, or other endocrinopathies**

- **Sedentary lifestyle with a high fat, high calorie diet**

- **African American, Hispanic, Native American, Asian American, or Pacific Islander**

---

impairs the ability of insulin to do its job properly. Interestingly, it may also cause or contribute to high blood pressure, abnormal lipid levels, and obesity.[34]

PREVENTION

Maintaining ideal body weight and an active lifestyle in individuals at risk may prevent the onset of type 2 diabetes. Currently there is no way to prevent type 1 diabetes.[35]

SIGNS & SYMPTOMS

Diabetes mellitus may present initially in a number of different ways. Type 1 DM usually presents with symptomatic hyperglycemia or diabetic ketoacidosis (DKA). Symptomatic hyperglycemia is characterized by polyuria followed by polydipsia and weight loss. Type 2 DM patients may present with symptomatic hyperglycemia or rarely with NKHHC. However, type 2 diabetes is frequently diagnosed in asymptomatic patients during routine medical examination or blood tests or when patients present with clinical manifestations of a late stage complication. Late stage complications are discussed below.

DIFFERENTIAL DIAGNOSIS

Diabetes mellitus must be differentiated from the following conditions which may present similar signs and symptoms. In the case of polydipsia, one must first rule out that this is due to medication side effect, psychogenic factors, or diabetes insipidus. For instance, many Western drugs cause oral dryness resulting in increased drinking. In the case of polyuria, one must rule out spastic bladder, urinary tract infection, hypercalcemia, medication side effect, renal wasting, and urologic or prostate conditions. For instance, benign prostatic hypertrophy and chronic prostatitis both cause frequent urination. Blurred vision may be due to myopia or presbyopia, while fatigue or weakness may be due to thyroid disorder, cardiovascular disease, pulmonary disease, autoimmune disease, anemia, adrenal insufficiency, or depression. And pruritus may be due to allergy, lymphoma, polycythemia, or renal failure. In addition, one must also rule out Cushing's disease and corticosteroid use.

DIFFERENTIAL DIAGNOSIS

- **Polydipsia: Medication side effect, psychogenic factors, diabetes insipidus**

- **Polyuria: Hypercalcemia, medication side effect, renal wasting, urologic or prostate conditions**

- **Blurred vision: Myopia, presbyopia, cataracts, macular degeneration, hypoglycemia, etc.**

- **Fatigue &/or weakness: Thyroid disorder, anemia, adrenal insufficiency, depression, etc.**

- **Pruritus: Allergy, renal failure, lymphoma, polycythemia**

- **Cushing's disease**

- **Corticosteroid use**

DIAGNOSIS

PHYSICAL EXAMINATION

Physical examination may reveal "stocking glove" neuropathy, cataracts, central obesity, acanthosis nigricans, carpal tunnel syndrome, mucocutaneous candidiasis, foot ulceration, elevated blood glucose levels with weight loss, decreased blood pressure, nonhealing wounds (especially on the extremities), recurrent cutaneous infections, retinal abnormalities or cataract formation, carotid bruits, abdominal tenderness, fatty liver, dry skin, hair loss over the lower leg and foot, and/or coolness of the extremities.

SYMPTOMS

The patient may present with fatigue, lethargy, poor concentration, and atypical thirst for liquids.

LABORATORY TESTS

The following laboratory test vales are those promulgated by the American Diabetes Association. These are somewhat more stringent than those of the National Diabetes Data Group (NDDG) and World Health Organization (WHO).

Two or more fasting blood glucose (FBG) levels over 126mg/dL (>6.99mmol/L)
(FBG between 111-125mg/dL = glucose intolerance)

Random, *i.e.*, non-fasting, blood glucose over 200mg/dL (>11.1mmol/L) plus other signs and symptoms

Oral glucose tolerance test (OGTT) over 200mg/dL (>11.1mmol/L)
(OGTT between 140-199mg/dL = glucose intolerance)

An oral glucose tolerance test may be helpful in diagnosing type 2 diabetes in those whose FBG is between 115-140mg/dL (6.38-7.77mmol/L). However, other conditions than DM can cause abnormalities in OGTT, such as the effects of drugs and normal aging, and not all patients with an abnormal OGTT will develop diabetes.

However, only half of adults with type 2 DM are symptomatic at the time of diagnosis, and only approximately 25% of previously undiagnosed adults with type 2 have a FBG equal to or over 140mg/dL.[36]

TREATMENT

GOALS OF TREATMENT

The goals of treatment with Western medicine are to relieve the patient's symptoms, improve their quality of life, prevent acute and chronic complications associated with diabetes, and correct metabolic abnormalities if that can be done safely.[37]

GENERAL CONSIDERATIONS

The Diabetes Control & Complications Trial (DCCT) has proven that hyperglycemia is responsible for most of the long-term microvascular complications of DM. This study has demonstrated that there is a linear relationship between levels of glycosylated hemoglobin (HbA1c) and the rate at which these complications develop.[38] Therefore, therapy for type 1 DM is aimed at metabolic control to lower levels of HbA1c while avoiding hypoglycemic episodes. This means that treatment must be individualized and modified when circumstances make any risk of hypoglycemia unacceptable, such as in those with short life expectancy or in those with cerebrovascular and/or cardiac disease.

DIET & EXERCISE

Diet and exercise to achieve weight reduction are the first

and most important management strategies in overweight patients with type 2 DM. If improvement in hyperglycemia is not achieved by diet and exercise, then trial treatment with one or more oral antidiabetic drugs is typically initiated. A separate chapter is devoted to dietary therapy for diabetes below.

PATIENT EDUCATION

Patient education is recognized as one of the pillars of the Western medical treatment of diabetes. It is regarded as essential to ensure the effectiveness of the prescribed therapy, to help the patient recognize the indications for seeking immediate medical attention, and to ensure appropriate foot care. On each physician visit, the patient is checked for signs and symptoms of complications. In addition, routine periodic laboratory evaluation includes lipid profile, blood urea nitrogen (BUN) and serum creatinine levels, ECG, and annual complete ophthalmologic examination.

BLOOD GLUCOSE MONITORING

Patients are taught how to monitor their own blood glucose levels, and patients being treated with insulin are taught to adjust their insulin doses accordingly. At least quarterly, HbA1c is checked to estimate blood glucose control over the preceding 1-3 months.

URINE KETONE MONITORING

Patients with type 1 DM are taught how to monitor their own urine for ketones and are advised to implement this test whenever they develop symptoms of a cold, flu, or other concurrent illness, nausea, vomiting, or abdominal pain, polyuria, or whenever their blood glucose levels are unexpectedly high.

DRUG THERAPIES

Western medications for diabetes mellitus are of two main types: insulin and oral antidiabetic drugs.

INSULIN

Insulin is used for type 1 and occasionally for type 2 diabetes (30-40%).[39] Because it is a polypeptide, it cannot be administered orally since it would be destroyed in the gastrointestinal tract. Therefore, insulin is injected subcutaneously, with the dose and type individualized for the patient's condition. Although it cannot be taken orally, a nasal inhalant form is currently under development. There are long-acting, intermediate-acting and short or rapid acting forms of insulin (the latter taken at meals) in order to stabilize glucose levels. Most patients with no endogenous insulin production inject themselves up to four times per day, with the dose of each injection dependent on the pattern of their glucose self-monitoring. Those with some pancreatic function may only require one injection per day. However, it is preferable to use split doses in type 1 DM patients and use a mixed regimen of short and long-acting insulins. There are also insulin pumps for so-called tight control.

ORAL ANTIDIABETIC DRUGS

Oral antidiabetic drugs are only used for type 2 diabetes. They cannot prevent symptomatic hyperglycemia or DKA in type 1 DM patients. Oral antidiabetic drugs are divided into two subgroups: oral hypoglycemic agents and oral antihyperglycemic agents.

ORAL HYPOGLYCEMIC AGENTS

Oral hypoglycemic agents are the sulfonylureas. The sulfonylureas lower blood glucose primarily by stimulating insulin secretion. Secondary effects include improving peripheral and hepatic insulin senstivity. There are a number of sulfonylurea drugs currently in use. Oral hypoglycemic agents are used when diet and exercise are ineffective or in conjunction wth diet and exercise. These include:

First generation:

> Tolbutamide (Orinase)
> Chlorpropamide (Diabinese, Glucamide)
> Acetohexamide (Dymelor)
> Tolazamide (Tolinase)

Second generation:

> Glyburide (Diabeta, Micronase)
> Glipizide (Glucotrol)
> Glimepiride (Amyril)
> Micronized glyburide (Glynase)
> Glipizide-GITS (Glucotrol XL)

These are applied in type 2 DM as monotherapy or in combination therapy with other oral agents and insulin if blood sugar levels are poorly controlled with monotherapy or during intercurrent illness. The cardiovascular safety of sulfonylureas is held in question due to increased risk of atheroslcerosis, vasoconstrictive action, dysrhythmias, and myocardial depression.

ORAL ANTIHYPERGLYCEMIC AGENTS

There are several different antihyperglycemic drugs currently in use. These are divided into the biguanides, the alpha-glucosidase inhibitors, and the thiazolidinediones or insulin sensitizers. Common antihyperglycemic drugs include:

> Metformin (Glucophage), a biguanide
> Acarbose (Precose), an alpha-glucosidase inhibitor
> Troglitazone (Rezulin), an insulin sensitizer
> Repaglinide (Prandin), an insulin sensitizer

These antihyperglycemic drugs are prescribed singly and in combination therapy. For instance, troglitazone is only used in combination with insulin or metformin, while repaglinide is only used in monotherapy. Metformin is used to prevent progression of glucose intolerance and to avoid atherogenic dyslipidemia.

BENEFITS OF DRUG THERAPY

Drug therapies aim to maintain average blood glucose levels at around 130mg/dL so as to:

1. Reduce, slow, and/or prevent miscrovascular damage and deterioration
2. Decrease symptoms
3. Prevent infection/accelerate wound or ulcer healing
4. Improve vision (by correcting error of refraction acutely and glaucoma long-term)
5. Decrease risk of comorbidities (primarily end organ damage, such as nephropathy, neuropathy, retinopathy, and macrovascular [i.e. cardiac] complications)

RISKS OF DRUG THERAPY

INSULIN THERAPY

Due to error in insulin dosage, a small or missed meal, or unplanned exercise, insulin therapy may result in hypoglycemia requiring emergency care. Insulin therapy may also cause rebound hyperglycemia in the early morning hours before breakfast, the so-called dawn phenomenon. In this case, those with type 1 DM may have to wake each night between 2-4 AM to monitor blood glucose levels. Insulin may also provoke both localized and generalized allergic reactions. Localized allergic reactions include immediate pain and burning followed, after several hours, by erythema, pruritus, and induration. Generalized aller-

gic reactions are rare, but may result in urticaria, angioedema, pruritus, bronchospasm, and even circulatory collapse. In addition, insulin therapy may result in insulin resistance (defined as the use of more than 200 units of insulin per day). Other local reactions to insulin injections include local fat atrophy or hypertrophy. Further, most patients treated with insulin for two or more months develop IgG antibodies to insulin. Of these, 20-30% of patients have insulin (IgE) allergy which may require switching types of insulin, desensitization, or administration of prednisone for many months.

ORAL ANTIDIABETIC THERAPY

Oral hypoglycemic agents carry the risk of hypoglycemia, especially in those with impaired renal function or the elderly. In a few cases, these drugs may cause allergic reactions, such as cholestatic jaundice. In particular, chlorpropamide may cause hypernatremia and a deterioration in mental status. In terms of antihyperglycemic drugs, gastrointestinal side effects are common with metformin, although these are often transient and may be prevented if the drug is taken with meals. Metformin is also contraindicated in patients with dehydration, congestive heart failure, liver and kidney disease (due to increase risk of lactic acidosis), or alcoholism. Gastrointestinal side effects are also common with acarbose. However, as with metformin, these are often transient. Troglitazone is potentially hepatotoxic in some idiosyncratic patients.

COMPLICATIONS OF DIABETES

The main complications of diabetes are neurovascular. In terms of microvascular complications, long-term diabetes may lead to small blood vessel disease or microangiopathy and thickening of capillary walls. Leakage from the capillaries leads to changes in the retina (i.e., retinopathy) causing decreased visual acuity and even blindness. Similar changes in the kidneys (nephropathy) causes impairment of renal function and even complete failure. In terms of macrovascular complications, atherosclerosis may occur earlier and progress faster in patients with diabetes. This may lead to cerebral vascular disease, coronary artery disease, and peripheral vascular disease. Cerebral vascular and coronary artery disease may lead to death, and peripheral vascular disease may lead to gangrene and amputation of affected limbs.

Chronic hyperglycemia causes chemical changes in the nerves which impair their transmission of signals or communication. This results in autonomic, focal, and/or peripheral neuropathy. Sixty percent of those with diabetes have some form of neuropathy, whether symptomatic or asymptomatic.[40] Autonomic nervous system dysfunction may manifest as gastric paresis, chronic diarrhea, incomplete emptying of the bladder, impotence, and/or orthostatic hypotension. Peripheral neuropathy may cause loss of sensitivity, burning, itching, or aching and pain, mostly in the lower extremities and, in contradistinction to compressive neuropathies, mostly in a "stocking-glove" pattern.

Other complications may include skeletal changes as a result of calcium deficiency and aging and skin diseases due to impaired sweat gland function. In addition, wounds and infections due to impaired immune system function and capillary damage may occur. The complications of diabetes mellitus are dealt with in separate chapters below.

PROGNOSIS

Prognosis in diabetes mellitus is dependent on the type of diabetes, 1 or 2, and the presence and severity of any complications. Complications usually begin 10-20 years after onset of disease. However, they also typically occur 4-7 years *before* diagnosis.[41] For many years, it was thought that the long-term complications of diabetes were inevitable. We now know that those may not occur with proper management. The Diabetes Control & Complications Trial showed that, in a group of 1,440 DM patients, those treated intensively (*i.e.*, tight control or HbA1c under 7%) had a 76% decreased risk of retinopathy, a 65% decreased risk of nephropathy, and a 55% decreased risk of neuropathy after eight years. In fact, the results were so dramatic that the study was stopped early so that all participants could benefit from intensive management.[42] Another survey, the United Kingdom Prospective Diabetes Study (UKPDS), was completed in 1997. This study followed close to 4,000 people with type 2 diabetes for 10 years. The study monitored how tight control of blood glucose (meaning HbA1c of 7%) and tight control of blood pressure (meaning a blood pressure of less than 144 over less than 82mmHg) could protect a person from the long-term complications of diabetes. At the end of the 10 years, the study showed that those people with tight control of blood glucose and blood pressure had a 32% decreased risk of all diabetes-related deaths, a 44% decreased risk of stroke, a 56% decreased risk of heart

failure, and a 37% decreased risk for microvascular complications. The study also found that for every one percentage point decrease in HbA1c, a person could decrease his or her risk for all complications by 25%. The UKPDS dramatically demonstrated that, with good self-care skills, blood glucose control, and blood pressure control, the complications of diabetes are not an inevitable course of the disease.

ENDNOTES:

1 www.healthlibrary.com/reading/vhai/mar-apr98/Dia-his.htm
2 *Ibid.*
3 www.vsbl.york.ac.uk/~mgwt/thesis-tth.chapter1.html
4 www.diabetes.ca/about_diabetes/timeline.html
5 Http://journal.diabetes.org/FullText/ClinicalDiabetes/V19N101/pg13.htm
6 www.diabetesinstitute.org/articles/brochure.html
7 www.healthlibrary.com, *op. cit.*
8 www.unigene.com/ireye/irsite.html
9 http://familydoctor.org/handouts/388.html
10 www.cdc.gov/diabetes/pubs/facts98.htm
11 Gates, Judy, *Diabetes: Etiology, Management Advances, and Early Interventions*, EDA 201-0438, Health & Sciences Television Network, Primedia Healthcare, Carrollton, TX, 2001, p. 3
12 www.cdc.gov/diabetes, *op. cit.*
13 http://diabetes-in-america.s-3.com/adobe/chpt2.pdf
14 www.britannica.com/news/reuters/article/story_id=167113
15 www.alternativedr.com/IMCAccess/ProfConditions/DiabetesMellituspc.htm
16 www.chebucto.ns.ca/Health/CPRC/diabetes.html
17 www.healthlibrary.com, *op. cit.*
18 www.bmj.com/cgi/content/full/316/7139/1221
19 www.cdc.gov/diabetes, *op. cit.*
20 www.britannica.com/news/reuters/article/story_id=169691
21 http://diabetes-in-america.s-3.com/adobe/chpt11.pdf
22 *Ibid.*
23 *Ibid.*
24 www.cdc.gov/diabetes, *op. cit.*
25 www.aace.com/clinicguideindex.html
26 www.cdc.gov/diabetes, *op. cit.*
27 Beers, Mark H. & Berkow, Robert, *The Merck Manual*, 17th edition, Merck Research Laboratories, Rahway, NJ, 1999, p. 165
28 American Diabetes Association, *Complete Guide to Diabetes*, Bantam Books, NY, 1999, p. 19
29 *Ibid.*, p. 22
30 Beers & Berkow, *op. cit.*, p. 165
31 www.itmonline.org/arts/diabacu.htm
32 http://diabetes.medscape.com/40567.rhtml?srcmp=endo_072001
33 Saudek, Christopher D. & Daly, Anne E., "Diabetes Update," *Newsweek*, Aug. 27, 2001, special advertising section, p. 8
34 www.nlm.nih.gov/medlineplus/ency/article/001214.htm#causesAndRisk
35 http://diabetes-in-america.s-3.com/adobe/chpt2.pdf, *op. cit.*
36 www.healthlibrary.com, *op. cit.*
37 *Ibid.*, p. 169
38 www.alternativedr.com, *op. cit.*
39 Gates, *op. cit.*, p. 4
40 www.uic.edu/depts/mcfp/geriatric/endocrine/sldoo5.htm
41 www.nlm.nih.gov/medlineplus/ency/article/001214.htm#prognosis
42 *Ibid.*

2

THE HISTORY OF DIABETES
IN CHINESE MEDICINE

Diabetes mellitus is a modern Western disease category which has been adopted by Chinese medicine in the 20th century under the Chinese translation, *tang niao bing* (sugar urine disease). However, Chinese doctors have long recognized the clinical manifestations of diabetes mellitus as a specific disorder under the name *xiao ke*, wasting and thirsting. Below is a brief history of the development of Chinese medical ideas on what is now most commonly referred to as diabetes mellitus.

SPRING & AUTUMN, WARRING STATES, AND HAN DYNASTY

The *Nei Jing (Inner Classic)*, the pre-eminent classic of Chinese medicine, was compiled in either the Spring and Autumn or Warring States period. Like so many other Chinese disease categories and seminal concepts, the name *xiao ke* first appears in the *Nei Jing* where there is mention to several different though related conditions: *xiao ke*, wasting and thirsting, *xiao dan*, pure heat wasting, *ge xiao*, diaphragm wasting, and *xiao zhong*, central wasting. References in the *Nei Jing* to wasting and thirsting are scattered through 14 *juan* or books of this classic which discuss its disease causes and mechanisms, clinical manifestations, and treatment.

In terms of disease causes, the authors of the *Nei Jing* recognized that overeating of sweets and fats, emotional stress, weakness of the five viscera, and obesity are all closely related to this disease. For instance, the *Su Wen (Simple Questions)*, "Treatise on Strange Diseases," says:

> This [condition] occurs in those who are fat and beautiful. This person must [eat] many sweet, fine [foods] and too many fats. Fats all cause heat inside humans, and sweets all cause center full-

ness. Therefore, the qi spills over above, transforming into wasting and thirsting.

The *Ling Shu (Spiritual Axis)*, "The Five Changes," says:

> Anger leads the qi to counterflow upward where it amasses and accumulates in the center of the chest. The qi and blood [thus] counterflow and lodge, and the hip skin [*i.e.*, fat] fills the muscles. The blood vessels do not move, and this transforms to make heat. Heat [then] leads to wasting of the muscles and skin. Therefore, this is called pure heat wasting.

It also says, "[If] the five viscera are all soft and weak, there is the susceptibility to the disease of pure heat wasting." While the *Su Wen*, "The Treatise on Understanding the Appraisal of Vacuity & Repletion," says, "[In] attack of pure heat wasting, [being] fat and [eating] rich foods lead to the accumulation of fat [meats] and fine [foods]."

In terms of disease mechanisms, the authors of the *Nei Jing* identified visceral yin insufficiency as the basic mechanism of this condition. If intestinal and stomach heat binds, it consumes and damages fluids and humors. This then leads to the onset of the main symptoms of this disease. In the *Su Wen*, "Divergent Treatise on Yin & Yang," it says, "Two yangs binding is called wasting." "Two yangs" refers to yang ming heat and binding. In the *Ling Shu*, "The Five Changes," it says:

> An indomitable heart leads to much anger, and anger leads to qi counterflowing upward... [Hence,] the blood vessels do not move, and this transforms to make heat. Heat [then] leads to

wasting of the muscles and skin [or flesh]. Therefore, this causes pure heat wasting.

The main symptoms of wasting and thirsting are polydipsia, polyphagia, polyuria, and bodily emaciation. In terms of these, the *Su Wen*, "Treatise on Qi Reversal," says, "[In] lung wasting, [if there are] one drink [and] two urinations, [this is] death and [the condition] cannot be treated." Likewise, the author says, "[If] the large intestine shifts heat to the stomach, [there will be] a predilection for eating and emaciation." In the *Ling Shu*, "The Teacher's Transmission," it says:

Stomach center heat leads to wasting of grains. Therefore, the person has a hanging heart [*i.e.*, feels anxious] and a predilection to hunger.

In terms of the treatment of this disease, it was believed at this time that people with wasting and thirsting should eat and be treated by things which are sweet in flavor and cold in nature. This was believed to enable the engenderment of fluids and thus stop thirst. However, one should also not eat fatty, rich foods, use penetrating, aromatic herbs, or take mineral medicinals which are dry and hot and damage fluids. The authors of the *Su Wen*, "Treatise on the Abdomen & Center," say, "[For] heat in the center/center wasting, it is not ok to administer rich, fatty [foods], penetrating herbs, or stone medicinals."

As for prognosis, the *Su Wen*, "Treatise on Understanding the Appraisal of Vacuity & Repletion," says:

Pure heat wasting… [if] the pulse is replete and large, [even if] the disease is enduring it can be treated. [If] the pulse is hanging,[1] small, and hard and the disease is enduring, it cannot be treated.

The *Ling Shu*, "Evil Qi, the Viscera & Bowels, and Disease & Form," speaking in terms of the heart, liver, spleen, lung, and kidney pulses says, "Faint and small makes for pure heat wasting." Additionally, the *Su Wen*, "Treatise on the Living Qi Communicating with Heaven," says, "The changes of rich, fatty [foods are] the engenderment of large clove sores on the feet."

In the late Han dynasty, Zhang Zhong-jing, in his *Jin Gui Yao Lue* (*Essentials of the Golden Cabinet*), also wrote about thirsting and wasting. According to Zhang, its main disease mechanisms are stomach heat and kidney vacuity.

[If] yang floats, the pulse is floating and rapid. Floating refers to the qi, [while] rapidity refers to the dispersion of grains. [If the pulse is] also large and hard, [this is because] qi exuberance has led to

many urinations. Many urinations result in hardness. [When] hardness and rapidity beat together, this is referred to as wasting and thirsting.

Zhang also says:

[If] the *fu yang* [or tarsal] pulse is rapid, the stomach has heat within it. This is referred to as dispersion of grains drinking and eating. The stools are constipated and hard, and urination is numerous.

Likewise, Zhang says:

[If] a man has wasting and thirsting, urination is contrarily numerous. [If] he drinks one *tou*, he urinates one *tou*.

Based on the coordination of pulse signs and symptoms, Zhang divided wasting and thirsting into lung, stomach, and kidney varieties for which he prescribed different formulas and medicinals – *Bai Hu Jia Ren Shen Tang* (White Tiger Plus Ginseng Decoction), *Wen Ge San* (Gecko Powder), and *Shen Qi Wan* (Kidney Qi Pills) respectively. Based on Zhang's location of this disease in the lungs, stomach, and kidneys, later writers called this condition the *san xiao* or three wastings and divided it into upper, middle, and lower wastings as we will see below.

JIN, SUI & TANG DYNASTIES

During the Jin, Sui, and Tang dynasties, taking longevity or immortality elixirs made from minerals was very popular, and this caused many people to develop wasting and thirsting due to this self-poisoning. In the Sui dynasty, Chao Yuan-fang, in his *Zhu Bing Yuan Hou Lun* (*Treatise on the Origins & Symptoms of Diseases*), says that wasting and thirsting is due to "administration of the five stones in various pills and powders." Likewise, Sun Si-miao, in his *Qian Jin Fang* (*Formulas [Worth] a Thousand [Pieces of] Gold*) published in the Tang dynasty, says wasting and thirsting may be due to taking powders of the five stones. After taking such stones, Sun says the lower burner develops vacuity heat, the kidneys become dry, and yin becomes depleted. This is the origin of *dryness* and heat as the disease mechanism of wasting and thirsting in Chinese medicine. However, Sun also recognized that overconsumption of alcohol could also cause wasting and thirsting: "Enduring accumulation [*i.e.*, consumption] of alcohol cannot but produce wasting and thirsting." Since alcohol's nature is hot, its consumption leads to the exuberance of heat in the three burners which then leads to dryness and parching of the five viscera. "Hence the person is not able not to drink." As Sun observed:

> Three things must be renounced: wine, sex, and eating salted, starchy cereal products. If this regimen can be observed, cure may follow without medicines.

Also in the Tang dynasty, Wang Tao, in his *Wai Tai Mi Yao (Secret Essentials of the External Platform)*, wrote that, "[If] the kidney qi becomes insufficient, [this may lead to] vacuity detriment wasting and thirsting with polyuria and low back pain." He also pointed out that, "Every time the disease comes on, the urine must be sweet," and that, "Those with wasting and thirsting become emaciated." In addition, Wang recognized that patients with wasting and thirsting have scanty qi, are not able to talk much, have vexatious heat within the heart, soreness of the lower legs, and lack of strength. If extreme, such patients may exhibit essence spirit abstraction. Wang also knew that this disease is relatively difficult to treat and may relapse. Further, Wang knew that, "[Those with] this disease have many welling and flat abscesses," and that their "skin engenders sores." It was Wang Tao who emphasized that the kidneys are the root of the onset of wasting and thirsting.

During the seventh century, the physician and bureaucrat Li Xuan wrote an entire monograph on wasting and thirsting in which he attempted to explain why the urine is sweet in such patients:

> This disease is due to weakness of the kidneys and bladder. In such cases, the urine is always sweet. Many physicians do not recognize this symptom... the cereal food of the farmers are the precursors of sweetness... the methods of making cakes and sweetmeats... mean that they all very soon turn to sweetness... It is the nature of the saltiness to descend [or be excreted]. But since the kidneys and bladder in the lumbus are weak, they cannot distill the finest essence. [Instead,] all is excreted as urine. Therefore, the sweetness in the urine comes forth, and the latter does not acquire its normal color.

In terms of treatment during this time, Sun Si-miao lists 52 formulas for wasting and thirsting disease. Among these, the main ingredients for clearing heat and engendering fluids are Radix Trichosanthis Kirlowii (*Tian Hua Fen*), Tuber Ophiopogonis Japonici (*Mai Men Dong*), Radix Rehmanniae (*Di Huang*), and Rhizoma Coptidis Chinensis (*Huang Lian*). However, practitioners of this time, such as Sun and Wang, were of the opinion that

Chinese medicinals for the treatment of this condition were not entirely satisfactory. Therefore, they also paid attention to the treatment and prevention of wasting and thirsting through dietary therapy. For instance, Sun Si-miao said that, if one was able to forego drinking alcohol, having sex, and eating salt, one can cure this condition without taking medicinals. According to Wang, "[In terms of] eating, it is desirable to take less but several times; it is not desirable to be satiated and [eat] too much." It was during this period that practitioners were taught that patients with this condition should take a walk after eating—the so-called thousand steps. Patients with wasting and thirsting should not go to sleep after eating and drinking till full.

Interestingly, during the Tang dynasty, acupuncture and moxibustion were prohibited in those with wasting and thirsting. As Sun saw:

> Moxibustion and piercing may lead to sores with suppuration of pussy water that cannot be checked. This may eventually develop into welling and flat abscesses which may even lead to emaciation and death.

Similarly Sun said, "It is also prohibited to do anything which might damage the skin and flesh." This prohibition against acupuncture and moxibustion in those with wasting and thirsting was obviously an attempt to prevent opportunistic infections and gangrene.

Thus, as Robert Temple points out in *The Genius of China*, "By the seventh century AD, the Chinese had published their observations on the sweetness of urine of diabetics, tried to come up with an explanation for it, and proposed a dietary regimen for control of diabetes which was not far from the modern method of avoiding alcohol and starchy foods."[2]

Song, Jin & Yuan dynasties

The Song, Jin, and Yuan dynasties are seen as a sort of renaissance within Chinese medicine. This was a time of great intellectual ferment, and a number of new ideas on wasting and thirsting entered Chinese medicine during these three dynasties. In the Song dynasty, Wang Huai-yin *et al.*, the compilers of the *Tai Ping Sheng Hui Fang (Tai Ping [Era] Imperial Grace Formulary)*, divided the treatment of wasting and thirsting into the three wastings. They said, "In terms of the three wasting, the first is called wasting and thirsting, the second is called central wasting, and the third is called kidney wasting."

The first leads to drinking lots of water but urinating less. This is wasting and thirsting. The second leads to eating lots of food but drinking less water. The urine is scanty and reddish yellow. This is central wasting. The third leads to drinking water followed by urinating what was [just] drunk. The urine is sweet in flavor, white, and turbid. The low back and lower limbs are wasted and emaciated. This is kidney wasting.

Each of these three species of wasting was correlated to one of the three burners, upper, middle, and lower. Li Min-shou, in his *Jian Yi Fang (Simple, Easy Formulas)*, "Wasting & Thirsting," says:

> If heat qi soars upwards, the heart suffers vacuity. Fire qi scatters and floods and is not restrained and contained... This is called wasting and thirsting and pertains to the upper burner. The disease is located in the tips [or branches]. If heat amasses in the center, the spleen suffers vacuity and hidden yang brews internally... This is called central wasting. It is also called spleen wasting. It pertains to the middle burner and the disease is located in the sea of water and grains. If heat is deep-lying in the lower burner, the kidneys suffer vacuity... This is called kidney wasting. It is also called acute wasting. It pertains to the lower burner, and the disease is located in the root.

Although the writers of the Song dynasty divided this condition into three subtypes, they knew these were only three different manifestations of a single disease. As the authors of the *Sheng Ji Zong Lu (Imperial Aid Assembled Records)* state: "Its basis is one even though it has three tips."

In 1189, Zhang Gao, writing in his *Yi Lun (Medical Discourses)*, noted the importance of skin care in those with wasting and thirsting and the danger of the slightest skin lesions.

> Whether or not such patients are cured, one must be on the watch for the development of large boils and carbuncles. Should such develop near the joints, the prognosis is very bad. I myself witnessed my friend Shao Ren-tao suffering from this disease for several years, and he died of the ulcers.

During the Jin and Yuan dynasties, there were four dominant schools of medicine, called the *Si Da Jia*, the Four Great Schools, and two of these schools added an evolutionary step to the understanding and treatment of wasting and thirsting. Liu He-jian, also called Liu Wan-su, was the founder of the School of Cold and Cool [Medicines]. In his *San Xiao Lun (Treatise on the Three Wastings)*, Liu emphasized dryness and heat as the main disease mechanisms of this condition.

> If drinking and eating and taking of cakes and candies are not proper, the intestines and stomach become dry and desiccated and qi and fluids do not obtain normal diffusion. There may [also] be consumption and chaos of the essence spirit and overstepping prohibitions [regarding sex]. Or, due to great disease, yin and qi [may suffer] detriment and blood and fluids may decline and become vacuous. Thus yang qi becomes bold and dryness and heat become severely depressed.

Liu points out that a number of different types of heat evils all produce thirst. For instance, heart shifting heat to the lungs produces thirst, kidney heat produces thirst, and stomach and large intestine heat produce thirst. As Liu points out in his *Huang Ti Su Wen Xuan Ming Lun Fang (Treatise Making Clear The Yellow Emperor's Simple Questions Plus Formulas)*, "Assembled Treatise on Wasting & Thirsting," although there are three wastings, "all are the result of heat." Based on this emphasis on heat as the main disease mechanism of wasting and thirsting, Liu recommended "supplementing the vacuity of kidney water and yin cold, draining the repletion of heart fire and yang heat, and eliminating dryness and heat from the intestines and stomach." Hence Liu Wan-su used a combination of supplementing and filling with cold and cool draining medicinals in the treatment of this disease, creating eight new formulas recorded in his *San Xiao Lun*.

Zhu Zhen-heng, a.k.a. Dan-xi, chronologically the last of the four great masters of the Jin-Yuan and founder of the School of Enriching Yin, elaborated on Liu Wan-su's ideas on the three wastings and dryness and heat. The treatment principles Zhu suggests for upper wasting in his *Dan Xi Xin Fa Zhi Yao (The Heart & Essence of Dan-xi's Methods of Treatment)* are to disinhibit dampness so that it can automatically moisten dryness. For middle wasting, Zhu advocated precipitating "till [excessive] drinking of water is discontinued." And for lower wasting, he thought that one should nurture the blood and depurate heat. In general, Zhu said, "The great method is to nourish the lungs, downbear fire, and engender the blood as the ruling [measures]." Zhu also recognized thirst and an excessive desire for water during pregnancy as a type of wasting and thirsting disease.

Although Li Gao, a.k.a. Dong-yuan, founder of the School of Supplementing Earth and arguably the greatest of the four great masters of the Jin-Yuan, did not write extensively on wasting and thirsting, he did describe the following characteristics of wasting and thirsting in his *Lan Shi Mi Cang (Orchid Chamber Secret Treasury)*, "Dry mouth, parched tongue, frequent, numerous urination, blocked, astringent defecation, with dry, bound stools," and "the ability to eat but emaciation." He also said there may be, "numbness of the upper and lower teeth, hardening of the gums with swelling and pain, wilting and weakness of the four limbs, front yin [*i.e.*, the genitalia] as if ice, and a susceptibility to anger and impaired memory." Likewise, Zhang Zi-he, founder of the School of Attack and Precipitation, correctly observed that, "Many patients with wasting and thirsting become deaf and blind and have sores and lichen, welling and flat abscesses."

In addition, the *Dong Yuan Shi Xiao Fang (Dong-yuan's Proven Effective Formulas)*, arranged and published by Ni Wei-de in the Ming dynasty, gives seven formulas attributed to Li for the treatment of wasting and thirsting. Like most of Li's formulas based on yin fire theory, all of these formulas contain a combination of supplementing and draining, warm and cold ingredients. Most of them contain spleen and yin supplements combined with heat-clearers and qi-rectifiers. Several also simultaneously address blood stasis. *Sheng Jin Gan Lu Yin Zi* (Engender Fluids Sweet Dew Drink) and *Qing Shen Bu Qi Tang* (Clear the Spirit & Supplement the Qi Decoction) are two representative formulas from this collection. The ingredients of *Sheng Jin Gan Lu Yin Zi* include Gypsum Fibrosum (*Shi Gao*), Radix Panacis Ginseng (*Ren Shen*), uncooked and mix-fried Radix Glycyrrhizae (*Gan Cao*), Fructus Gardeniae Jasminoidis (*Zhi Zi*), Fructus Cardamomi (*Bai Dou Kou*), Cortex Phellodendri (*Huang Bai*), Radix Angelicae Dahuricae (*Bai Zhi*), Fructus Forsythiae Suspensae (*Lian Qiao*), Semen Pruni Armeniacae (*Xing Ren*), Tuber Ophiopogonis Japonici (*Mai Men Dong*), Rhizoma Coptidis Chinensis (*Huang Lian*), Radix Auklandiae Lappae (*Mu Xiang*), Radix Platycodi Grandiflori (*Jie Geng*), Rhizoma Cimicifugae (*Sheng Ma*), Rhizoma Curcumae Longae (*Jiang Huang*), Rhizoma Anemarrhenae Aspheloidis (*Zhi Mu*), Radix Angelicae Sinensis (*Dang Gui*), Buthus Martensis (*Quan Xie*), Herba Agastachis Seu Pogostemi (*Huo Xiang*), Radix Bupleuri (*Chai Hu*), Herba Eupatorii Fortunei (*Pei Lan*), Flos Helianthi Annui (*Bai Kui Hua*), and Fructus Cubebae (*Bi Cheng Qie*). *Qing Shen Bu Qi Tang* is composed of Rhizoma Cimicifugae (*Sheng Ma*), Radix Bupleuri (*Chai Hu*), uncooked Radix Glycyrrhizae (*Gan Cao*), Cortex Phellodendri (*Huang Bai*), Rhizoma Coptidis Chinensis (*Huang Lian*), Rhizoma Anemarrhenae Aspheloidis (*Zhi Mu*), Gypsum Fibrosum (*Shi Gao*), Semen Pruni

Armeniacae (*Xing Ren*), Semen Pruni Persicae (*Tao Ren*), Radix Angelicae Sinensis (*Dang Gui*), Flos Carthami Tinctorii (*Hong Hua*), Radix Ledebouriellae Divaricatae (*Fang Feng*), Herba Seu Flos Schizonepetae Tenuifoliae (*Jing Jie Sui*), cooked Radix Rehmanniae (*Shu Di*), uncooked Radix Rehmanniae (*Sheng Di*), Fructus Zanthoxyli Bungeani (*Chuan Jiao*), and Herba Asari Cum Radice (*Xi Xin*). Anyone familiar with Li's formulas will immediately recognize their characteristic composition. They are models of complexity and sophistication which reflect the complexity of this condition.

MING DYNASTY

In the Ming dynasty, practitioners and authors continued to build on the basis laid down by their predecessors, recognizing more and more complicating symptoms of this disease entity. For instance, Tai Si-gong, in his *Mi Chuan Zheng Zhi Yao Lue (Essentials of the Secret Transmission of Proven Treatments)*, says, "[In] the three wastings, urination is excessive and there is constipation." The authors of the *Pu Ji Fang (Universal Aid Formulas)* noted that those with wasting and thirsting may have "restless sleep and the four limbs may be exhausted and fatigued," while Miao Xi-yong saw that those with thirsting and wasting often had "toothache and missing teeth."

In terms of disease mechanism theory, more emphasis was placed on fortifying the spleen and boosting the qi. For instance, in the *Mi Chuan Zheng Zhi Yao Lue*, "Wasting & Thirsting," it says:

> [When] the three wastings are [first] obtained, the qi is replete and the blood is vacuous. [However, if this] endures and endures and is not treated, qi vacuity takes priority, leading to inability to produce strength."

Likewise, Tai says: "[If] the three wastings endure and the urination is not foul-smelling but, contrarily, becomes sweet, the qi is thrown out in the urine bucket and the disease gets worse." Similarly, it was increasingly recognized that, as this condition worsens, it also involves decline of the lifegate fire which becomes unable to rotten and ripen the water and grains. Hence the qi of water and grains is unable to steam and ascend to moisten the lungs. The canopy becomes dry and parched, and thus there is yet another mechanism of thirst. Hence, in the Ming, the saying was created:

> Do not divide upper, middle, and lower. First, quickly treat the kidneys, promptly administering *Liu Wei Wan* (Six Flavors [Rehmannia] Pills)

or additions and subtractions to *Ba Wei Wan* (Eight Flavors Pills) following the symptoms. By downbearing heart fire and enriching kidney water, thirst is automatically stopped.

This became the root principle for treating wasting and thirsting in this period, and practitioners asked themselves, "[If] a person's water and fire obtain levelness [or balance] and qi and blood obtain nourishment, how can there be wasting?" Li Ding, author of the famous *Yi Xue Ru Men* (*Entering the Door of the Study of Medicine*), "Thirsting & Wasting," expressed these treatment principles by saying:

> [When] treating thirst, initially one should nourish the lungs and downbear the heart. [However, if the condition] endures, this leads to enriching the kidneys and nourishing the spleen. Because the root is in the kidneys and the branch is in the lungs, warming the kidneys leads the qi to ascend and upbear, thus moistening the lungs. Kidney chill leads to qi not being upborne and the lungs being scorched. Therefore, *Shen Qi Wan* (Kidney Qi Pills) is a fine formula for wasting and thirsting. Further, [since] the heart and kidneys both connect with the spleen, nourishing the spleen leads to fluids and humors automatically being engendered. *Shen Ling Bai Zhu San* (Ginseng, Poria & Atractylodes Powder) does this.

Hence the combination of *Shen Qi Wan* and *Shen Ling Bai Zhu San* became the main formula for the treatment of wasting and thirsting at this time.

Zhang Jing-yue, also known as Zhang Jie-bin, was one of the founders of the Ming dynasty School of Warm Supplementation. In his *Jing Yue Quan Shu* (*Jing-yue's Complete Book*), he says that wasting and thirsting is due to kidney qi insufficiency and decline and receding of the original yang. Hence the qi does not contain or manage the essence, nor does it transform fluids. Therefore, treatment should include *Zuo Gui Yin* (Restore the Left [Kidney] Pills) to seek yang within yin and *You Gui Wan* (Restore the Right [Kidney] Pills) to seek yin within yang. This then results in yin and yang becoming regulated and integrated.

QING DYNASTY

In the Qing dynasty, practitioners continued refining the teachings of the past concerning wasting and thirsting as well as created some new concepts and techniques. Qin Chang-yu, in his *Zheng Yin Mai Zhi* (*The Causes, Pulses & Treatment of Conditions*), identified the three great symp-

toms of wasting and thirsting thusly, "[In] this condition, following drinking, there is thirst; following eating, there is hunger; following urination, there is urination." Chen Shi-duo, in his *Bian Zheng Bing Jian* (*The Ice Mirror of Pattern Discrimination*) recognized that this condition is often complicated by gangrene of the lower extremities and that this indicated a poor prognosis.

Also during the Qing, practitioners began to appreciate the role of the liver in the mechanisms of this disease. Huang Yuan-yu, in his *Si Sheng Xin Yuan* (*Four Sage's Heart Origin*), "Wasting & Thirsting," says:

> Wasting and thirsting is a disease of the foot *jue yin*. *Jue yin* wind wood and *shao yang* ministerial fire make an exterior-interior [relationship]... The nature of wood is to desire coursing and discharge... [If] coursing and discharging are not fulfilled... this may lead to ministerial fire losing its hibernation and storage.

What this means is that liver depression qi stagnation may lead to depressive heat. Because of the close connection between the liver and kidneys or the liver and lifegate/ministerial fire, liver depression transforming heat may mutually inflame ministerial fire and cause heat or hyperactivity in any of the viscera and bowels connected to the lifegate fire—for instance, the stomach. If liver and stomach heat and hyperactivity flame upward, they will eventually accumulate in and damage the yin fluids of the lungs and heart. Ye Tian-shi, one of the greatest doctors of the Qing dynasty recommended the formula, *Shi Gao E Jiao Tang* (Gypsum & Donkey Skin Glue Decoction) for just this scenario of liver yang assailing the stomach resulting in dryness damaging the lungs.[3] Therefore, the author of the *Su Ling Wei Yun* (*An Accumulation of the Finest [Points] of the Simple [Questions &] Spiritual [Axis]*), in "Thirsting & Wasting Explained," says, "Wasting and thirsting disease is solely due to punishment by liver wood, not by punishment by lung metal." This Qing dynasty emphasis on the role of the liver in the engenderment of wasting and thirsting disease is summed up by Wu Qian *et al.*, the compilers of the *Yi Zong Jin Jian* (*The Golden Mirror of Ancestral Medicine*) when they say, "Wasting and thirsting condition is a *jue yin* diease."

However, this does not mean that this teaching concerning the liver supplanted the Ming dynasty's emphasis on the kidneys. Li Zhong-zi, in his *Zheng Zhi Hui Bu* (*Proven Treatments Collected Supplements*) said:

> [In] the treatment of wasting and thirsting... ini-

tially one should nourish the lungs and clear the heart. [If the condition] endures, this leads to the necessity of supplementing the kidneys and nourishing the spleen. The root of engenderment of the fluids and humors of the five viscera is located in the kidneys. Therefore, warming the kidneys and ascending and upbearing the qi leads to the lungs being moistened.

Likewise, other Chinese doctors, such as Chen Shi-duo, in his *Shi Shi Mi Lu (Stone Chamber Secret Teachings)*, continued to emphasize the kidneys as the root of the treatment of wasting and thirsting. Ultimately, Chinese practitioners began more and more to think in terms of simultaneously treating the liver and kidneys. This meant nourishing and emolliating the liver at the same time as supplementing kidney yin and possibly also invigorating kidney yang.

Also in the Qing dynasty, Chinese doctors began discussing the role of transforming phlegm and eliminating dampness in the treatment of wasting and thirsting. For instance, Fei Bo-xiong thought that clearing and moistening for upper wasting should be assisted by seeping dampness and transforming phlegm and that clearing the yang ming for middle wasting should be assisted by moistening dryness and transforming phlegm. This attention to phlegm was no doubt partly due to the fact that wasting and thirsting has long been associated with obesity in Chinese medicine, and adipose tissue is seen as phlegm, dampness, and turbidity. It is also partly due to the physiological characteristics of the spleen that it likes dryness and is averse to dampness. This is the argument Chen Xiu-yuan makes in his *Yi Xue Shi Zai Yi (The Study of Medicine is Truly Easy)*, "The Three Wasting Conditions," where he advocates "treating [this condition] with spleen-drying medicinals."

MODERN CHINESE MEDICINE

Perhaps the single most important development of the treatment of wasting and thirsting in Chinese medicine during the 20th century was the identification of wasting and thirsting with the modern Western disease category of diabetes mellitus. For instance, Lin Zhi-gang simply and unambiguously states, "Diabetes is categorized in Chinese medicine as 'wasting and thirsting' disease,"[4] and this is not just the opinion of a single practitioner. Such specific and unambiguous identification of diabetes mellitus with wasting and thirsting is corroborated by Yang Lian-de,[5] Cheng Can-ruo,[6] and Lin Yun-gui,[7] just to name several other famous contemporary Chinese

practitioners cited from a single anthology of acupuncture case histories. In fact, such identification of DM with wasting and thirsting commonly forms the opening statement of concluding discussion sections of Chinese research reports on the treatment of diabetes. Clinicians familiar with the Western medical signs and symptoms of diabetes will have no trouble recognizing the salient features of DM in the above traditional descriptions of wasting and thirsting and the correspondence between wasting and thirsting and diabetes mellitus is closer than that of most other traditional Chinese and their putative modern Western disease categories. In fact, as a review of our Chinese language bibliography shows, most modern Chinese clinicians primarily refer to diabetes mellitus and only occasionally speak about wasting and thirsting in other than in an historical context. Most importantly, because of the close correspondence between these two disease categories, we can now use Western laboratory examinations, such as blood glucose and urine glucose and ketones, to help us diagnose this disease and track the patient's progress or lack thereof. Since routine blood and urine examinations are part of most people's annual physical exams, these modern methods can help detect this potentially crippling and life-threatening condition early on when it is still treatable with Chinese medicine.

In terms of building on the past, modern Chinese medicine recognizes and preserves the truth in all the foregoing teachings on wasting and thirsting presented above through the various dynasties of Chinese history. As should be apparent from the copious quotes above, modern Chinese doctors are not cut off from and we continue to study all of the ancient texts regardless of school. However, based on the sum of knowledge and experience gained from these texts, we now know that wasting and thirsting or diabetes may involve the lungs, heart, spleen, liver, and kidneys, both yin and yang, as well as the stomach and intestines. It may also be associated with dryness and heat as well as phlegm and dampness (even at one and the same time). That being said, most modern practitioners believe that the main mechanisms and, therefore, patterns of diabetes mellitus are qi and yin vacuity. For instance, Feng Ming-qing, a professor at the Henan College of Chinese Medicine, says, "In terms of diagnosis, the qi and yin vacuity pattern is the main one in most [diabetes] patients."[8]

In addition, modern practitioners have come to realize the importance of the role of blood stasis, especially in the many complications of diabetes. Feng Ming-qing gives voice to this contemporary teaching as well when he says, "[In diabetes,] vacuity and stasis are mixed – vacuity is the root and stasis is the tip [or branch]."[9] Blood and fluids share a common source. Therefore, fluid insufficiency may lead to blood vacuity. If the blood is too vacuous to nourish the heart and its vessels, these cannot stir the blood properly, thus leading to blood stasis. Similarly, if blood does not nourish the liver, the liver cannot maintain its control over coursing and discharge. Hence, qi stagnation eventually may lead to blood stasis. Likewise, because the blood and fluids flow together and phlegm is nothing other than congealed fluids, phlegm and dampness may hinder and obstruct the free flow of the blood, leading to blood stasis. On the other hand, static blood impedes the engenderment of new or fresh blood and is also called dry blood. Therefore, it is easy to see that there are multiple disease mechanisms for the creation of blood stasis in patients with wasting and thirsting. As another example of this modern thinking on the role of blood stasis in diabetes, Hu Jian-hua, a professor at the Shanghai University of Chinese Medicine, has written:

> [If] wasting and thirsting endure for [many] days, yin detriment reaches yang resulting in yin and yang dual vacuity. Yang vacuity leads to cold congelation, and this can lead to blood stasis.[10]

Because we now know there are multiple disease mechanisms at work in this condition and individual patients may have individual combinations of these mechanisms, modern practitioners of Chinese medicine emphasize that treatment of this condition should be individually tailored on the basis of each patient's personal pattern discrimination. Although different contemporary Chinese doctors may use slightly different schemes for the pattern discrimination of this condition, there is broad agreement between contemporary practitioners of Chinese medicine on the main patterns of this condition and the main signs and symptoms of these patterns. Thus the standard for the contemporary professional Chinese medical treatment of this condition is summed up in the four Chinese words, *bian zheng lun zhi*, treatment should be based on pattern discrimination.

Another new development within Chinese medicine is broad-based outcomes research. During the last fifty years, researchers in the People's Republic of China have conducted scores of clinical audits of a host of treatment approaches for this condition. These clinical audits help substantiate the efficacy of Chinese medicine in the treatment of diabetes as well as help assess the relative merits and effectiveness of these different protocols. Because of the clinical importance of these outcomes studies, we have included numerous abstracts of such studies in this book. Further, modern pharmacodynamic research on Chinese medicinals is helping explain why Chinese medicinals have the effects they do on this disorder. Although, such pharmacodynamic research cannot and should not replace the wisdom of selecting these medicinals on the basis of each patient's personal pattern(s), they can help build trust in these medicinals on the part of both practitioners and patients alike. Since placebo plays a large part in every healing encounter, such increased trust, or faith, cannot but benefit our patients.

And finally, modern practitioners are learning how to integrate the precision, power, and speed of modern Western medicine with the safety and holism of Chinese medicine. As we have seen, wasting and thirsting, or what we now refer to as diabetes, has traditionally been considered a potentially difficult to treat disease within Chinese medicine. Many of the complications of this disorder are severely disabling and even life-threatening. When Chinese medicine is used in tandem with modern Western medicine, Chinese comparative research suggests that both benefit. Using such a combination, Chinese medicine typically improves the therapeutic efficacy of Western antidiabetic medications, helps reduce necessary dosages of such Western medications, and helps prevent or eliminate the side effects of such medications. On the other hand, Western medicines often are able to achieve therapeutic results in cases that are recalcitrant to Chinese medicine alone. This includes both serious, debilitating conditions, such as retinopathy and gangrene, as well as life-threatening emergency conditions, such as stroke, myocardial infarction, and ketoacidosis.

Hopefully, the reader will see from this brief history of the Chinese disease category of wasting and thirsting that Chinese medicine is a continuously evolving body of knowledge and practice. Although rooted in classics written more than 2,000 years ago, advances in the Chinese knowledge about and treatment of this condition have been made in every dynasty and continue to be made to this very day.

ENDNOTES:

[1] *Xuan*, or hanging, also describes something that is spaced far apart. In terms of the pulse, this seems the most likely interpretation – that the beats are relatively spaced farther apart than normal, *i.e.*, a slow pulse.
[2] Temple, Robert, *The Genius of China*, Simon & Schuster, Inc., NY, 1986, p. 133
[3] This formula is comprised of: Gypsum Fibrosum (*Shi Gao*), Rhizoma Anemarrhenae Aspheloidis (*Zhi Mu*), Gelatinum Corii Asini (*E Jiao*), uncooked Radix Rehmanniae (*Sheng Di*), uncooked Radix Glycyrrhizae (*Gan Cao*), and uncooked Radix Albus Paeoniae Lactiflorae (*Bai Shao*).
[4] Lin Zhi-gang, "A Study of the Efficacy of Treating Type II Diabetes with Integrated Acupuncture & Medicinals," *Fu Jian Zhong Yi Yao*

(*Fujian Chinese Medicine & Medicinals*), #2, 2000, p. 20
[5] Yang Lian-de, quoted in *Zhong Guo Dang Dai Zhen Jiu Ming Jia Yi An* (*Contemporary Chinese National Acupuncture & Moxibustion Famous Masters Case Histories*), compiled by Wang Xue-tai & Liu Guan-jun, Jilin Science & Technology Publishing Co., Changchun, 1991, p.361
[6] Cheng Can-ruo, *Ibid.*, p. 636
[7] Lin Yun-gui, *Ibid.*, p. 715
[8] Feng Ming-qing, as reported by Liang Guang-yu in "A Brief Introduction to Professor Feng Ming-qing's Theory & Understanding of the Treatment of Diabetes," *He Nan Zhong Yi* (*Henan Chinese Medicine*), # 1, 2000, p. 15
[9] *Ibid.*, p. 15
[10] Hu Jian-hua, as anthologized in Dan Shu-jian & Chen Zi-hua's *Xiao Ke Juan* (*The Wasting & Thirsting Book*), Chinese National Chinese Medicine & Medicinals Publishing Co., Beijing, 1999, p. 263

3

The Disease Causes & Mechanisms of Diabetes

Most Chinese sources consider dryness and heat leading to qi and yin vacuity as the main disease mechanisms of diabetes mellitus. This dryness and heat may be due to any of five main causes: 1) natural endowment exuberance *or* insufficiency, 2) dietary irregularity, 3) psychoemotional stress, 4) unregulated stirring and stillness, and 5) unregulated sexual activity. A sixth disease cause may be iatrogenesis, and a seventh may be gu worms.

FORMER HEAVEN NATURAL ENDOWMENT

When it comes to former heaven natural endowment as a disease cause of diabetes, most Chinese authors stress former heaven insufficiency. This may mean either a former heaven qi and/or yin insufficiency. For instance, Prof. Zhang Su-qing of Xian stresses an original yin depletion and vacuity as the main type of natural endowment insufficiency.[1] Some people are simply born with less yin than others. The act of living is the transformation of yin into yang and the consumption of yin by yang in the same way a candle's flame transforms wax into light and also consumes that wax. The *Nei Jing (Inner Classic)* says, "[By] 40 years, yin is automatically half." This statement alone helps explain why diabetes is primarily a condition associated with aging. If yin is insufficient to moisten and enrich, this leads to symptoms of dryness. If yin is insufficient to control yang, this leads to hyperactivity of yang and the engenderment of internal heat. If a person is born with less yin, such symptoms of yin fluid dryness and insufficiency may appear earlier than in another person born with more yin. In addition, once yin vacuity gives rise to yang hyperactivity and internal heat, such internal heat damages and consumes yin fluids all the more.

However, the *Ling Shu (Spiritual Axis)*, "Five Changes," also notes, "[If] the five viscera are soft and weak, [there will be] susceptibility to pure heat wasting disease." The word *ruo* or weak primarily implies qi vacuity in Chinese medicine. If any of the five viscera are fragile or weak, they cannot perform their various functions. These functions include the transformation and engenderment of qi, blood, and fluids. They include the movement and transformation of food and liquids as well as the movement of the blood. They also include the transformation of excess qi and blood into latter heaven essence. Impairment in any of these functions may lead to further qi and yin vacuity or the engenderment of heat evils, phlegm rheum, qi stagnation, and blood stasis. Thus, the *Ling Shu*, "Root Treasuries," states that heart fragility, lung fragility, liver fragility, spleen fragility, and/or kidney fragility leads to "susceptibility to pure heat wasting disease and easy damage." This means that the qi and yin of persons with inherently weak viscera may be more easily damaged than others whose viscera are inherently stronger.

However, diabetes may also be associated with former heaven, or at least habitual, bodily exuberance. Just as some people have a inherent tendency to qi or yin vacuity, others have an inherent tendency to yang exuberance. People with yang exuberance easily develop internal heat. They also commonly have exuberant stomach yang. When one has exuberant stomach yang, they tend to disperse and transform foods and liquids more quickly than others. Thus they develop large appetites and frequently overeat. If overeating leads to gaining weight and developing adipose tissue, such adipose tissue itself aggravates internal heat. This is based on the saying, "[If one is] fat, [they] must have internal heat." In addition, people with habitual bodily yang exuberance also tend to overwork. During their youth, they have a greater capacity for work and exertion. However, as the aging process begins to take its toll, these people may still habitually overwork, failing to conserve their qi and yin, thus damaging and consuming both through overtaxation.

In real life, people are not entirely habitually qi and/or yin vacuous and insufficient or habitually yang exuberant. Most people are born with a complex assortment of innate vacuities and repletions. It is common to find persons with a strong spleen having weak kidneys or vice versa. Similarly, it is also common to find people with a hot, exuberant stomach and a cold, damp spleen. In any case, Chinese medicine does recognize that inherited tendencies, bodily constitution, and age all play a large part in the development of diabetes.

DIETARY IRREGULARITIES

From as early as the Spring and Autumn and Warring States periods, Chinese doctors have understood that diet plays a very large part in the causation of this disease. The Chinese medical literature identifies three main groups of foods which may cause diabetes. The first are sugars and sweets. Sweet is the flavor of the earth phase and is, therefore, inherently damp. This means that sweet-flavored foods engender fluids in the body. Because the sweet flavor homes to the spleen, sweet-flavored foods especially engender fluids in the spleen. However, the spleen likes dryness and is averse to dampness. Dampness in the spleen damages it, leading to both its encumbrance and vacuity. In Chinese medicine, it is believed that the sweet flavor is moderating or relaxing. Therefore, persons experiencing liver depression qi stagnation typically crave sweets as a sort of self-medication of their tension and depression. While sweet-flavored foods may temporarily relax this tension and depression, ultimately they damage the spleen.

The second group of foods Chinese medicine believes may cause DM are fats and oils. Fats and oils are both inherently damp and inherently hot in Chinese medicine. This means that fats and oils engender fluids. If fats and oils are excessively consumed, an overabundance of fluids will transform into damp evils. These damp evils may give rise to damp heat, they may damage the spleen, resulting in spleen encumbrance and vacuity, and they may eventually congeal into phlegm.

The third group of foods Chinese medicine implicates in the etiology of this condition is alcohol. Alcohol is described in Chinese medicine as being acrid, bitter, sweet, and hot. The heat, acridity, and bitterness of alcohol all damage and consume yin and engender internal heat, while the sweetness of alcohol engenders dampness and damages the spleen which is averse to dampness.

Therefore, long-term and/or excessive consumption of alcohol easily leads to dampness and heat. If this damp heat endures, it eventually leads to qi and yin vacuities.

In addition, overeating acrid, warm or hot foods may exacerbate any tendency for any of the above three dietary irregularities to result in damp heat and damage and consumption of yin fluids.

PSYCHOEMOTIONAL STRESS

Zhang Zi-he, in his *Ru Men Shi Qin (A Confucian's Responsibility for One Parent's)*, "Treatise on the Three Wastings," says, "Wasting and thirsting... is produced by excessive consumption and chaos of the essence spirit [or psyche] and dryness, heat, depression, and exuberance." This underscores the importance of psychoemtional stress as one of the contributory causes of diabetes in Chinese medicine. Stress, no matter what kind, always involves some sort of unfulfilled desire. Either we desire something which we positively want but cannot have or, at least cannot have as much of as we want, such as time or money, or we desire to be rid of something which we negatively do not want, such as trouble, pain, suffering, and disease. In either case, unfulfilled desires leads to liver depression qi stagnation, since every desire, whether positive or negative is nothing other than the subjective sensation of the flow of qi towards or away from something. Because the liver governs coursing and discharge, any thwarting of the movement of qi may damage the liver, causing it to become depressed.

When the liver becomes depressed, any of several things may happen. One, the liver may counterflow horizontally and invade the earth phase. In that case, the spleen typically becomes vacuous and weak, while the stomach may either become vacuous and weak or hot and hyperactive. Secondly, liver depression may transform heat. If this heat endures, it may damage yin fluids. Since heat, due to its yang nature, always tends to move upwards, this heat not only accumulates in and damages the yin of the liver-gallbladder but also accumulates in and damages the yin of the stomach, lungs, and heart. Third, since the qi moves the blood and body fluids, liver depression may give rise to blood stasis on the one hand and phlegm dampness on the other.

In addition, specific emotions may damage specific viscera and cause specific types of damage to the flow of qi. For instance, overthinking and worry damage the spleen, causing the qi to bind in the middle, while anger damages the liver and leads the qi to rise. When anger damages the liver, this means that, subsequent to the anger, liver depression qi stagnation become even worse. When anger leads the qi to rise, this aggravates any tendency of the liver, stomach, lungs, or heart to counterflow upward. Fear damages the kidneys and leads the qi to descend. Thus continuous or excessive fear may lead to kidney qi vacuity and polyuria. Excessive sorrow damages the lungs and scatters the qi. If the lung qi is scattered, the defensive qi cannot densely pack the interstices and prevent entry by external evils. Likewise, it cannot downbear and depurate. This means that the lungs cannot rid themselves of the heat that tends to accumulate in them, nor can they rid themselves of phlegm and rheum which may back up within them. Excessive joy may be interpreted in either of two ways. On the one hand, it may be interpreted as excitement and agitation which easily give rise to heat which then harasses the heart and consumes yin. On the other, it may be interpreted as happiness. When interpreted this way, joy is relaxing and is the antidote to all the other pathological affects. However, if happiness leads to complacency and lethargy, these may then lead to qi vacuity and stasis and stagnation as described below.

UNREGULATED STIRRING & STILLNESS

In Chinese medicine, stirring refers to any movement or activity in the body since all activities are dependent on, and a manifestation of, the movement of the qi. This can be mental-emotional stirring, verbal stirring, or physical stirring. Every stirring or movement in the body is empowered by qi. Therefore, it is easy to see that overtaxation may consume and damage the qi. Further, because the spleen is the latter heaven root of the engenderment and transformation of qi, fatigue and overtaxation first and foremost damage the spleen. This can then lead to any of the complications associated with a vacuous, weak spleen. However, as explained above, life is the transformation and consumption of yin blood by yang qi. Thus, fatigue and overtaxation do not just result in qi vacuity but also in yin vacuity.

Stillness is the absence of stirring. It can mean mental-emotional stillness, verbal stillness, or physical stillness. However, as a cause of disease, stillness primarily refers to too much physical inactivity. Physical activity promotes the function of the spleen and stomach, stomach and intestines vis à vis the upbearing of the clear and downbearing of the turbid. In other words, although overtaxation consumes and damages the qi, adequate physical activity promotes the spleen's engenderment of the qi. Thus it is said, "Excessive lying damages the spleen." Therefore, insufficient physical exercise may cause or aggravate spleen vacuity. Physical activity also promotes the movement of the qi, blood, and fluids throughout the body. Hence physical inactivity contributes to the depression of the qi, blood, dampness, and phlegm. For instance, physical activity is one way of dealing with liver depression qi stagnation. It is also a way to remedy obesity due to accumulation of phlegm turbidity and poor circulation due to blood stasis.

It is easy to see that, when it comes to stirring and stillness, too much or too little of either may contribute to the causation of diabetes mellitus. As in all things having to do with Chinese medicine, the key is the Doctrine of the Mean— exercise and rest in the right, i.e., moderate, amounts.

UNREGULATED SEXUAL ACTIVITY

According to Chinese medical theory, sexual desire is the subjective experience of the flaming and exuberance of the lifegate fire. If one indulges this desire by engaging in a sexual activity that leads to orgasm, yang reaches its apogee or extreme and transforms into yin. In terms of qi, blood, yin, and yang, this means that qi and yang are both discharged, while yin essence is lost and/or consumed. Because the kidneys govern the genitalia, excessive sexual activity is believed to lead to kidney qi and essence consumption and vacuity. Thus Wang Tao, in his *Wai Tai Mi Yao (Secret Essentials of the External Platform)*, "Wasting & Thirsting and Middle Wasting," says:

> Excessive bedroom affairs must result in kidney qi vacuity and consumption and the engenderment of heat in the lower burner. [This] heat leads to kidney dryness, and kidney dryness leads to thirst.

Interestingly, in our experience it is people with habitual yang exuberance who have the most sexual desire. These typically are also people who hunger rapidly, easily transform depression into heat, and tend to overwork. Further, stirring of the lifegate or ministerial fire causes it to counterflow upward, leaving its source in the lower burner and harassing above. According to Li Dong-yuan, upward stirring of the ministerial fire damages the spleen and leads to qi vacuity based on the saying, "Strong fire eats the qi." Thus excessive sexual activity may lead to both spleen and kidney vacuity.

IATROGENESIS

Traditionally, it was believed that overadministration of mineral medicinals in the form of longevity tonics or elixirs of immortality may damage yin due to these mineral medicinals' warm, acrid nature. Both Sun Si-miao and Wang Tao, living and writing in the Tang dynasty, emphasized such mineral medicinals as causes of wasting and thirsting. In a modern context, certain Western medicinals may cause or aggravate insulin resistance and thus lead to or aggravate diabetes. For instance, both thiazide diuretics and beta-blockers administered to lower and control the blood pressure may cause or aggravate diabetes, while lithium, administered to control bipolar affective disorder, may cause or aggravate the nephropathy often associated with long-term diabetes.

According to the logic of Chinese medicine, other Western drugs which might cause or contribute to the development of diabetes include antibiotics and corticosteroids, such as prednisone. Long-term or excessive use of antibiotics may damage the spleen. This leads proximally to spleen qi vacuity with all its attendant complications and, down the line, to the engenderment of turbid dampness or damp heat. Corticosteroids are very upbearing and out-thrusting. This is why they are so effective for dispersing inflammation. They clear heat the same way that Chinese exterior-resolving medicinals do, but thrusting it out of the body. However, their down-side is similar to that of other powerful acrid, out-thrusting, exterior-resolving medicinals—they consume yin and lead to yang hyperactivity. Since yin and yang are mutually rooted, ultimately, they lead to yin and yang vacuity with concomitant fire effulgence.

GU WORMS

While the Chinese literature does not, to the best of our knowledge, discuss worms or *chong* as a disease cause of wasting and thirsting, we believe that, in at least some cases, an understanding of gu worms may be helpful in understanding the pathophysiology of DM. In Chinese medicine, worms are divided into two broad categories: visible and invisible. Visible worms include tapeworms, roundworms, pinworms, and hookworms, the same parasitic worms recognized by modern Western medicine. However, Chinese medicine also recognizes a category of "invisible" worms called gu. *Gu* worms are disease-causing agents that somehow enter the body through the mouth with food. Once inside the body, they cause multisystem, complex, knotty disorders. These multisystem disorders always involve chronic digestive complaints, such as indigestion, flatulence, diarrhea, or alternating diarrhea and constipation. On top of such chronic digestive disorders, they also typically involve musculoskeletal disorders, dermatological disorders, and psychiatric disturbances as well as various endocrine dyscrasias, including reproductive disorders.

According to Zhu Dan-xi, gu worm disorders always involve great spleen vacuity complicated by dampness, qi stagnation, and blood stasis. Nowadays, we say that gu worm disorders always involve the triad of spleen vacuity, liver depression, and damp heat, with liver depression qi stagnation possibly giving rise to blood stasis. As we have seen above, spleen vacuity, liver depression, and damp heat are all potential disease mechanisms of diabetes. Further, *Candida albicans*, although categorized as a fungus in Western medicine, is categorized as one of the invisible "worms" of Chinese medicine, and, at least some modern Western clinicians believe that chronic candidiasis may give rise to polysystemic conditions which include diabetes. In this case, it is a diet heavy in sugars and sweets, refined carbohydrates, and alcohol and other fermented foods which causes or at least aggravates candidiasis. While one does not *have* to consider gu worms as a cause of diabetes (since spleen vacuity, damp heat, and liver depression are adequate disease mechanisms on their own), it is our experience that taking gu worms into account helps to clarify both the Chinese herbal and dietary therapy of DM patients with obvious polysystemic chronic candidiasis.

DISEASE MECHANISMS

Above we have presented the main Chinese medical disease causes of diabetes. Such disease causes then initiate a train of disease mechanisms. In our experience, most DM patients' conditions are the result of a number of factors causing a conjunction of several mechanisms, any or all of which lead to qi and yin vacuity with dryness and heat. For instance, we have seen above that any of a number of factors may cause spleen vacuity – overeating sweets and fats, psychoemotional stress causing liver depression, overtaxation and fatigue, etc. If spleen vacuity fails to move and transform fluids and these collect and accumulate, transforming into dampness, this dampness (or phlegm dampness) may itself lead directly to yin vacuity. This is because evil dampness is nothing other than righteous fluids which are bound up in a way which makes them unavailable to moisten and enrich the body tissues. Thus dampness and phlegm can themselves lead directly to yin vacuity. Similarly, both dampness and phlegm may hinder and obstruct the free flow of yang qi. Since yang qi is inherently warm, if it becomes backed up behind depressed phlegm and dampness, it may transform into heat, thus turning dampness into damp heat and phlegm into phlegm heat. In either case, the heat of damp heat or phlegm heat may damage and consume yin fluids. Further, since blood and fluids flow together, if dampness and/or phlegm cause blood stasis, static blood may impede the engenderment of new or fresh blood. In that case, dry blood may lead to or aggravate yin vacuity.

In the same way, there are a number of pathological disease mechanisms involved in DM shared between two or more viscera and bowels. We have already seen above how liver depression may invade the spleen and stomach. If the stomach becomes hot and, therefore, hyperactive, it will disperse foods and liquids more quickly than normal. It is said in Chinese medicine, "The kidneys are the bar of the stomach." This saying has to do with the fact that, at least from one perspective, it is the stomach which sends turbid fluids down to the kidneys for eventual excretion by the bladder. Therefore, polyuria may be due at first solely to a stomach heat repletion. However, over time, the kidney qi may become exhausted by this polyuria since some kidney-bladder qi is used up by the expulsion of, and exits with, the urine. This is the mechanism which explains how stomach heat repletion results in eventual kidney qi vacuity. However, damp heat pouring downward from the middle burner may also damage the liver and kidneys below, leading to either or both yin and yang vacuities.

As stated above, heat is yang in nature and, therefore, has an innate tendency to rise. In addition, all the yang qi in the body is connected to and rooted in the lifegate fire. Damp heat pouring downward may stir lifegate fire, resulting in hyperactivity of ministerial fire. Such hyperactivity and upward flaming of ministerial-lifegate fire may then cause or aggravate any evil heat or yang hyperactivity in any of the viscera and bowels of the body, but especially in the liver-gallbladder, stomach, heart, and lungs. The lungs are the florid canopy, and the heart is the tai yang of yang. Both are located in the upper burner. Therefore, all heat will tend to ascend to accumulate in and damage lung yin and accumulate in and harass the heart spirit.

On the other hand, the heart and lungs both primarily get their qi and, in the case of the heart, their blood from the spleen. It is the spleen which upbears the clear to become the qi in the lungs and the blood in the heart. Therefore, anything which causes a spleen qi vacuity may also cause a heart and/or lung vacuity. Since the lungs govern the defensive qi, a spleen-lung qi vacuity may lead to easy contraction of external evils and/or nondepuration and downbearing of the qi and fluids. Since it is the heart qi which constructs and the heart blood which nourishes the spirit, a spleen-heart vacuity may lead to nonconstruction and malnourishment of the heart spirit with attendant restless and disquietude. It may also lead to the heart failing to stir the vessels and thus the engenderment of blood stasis in the chest, causing heart pain and loss of consciousness.

According to the *Nei Jing*, the spleen typically becomes vacuous and weak in the mid 30s (if not before). As the authors of the *Nei Jing* would have it, this is why we begin to develop wrinkles on our faces at around this time, *i.e.*,

the blood is not nourishing the skin above. According to Yan De-xin, the modern Chinese geriatrics specialist, this spleen vacuity in the mid 30s is due to liver depression and other impediments to the free flow of qi developed earlier. By 40, half our yin is automatically half used up by the simple act of living. Those of us who have lived more intensely, may have used up more than half our yin by that age. Now, grey hair begins to show on our heads, due to liver blood and kidney yin declining and becoming insufficient. If spleen qi vacuity reaches the kidneys, this may give rise to spleen-kidney qi or yang vacuity. A yin and blood vacuity may fail to nourish and emolliate the liver and hence the liver may not be able to control its function of coursing and discharging. This may then cause or aggravate liver depression. Likewise, if yang vacuity becomes vacuous and insufficient, ministerial fire may not adequately warm and steam the liver. Again, the liver may not be able to manage its function of coursing and discharging, with the causation and aggravation of liver depression.

If spleen vacuity and/or enduring heat evils lead to yin and blood vacuity, the sinews and vessels may lack adequate nourishment. The sinews may become numb and the skin insensitive, or they may contract, giving rise to spasms and contractures. It is also possible for the sinews and vessels to lose their nourishment due to blockage and obstruction by blood stasis and phlegm. In either case, the channels and vessels will fail to move and stir the qi and blood throughout the body, and any number of viscera, bowels, orifices, and body tissues may fail to perform their functions.

If dampness is engendered internally, being heavy and turbid, it tends to sink downward to the lower half of the body where it obstructs the free flow of qi and blood. If damp depression transforms heat or internal heat mixes with dampness, damp heat may be engendered. If this damp heat stews and smolders, it may brew toxins. These toxins may then cause various types of toxic swelling and ulcers on the skin, especially on the lower half of the body. Since these toxic swellings impede not only the free flow of yang qi but also that of yin blood, frequently these heat toxins become bound with blood stasis, thus giving rise to stasis heat, *i.e.*, blood stasis and heat. If heat and toxins putrefy the flesh and blood stasis deprives the flesh of its nourishment, this may give rise to necrosis.

Hence it is easy to see why Chinese doctors consider diabetes a "knotty" disease. A knotty disease means a disease caused by a number of intertwined disease mechanisms, and the disease mechanisms of diabetes in real-life patients are nothing if not intertwined. However, in an attempt to keep things simple, we agree with Quan Xiao-

The Disease Causes and Disease Mechanisms of Diabetes — Table A

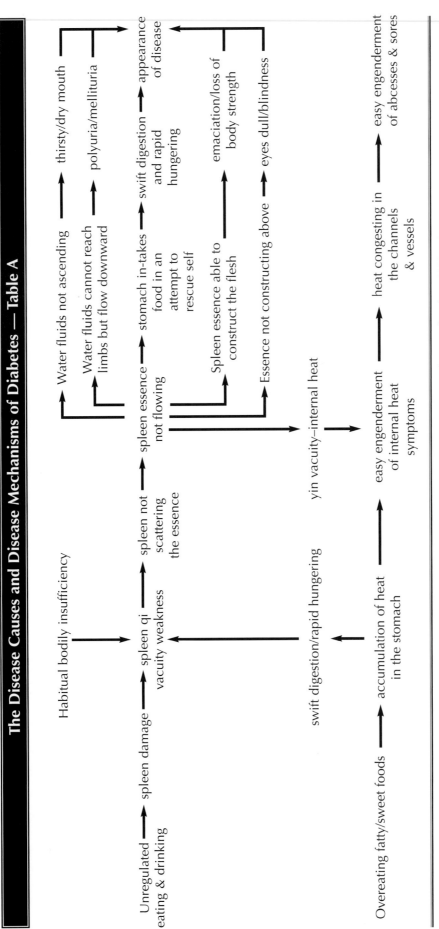

From Pan Zhao-xi, "The Disease Causes, Disease Mechanisms, & Treatment Methods for Diabetes," *Jiang Su Zhong Yi (Jiangsu Chinese Medicine)*, #1, 2000, p. 2

The Disease Causes and Disease Mechanisms of Diabetes —Table B

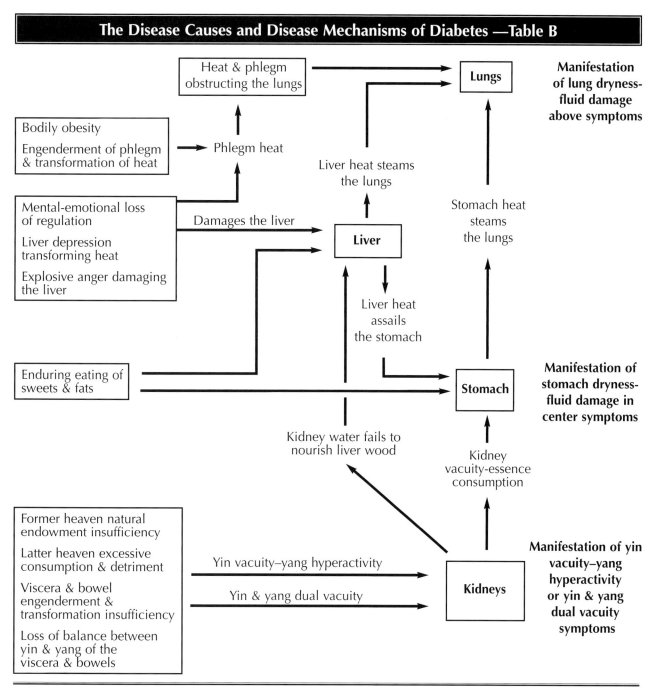

From Gan Rui-feng & Lü Ren-he, *Tang Niao Bing (Diabetes)*, People's Health & Hygiene Publishing Co., Beijing, 1985, p. 9

lin that the four great mechanisms of diabetes are depression, heat, vacuity, and detriment.[2] Depression here means liver depression. Heat primarily means liver and stomach heat. Vacuity means spleen and lung qi vacuity, lung-stomach fluid damage, qi and yin vacuity, liver-kidney yin vacuity, and spleen-kidney yang vacuity. And detriment means detriment to the vessels. This includes detriment to the large blood vessels of the heart, brain, and lower extremities and the small blood vessels of the eyes, kidneys, and nerves.

BODY TYPE & DISEASE MECHANISMS

According to Quan Xiao-lin, there are different disease mechanisms typically at work in obese and nonobese patients with type 2 diabetes. For those who are obese, Quan emphasizes the overeating of fats and oils and sugars and sweets. These damage the spleen, create phlegm turbidity internally, and lead to the engenderment of heat. In those who are not obese, Quan emphasizes inherent softness and weakness of the five viscera predisposing a person to easy injury by profuse anger. Anger leads the qi to counterflow upward to amass and accumulate within the chest. The blood and qi counterflow and lodge in the skin and muscles, and the blood vessels do not move. Eventually, stasis and stagnation transforms heat which then wastes the muscles and skin. Therefore, in those with diabetes who are not obese, Quan believes the main disease mechanisms are psychoemotional damage to the liver resulting in qi depression and blood stasis, with depression transforming heat.

In addition, Quan believes that the disease mechanisms in those who are obese must be further divided into repletion and vacuity types. In obese women who actually eat less than normal, Quan thinks the main mechanism is spleen vacuity not moving or transporting. Thus phlegm turbidity accumulates, eventually transforming heat. In these patients, there is a lusterless facial complexion, puffy, atonic flesh, fatigue, lack of strength, scanty qi, and a deep, fine pulse. These patients typically do not prominently display the three polys – polydipsia, polyphagia, and polyuria. In those who are obese with a red facial complexion, firm muscles and flesh, undepleted strength, no fatigue, and a surging, large, forceful pulse, the main disease mechanism is overeating leading to spleen qi depression and stagnation, with depression engendering heat. In the first case, there is mainly spleen vacuity, while in the second, there is mainly stomach repletion.[3]

FROM CRADLE TO GRAVE

Many medical authorities believe, "Diabetes is one of the fastest growing health problems today."[4] Although Chinese practitioners recognized this disease as a discrete medical condition more than 2,000 years ago, its incidence appears to be rising in relationship to a group of factors associated with modern and postmodern lifestyle. Some of these factors are obvious and others are not so obvious. Obvious factors include increased consumption of sugars and sweets and fats and oils, decreased physical activity, and increased psychoemotional stress. Less obvious factors include improper feeding of newborns and tod-

dlers and overuse of antibiotics in early childhood. We have seen that spleen vacuity plays a central role in the disease mechanisms of diabetes, and we know that spleen vacuity may be due to overeating sweets, too little physical exercise, overtaxation, and excessive thinking and worrying – all frequently encountered disease causes in Western and other developed countries. However, it is our observation that spleen vacuity in the West is often set in motion in the earliest days and weeks after birth.

It is a statement of fact that the spleen is inherently vacuous and weak in infants and toddlers. Therefore, they easily develop food stagnation. Milk, even mother's milk but especially cow's milk, is very high in *wei* or flavor. Foods high (Chinese say thick) in flavor are highly nutritious, meaning they nourish yin. However, they are also relatively hard to digest and easily create a surplus of dampness and turbidity if overconsumed. This evil dampness and turbidity inhibits the free flow of the qi mechanism and damages the spleen, aggravating the baby's inherent spleen weakness. This situation is commonly created in real-life Western babies by feeding on demand. This means feeding the child, usually with breast milk, any time he or she cries, based on the naive assumption that hunger is the only reason for a baby to cry. Although milk, and especially mother's milk, is the single best food for newborn babies to eat, eating even too much of this wonderful food can cause medical problems, *i.e.*, food stagnation and spleen vacuity. Because food stagnation hinders and obstructs the movement of qi, food stagnation may also give rise to liver depression. In that case, liver depression may also aggravate spleen vacuity. Further, because food and qi stagnation may transform heat, heat in the stomach may be engendered, developing a lifelong tendency to spleen vacuity and stomach heat.

To make matters worse, antibiotics are considered extremely cold and heat-clearing in Chinese medicine. In the People's Republic of China, many Chinese doctors now recognize a new disease entity called "post-antibiotic spleen vacuity syndrome." This refers to the sequelae of excessive or long-term antibiotic use primarily in children. It is a well known fact that antibiotics are routinely mis- and overprescribed. This is so both in China and in the West. Often, infants' first exposure to antibiotics comes in response to food stagnation from overfeeding which has given rise to heat in the stomach and intestines. This heat is often exacerbated at the time of teething due to a global periodic hyperactivity in lifegate fire associated with growth and development. This periodic hyperactivity is a normal physiologic event. However, when lifegate fire becomes periodically hyperactive, because it is connected to the yang qi of all the other viscera and bowels and body tissues, it may cause mutual inflammation of any smoldering, subclinical heat evils anywhere in the body. Since the yang ming has a lot of qi, this periodic lifegate fire hyperactivity may especially cause inflammation of any heat in the stomach and intestines. The stomach and intestines have internal network vessels that go to the inner ear. If heat evils travel up these internal pathways, it may become trapped in the bony box of the ear where it brews and putrifies the blood and fluids there, thus engendering pus. Hence the Western physician prescribes antibiotics for otitis media. This eliminates the inflammation, but often damages the baby's already weak spleen. Because the antibiotics have done nothing to eliminate the dampness, turbidity, and stagnant food which caused the transformative heat evils in the first place, these may return over time, especially since their root disease mechanism is spleen vacuity. Hence a vicious cycle is created of heat evils due to spleen vacuity leading to the prescription of antibiotics leading to more spleen vacuity.

On top of this vicious cycle, we then commonly feed our children foods which only aggravate heat in the stomach and dampness and vacuity in the spleen. For instance, fried, fatty foods, such as potato chips, french fries, hamburgers and hot dogs all engender heat and dampness internally. Other less obvious foods which damage children's spleens are fruit juices, uncooked vegetables, and chilled and iced foods. Fruit juices are intensely sweet. They are the concentrated sweetness of many pieces of fruit. While a little sweet fortifies the spleen, excessive sweetness damages the spleen and engenders dampness. Likewise, while uncooked vegetables, such as celery, carrots, cucumbers, and lettuce have lots of vitamins, they tend to be cool or cold. Cooking helps mitigate this cool nature. However, if eaten raw or uncooked by those with a weak spleen, such uncooked vegetables may also damage the spleen. This is even more likely if one fills the raw celery stalk with cream cheese or peanut butter, staple snacks at many American daycare centers. When children develop hot stomachs, as is all too common among Western

toddlers, they will tend to crave cold foods and drinks. However, cold, chilled, iced foods and drinks have two seemingly opposite effects on children's (and adults') middle burners. The coldness damages the spleen at the same time as it actually heats the stomach. This is because, when something very cold lands in the stomach, the stomach's first response, in terms of Chinese medicine, is for its yang qi to become hyperactive in order to transform and disperse this coldness. Therefore, habitual consumption of chilled and iced foods and drinks creates habitual stomach heat which then becomes its own vicious cycle.

The point of this discussion is that, in many Westerners and those living in developed countries, the beginnings of the disease mechanisms of diabetes mellitus are initiated almost immediately after birth due to improper feeding and iatrogenesis – spleen vacuity and dampness, liver depression qi stagnation, and stomach heat. When one adds on top of this pediatric scenario the modern Western diet and lifestyle of adults, it seems to us no wonder that the incidence of this condition is increasing in developed countries adopting the diet and lifestyle of the U.S.A. and Western Europe. Interestingly, these same disease mechanisms also often result in allergies, allergies can lead to autoimmune diseases, and diabetes may be, at least in part, an autoimmune disease. Therefore, in order to prevent the growth in incidence of diabetes in the developed and developing world, we not only need to be careful of diet and lifestyle in adults but also need to reform our thinking about the feeding and health care of the very young.[5]

ENDNOTES:

[1] Zhao Kun *et al.*, "Professor Zhang Su-qing's Experience of the Diagnosis & Treatment of Diabetes," *Xin Zhong Yi (New Chinese Medicine)*, #5, 2001, p. 14
[2] Quan Xiao-lin, "Six Treatises on Wasting & Thirsting," *Zhong Yi Za Zhi (Journal of Chinese Medicine)*, #4, 2001, p. 252-253
[3] *Ibid.*, p. 252
[4] www.phcg.com/library/summaries/hstn/jan2001/201-0438.htm
[5] For more information on the feeding of infants and post-antibiotic spleen vacuity syndrome, see Bob Flaws's *A Handbook of TCM Pediatrics*, Blue Poppy Press, Boulder, CO, 1997

DIABETES MATERIA MEDICA

Most patients with diabetes mellitus exhibit some combination of qi and yin vacuity, dryness, and heat. Therefore, the main treatment principles for the treatment of DM are to 1) fortify the spleen and supplement the qi, 2) supplement the kidneys and enrich yin, and 3) clear heat and engender fluids. If yin disease reaches yang, one will also have to invigorate yang. If spleen vacuity has given rise to dampness, one will also have to dry dampness and eliminate turbidity, while if enduring disease has resulted in blood stasis, one will also have to quicken the blood and transform or dispel stasis. Because there is a fairly circumscribed group of treatment principles, we can also identify the most commonly used Chinese medicinals in the treatment of diabetes. Most formulas for diabetes and its complications will include at least several of the medicinals described below.

RADIX PANACIS GINSENG (REN SHEN)

NATURE & FLAVOR: Sweet, slightly bitter, and level (or neutral)

CHANNEL GATHERING: Spleen, lungs & heart

FUNCTIONS & INDICATIONS:

1. Greatly supplements the original qi: Used for vacuity desertion conditions either alone or with Radix Lateralis Praeparatus Aconiti Carmichaeli (*Fu Zi*), as in *Du Shen Tang* (Solitary Ginseng Decoction) and *Shen Fu Tang* (Ginseng & Aconite Decoction) respectively.

2. Engenders fluids: Used for spleen vacuity transforming fluids insufficiency or heat diseases damaging fluids conditions. It is often combined with Radix Trichosanthis

Kirlowii (*Tian Hua Fen*) and Radix Dioscoreae Oppositae (*Shan Yao*) for this purpose.

3. Supplements the spleen and lungs and supports the righteous qi: Used for spleen vacuity and lung weakness conditions, such as diarrhea and cough. It is also used in global asthenic conditions.

DOSE: 6-9g; up to 30g when used alone

CONTRAINDICATIONS: Do not use with radishes. Use cautiously if dryness and heat are severe.

RADIX DIOSCOREAE OPPOSITAE (SHAN YAO)

NATURE & FLAVOR: Sweet and neutral

CHANNEL GATHERING: Kidneys, lungs & spleen

FUNCTIONS & INDICATIONS:

1. Fortifies the spleen and supplements the lungs: Used for spleen and/or lung vacuity. This medicinal can be combined with Rhizoma Atractylodis Macrocephalae (*Bai Zhu*) and Sclerotium Poriae Cocos (*Fu Ling*) for spleen vacuity diarrhea and fatigue. It can also be combined with Tuber Ophiopogonis Japonici (*Mai Men Dong*) and Fructus Schisandrae Chinensis (*Wu Wei Zi*) for lung vacuity cough.

2. Secures the kidneys and boosts the essence: Used for kidney yin vacuity. It can be combined with cooked Radix Rehmanniae (*Shu Di*) for night sweats or with Radix Codonopsitis Pilosulae (*Dang Shen*) for fatigue and watery stools due to spleen-kidney qi vacuity. Also used with

Semen Euryalis Ferocis (*Qian Shi*) for diarrhea, spermatorrhea, and vaginal discharge due to kidneys not securing the essence.

DOSE: 9-30g

CONTRAINDICATIONS: Do not use for replete dampness, stagnation, or accumulation.

Shan Yao can be used decocted and administered as a tea in high dosages (250g) for vacuities of the spleen, lungs, and kidneys in wasting and thirsting disease.

UNCOOKED RADIX REHMANNIAE (*SHENG DI*)

NATURE & FLAVOR: Sweet, bitter, cold

CHANNEL GATHERING: Heart, liver & kidneys

FUNCTIONS & INDICATIONS:

1. Clears heat, nourishes yin, and engenders fluids: Used for wasting and thirsting disease, oral thirst, and polydipsia. For these purposes, commonly combined with Radix Dioscoreae Oppositae (*Shan Yao*) and Fructus Corni Officinalis (*Shan Zhu Yu*).

2. Clears heat and cools the blood: Used for warm heat entering the constructive and blood resulting in various conditions, such as a crimson tongue, body heat (or generalized fever), hematemesis, hemafecia, etc. Commonly combined with Cortex Radicis Moutan (*Dan Pi*) and Radix Rubrus Paeoniae Lactiflorae (*Chi Shao*), as in *Xi Jiao Di Huang Tang* (Rhinoceros Horn & Rehmannia Decoction).

3. Enriches yin and clears heat: Used for heat diseases damaging yin and yin vacuity-internal heat conditions. Commonly combined with Herba Artemisiae Apiaceae (*Qing Hao*) and Carapax Amydae Sinensis (*Bie Jia*), as in *Qing Hao Bie Jia Tang* (Artemisia Apiacea & Carapax Amydae Decoction).

DOSE: 9-30g

CONTRAINDICATIONS: Do not use in cold patterns

Modern research has shown that *Sheng Di* has a hypoglycemic effect.

RADIX CODONOPSITIS PILOSULAE (*DANG SHEN*)

NATURE & FLAVOR: Sweet, level

CHANNEL GATHERING: Spleen & lungs

FUNCTIONS & INDICATIONS:

1. Fortifies the spleen and supplements the qi: Used for spleen qi vacuity weakness with loss of control over the origin (of qi and blood) and movement and transformation, with symptoms such as torpid intake and fatigue. Commonly combined with Radix Dioscoreae Oppositae (*Shan Yao*), Rhizoma Atractylodis Macrocephalae (*Bai Zhu*), and Sclerotium Poriae Cocos (*Fu Ling*), as in *Si Jun Zi Tang* (Four Gentlemen Decoction) and *Shen Ling Bai Zhu San* (Ginseng [or Codonopsis], Poria & Atractylodes Powder).

2. Supplements the center: Used for spleen vacuity with insufficiency of engenderment and transformation of the qi and blood, fluids and humors. Commonly combined with Radix Astragali Membranacei (*Huang Qi*) to boost the qi and engender fluids.

DOSE: 9-20g

CONTRAINDICATIONS: Internal heat exuberance. Do not use with radishes.

RADIX ASTRAGALI MEMBRANACEI (*HUANG QI*)

NATURE & FLAVOR: Sweet, slightly warm

CHANNEL GATHERING: Spleen & lungs

FUNCTIONS & INDICATIONS:

1. Supplements the qi and upbears yang: Used for a variety of qi vacuity conditions where there is mainly lung-spleen vacuity with fatigue, lack of strength, shortness of breath, poor appetite, diarrhea, and downward sagging of the internal organs. Commonly combined with Radix Panacis Ginseng (*Ren Shen*) and Rhizoma Atractylodis Macrocephalae (*Bai Zhu*).

2. Boosts the qi and stops thirst: Used for spleen vacuity not ordering the fluids upward causing thirst, and qi and blood vacuity causing lack of strength and emaciation. Commonly combined with Radix Dioscoreae Oppositae

(*Shan Yao*), Tuber Ophiopogonis Japonici (*Mai Men Dong*), Radix Trichosanthis Kirlowii (*Tian Hua Fen*), and Rhizoma Atractylodis (*Cang Zhu*).

3. Secures the exterior and out-thrusts toxins: Used for exterior vacuity spontaneous perspiration and righteous vacuity without the power to out-thrust and exit toxins externally.

DOSE: 9-30g and up to as much as 60g

CONTRAINDICATIONS: Use a smaller dose in internal heat exuberance.

Huang Qi raises the body's immunity. It has also been demonstrated to lower blood sugar in living beings.

RHIZOMA COPTIDIS CHINENSIS (HUANG LIAN)

NATURE & FLAVOR: Bitter, cold, without toxins

CHANNEL GATHERING: Heart, liver, stomach & large intestine

FUNCTIONS & INDICATIONS:

1. Clears heat and drains fire: Used for middle burner fire exuberance with oral thirst, rapid hungering, and high fever. Commonly combined with Radix Scutellariae Baicalensis (*Huang Qin*), Radix Trichosanthis Kirlowii (*Tian Hua Fen*), and Rhizoma Anemarrhenae Aspheloidis (*Zhi Mu*).

2. Dries dampness and resolves toxins: Used for dysentery, enteritis, and fire toxins causing sores and welling abscesses.

DOSE: 3-15g, added to decoctions later

CONTRAINDICATIONS: Spleen-stomach vacuity cold conditions

RHIZOMA ANEMARRHENAE ASPHELOIDIS (ZHI MU)

NATURE & FLAVOR: Bitter, sweet, cold

CHANNEL GATHERING: Lungs, stomach & kidneys

FUNCTIONS & INDICATIONS:

1. Clears heat and drains fire, enriches yin and supplements the lungs and kidneys: Used for lung-kidney yin vacuity with tidal heat, night sweats, vexatious heat in the five hearts, dry mouth, oral thirst, polydipsia, and polyuria. Commonly combined with Radix Trichosanthis Kirlowii (*Tian Hua Fen*), Cortex Phellodendri (*Huang Bai*), Fructus Lycii Chinensis (*Gou Qi Zi*), and Fructus Schisandrae Chinensis (*Wu Wei Zi*).

2. Drains fire and eliminates vexation: Used for warm disease evils existing in the qi aspect or division with high fever and vexatious thirst. Commonly combined with Gypsum Fibrosum (*Shi Gao*), as in *Bai Hu Tang* (White Tiger Decoction).

DOSE: 6-15g

CONTRAINDICATIONS: Diarrhea

Modern research has shown that the combination of *Zhi Mu* and Radix Trichosanthis Kirlowii (*Tian Hua Fen*) can lower blood glucose.

RADIX TRICHOSANTHIS KIRLOWII (TIAN HUA FEN)

NATURE & FLAVOR: Bitter, slightly sweet, cold

CHANNEL GATHERING: Lungs & stomach

FUNCTIONS & INDICATIONS:

1. Clears heat and engenders fluids: Used for heat diseases which have damaged fluids with oral thirst and wasting and thirsting. Commonly combined with Radix Dioscoreae Oppositae (*Shan Yao*), Rhizoma Anemarrhenae Aspheloidis (*Zhi Mu*), Fructus Schisandrae Chinensis (*Wu Wei Zi*), and Folium Lophatheri Gracilis (*Dan Zhu Ye*).

2. Moistens the lungs and stops cough: Used for lung dryness cough and dry throat. Commonly combined with Tuber Ophiopogonis Japonici (*Mai Men Dong*) and Tuber Asparagi Cochinensis (*Tian Men Dong*).

3. Disperses swelling and expels pus: Used for sores, ulcers, swellings, and toxins.

DOSE: 6-20g

CONTRAINDICATIONS: Do not use during pregnancy.

TUBER OPHIOPOGONIS JAPONICI (MAI MEN DONG)

NATURE & FLAVOR: Sweet, slightly bitter, slightly cold

CHANNEL GATHERING: Heart, lungs & stomach

FUNCTIONS & INDICATIONS:

1. Enriches yin and engenders fluids: Used for heat diseases which have damaged fluids with oral thirst, dry tongue, and wasting and thirsting. Commonly combined for these purposes with uncooked Radix Rehmanniae (*Sheng Di*) and Radix Glehniae Littoralis (*Sha Shen*).

2. Moistens the lungs and clears the heart, drains heat and eliminates vexation: Used for yin vacuity and lung dryness with cough and for heart yin insufficiency with fright palpitations and fearful throbbing.

DOSE: 6-20g

FRUCTUS SCHISANDRAE CHINENSIS (WU WEI ZI)

NATURE & FLAVOR: Sour, sweet, warm

CHANNEL GATHERING: Lungs, heart & kidneys

FUNCTIONS & INDICATIONS:

1. Boosts the qi, engenders fluids, and stops thirst: Used for lung-spleen qi vacuity with non-engenderment of fluids and humors resulting in oral thirst, fatigue, and cough. Commonly combined with Tuber Ophiopogonis Japonici (*Mai Men Dong*), Radix Codonopsitis Pilosulae (*Dang Shen*), Radix Astragali Membranacei (*Huang Qi*), and Sclerotium Poriae Cocos (*Fu Ling*).

2. Supplements the kidneys and nourishes the heart: Used for kidney yin debility and vacuity with simultaneous lung vacuity manifest by cough. Commonly combined with dry Rhizoma Zingiberis (*Gan Jiang*), Rhizoma Pinelliae Ternatae (*Ban Xia*), and Fructus Corni Officinalis (*Shan Zhu Yu*).

DOSE: 6-20g

HERBA DENDROBII (SHI HU)

NATURE & FLAVOR: Sweet, bland, slightly cold

CHANNEL GATHERING: Lungs, stomach & kidneys

FUNCTIONS & INDICATIONS:

1. Nourishes yin and engenders fluids: Used for stomach yin insufficiency with vexatious thirst. Commonly combined with Tuber Ophiopogonis Japonici (*Mai Men Dong*), Radix Trichosanthis Kirlowii (*Tian Hua Fen*), Radix Scrophulariae Ningpoensis (*Xuan Shen*), and uncooked Radix Rehmanniae (*Sheng Di*).

2. Enriches yin and clears heat: Used for heat diseases which have damaged yin with dry mouth and spontaneous perspiration. Commonly combined with Rhizoma Anemarrhenae Aspheloidis (*Zhi Mu*), Radix Stellariae Dichotomae (*Yin Chai Hu*), and Rhizoma Picrrorhizae (*Hu Huang Lian*).

DOSE: 6-20g

FRUCTUS LYCII CHINENSIS (GOU QI ZI)

NATURE & FLAVOR: Sweet, level

CHANNEL GATHERING: Liver & kidneys

FUNCTIONS & INDICATIONS:

1. Supplements yin and blood, stops wasting and thirsting: Used for kidney vacuity and blood debility with low back and knee soreness and limpness, dry mouth with desire to drink, and polyuria. Commonly combined with uncooked Radix Rehmanniae (*Sheng Di*), Fructus Schisandrae Chinensis (*Wu Wei Zi*), and Semen Cuscutae Chinensis (*Tu Si Zi*).

2. Nourishes the liver and brightens the eyes: Used for liver-kidney insufficiency and essence blood debility and vacuity with dizziness, blurred vision, and decreased visual acuity. Commonly combined with Flos Chrysanthemi Morifolii (*Ju Hua*), Fructus Corni Officinalis (*Shan Zhu Yu*) uncooked Radix Rehmanniae (*Sheng Di*), cooked Radix Rehmanniae (*Shu Di*), Radix Dioscoreae Oppositae (*Shan Yao*), and Cortex Eucommiae Ulmoidis (*Du Zhong*).

DOSE: 6-20g

CONTRAINDICATIONS: Spleen vacuity diarrhea and replete evils

Gou Qi Zi has both hypoglycemic and blood lipid lowering effects.

RADIX PUERARIAE (GE GEN)

NATURE & FLAVOR: Acrid, sweet, level

CHANNEL GATHERING: Spleen & stomach

FUNCTIONS & INDICATIONS:

1. Resolves heat and engenders fluids: Used for bodily heat and wasting and thirsting conditions. Commonly combined with Radix Trichosanthis Kirlowii (*Tian Hua Fen*), Radix Scrophulariae Ningpoensis (*Xuan Shen*), and Cortex Radicis Moutan (*Dan Pi*).

2. Resolves the muscles and out-thrusts rashes: Used for external contraction wind cold or wind heat with stiff neck. Commonly combined with Herba Ephedrae (*Ma Huang*) and Ramulus Cinnamomi Cassiae (*Gui Zhi*) for wind cold. Used for the initial stage of measles (*i.e.*, wind heat), commonly combined with Rhizoma Cimicifugae (*Sheng Ma*).

DOSE: 6-20g

Ge Gen has hypoglycemic, hypotensive, and blood lipid lowering effects.

FRUCTUS TRICHOSANTHIS KIRLOWII (GUA LOU)

NATURE & FLAVOR: Sweet, cold

CHANNEL GATHERING: Lungs, stomach & large intestine

FUNCTIONS & INDICATIONS:

1. Moistens lung dryness and stops wasting and thirsting: Used for lung heat cough with thick, sticky phlegm. Commonly combined with Rhizoma Pinelliae Ternatae (*Ban Xia*), Rhizoma Anemarrhenae Aspheloidis (*Zhi Mu*), Bulbus Fritillariae (*Bei Mu*), and Rhizoma Arisaematis (*Nan Xing*). When used for wasting and thirsting, commonly combined with Radix Scrophulariae Ningpoensis (*Xuan Shen*), Tuber Ophiopogonis Japonici (*Mai Men Dong*), Rhizoma Anemarrhenae Aspheloidis (*Zhi Mu*), and Radix Scutellariae Baicalensis (*Huang Qin*).

2. Loosens the chest and rectifies the qi: Used for chest impediment, chest oppression, and discomfort under the heart. Commonly combined with Fructus Immaturus Citri Aurantii (*Zhi Shi*) and Bulbus Allii Fistulosi (*Cong Bai*).

3. Moistens the intestines and frees the flow of the stools: Used for intestinal dryness constipation. Commonly combined with Semen Cannabis Sativae (*Huo Ma Ren*) and Semen Pruni (*Yu Li Ren*).

DOSE: 6-20g

CONTRAINDICATIONS: Spleen-stomach vacuity cold with vomiting or diarrhea

Gua Lou has hypoglycemic, hypotensive, and blood lipid lowering effects.

HERBA EUPATORII FORTUNEI (PEI LAN)

NATURE & FLAVOR: Acrid, level

CHANNEL GATHERING: Spleen & stomach

FUNCTIONS & INDICATIONS:

1. Engenders fluids and stops thirst: Used for summerheat heat damaging fluids and wasting and thirsting.

2. Resolves summerheat and scatters dampness: Used for summerheat dampness encumbering the spleen with ductal oppression, torpid intake, emission of heat, and slimy tongue fur. Commonly combined with Herba Agastachis Seu Pogostemi (*Huo Xiang*), Fructus Amomi (*Sha Ren*), and Folium Perillae Frutescentis (*Zi Su Ye*).

DOSE: 6-30g

SCLEROTIUM PORIAE COCOS (FU LING)

NATURE & FLAVOR: Sweet, bland, level

CHANNEL GATHERING: Heart, lungs, spleen & bladder

FUNCTIONS & INDICATIONS:

1. Fortifies the spleen and supplements the center: Used for spleen vacuity with reduced appetite and fluids and humors collecting internally. Commonly combined with Radix Codonopsitis Pilosulae (*Dang Shen*), Radix Astragali Membranacei (*Huang Qi*), Rhizoma Atractylodis Macrocephalae (*Bai Zhu*), and Radix Dioscoreae Oppositae (*Shan Yao*).

2. Disinhibits water and seeps dampness: Used for water dampness collecting internally, inhibited urination, super-

ficial edema, and phlegm rheum conditions. Commonly combined with Sclerotium Polypori Umbellati (*Zhu Ling*), Rhizoma Alismatis (*Ze Xie*), Rhizoma Atractylodis Macrocephalae (*Bai Zhu*), and Semen Plantaginis (*Che Qian Zi*).

3. Nourishes the heart and quiets the spirit: Used for heart spirit restlessness, insomnia, and profuse dreams. Commonly combined with Semen Zizyphi Spinosae (*Suan Zao Ren*), Radix Polygalae Tenuifoliae (*Yuan Zhi*), and Flos Albizziae Julibrissinis (*He Huan Hua*).

DOSE: 6-20g

Fu Ling has been shown to have both hypoglycemic and sedative effects.

RHIZOMA ALISMATIS (ZE XIE)

NATURE & FLAVOR: Sweet, bland, cold

CHANNEL GATHERING: Kidneys & bladder

FUNCTIONS & INDICATIONS:

1. Disinhibits water and seeps dampness: Used for water dampness collecting internally, inhibited urination, edema, etc. Commonly combined with Rhizoma Atractylodis Macrocephalae (*Bai Zhu*), Sclerotium Poriae Cocos (*Fu Ling*), and Sclerotium Polypori Umbellati (*Zhu Ling*) in the treatment of nephritis.

2. Clears heat and protects yin: Used for lower burner damp heat with red, choppy urination. Commonly combined with Semen Plantaginis (*Che Qian Zi*), Semen Dolichoris Lablab (*Bai Bian Dou*), and Herba Dianthi (*Qu Mai*) in the treatment of diabetes complicated by urinary tract infections.

DOSE: 6-20g

Ze Xie has hypoglycemic, hypotensive, and blood lipid lowering effects.

SEMEN CUSCUTAE CHINENSIS (TU SI ZI)

NATURE & FLAVOR: Acrid, sweet, level

CHANNEL GATHERING: Liver & kidneys

FUNCTIONS & INDICATIONS:

1. Supplements the kidneys and boosts the essence: Used for kidney yang vacuity and decline with low back soreness, seminal emission, etc. Commonly combined with Fructus Lycii Chinensis (*Gou Qi Zi*), Semen Astragali Complanati (*Sha Yuan Zi*), Fructus Rubi Chingii (*Fu Pen Zi*), and Rhizoma Polygonati (*Huang Jing*). Commonly combined with Gecko (*Ge Jie*), Cordyceps Sinensis (*Dong Chong Xia Cao*), and Fructus Ligustri Lucidi (*Nu Zhen Zi*).

2. Nourishes the liver and brightens the eyes: Used for liver-kidney insufficiency with bilateral blurred vision. Commonly combined with Fructus Lycii Chinensis (*Gou Qi Zi*), Flos Chrysanthemi Morifolii (*Ju Hua*), cooked Radix Rehmanniae (*Shu Di*), and uncooked Radix Rehmanniae (*Sheng Di*).

DOSE: 6-20g

GECKO (GE JIE)

NATURE & FLAVOR: Salty, level

CHANNEL GATHERING: Lungs & kidneys

FUNCTIONS & INDICATIONS:

1. Supplements the kidneys: Used for kidney vacuity impotence and wasting and thirsting. Commonly combined with Fructus Psoraleae Corylifoliae (*Bu Gu Zhi*), Semen Cuscutae Chinensis (*Tu Si Zi*), and Herba Cistanchis Deserticolae (*Rou Cong Rong*).

2. Supplements the lungs: Used for lung vacuity panting and coughing and hacking of blood. Commonly combined with Rhizoma Anamarrhenae Aspheloidis (*Zhi Mu*), Bulbus Fritillariae (*Bei Mu*), and Rhizoma Bletillae Striatae (*Bai Ji*).

DOSE: 3-5g when taken powdered; more when added to a decoction

COOKED RADIX REHMANNIAE (SHU DI)

NATURE & FLAVOR: Sweet, slightly warm

CHANNEL GATHERING: Liver & kidneys

FUNCTIONS & INDICATIONS:

1. Enriches and supplements kidney yin: Used for kidney yin debility and vacuity with low back soreness, dizziness, tinnitus, and wasting and thirsting. Commonly combined with Fructus Corni Officinalis (*Shan Zhu Yu*), Radix Dioscoreae Oppositae (*Shan Yao*), and uncooked Radix Rehmanniae (*Sheng Di*).

2. Supplements the blood: Used for various blood vacuity conditions and commonly used in gynecology. Commonly combined with Radix Angelicae Sinensis (*Dang Gui*), Radix Albus Paeoniae Lactiflorae (*Bai Shao*), and Caulis Milletiae Seu Spatholobi (*Ji Xue Teng*).

DOSE: 6-30g

CONTRAINDICATIONS: Due to this medicinal's enriching, slimy nature, over time, it hinders the spleen and causes lodging of evils. Therefore, it is contraindicated in the case of evil repletions and diarrhea.

Shu Di has only a slight hypoglycemic effect by itself.

TUBER ASPARAGI COCHINENSIS (TIAN MEN DONG)

NATURE & FLAVOR: Sweet, bitter, cold

CHANNEL GATHERING: Lungs & kidneys

FUNCTIONS & INDICATIONS:

1. Enriches and supplements lung-kidney yin: Used for yin vacuity with tidal heat, night sweats, cough, and dry mouth. For lung vacuity, commonly combined with Tuber Ophiopogonis Japonici (*Mai Men Dong*) and Bulbus Fritillariae Cirrhosae (*Chuan Bei Mu*). For kidney vacuity, commonly combined with uncooked Radix Rehmanniae (*Sheng Di*), Rhizoma Anemarrhenae Aspheloidis (*Zhi Mu*), and Radix Glehniae Littoralis (*Sha Shen*).

2. Clears vacuity heat: Used for yin vacuity with dryness and heat internally exuberant, dry cough, hacking blood, etc. Commonly combined with Tuber Ophiopogonis Japonici (*Mai Men Dong*), Radix Stemonae (*Bai Bu*), Rhizoma Bletillae Striatae (*Bai Ji*), and Radix Pseudoginseng (*San Qi*).

DOSE: 6-30g

CONTRAINDICATIONS: Spleen vacuity diarrhea

SEMEN NELUMBINIS NUCIFERAE (LIAN ZI)

NATURE & FLAVOR: Sweet, astringent, level

CHANNEL GATHERING: Spleen, kidneys & heart

FUNCTIONS & INDICATIONS:

1. Boosts the kidneys and secures the essence: Used for seminal emission, frequent urination, etc. Commonly combined with Semen Astragali Complanati (*Sha Yuan Zi*), Semen Euryalis Ferocis (*Qian Shi*), Concha Ostreae (*Mu Li*), Os Draconis (*Long Gu*), and Rhizoma Polygonati (*Huang Jing*). For wasting and thirsting, commonly combined with uncooked Radix Rehmanniae (*Sheng Di*), Radix Scrophulariae Ningpoensis (*Xuan Shen*), and Rhizoma Coptidis Chinensis (*Huang Lian*), as in *Qing Xin Lian Zi Yin* (Clear the Heart Lotus Seed Drink).

2. Supplements the spleen and stops diarrhea: Used for spleen vacuity diarrhea. Commonly combined with Radix Codonopsitis Pilosulae (*Dang Shen*), Rhizoma Atractylodis Macrocephalae (*Bai Zhu*), Sclerotium Poriae Cocos (*Fu Ling*), and Fructus Rosae Laevigatae (*Jin Ying Zi*).

3. Nourishes the heart and calms the spirit: Used for heart vexation and insomnia. Commonly combined with Semen Biotae Orientalis (*Bai Zi Ren*), Arillus Euphoriae Longanae (*Long Yan Rou*), and Radix Polygalae Tenuifoliae (*Yuan Zhi*).

DOSE: 6-20g

HERBA EPIMEDII (XIAN LING PI, A.K.A. YIN YANG HUO)

NATURE & FLAVOR: Acrid, cold

CHANNEL GATHERING: Liver & kidneys

FUNCTIONS & INDICATIONS:

1. Supplements the kidneys: Used for impotence, penile pain, wasting and thirsting. Commonly combined with Rhizoma Polygonati (*Huang Jing*), Fructus Corni Officinalis (*Shan Zhu Yu*), and Gecko (*Ge Jie*).

2. Dispels wind and eliminates dampness: Used for wind damp impediment pain and numbness of the four limbs. Commonly combined with Radix Clematidis Chinensis (*Wei Ling Xian*), Cortex Eucommiae Ulmoidis (*Du Zhong*), and Radix Dipsaci (*Xu Duan*).

3. Stops cough and levels panting: Used for kidney vacuity loss of gathering and grasping panting. Commonly combined with Semen Juglandis Regiae (*Hu Tao Ren*), Fructus Psoraleae Corylifoliae (*Bu Gu Zhi*), and Gecko (*Ge Jie*).

DOSE: 6-20g

Xian Ling Pi has a definite hypoglycemic effect.

FRUCTUS CORNI OFFICINALIS (SHAN ZHU YU)

NATURE & FLAVOR: Sweet, sour, warm

CHANNEL GATHERING: Liver & kidneys

FUNCTIONS & INDICATIONS:

1. Supplements the liver and kidneys: Used for liver-kidney yin vacuity, low back soreness, impotence, frequent urination. Commonly combined with Radix Dioscoreae Oppositae (*Shan Yao*), cooked Radix Rehmanniae (*Shu Di*), uncooked Radix Rehmanniae (*Sheng Di*), and Radix Polygoni Multiflori (*He Shou Wu*).

2. Restrains and contains, secures and gathers: Used for essence, fluid, humor, and/or blood desertion conditions. Commonly combined with Semen Euryalis Ferocis (*Qian Shi*), Fructus Rosae Laevigatae (*Jin Ying Zi*), and Fructus Schisandrae Chinensis (*Wu Wei Zi*).

DOSE: 6-30g

FRUCTUS MORI ALBI (SANG SHEN)

NATURE & FLAVOR: Sweet, slightly cold

CHANNEL GATHERING: Heart, liver & kidneys

FUNCTIONS & INDICATIONS:

1. Enriches yin and engenders fluids. Used for yin vacuity and scanty fluids wasting and thirsting. Commonly com-

bined with Herba Dendrobii (*Shi Hu*), Rhizoma Polygonati Odorati (*Yu Zhu*), Radix Trichsanthis Kirlowii (*Tian Hua Fen*), uncooked Radix Rehmanniae (*Sheng Di*), and Radix Scrophulariae Ningpoensis (*Xuan Shen*).

2. Supplements the blood and moistens dryness: Used for yin and blood insufficiency headache, dizziness, tinnitus, and premature greying of the hair. Commonly combined with Fructus Ligustri Lucidi (*Nu Zhen Zi*), Herba Ecliptae Prostratae (*Han Lian Cao*), and Radix Polygoni Multiflori (*He Shou Wu*).

DOSE: 6-20g

FRUCTUS LIGUSTRI LUCIDI (NU ZHEN ZI)

NATURE & FLAVOR: Sweet, bitter, cool

CHANNEL GATHERING: Liver & kidneys

FUNCTIONS & INDICATIONS:

Enriches and supplements liver-kidney yin. Used for various liver-kidney yin vacuity conditions, such as low back and knee soreness and limpness, dizziness, and blurred vision. Commonly combined with Herba Ecliptae Protratae (*Han Lian Cao*), Semen Cuscutae Chinensis (*Tu Si Zi*), Flos Chrysanthemi Morifolii (*Ju Hua*), and Fructus Rubi Chingii (*Fu Pen Zi*).

DOSE: 6-20g

Nu Zhen Zi has been shown to have a definite hypoglycemic effect.

RADIX PSEUDOGINSENG (SAN QI, A.K.A. TIAN QI)

NATURE & FLAVOR: Sweet, slightly bitter, warm

CHANNEL GATHERING: Liver & stomach

FUNCTIONS & INDICATIONS:

Quickens the blood and transforms stasis: Used for various types of static blood obstruction and stagnation, fall and strike, detriment and damage. Can be used alone or with Crinis Carbonisatus (*Xue Yu Tan*) and Rhizoma Bletillae Striatae (*Bai Ji*).

DOSE: 3-9g

CONTRAINDICATIONS: Do not use for excessive bleeding with qi following blood desertion.

This medicinal has shown hypoglycemic effects on high blood glucose in mice.

FRUCTUS PRUNI MUME (WU MEI)

NATURE & FLAVOR: Sour, astringent, level

CHANNEL GATHERING: Liver, spleen, lungs & large intestine

FUNCTIONS & INDICATIONS:

1. Constrains the lungs and astringes the intestines: Used for cough and enduring dysentery conditions. For cough, commonly combined with Semen Pruni Armeniacae (*Xing Ren*), Pericarpium Papaveris Somniferi (*Ying Su Ke*), and Rhizoma Pinelliae Ternatae (*Ban Xia*). For enduring dysentery and diarrhea that will not stop, commonly combined with Fructus Terminaliae Chebulae (*He Zi*), Semen Myristicae Fragrantis (*Rou Dou Kou*), and Fructus Schisandrae Chinensis (*Wu Wei Zi*).

2. Engenders fluids and stops thirst: Used for vacuity heat leading to wasting and thirsting. Commonly combined with Radix Trichosanthis Kirlowii (*Tian Hua Fen*), Radix Puerariae (*Ge Gen*), and Tuber Ophiopogonis Japonici (*Mai Men Dong*).

3. Quiets roundworms: Used for the treatment of roundworms in the presence of hot and cold, vacuity and repletion. Commonly combined with dry Rhizoma Zingiberis (*Gan Jiang*) and Cortex Phellodendri (*Huang Bai*), as in *Wu Mei Wan* (Mume Pills).

DOSE: 6-20g

FRUCTUS ROSAE LAEVIGATAE (JIN YING ZI)

NATURE & FLAVOR: Sweet, astringent, level

CHANNEL GATHERING: Kidneys, bladder & large intestine

FUNCTIONS & INDICATIONS:

1. Secures the kidneys and shuts off the spring: Used for kidney vacuity frequent, numerous urinations. Commonly combined with Fructus Alpiniae Oxyphyllae (*Yi Zhi Ren*) and Fructus Rubi Chingii (*Fu Pen Zi*).

2. Restrains, constrains, and stops diarrhea: Used for enduring diarrhea. Commonly combined with Pericarpium Papaveris Somniferi (*Ying Su Ke*).

DOSE: 6-20g

CORTEX PHELLODENDRI (HUANG BAI)

NATURE & FLAVOR: Bitter, cold

CHANNEL GATHERING: Kidneys, bladder & large intestine

FUNCTIONS & INDICATIONS:

1. Clears heat and dries dampness: Used for damp heat internally brewing conditions, such as diarrhea and dysentery, abnormal vaginal discharge, and heat strangury. Commonly combined with Rhizoma Coptidis Chinensis (*Huang Lian*), Radix Scutellariae Baicalensis (*Huang Qin*), and Fructus Gardeniae Jasminoidis (*Zhi Zi*).

2. Drains fire and resolves toxins: Used for damp heat toxins internally brewing conditions, such as sores and ulcers, eczema, and lichen. Commonly combined with Fructus Gardeniae Jasminoidis (*Zhi Zi*), Radix Sophorae Flavescentis (*Ku Shen*), and Radix Gentianae Scabrae (*Long Dan Cao*).

3. Recedes vacuity heat: Used for seminal emission, night sweats, bone-steaming, and tidal heat. Commonly combined with Rhizoma Anemarrhenae Aspheloidis (*Zhi Mu*), as in *Zhi Bai Di Huang Wan* (Anemarrhena & Phellodendron Rehmannia Pills).

DOSE: 6-20g

CONTRAINDICATIONS: Spleen vacuity

Huang Bai has a hypoglycemic effect.

CORTEX RADICIS MOUTAN (DAN PI)

NATURE & FLAVOR: Bitter, acrid, slightly cold

CHANNEL GATHERING: Heart, liver & kidneys

FUNCTIONS & INDICATIONS:

1. Clears heat and cools the blood: Used for blood heat hematemesis, macular rashes, etc., due to heat entering the yin aspect or division. Commonly combined with Rhizoma Anemarrhenae Aspheloidis (*Zhi Mu*), Cortex Phellodendri (*Huang Bai*), and Radix Rubrus Paeoniae Lactiflorae (*Chi Shao*).

2. Quickens the blood and dispels stasis: Used for blood stasis and channel blockage, concretions and conglomerations, etc. Commonly combined with Ramulus Cinnamomi Cassiae (*Gui Zhi*), Semen Pruni Persicae (*Tao Ren*), Resina Olibani (*Ru Xiang*), and Resina Myrrhae (*Mo Yao*).

DOSE: 6-20g

CONTRAINDICATIONS: Use cautiously during pregnancy.

RHIZOMA ATRACTYLODIS (CANG ZHU)

NATURE & FLAVOR: Acrid, bitter, warm

CHANNEL GATHERING: Spleen & stomach

FUNCTIONS & INDICATIONS:

1. Dries dampness and fortifies the spleen: Used for spleen vacuity with damp encumbrance torpid intake and diarrhea. Commonly combined with Rhizoma Atractylodis Macrocephalae (*Bai Zhu*).

2. Dispels wind and eliminates dampness: Used for damp impediment and aching and numbness of the four limbs. Commonly combined with Cortex Phellodendri (*Huang Bai*) and Radix Achyranthis Bidentatae (*Niu Xi*), as in *San Miao San* (Three Wonders Powder).

DOSE: 6-20g

Cang Zhu has a marked hypoglycemic effect.

RADIX SALVIAE MILTIORRHIZAE (DAN SHEN)

NATURE & FLAVOR: Bitter, slightly cold

CHANNEL GATHERING: Heart, pericardium & liver

FUNCTIONS & INDICATIONS:

1. Quickens the blood and transforms stasis: Used for various types of static blood obstruction and stagnation in the lower abdomen, chest, and hypochondrium. Can be used alone or with Radix Rubrus Paeoniae Lactiflorae (*Chi Shao*), Radix Ligustici Wallichii (*Chuan Xiong*), or Radix Angelicae Sinensis (*Dang Gui*).

2. Calms the spirit and quiets the heart: Used for insomnia, irritability, and palpitations. It is often combined with Semen Biotae Orientalis (*Bai Zi Ren*) or Semen Zizyphi Spinosae (*Suan Zao Ren*).

3. Expesl pus and stops pain: Used for blood stasis complications of diabetes and for treating wounds and sores of the limbs. Can be combined with Resina Olibani (*Ru Xiang*) and Squama Manitis Pentadactylis (*Chuan Shan Jia*) for painful swellings and sores of the skin.

DOSE: 6-15g; up to 30g when used alone

CONTRAINDICATIONS: Use only when blood stasis is present.

This medicinal has shown hypoglycemic effects on high blood glucose. It also lowers serum cholesterol levels, inhibits dermatomycoses, has the ability to lower blood viscosity, inhibits platelet aggregation, and prevents thrombosis.

RADIX ET RHIZOMA POLYGONATI CUSPIDATI (HU ZHANG)

NATURE & FLAVOR: Bitter, cold

CHANNEL GATHERING: Liver, gallbladder & lungs

FUNCTIONS & INDICATIONS:

1. Dispels wind and disinhibits dampness: Used for wind dampness in the channels affecting the skin. Can be combined with Flos Lonicerae Japonicae (*Jin Yin Hua*) and Radix Salviae Miltiorrhizae (*Dan Shen*) for psoriasis or skin sores.

2. Disinhibits dampness and clears heat: Used for damp heat in the liver and gallbladder. Can be combined with Herba Artemisiae Capillaris (*Yin Chen Hao*) for jaundice or with Herba Lysimachiae Seu Desmodii (*Jin Qian Cao*) for biliary or urinary stones.

3. Breaks stasis and frees the flow of the channels: Used for the complications of blood stasis in gynecology and traumatology. Can be combined with Resina Olibani (*Ru Xiang*), Herba Leonuri Heterophylli (*Yi Mu Cao*), Radix Salviae Miltiorrhizae (*Dan Shen*), Caulis Millettiae Seu Spatholobi (*Ji Xue Teng*), or Flos Carthami Tinctorii (*Hong Hua*).

DOSE: 9-30g

CONTRAINDICATIONS: Do not use during pregnancy.

This medicinal has shown hypoglycemic effects on high blood glucose as well as antiviral and antibacterial effects. In the treatment of wasting and thirsting, it is reported that *Hu Zhang* may be used even as a single medicinal. In the *Ben Cao Gang Mu (Materia Medica, Outline & Details)*, *Hu Zhang* is used "for the treatment of great heat leading to dryness, stops thirst, disinhibits urination, and eliminates all heat toxins." When diabetes is complicated by high blood pressure and coronary heart disease, the use of this medicinal has very good results.

5

COMMONLY USED CHINESE MEDICINAL FORMULAS IN DIABETES

Because there is a core group of patterns which present in patients with diabetes, one can also identify the most commonly prescribed standard guiding formulas. These formulas mostly clear heat and engender fluids, supplement the qi and yin, supplement yin and yang when yin disease has reached yang, secure and astringe the kidney qi, quicken the blood, and/or transform phlegm and eliminate dampness. However, because each patient is unique and will typically present with several patterns coterminously, these formulas are used with any number of additions and subtractions in real life.

1. HEAT-CLEARING, YIN-ENRICHING, FLUID-ENGENDERING FORMULAS

BAI HU TANG (WHITE TIGER DECOCTION)

INGREDIENTS: Uncooked Gypsum Fibrosum (*Shi Gao*), 20-30g, Semen Oryzae Sativae (*Jing Mi*), 15-30g, Rhizoma Anemarrhenae Aspheloidis (*Zhi Mu*), 9-12g, and Radix Glycyrrhizae (*Gan Cao*), 3-6g

FUNCTIONS: Clears heat from the qi aspect or division, engenders fluids, and stops thirst

INDICATIONS: Heat in the yang ming damaging fluids and causing thirst

YU NU JIAN (JADE MAIDEN DECOCTION)

INGREDIENTS: Uncooked Gypsum Fibrosum (*Shi Gao*), 20-30g, cooked Radix Rehmanniae (*Shu Di*) and Tuber Ophiopogonis Japonici (*Mai Men Dong*), 12g each, Rhizoma Anemarrhenae Aspheloidis (*Zhi Mu*), 9-12g, and Radix Achyranthis Bidentatae (*Niu Xi*), 9g

FUNCTIONS: Clears heat and enriches yin, engenders fluids and stops thirst

INDICATIONS: Heat in the yang ming damaging fluids and causing thirst

GAN LU YIN (SWEET DEW DRINK)

INGREDIENTS: Uncooked Radix Rehmanniae (*Sheng Di*), Tuber Ophiopogonis Japonicae (*Mai Men Dong*), Tuber Asparagi Cochinensis (*Tian Men Dong*), Herba Dendrobii (*Shi Hu*), Herba Artemisiae Capillaris (*Yin Chen Hao*), Radix Scutellariae Baicalensis (*Huang Qin*), Folium Eriobotryae Japonicae (*Pi Pa Ye*), and Fructus Immaturus Citri Aurantii (*Zhi Shi*), 9g each, and Radix Glycyrrhizae (*Gan Cao*), 6g

FUNCTIONS: Clears heat and eliminates dampness, nourishes the stomach and rectifies the qi

INDICATIONS: Dampness and heat in the liver and stomach with yin vacuity

HUANG LIAN DI HUANG TANG (COPTIS & REHMANNIA DECOCTION)

INGREDIENTS: Rhizoma Coptidis Chinensis (*Huang Lian*), uncooked Radix Rehmanniae (*Sheng Di*), Radix Trichosanthis Kirlowii (*Tian Hua Fen*), Fructus Schisandrae Chinensis (*Wu Wei Zi*), Radix Angelicae Sinensis (*Dang Gui*), Radix Panacis Ginseng (*Ren Shen*), Radix Puerariae (*Ge Gen*), Sclerotium Poriae Cocos (*Fu Ling*), Tuber Ophiopogonis Japonicae (*Mai Men Dong*), and Radix Glycyrrhizae (*Gan Cao*), 9g each, uncooked Rhizoma Zingiberis (*Sheng Jiang*) and Folium Lophatheri

Gacilis (*Dan Zhu Ye*), 6g each, and Fructus Zizyphi Jujubae (*Da Zao*), 5-7 pieces

FUNCTIONS: Clears heat and engenders fluids, boosts the qi and enriches yin

INDICATIONS: Qi and yin vacuity with fire effulgence

QING WEI ZI ZAO YIN (CLEAR THE STOMACH & ENRICH DRYNESS DRINK)

INGREDIENTS: Uncooked Gypsum Fibrosum (*Shi Gao*), 30g, Tuber Ophiopogonis Japonici (*Mai Men Dong*), Tuber Asparagai Cochinensis (*Tian Men Dong*), Radix Trichosanthis Kirlowii (*Tian Hua Fen*), and Semen Oryzae Sativiae (*Geng Mi*), 20g each, Fructus Gardeniae Jasminoidis (*Zhi Zi*) and Radix Scrophulariae Ningpoensis (*Xuan Shen*), 15g each, wine-processed Radix Et Rhizoma Rhei (*Da Huang*) and Radix Scutellariae Baicalensis (*Huang Qin*), 9g each, and mix-fried Radix Glycyrrhizae (*Gan Cao*), 6g

FUNCTIONS: Clears the stomach and strongly engenders fluids

INDICATIONS: Heat and dryness in the yang ming damaging fluids and causing thirst

LIANG GE JIU FEI YIN (COOL THE DIAPHRAGM & RESCUE THE LUNGS DRINK)

INGREDIENTS: Uncooked Gypsum Fibrosum (*Shi Gao*), Tuber Asparagi Cochinensis (*Tian Men Dong*), Tuber Ophiopogonis Japonici (*Mai Men Dong*), Radix Trichosanthis Kirlowii (*Tian Hua Fen*), and Semen Oryzae Sativiae (*Geng Mi*), 30g each, Cortex Radicis Lycii Chinensis (*Di Gu Pi*) and Rhizoma Anemarrhenae Aspheloidis (*Zhi Mu*), 15g each, Radix Scutellariae Baicalensis (*Huang Qin*), 9g, and uncooked Radix Glycyrrhizae (*Gan Cao*), 6g

FUNCTIONS: Clears the lungs and stomach, engenders fluids and stops thirst

INDICATIONS: Lung-stomach heat damaging fluids and causing thirst

HE CHEN TANG (CLOSE & DEEPEN DECOCTION)

INGREDIENTS: Radix Scrophulariae Ningpoensis (*Xuan Shen*), 15g, cooked Radix Rehmanniae (*Shu Di*), 12-15g, Tuber Ophiopogonis Japonici (*Mai Men Dong*), 12g, Fructus Corni Officinalis (*Shan Zhu Yu*), 9-15g, and Semen Plantaginis (*Che Qian Zi*), 9g

FUNCTIONS: Enriches water and clears heat

INDICATIONS: Yin vacuity with heat

ZHI BAI DI HUANG WAN (ANEMARRHENA & PHELLODENDRON REHMANNIA PILLS)

INGREDIENTS: Uncooked Radix Rehmanniae (*Shu Di*), 12-15g, Radix Dioscoreae Oppositae (*Shan Yao*), Fructus Corni Officinalis (*Shan Zhu Yu*), Rhizoma Anemarrhenae Aspheloidis (*Zhi Mu*), and Sclerotium Poriae Cocos (*Fu Ling*), 9-15g each, Cortex Phellodendri (*Huang Bai*), 9g, and Rhizoma Alismatis (*Ze Xie*) and Cortex Radicis Moutan (*Dan Pi*), 6-9g each

FUNCTIONS: Supplements the kidneys and enriches yin, clears heat and drains fire

INDICATIONS: Yin vacuity with fire effulgence

DA BU YIN WAN (GREAT SUPPLEMENT YIN PILLS)

INGREDIENTS: Cooked Radix Rehmanniae (*Shu Di*) and Plastrum Testudinis (*Gui Ban*), 15g each, and Rhizoma Anemarrhenae Aspheloidis (*Zhi Mu*) and Cortex Phellodendri (*Huang Bai*), 12g each

FUNCTIONS: Enriches yin and downbears fire

INDICATIONS: Yin vacuity with internal heat

SHENG DI BA WEI TANG (UNCOOKED REHMANNIA EIGHT FLAVORS DECOCTION)

INGREDIENTS: Uncooked Radix Rehmanniae (*Sheng Di*) and Tuber Ophiopogonis Japonici (*Mai Men Dong*), 15g each, Radix Dioscoreae Oppositae (*Shan Yao*), Rhizoma Anemarrhenae Aspheloidis (*Zhi Mu*), Cortex Radicis Moutan (*Dan Pi*), and Folium Nelumbinis Nuciferae (*Ou Ye*), 9g each, Radix Scutellariae Baicalensis (*Huang Qin*) and Cortex Phellodendri (*Huang Bai*), 6-9g each, and Rhizoma Coptidis Chinensis (*Huang Lian*), 3-6g

FUNCTIONS: Enriches yin and clears heat

INDICATIONS: Yin vacuity with fire effulgence

QING XIN LIAN ZI YIN (CLEAR THE HEART LOTUS SEED DRINK)

INGREDIENTS: Semen Nelumbinis Nuciferae (*Lian Zi*), Sclerotium Poriae Cocos (*Fu Ling*), and Radix Astragali

Membranacei (*Huang Qi*), 20g each, Radix Scutellariae Baicalensis (*Huang Qin*), Tuber Ophiopogonis Japonici (*Mai Men Dong*), Cortex Radicis Lycii Chinensis (*Di Gu Pi*), Semen Plantaginis (*Che Qian Zi*), and mix-fried Radix Glycyrrhizae (*Gan Cao*), 15g each, and Radix Panacis Ginseng (*Ren Shen*), 6-9g

FUNCTIONS: Supplements the qi and yin and clears heart fire

INDICATIONS: Qi & dual vacuity with heart fire

YI TANG TANG (REPRESS SUGAR DECOCTION)

INGREDIENTS: Uncooked Gypsum Fibrosum (*Shi Gao*), 20-30g, Fructus Alpiniae Oxyphyllae (*Yi Zhi Ren*), 15g, cooked Radix Rehmanniae (*Shu Di*) and Tuber Ophiopogonis Japonici (*Mai Men Dong*), 12g each, and Radix Dioscoreae Oppositae (*Shan Yao*), Radix Trichosanthis Kirlowii (*Tian Hua Fen*), Herba Dendrobii (*Shi Hu*), Rhizoma Dioscoreae Hypoglaucae (*Bie Xie*), Semen Euryalis Ferocis (*Qian Shi*), Fructus Rubi Chingii (*Fu Pen Zi*), Semen Cuscutae Chinensis (*Tu Si Zi*), Ootheca Mantidis (*Sang Piao Xiao*), and Galla Rhois (*Wu Bei Zi*), 9g each

FUNCTIONS: Nourishes yin, clears heat, secures and astringes

INDICATIONS: Yin vacuity with heat in the yang ming damaging fluids complicated by kidney qi loss of securing and astringing

SHA SHEN MAI DONG TANG (GLEHNIA & OPHIOPOGON DECOCTION)

INGREDIENTS: Radix Glehniae Littoralis (*Sha Shen*) and Tuber Ophiopogonis Japonici (*Mai Men Dong*), 20g each, Radix Trichosanthis Kirlowii (*Tian Hua Fen*), 15g, and Rhizoma Polygonati Odorati (*Yu Zhu*), uncooked Semen Dolichoris Lablab (*Bai Bian Dou*), uncooked Radix Glycyrrhizae (*Gan Cao*), and Folium Mori Albi (*Sang Ye*), 10g each

FUNCTIONS: Engenders fluids and increases humors

INDICATIONS: Yin fluid damage with oral thirst

2. HEAT-CLEARING, FLUID-ENGENDERING, QI-SUPPLEMENTING FORMULAS

BAI HU JIA REN SHEN TANG (WHITE TIGER PLUS GINSENG DECOCTION)

INGREDIENTS: Same as above plus Radix Panacis Ginseng (*Ren Shen*), 6-9g

FUNCTIONS: Clears heat and engenders fluids, fortifies the spleen and supplements the qi

INDICATIONS: Heat in the yang ming with damaged fluids and concomitant spleen qi vacuity

ZHU YE SHI GAO TANG (LOPHATHERUM & GYPSUM DECOCTION)

INGREDIENTS: Uncooked Gypsum Fibrosum (*Shi Gao*), 20-30g, Semen Oryzae Sativae (*Geng Mi*), 15-30g, Tuber Ophiopogonis Japonici (*Mai Men Dong*), 12g, Herba Lophatheri Gracilis (*Dan Zhu Ye*), Rhizoma Pinelliae Ternatae (*Ban Xia*), and Radix Panacis Ginseng (*Ren Shen*), 9g each, and mix-fried Radix Glycyrrhizae (*Gan Cao*), 6g

FUNCTIONS: Clears heat and engenders fluids, supplements the qi and harmonizes the stomach

INDICATIONS: Heat in the yang ming with damaged fluids, spleen vacuity, and stomach disharmony or an element of phlegm and dampness

MAI MEN DONG YIN ZI (OPHIOPOGON DRINK)

INGREDIENTS: Tuber Ophiopogonis Japonici (*Mai Men Dong*) and uncooked Radix Rehmanniae (*Sheng Di*), 12g each, Rhizoma Anemarrhenae Aspheloidis (*Zhi Mu*), 9-12g, Fructus Trichosanthis Kirlowii (*Gua Lou*), Radix Puerariae (*Ge Gen*), and Sclerotium Pararadicis Poriae Cocos (*Fu Shen*), 9g each, Radix Panacis Ginseng (*Ren Shen*), 6-9g, and mix-fried Radix Glycyrrhizae (*Gan Cao*), 6g

FUNCTIONS: Clears heat at the same time as it fortifies the spleen, engenders fluids and stops thirst

INDICATIONS: *Yang ming* heat with damaged fluids and oral thirst accompanied by spleen qi vacuity

SHENG MAI SAN (ENGENDER THE PULSE POWDER)

INGREDIENTS: Tuber Ophiopogonis Japonici (*Mai Men Dong*), 12-15g, Fructus Schisandrae Chinensis (*Wu Wei Zi*), 9g, and Radix Panacis Ginseng (*Ren Shen*), 6-9g

FUNCTIONS: Supplements the qi and nourishes yin

INDICATIONS: Qi and yin vacuity profuse perspiration, lack of strength, oral thirst, and polydipsia

YU QUAN WAN (JADE SPRING PILLS)

INGREDIENTS: Radix Astragali Membranacei (*Huang Qi*), 15-30g, Tuber Ophiopogonis Japonici (*Mai Men Dong*), 12g, Radix Puerariae (*Ge Gen*), Radix Trichosanthis Kirlowii (*Tian Hua Fen*), Fructus Pruni Mume (*Wu Mei*), and Sclerotium Poriae Cocos (*Fu Ling*), 9g each, Radix Panacis Ginseng (*Ren Shen*), 6-9g, and Radix Glycyrrhizae (*Gan Cao*), 6g

FUNCTIONS: Fortifies the spleen and boosts the qi, clears heat and engenders fluids

INDICATIONS: Qi vacuity and fluid insufficiency with heat in the heart, lungs, and stomach

WU ZHI YU QUAN WAN (FIVE JUICES JADE SPRING PILLS)

INGREDIENTS: Uncooked Radix Rehmanniae (*Sheng Di*) and Tuber Ophiopogonis Japonici (*Mai Men Dong*), 12g each, Radix Puerariae (*Ge Gen*), Radix Trichosanthis Kirlowii (*Tian Hua Fen*), Fructus Schisandrae Chinensis (*Wu Wei Zi*), Fructus Pruni Mume (*Wu Mei*), and Radix Angelicae Sinensis (*Dang Gui*), 9g each, Radix Panacis Ginseng (*Ren Shen*), 6-9g, Radix Glycyrrhizae (*Gan Cao*), 6g, and Plumula Nelumbinis Nuciferae (*Lian Zi Xin*) and Rhizoma Coptidis Chinensis (*Huang Lian*), 3-6g each

FUNCTIONS: Fortifies the spleen and boosts the qi, clears the heart and engenders fluids

INDICATIONS: Spleen qi vacuity with heat in the heart and fluid damage causing oral thirst

YU YE TANG (JADE HUMOR DECOCTION)

INGREDIENTS: Radix Astragali Membranacei (*Huang Qi*), 15-30g, Radix Dioscoreae Oppositae (*Shan Yao*), 9-15g, Rhizoma Anemarrhenae Aspheloidis (*Zhi Mu*), 9-12g, and Endothelium Corneum Gigeriae Galli (*Ji Nei Jin*), Radix Puerariae (*Ge Gen*), Fructus Schisandrae Chinensis (*Wu Wei Zi*), and Radix Trichosanthis Kirlowii (*Tian Hua Fen*), 9g each

FUNCTIONS: Fortifies the spleen and boosts the qi, clears heat, engenders fluids, and stops thirst

INDICATIONS: Spleen qi vacuity with heat and dryness damaging fluids and causing oral thirst

DI HUANG YIN ZI (REHMANNIA DRINK)

INGREDIENTS: Radix Astragali Membranacei (*Huang Qi*), 15-30g, cooked Radix Rehmanniae (*Shu Di*), uncooked Radix Rehmanniae (*Sheng Di*), Tuber Asparagi Cochinensis (*Tian Men Dong*), and Tuber Ophiopogonis Japonici (*Mai Men Dong*), 12g each, Rhizoma Alismatis (*Ze Xie*), Herba Dendrobii (*Shi Hu*), and Folium Eriobotryae Japonicae (*Pi Pa Ye*), 9g each, Radix Panacis Ginseng (*Ren Shen*) and stir-fried Fructus Citri Aurantii (*Zhi Ke*), 6-9g each, and mix-fried Radix Glycyrrhizae (*Gan Cao*), 6g

FUNCTIONS: Fortifies the spleen and boosts the qi, clear s heat from the stomach and lungs, engenders fluids and stops thirst

INDICATIONS: Lung-stomach heat damaging and causing detriment to yin fluids with concomitant spleen qi vacuity

WU MEI TANG (MUME DECOCTION)

INGREDIENTS: Fructus Pruni Mume (*Wu Mei*), 15g, Radix Rubiae Cordifoliae (*Qian Cao Gen*), 12g, Radix Scutellariae Baicalensis (*Huang Qin*), Radix Puerariae (*Ge Gen*), and Sclerotium Poriae Cocos (*Fu Ling*), 9g each, Radix Panacis Ginseng (*Ren Shen*), 6-9g, and mix-fried Radix Glycyrrhizae (*Gan Cao*), 6g

FUNCTIONS: Fortifies the spleen and supplements the qi, clears heat, engenders fluids, and stops thirst

INDICATIONS: Spleen qi vacuity with lung-stomach heat damaging the fluids

HUANG QI YIN (ASTRAGALUS DRINK)

INGREDIENTS: Radix Astragali Membranacei (*Huang Qi*), 15-30g, uncooked Radix Rehmanniae (*Sheng Di*), 12-15g, Radix Trichosanthis Kirlowii (*Tian Hua Fen*) and Tuber Ophiopogonis Japonici (*Mai Men Dong*), 9-12g each, Sclerotium Pararadicis Poriae Cocos (*Fu Shen*), 9g, and mix-fried Radix Glycyrrhizae (*Gan Cao*), 6g

FUNCTIONS: Fortifies the spleen and supplements the qi, clears heat, engenders fluids, and stops thirst

INDICATIONS: Spleen qi vacuity with lung-stomach heat damaging the fluids

JIANG XIN TANG (DOWNBEAR THE HEART DECOCTION)

INGREDIENTS: Honey mix-fried Radix Astragali Membranacei (*Huang Qi*) and cooked Radix Rehmanniae (*Shu Di*), 15g each, Radix Polygalae Tenuifoliae (*Yuan Zhi*), Radix Angelicae Sinensis (*Dang Gui*), Radix

Ligustici Wallichii (*Chuan Xiong*), Sclerotium Poriae Cocos (*Fu Ling*), Fructus Schisandrae Chinensis (*Wu Wei Zi*), and Radix Trichosanthis Kirlowii (*Tian Hua Fen*), 9g each, and Radix Panacis Ginseng (*Ren Shen*) and mix-fried Radix Glycyrrhizae (*Gan Cao*), 6-9g each

FUNCTIONS: Boosts the qi and engenders fluids, enriches and supplements yin and blood, calms the heart and quiets the spirit

INDICATIONS: Heart qi and blood vacuity with concomitant yin vacuity and fluid dryness and a disquieted spirit

3. LIVER BLOOD-KIDNEY YIN NOURISHING & ENRICHING FORMULAS

YI GUAN JIAN (ONE LINK DECOCTION)

INGREDIENTS: Tuber Ophiopogonis Japonici (*Mai Men Dong*) and uncooked Radix Rehmanniae (*Sheng Di*), 12g each, and Radix Glehniae Littoralis (*Sha Shen*), Radix Angelicae Sinensis (*Dang Gui*), Fructus Lycii Chinensis (*Gou Qi Zi*), and Fructus Meliae Toosandan (*Chuan Lian Zi*), 9g each

FUNCTIONS: Nourishes the blood and enriches yin at the same time as it emolliates and harmonizes the liver

INDICATIONS: Liver blood-kidney yin vacuity with concomitant liver depression

LIU WEI DI HUANG WAN (SIX FLAVORS REHMANNIA PILLS)

INGREDIENTS: Cooked Radix Rehmanniae (*Shu Di*), 12-15g, Radix Dioscoreae Oppositae (*Shan Yao*), Fructus Corni Officinalis (*Shan Zhu Yu*), and Sclerotium Poriae Cocos (*Fu Ling*), 9-15g each, and Rhizoma Alismatis (*Ze Xie*) and Cortex Radicis Moutan (*Dan Pi*), 6-9g each

FUNCTIONS: Supplements the kidneys and enriches yin

INDICATIONS: Kidney yin vacuity

QI JU DI HUANG WAN (LYCIUM & CHRYSANTHEMUM REHMANNIA PILLS)

Ingredients: Cooked Radix Rehmanniae (*Shu Di*), 12-15g, Radix Dioscoreae Oppositae (*Shan Yao*), Fructus Corni Officinalis (*Shan Zhu Yu*), Radix Lycii Chinensis (*Gou Qi Zi*), and Sclerotium Poriae Cocos (*Fu Ling*), 9-15g each, Flos Chrysanthemi Morifolii (*Ju Hua*), 9g, and Rhizoma Alismatis (*Ze Xie*) and Cortex Radicis Moutan (*Dan Pi*), 6-9g each

FUNCTIONS: Nourishes the liver and enriches the kidneys, clears the liver and brightens the eyes

INDICATIONS: Liver blood-kidney yin vacuity with possible liver heat and decreased visual acuity

ZUO GUI YIN (RESTORE THE LEFT [KIDNEY] DRINK)

INGREDIENTS: Cooked Radix Rehmanniae (*Shu Di*), 12-15g, Radix Dioscoreae Oppositae (*Shan Yao*), Fructus Corni Officinalis (*Shan Zhu Yu*), and Fructus Lycii Chinensis (*Gou Qi Zi*), 9-15g each, Sclerotium Poriae Cocos (*Fu Ling*), 9-12g, and mix-fried Radix Glycyrrhizae (*Gan Cao*), 6-9g

FUNCTIONS: Supplements the kidneys and enriches yin

INDICATIONS: Kidney yin vacuity

ZI SHUI CHENG JIN YIN (ENRICH WATER & ORDER METAL DRINK)

INGREDIENTS: Uncooked Radix Astragali Membranacei (*Huang Qi*), 25g, uncooked Radix Rehmanniae (*Sheng Di*), Fructus Ligustri Lucidi (*Nu Zhen Zi*), Fructus Mori Albi (*Sang Shen*), and Tuber Ophiopogonis Japonici (*Mai Men Dong*), 20g each, Fructus Corni Officinalis (*Shan Zhu Yu*), Fructus Lycii Chinensis (*Gou Qi Zi*), Radix Codonopsitis Pilosulae (*Dang Shen*), and Radix Dioscoreae Oppositae (*Shan Yao*), 15g each, and Fructus Schisandrae Chinensis (*Wu Wei Zi*),10g

FUNCTIONS: Nourishes the liver and enriches the kidneys, fortifies the spleen and boosts the qi

INDICATIONS: Qi & yin dual vacuity

YI GAN ZI SHEN XIAO KE YIN (REPRESS THE LIVER & ENRICH YIN WASTING & THIRSTING DRINK)

INGREDIENTS: Uncooked Radix Albus Paeoniae Lactiflorae (*Bai Shao*), uncooked Os Draconis (*Long Gu*), uncooked Concha Ostreae (*Mu Li*), Radix Dioscoreae Oppositae (*Shan Yao*), and cooked Radix Rehmanniae (*Shu Di*), 30g each, Rhizoma Polygonati Odorati (*Yu Zhu*), Radix Puerariae (*Ge Gen*), and Radix Trichosanthis Kirlowii (*Tian Hua Fen*), 20g each, Tuber Ophiopogonis Japonici (*Mai Men Dong*) and Radix Polygoni Multiflori (*He Shou Wu*), 15g each, and Rhizoma Polygonati (*Huang Jing*) and

Herba Cistanchis Deserticolae (*Rou Cong Rong*), 12g each

FUNCTIONS: Enriches yin, engenders fluids, and represses the liver

INDICATIONS: Liver-kidney yin vacuity with liver fire tending to effulgence

SUAN XIE GAN MU FANG (SOURLY DRAIN LIVER WOOD FORMULA)

INGREDIENTS: Radix Albus Paeoniae Lactiflorae (*Bai Shao*), Fructus Pruni Mume (*Wu Mei*), Radix Trichosanthis Kirlowii (*Tian Hua Fen*), Rhizoma Polygonati Odorati (*Yu Zhu*), Herba Dendrobii (*Shi Hu*), and uncooked Radix Rehmanniae (*Sheng Di*), 15g each, Cortex Radicis Moutan (*Dan Pi*) and Radix Bupleuri (*Chai Hu*), 9g each, and Rhizoma Coptidis Chinensis (*Huang Lian*) and Radix Glycyrrhizae (*Gan Cao*), 3-6g each

FUNCTIONS: Sourly and sweetly transforms yin, represses the liver and engenders fluids

INDICATIONS: Liver-kidney yin vacuity with liver depression transforming heat

ZI SHUI QING GAN YIN (ENRICH WATER & CLEAR THE LIVER DRINK)

INGREDIENTS: Cooked Radix Rehmanniae (*Shu Di*) and Radix Dioscoreae Oppositae (*Shan Yao*), 30g, Radix Trichosanthis Kirlowii (*Tian Hua Fen*) and Radix Puerariae (*Ge Gen*), 15g each, Radix Albus Paeoniae Lactiflorae (*Bai Shao*) and Fructus Lycii Chinensis (*Gou Qi Zi*), 12g each, Semen Zizyphi Spinosae (*Suan Zao Ren*), Tuber Ophiopogonis Japonici (*Mai Men Dong*), Fructus Corni Officinalis (*Shan Zhu Yu*), and Cortex Radicis Moutan (*Dan Pi*), 9g each, and Radix Bupleuri (*Chai Hu*) and Fructus Gardeniae Jasminoidis (*Zhi Zi*), 6g each

FUNCTIONS: Enriches and nourishes the liver and kidneys, clears heat and engenders fluids

INDICATIONS: Liver-kidney yin vacuity with liver depression transforming heat

4. YANG-SUPPLEMENTING FORMULAS

SHEN QI WAN (KIDNEY QI PILLS)

INGREDIENTS: Cooked Radix Rehmanniae (*Shu Di*), 12-

15g, Radix Dioscoreae Oppositae (*Shan Yao*), Fructus Corni Officinalis (*Shan Zhu Yu*), and Sclerotium Poriae Cocos (*Fu Ling*), 9-15g each, and Ramulus Cinnamomi Cassiae (*Gui Zhi*), Radix Lateralis Praeparatus Aconiti Carmichaeli (*Fu Zi*), Rhizoma Alismatis (*Ze Xie*), and Cortex Radicis Moutan (*Dan Pi*), 6-9g each

FUNCTIONS: Supplements the kidneys and warms yang

INDICATIONS: Yin and yang dual vacuity

YOU GUI YIN (RESTORE THE RIGHT [KIDNEY] DRINK)

INGREDIENTS: Cooked Radix Rehmanniae (*Shu Di*), 12-15g, Radix Dioscoreae Oppositac (*Shan Yao*), Fructus Corni Officinalis (*Shan Zhu Yu*), Cortex Eucommiae Ulmoidis (*Du Zhong*), and Fructus Lycii Chinensis (*Gou Qi Zi*), 9-15g each, Sclerotium Poriae Cocos (*Fu Ling*), 9-12g, and Cortex Cinnamomi Cassiae (*Rou Gui*), Radix Lateralis Praeparatus Aconiti Carmichaeli (*Fu Zi*), and mix-fried Radix Glycyrrhizae (*Gan Cao*), 6-9g each

FUNCTIONS: Supplements the kidneys and warms yang

INDICATIONS: Yin and yang dual vacuity

DAO HUO SHENG YIN TANG (ABDUCT FIRE & UPBEAR YIN DECOCTION)

INGREDIENTS: Radix Scrophulariae Ningpoensis (*Xuan Shen*), 30-60g, cooked Radix Rehmanniae (*Shu Di*) and Tuber Ophiopogonis Japonici (*Mai Men Dong*), 30g each, Radix Morindae Officinalis (*Ba Ji Tian*), 15g, Fructus Corni Officinalis (*Shan Zhu Yu*), 12g, and Fructus Schisandrae Chinensis (*Wu Wei Zi*) and Cortex Cinnamomi Cassiae (*Rou Gui*), 6g each

FUNCTIONS: Greatly supplements kidney water while simultaneously warming kidney yang

INDICATIONS: Yin and yang dual vacuity with vacuity fire flaming upward

YI QI FU YANG YIN (BOOST THE QI & SUPPORT YANG DRINK)

INGREDIENTS: Uncooked Radix Astragali Membranacei (*Huang Qi*), 25g, cooked Radix Rehmanniae (*Shu Di*) and stir-fried Radix Dioscoreae Oppositae (*Shan Yao*), 20g each, Fructus Rubi Chingii (*Fu Pen Zi*), Radix Morindae Officinalis (*Ba Ji Tian*), Semen Cuscutae Chinensis (*Tu Si Zi*), and Fructus Corni Officinalis (*Shan Zhu Yu*), 15g each, Fructus Schisandrae Chinensis (*Wu Wei Zi*), 9g,

Radix Lateralis Praeparatus Aconiti Carmichaeli (*Fu Zi*), 6g, and Fructus Amomi (*Sha Ren*), 4.5g

FUNCTIONS: Supplements and invigorates yin and yang, fortifies the spleen, secures and astringes

INDICATIONS: Qi, yin, and yang vacuity with kidney vacuity not securing and astringing

ZI YIN ZHU YANG FANG (ENRICH YIN & INVIGORATE YANG FORMULA)

INGREDIENTS: Radix Puerariae (*Ge Gen*) and Radix Scrophulariae Ningpoensis (*Xuan Shen*), 15g each, cooked Radix Rehmanniae (*Shu Di*) and uncooked Radix Rehmanniae (*Sheng Di*), 12-15g each, Radix Dioscoreae Oppositae (*Shan Yao*), Fructus Corni Officinalis (*Shan Zhu Yu*), and Radix Salviae Miltiorrhizae (*Dan Shen*), 9-15g each, Herba Cistanchis Deserticolae (*Rou Cong Rong*), 9g, and Cortex Cinnamomi Cassiae (*Rou Gui*), 6-9g

FUNCTIONS: Enriches yin, invigorates yang, and quickens the blood

INDICATIONS: Yin and yang dual vacuity complicated by blood stasis

5. SECURING & ASTRINGING FORMULAS

SUO QUAN WAN (REDUCE THE SPRING PILLS)

INGREDIENTS: Radix Dioscoreae Oppositae (*Shan Yao*), 9-15g, Fructus Alpiniae Oxyphyllae (*Yi Zhi Ren*), 9-12g, and Radix Linderae Strychnifoliae (*Wu Yao*), 6-9g

FUNCTIONS: Secures the essence and stops leakage

INDICATIONS: Kidney qi not securing polyuria

BU YIN GU SE TANG (SUPPLEMENT YIN, ASTRINGE & SECURE DECOCTION)

INGREDIENTS: Uncooked Radix Rehmanniae (*Sheng Di*), Radix Astragali Membranacei (*Huang Qi*), and Radix Scrophulariae Ningpoensis (*Xuan Shen*), 15g each, Concha Ostreae (*Mu Li*) and Os Draconis (*Long Gu*), 12g each, Cortex Radicis Moutan (*Dan Pi*), Fructus Schisandrae Chinensis (*Wu Wei Zi*), Fructus Corni Officinalis (*Shan Zhu Yu*), and Radix Trichosanthis Kirlowii (*Tian Hua Fen*), 9g each, and Plumula Nelumbinis Nuciferae (*Lian Zi Xin*), 3-6g

FUNCTIONS: Enriches the kidneys and clears the heart, secures and astringes

INDICATIONS: Yin vacuity, heat in the heart, and kidney qi not securing and astringing

TU SI ZI WAN (CUSCUTA PILLS)

INGREDIENTS: Concha Ostreae (*Mu Li*), 12g, Semen Cuscutae Chinensis (*Tu Si Zi*), Herba Cistanchis Deserticolae (*Rou Cong Rong*), Ootheca Mantidis (*Sang Piao Xiao*), Fructus Schisandrae Chinensis (*Wu Wei Zi*), and Endothelium Corneum Gigeriae Galli (*Ji Nei Jin*), 9g each, Cornu Cervi Parvum (*Lu Rong*), 6g, and Radix Lateralis Praeparatus Aconiti Carmichaeli (*Fu Zi*), 3-9g

FUNCTIONS: Secures and astringes the kidney qi at the same time as invigorating yang

INDICATIONS: Kidney yang vacuity with nonsecuring and nonastringing

SANG PIAO XIAO SAN (OOTHECA MANTIDIS POWDER)

INGREDIENTS: Os Draconis (*Long Gu*), 18g, Plastrum Testudinis (*Gui Ban*), 15g, vinegar mix-fried Ootheca Mantidis (*Sang Piao Xiao*), 12g, Rhizoma Acori Graminei (*Shi Chang Pu*), Radix Panacis Ginseng (*Ren Shen*), Sclerotium Pararadicis Poriae Cocos (*Fu Shen*), and Radix Angelicae Sinensis (*Dang Gui*), 9g each, and Radix Polygalae Tenuifoliae (*Yuan Zhi*), 6g

FUNCTIONS: Regulates and supplements the heart and kidneys, astringes the essence and stops loss

INDICATIONS: Heart and kidney dual vacuity

CONTRAINDICATIONS:

1. Do not use for incontinence due to exuberant heat in the lower burner.
2. Do not use for damp heat in the lower burner.

6. BLOOD-QUICKENING FORMULAS

XUE FU ZHU YU TANG (BLOOD MANSION DISPEL STASIS DECOCTION)

INGREDIENTS: Uncooked Radix Rehmanniae (*Sheng Di*), 12g, Semen Pruni Persicae (*Tao Ren*), Flos Carthami Tinctorii (*Hong Hua*), Radix Angelicae Sinensis (*Dang*

Gui), Radix Ligustici Wallichii (Chuan Xiong), Radix Rubrus Paeoniae Lactiflorae (Chi Shao), and Radix Achyranthis Bidentatae (Niu Xi), 9g each, Radix Bupleuri (Chai Hu), 3-9g, Radix Platycodi Grandiflori (Jie Geng), 6-9g, and Radix Glyycrrhizae (Gan Cao), 3-6g

FUNCTIONS: Quickens the blood and dispels stasis, especially in the chest

TAO HONG SI WU TANG (PERSICA & CARTHAMUS FOUR MATERIALS DECOCTION)

INGREDIENTS: Cooked Radix Rehmanniae (Shu Di), 12-15g, Semen Pruni Persicae (Tao Ren), Flos Carthami Tinctorii (Hong Hua), Radix Angelicae Sinensis (Dang Gui), and Radix Rubrus Paeoniae Lactiflorae (Chi Shao), 9g each, and Radix Ligustici Wallichii (Chuan Xiong), 6-9g

FUNCTIONS: Quickens the blood and transforms stasis

INDICATIONS: Blood stasis

DANG GUI HUO XUE TANG (DANG GUI QUICKEN THE BLOOD DECOCTION)

INGREDIENTS: Radix Salviae Miltiorrhizae (Dan Shen), Radix Scrophulariae Ningpoensis (Xuan Shen), and Caulis Lonicerae Japonicae (Ren Dong Teng), 15g each, and Radix Angelicae Sinensis (Dang Gui), Flos Carthami Tinctorii (Hong Hua), and Radix Rubrus Paeoniae Lactiflorae (Chi Shao), 9g each

FUNCTIONS: Quickens the blood, clears heat, and resolves toxins

INDICATIONS: Blood stasis and heat toxins

HUO XUE JIANG TANG FANG (QUICKEN THE BLOOD & LOWER SUGAR FORMULA)

INGREDIENTS: Radix Astragali Membranacei (Huang Qi), 15-30g, Radix Salviae Miltiorrhizae (Dan Shen) and Radix Scrophulariae Ningpoensis (Xuan Shen), 15g each, cooked Radix Rehmanniae (Shu Di) and uncooked Radix Rehmanniae (Sheng Di), 12g each, Radix Dioscoreae Oppositae (Shan Yao), 9-15g, Rhizoma Atractylodis (Cang Zhu), Radix Angelicae Sinensis (Dang Gui), Radix Rubrus Paeoniae Lactiflorae (Chi Shao), Radix Ligustici Wallichii (Chuan Xiong), Herba Leonuri Heterophylli (Yi Mu Cao), and Radix Puerariae (Ge Gen), 9g each, and Radix Auklandiae Lappae (Mu Xiang), 6-9g

FUNCTIONS: Quickens and cools the blood, boosts the qi

and nourishes the blood, fortifies the spleen and supplements the kidneys, moves and rectifies the qi

INDICATIONS: Blood stasis with qi and blood vacuity, spleen and kidney vacuity with possible blood heat

JIA WEI SI WU TANG (ADDED FLAVORS FOUR MATERIALS DECOCTION)

INGREDIENTS: Tuber Ophiopogonis Japonici (Mai Men Dong) and cooked Radix Rehmanniae (Shu Di), 12g each, Radix Angelicae Sinensis (Dang Gui), Radix Ligustici Wallichii (Chuan Xiong), Radix Albus Paeoniae Lactiflorae (Bai Shao), Radix Achyranthis Bidentatae (Niu Xi), Rhizoma Atractylodis (Cang Zhu), Cortex Phellodendri (Huang Bai), Fructus Schisandrae Chinensis (Wu Wei Zi), Rhizoma Anemarrhenae Aspheloidis (Zhi Mu), and Cortex Eucommiae Ulmoidis (Du Zhong), 9g each, Radix Panacis Ginseng (Ren Shen), 6-9g, and Rhizoma Coptidis Chinensis (Huang Lian), 3-6g

FUNCTIONS: Supplements the qi and nourishes the blood, supplements the kidneys and quickens the blood, clears (damp) heat and engenders fluids

INDICATIONS: Qi, blood, and yin vacuity with blood stasis and damp heat

SHEN QI TAO HONG TANG (CODONOPSIS, ASTRAGALUS, PERSICA & CARTHAMUS DECOCTION)

INGREDIENTS: Radix Codonopsitis Pilosulae (Dang Shen), Radix Astragali Membranacei (Huang Qi), uncooked Radix Rehmanniae (Sheng Di), Gypsum Fibrosum (Shi Gao), and Radix Salviae Miltiorrhizae (Dan Shen), 30g each, Rhizoma Anemarrhenae Aspheloidis (Zhi Mu), 20g, Rhizoma Atractylodis (Cang Zhu), 15g, and Semen Pruni Persicae (Tao Ren) and Flos Carthami Tinctorii (Hong Hua), 6-9g each

FUNCTIONS: Boosts the qi and quickens the blood, clears heat and nourishes yin

INDICATIONS: Qi and yin dual vacuity with blood stasis and marked heat damaging the fluids

HUA YU JIANG TANG TANG (TRANSFORM STASIS & LOWER SUGAR DECOCTION)

INGREDIENTS: Radix Salviae Miltiorrhizae (Dan Shen), Radix Angelicae Sinensis (Dang Gui), uncooked Radix

Rehmanniae (*Sheng Di*), Tuber Ophiopogonis Japonici (*Mai Men Dong*), Radix Trichosanthis Kirlowii (*Tian Hua Fen*), Herba Dendrobii (*Shi Hu*), and Cortex Radicis Moutan (*Dan Pi*), 20g each, and Semen Pruni Persicae (*Tao Ren*), Radix Rubrus Paeoniae Lactiflorae (*Chi Shao*), Radix Ligustici Wallichii (*Chuan Xiong*), Radix Achyranthis Bidentatae (*Niu Xi*), and Fructus Citri Aurantii (*Zhi Ke*), 15g each

FUNCTIONS: Quickens the blood and transforms stasis, nourishes yin and engenders fluids

INDICATIONS: Yin and fluid vacuity dryness with marked blood stasis

7. PHLEGM DAMPNESS TRANSFORMING & ELIMINATING FORMULAS

NEI JIN OU YE JIAN (CHICKEN GIZZARD & LOTUS LEAF DECOCTION)

INGREDIENTS: Rhizoma Atractylodis (*Cang Zhu*), Rhizoma Coptidis Chinensis (*Huang Lian*), and Endothelium Corneum Gigeriae Galli (*Ji Nei Jin*), 25g each, Folium Nelumbinis Nuciferae (*Ou Ye*), Herba Eupatorei Fortunei (*Pei Lan*), and Rhizoma Atractylodis Macrocephalae (*Bai Zhu*), 18g each, uncooked Radix Dioscoreae Oppositae (*Shan Yao*), Radix Trichosanthis Kirlowii (*Tian Hua Fen*), and Fructus Mori Albi (*Sang Shen*), 15g each, and Herba Lemnae Seu Spirodelae (*Fu Ping Ye*) and Fructus Schisandrae Chinensis (*Wu Wei Zi*), 6g each

FUNCTIONS: Fortifies the spleen and dries dampness, harmonizes the stomach and engenders fluids

INDICATIONS: Phlegm and dampness obstructing internally with spleen qi vacuity and fluid damage

JIA WEI ER CHEN TANG (ADDED FLAVORS TWO AGED [INGREDIENTS] DECOCTION)

INGREDIENTS: Radix Salviae Miltiorrhizae (*Dan Shen*) and Radix Puerariae (*Ge Gen*), 30g each, Sclerotium Poriae Cocos (*Fu Ling*), Rhizoma Atractylodis (*Cang Zhu*), and Rhizoma Atractylodis Macrocephalae (*Bai Zhu*), 15g each, Semen Cassiae Torae (*Cao Jue Ming*), 24g, Rhizoma Pinelliae Ternatae (*Ban Xia*), 9g, and Pericarpium Citri Reticulatae (*Chen Pi*), 6g

FUNCTIONS: Transforms phlegm and eliminates dampness, quickens the blood and engenders fluids

INDICATIONS: Phlegm dampness internally stagnating with spleen vacuity, blood stasis, and fluid damage

JING XUAN HUA SHI FANG (MILDLY DIFFUSING & TRANSFORMING DAMPNESS FORMULA)

INGREDIENTS: Ginger-processed Rhizoma Pinelliae Ternatae (*Ban Xia*), Concha Meretricis (*Wen Ge*), Sclerotium Poriae Cocos (*Fu Ling*), and Semen Coicis Lachryma-jobi (*Yi Yi Ren*), 20g each, Semen Pruni Armeniacae (*Xing Ren*) and Rhizoma Acori Graminei (*Shi Chang Pu*), 10g each and Fructus Cardamomi (*Bai Dou Kou*), Folium Lophatheri Gracilis (*Dan Zhu Ye*), and Cortex Magnoliae Officinalis (*Hou Po*), 6g each

FUNCTIONS: Mildly diffuses and transforms dampness

INDICATIONS: Damp evils obstructing and stagnating in the three burners inhibiting the transport of fluids and humors

BEI MU GUA LOU SAN (FRITILLARIA & TRICHOSANTHES POWDER)

INGREDIENTS: Fructus Trichosanthis Kirlowii (*Gua Lou*) and Radix Trichosanthis Kirlowii (*Tian Hua Fen*), 12g each, Bulbus Fritillariae Thunbergii (*Zhe Bei Mu*), Sclerotium Poriae Cocos (*Fu Ling*), and Radix Platycodi Grandiflori (*Jie Geng*), 9g each, and Exocarpium Citri Rubri (*Ju Hong*), 6g

FUNCTIONS: Moistens the lungs and clears heat, rectifies the qi and transforms phlegm

INDICATIONS: Lung dryness with phlegm

XIAO LUO WAN (DISPERSE SCROFULA PILLS)

INGREDIENTS: Radix Scrophulariae Ningpoensis (*Xuan Shen*), Concha Ostreae (*Mu Li*), and Bulbus Fritillariae Thunbergii (*Zhe Bei Mu*), 15g each
FUNCTIONS: Clears heat and transforms phlegm, softens hardness and scatters nodulation

INDICATIONS: Phlegm nodulation with yin vacuity and internal heat

6

ACUPUNCTURE, ACUPRESSURE & TUINA AND THE TREATMENT OF DIABETES

In the ancient Chinese medical literature, references to acupuncture's treatment of wasting and thirsting are relatively many. However, in the later literature, its mention is relatively scarce.[1] According to Xiao Shao-qing, a contemporary Chinese acupuncture expert, acupuncture and moxibustion are only adjunctive therapies for diabetes.[2] However, Yang Lian-de feels that acupuncture can get a good effect in the treatment of this disease.[3] According to Li and Meng, contemporary Chinese experts on the treatment of diabetes, acupuncture for mild to moderate type 2 diabetes with a short disease course gets relatively good results. They also say that, in order to get those results, the course of treatment must be long, i.e., more than three months. If treatment can be given regularly (in China, three times per week) for more than three months, the treatment effects can be quite high.[4] Conversely, it is their experience that it is difficult to get much result in a short period of time using acupuncture. As exemplified by various research and case histories included in this book, acupuncture can help patients reduce and even stop the use of oral hypoglycemics and antidiabetics. For instance, it is Cheng Can-ruo's experience that acupuncture can enable some patients to get off hypoglycemic medications.[5] In some cases, it may even stop the necessity of using insulin. However, it is difficult to get an effect from acupuncture if the islets of Langerhans have completely stopped secreting insulin. In addition, acupuncture gets the best effects in cases of type 2 diabetes uncomplicated by other disorders, such as neuropathy. Results are not so good in those with a long disease course or severe symptoms. Li and Meng also say that acupuncture should be used cautiously in patients with welling and flat abscesses and pruritus.

Yang Lian-de primarily recommends the use of the back transport points for this condition, with supplemention of *Pi Shu* (Bl 20) and *Shen Shu* (Bl 23) addressing the root vacuities and draining of other appropriate back transport points addressing the tip or branch repletions. For instance, for the treatment of polydipsia, vexatious thirst, and dry mouth, Yang recommends draining *Fei Shu* (Bl 13). For polyphagia, easy hungering, and constipation, he recommends draining *Wei Shu* (Bl 21) and omitting *Pi Shu*. For blurred vision, he suggests supplementing *Gan Shu* (Bl 18). If there is simultaneous qi stagnation and/or blood stasis, he recommends adding *Ge Shu* (Bl 17), and, for pruritus, he recommends adding *Xin Shu* (Bl 15) and *Ge Shu*. These points can then be combined with other points on the torso and extremities as necessary.

However, because of the lowered immunity of patients with diabetes, one must take care to use sterile needles and properly disinfect the skin when performing acupuncture on patients with diabetes. During the Tang dynasty, acupuncture and moxibustion were forbidden in patients with enduring diabetes. Wang Tao, in the *Wai Tai Mi Yao* (*Secret Essentials of the External Platform*) says, "[If] wasting and thirsting [have lasted] 100 days or more, acupuncture and moxibustion are prohibited." Because of the poor wound healing of most diabetic patients, direct moxibustion is generally considered contraindicated or prohibited. Instead, one should use indirect moxibustion, taking care not to create moxa sores which may then become infected. The practitioner should keep these precautions in mind while reading the clinical research and case histories and when treating diabetics with moxibustion. Cheng Can-ruo believes that, in general, moxibustion should not be used until the basic symptoms are controlled. Then it may be used in order to supplement the root kidney vacuity.[6]

It is possible to substitute acupressure at the same acupuncture points for those who are afraid of needles. Acupressure massage is very effective for reducing blood sugar levels especially when the acupressure sessions are administered frequently, for instance, daily for one week or more. Commonly used acupoints, such as *Tian Shu* (St 25), *Liang Men* (St 21), *Guan Yuan* (CV 4), *Zhong Wan* (CV 12), *Gan Shu* (Bl 18), *Dan Shu* (Bl 19), and *Wei Shu* (Bl 21), easily lend themselves to acupressure massage with good results.[7] Another acupressure prescription consists of *Fei Shu* (Bl 13), *Xue Hai* (Sp 10), *Pi Shu* (Bl 20), *Shen Shu* (Bl 23), and *Zhong Wan* (CV 12).[8]

ACUPUNCTURE AND MOXIBUSTION FORMULAS FOR THE TREATMENT OF WASTING AND THIRSTING DISEASE FROM FAMOUS CHINESE ACUPUNCTURE TEXTS, BOTH PREMODERN AND CONTEMPORARY:

A. *Pu Ji Fang (Universal Aid Formulas)*: Cheng Jiang (CV 24), Yi She (Bl 49), Guan Chong (TB 1), Ran Gu (Ki 2).

B. *Shen Ying Jing (Divinely Responding Classic)*: Shui Gou (GV 26), Cheng Jiang (CV 24), Jin Jin & Yu Ye (M-HN-20), Qu Chi (LI 11), Lao Gong (Per 8), Tai Chong (Liv 3), Xing Jian (Liv 2), Shang Qiu (Sp 5), Ran Gu (Ki 2), Yin Bai (Sp 1), Tai Xi (Ki 3).

C. *Bian Que Xin Shu (Bian Que's Heart Book)*: Guan Yuan (CV 4), moxa up to 200 cones

D. *Shen Jiu Jing Lun (Treatise on the Divine Moxibustion Classic)*: Moxa Cheng Jiang (CV 24), Tai Xi (Ki 3), Zhi Zheng (SI 7), Yang Chi (TB 4), Zhao Hai (Ki 6), Shen Shu (Bl 23), Xiao Chang Shu (Bl 27), and the tip of the large toe.

E. *Zhong Guo Zhen Jiu Xue (A Study of Chinese Acupuncture & Moxibustion)*: Needle Fei Shu (Bl 13), Gan Shu (Bl 18), Pi Shu (Bl 20), Shen Shu (Bl 23), Lian Quan (CV 23), Zhong Wan (CV 12), Guan Yuan (CV 4), Tai Yuan (Lu 9), Shen Men (Ht 7), San Yin Jiao (Sp 6), Ran Gu (Ki 2), once every other day with medium stimulation and moxa; treat Guan Yuan (CV 4) and Ming Men (GV 4) every day with a moxa roll.

F. *Zhong Hua Zhen Jiu Xue (A Study of Chinese Acupuncture & Moxibustion)*: For upper wasting, Fei Shu (Bl 13), Jin Jin & Yu Ye (M-HN-20, bleed), Nei Guan (Per 6), Yu Ji (Lu 10), Shao Fu (Ht 8). For middle wasting, Fei Shu (Bl 13), Pi Shu (Bl 20), Jin Jin & Yu Ye (M-HN-20, bleed), Zhong Wan (CV 12), Shao Shang (Lu 11), Da Du (Sp 2), Feng

Long (St 40). For lower wasting, Xin Shu (Bl 15), Shen Shu (Bl 23), Qi Hai (CV 6), Guan Yuan (CV 4), Ran Gu (Ki 2), Yong Quan (Ki 1).

G. *Zhen Jiu Da Quan (The Great Collection of Acupuncture & Moxibustion)*: Lie Que (Lu 7), Pi Shu (Bl 20), Zhong Wan (CV 12), Zhao Hai (Ki 6), Zu San Li (St 36), Guan Chong (TB 1).

H. *Zhen Jiu Da Cheng (The Great Compendium of Acupuncture & Moxibustion)*: Ren Zhong (GV 26), Lian Quan (CV 23), Qi Hai (CV 6), Shen Shu (Bl 23), Hai Quan (M-HN-37).

I. *Zhong Guo Zhen Jiu Chu Fang Xue (A Study of Chinese Acupuncture & Moxibustion Prescription-writing)*: Yi Shu (M-BW-12), Fei Shu (Bl 13), Pi Shu (Bl 20), Shen Shu (Bl 23), Zu San Li (St 36), Tai Xi (Ki 3). If there is oral thirst and severe polydipsia, add Shao Shang (Lu 11), Yu Ji (Lu 10), and Ge Shu (Bl 17). If there is polyphagia, rapid hungering, and emaciation, add Wei Shu (Bl 21) and Zhong Wan (CV 12). If there is polyuria, add Fu Liu (Ki 7) and Shui Quan (Ki 5).

J. *Zhen Jiu Yi Xue Yan Ji (An Examination & Assembly of Acupuncture & Moxibustion Medical Studies)*: Main points: Pi Shu (Bl 20), Ge Shu (Bl 17), Yi Shu (M-BW-12), Zu San Li (St 36), San Yin Jiao (Sp 6). Auxillary points: Fei Shu (Bl 13), Wei Shu (Bl 21), Gan Shu (Bl 18), Zhong Wan (CV 12), Guan Yuan (CV 4), Shen Men (Ht 7), Ran Gu (Ki 2), Yin Ling Quan (Sp 9).

K. *Zhen Jiu Da Ci Dian (The Great Dictionary of Acupuncture & Moxibustion)*: For upper wasting, Shao Fu (Ht 8), Xin Shu (Bl 15), Tai Yuan (Lu 9), Fei Shu (Bl 13), Yi Shu (M-BW-12). For middle wasting, Nei Ting (St 44), San Yin Jiao (Sp 6), Pi Shu (Bl 20), Wei Shu (Bl 21), Yi Shu (M-BW-12). For lower wasting, Tai Xi (Ki 3), Tai Chong (Liv 3), Gan Shu (Bl 18), Shen Shu (Bl 23), Yi Shu (M-BW-12). For blurry vision, add Guang Ming (GB 37), for dizziness, add Shang Xing (GV 23), for yang vacuity, moxa Ming Men (GV 4). Also recommended is Wei Guan Xia Shu; a group of three points, the first is located on the Governor Vessel at the lower border of the spinous process of the eighth thoracic vertebra; the other two points (Yi Shu, M-BW-12) are located 1.5 *cun* lateral to the first point. Needle obliquely 0.5-0.7 *cun* or moxa 100 times.

L. *Nei Ke Zhen Jiu Pei Xue Xin Bian (A New Compilation of Acupuncture & Moxibustion for Internal Medicine)*: For upper wasting, Fei Shu (Bl 13), He Gu (LI 4), Yu Ji (Lu

10), *Lian Quan* (CV 23). If there is lung and kidney qi vacuity, add *Shen Shu* (Bl 23), *Guan Yuan* (CV 4), *Tai Xi* (Ki 3), and *Fei Shu* (Bl 13), all with supplementing method. If lung and stomach heat is intense, add *Zu San Li* (St 36), *San Yin Jiao* (Sp 6), and *Nei Ting* (St 44), using a draining method. For middle wasting, *Qu Chi* (LI 11), *Yu Ji* (Lu 10), *San Yin Jiao* (Sp 6), and *Nei Ting* (St 44). For lower wasting, *Shen Shu* (Bl 23), *Zhong Ji* (CV 3), *Fu Liu* (Ki 7), *San Yin Jiao* (Sp 6). If kidney yin is insufficient, add *Shen Shu* (Bl 23), *Zhi Shi* (Bl 52), *Xin Shen* (Bl 15), *Shen Men* (Ht 7), *Tai Xi* (Ki 3), *San Yin Jiao* (Sp 6), with even-supplementing even-draining method. When the pattern is yin and yang dual vacuity, use *Shen Shu* (Bl 23), *Zhi Shi* (Bl 52), *Ming Men* (GV 4), *Tai Xi* (Ki 3), *San Yin Jiao* (Sp 6), with supplementing method and moxa on *Ming Men*. When liver and kidney essence qi is insufficient, add *Gan Shu* (Bl 18), *Ting Gong* (SI 19), with supplementing method. If welling abscesses and sores are present, use *Da Zhui* (GV 14), *Qu Chi* (LI 11), and *He Gu* (LI 4), with draining method.

M. *Zhen Jiu Ji Cheng (A Compilation of Acupuncture & Moxibustion):* For wasting and thirsting polydipsia needle and/or moxa *Ren Zhong* (GV 26), *Jin Jin & Yu Ye* (M-HN-20), *Cheng Jiang* (CV 24), *Qu Chi* (LI 11), *Lao Gong* (Per 8), *Tai Chong* (Liv 3), *Xing Jian* (Liv 2), *Ran Gu* (Ki 2), *Yin Bai* (Sp 1).

N. *Jin Zhen Wang Le Ting (Golden Needle Wang Le-ting):* For upper wasting, *Jin Jin & Yu Ye* (M-HN-20, bleed), *Shao Shang* (Lu 11), *Qu Ze* (Per 3), *Yu Ji* (Lu 10) and *Tai Xi* (Ki 3). For middle wasting: *Zhong Wan* (CV 12), *Tian Shu* (St 25), *Zu San Li* (St 36), and *Nei Guan* (Per 6). *Pi Shu* (Bl 20), *Wei Shu* (Bl 21), *Da Chang Shu* (Bl 25), *Da Du* (Sp 2), *Da Ling* (Per 7), *Zu San Li* (St 36), and/or *Yang Ling Quan* (GB 34) may be added. For lower wasting, *Fei Shu* (Bl 13), *Shen Shu* (Bl 23), *Pang Guang Shu* (Bl 28), *San Yin Jiao* (Sp 6), *Guan Yuan* (CV 4), and *Fu Liu* (Ki 7). In this case, *San Jiao Shu* (Bl 22), *Yin Ling Quan* (Sp 9), *Zu San Li* (St 36), *Ming Men* (GV 4), *Yong Quan* (Ki 1), and/or *Ran Gu* (Ki 2) may be added.

O. *Jia Yi Jing (The Systematic Classic of Acupuncture & Moxibustion):* For wasting and thirsting with general fever and yellowing of the face and eyes, *Yi She* (Bl 44). For polydipsia, *Cheng Jiang* (CV 24) and *Wan Gu* (SI 4). For counterflow qi penetrating the throat with cold hands and feet and yellowish urine, *Tai Xi* (Ki 3). For wasting and thirsting with jaundice, vexation, and fullness, *Ran Gu* (Ki 2).

P. *Tong Shi Zhen Jiu Zheng Jing Qi Xue Xue (A Study of Master Tong's Acupuncture & Moxibustion Regular Channel*

[&] *Extraordinary Points):* The Three Emperors, *i.e.*, *Yin Ling Quan* (Sp 9), *Lou Gu* (Sp 7), and *San Yin Jiao* (Sp 6).

WATER-NEEDLING

Water-needling refers to point injection therapy. For the treatment of diabetes, one can use 6ml of *Huang Qi Zhu She Ye* (Astragalus Injectable Liquid) at two points per day, once every day, choosing from *Gan Shu* (Bl 18), *Wei Guan Xia Shu* (Gastric Canal Lower Transport, located 1.5 *cun* lateral below the eighth thoracic vertebra spinous process), *Pi Shu* (Bl 20), and *Shen Shu* (Bl 23).

SKIN-NEEDLING

Skin-needling refers to tapping the skin with a seven star or plum blossom needle. For the treatment of diabetes, tap along both sides of the spinal column from T7-10 once every other day. In this case, 10 treatments equal one course, and a five day rest should be given between successive courses. Another approach divides the regions for treatment: For upper wasting, tap the nape of the neck, T5-10, and the sacrum. For middle wasting, tap the nape of the neck, the mastoid region, T8-12, and the sacrum. For lower wasting, tap both sides of the entire spine, the inferior border of the mandible, and the medial portion of the leg. When using skin-needling for the treatment of diabetes, tapping should be light since the skin of those with diabetes can be sensitive and the risk of infection is greater than for those without this condition.

EAR ACUPUNCTURE

Ear acupuncture may be done at Pancreas, Internal Secretion (or Endocrine), Triple Burner, Kidney, Vagus Root, Heart, and/or Liver. If there is polydipsia, add Lung and Thirst Point. If there is polyphagia, add Spleen and Stomach. If there is polyuria, add Urinary Bladder. If needling, choose 3-5 points each time and needle once every other day, retaining the needles for 20 minutes each time. One can also use press needles, ion pellets, magnets, or Semen Vaccariae Segetalis (*Wang Bu Liu Xing*) taped over the points and stimulated by finger pressure several times per day.

The authors of the *Er Xue Zhi Bai Bing (The Treatment of One Hundred Diseases with Ear Acupuncture)* suggest the following points: Pancreas, Pancreas Gland Point, Endocrine, Liver, *Shen Men*, Brain Point, Kidney, Urinary Bladder, Thirst Point, Hunger Point, Stomach, Lung, *Shen Bao*, and Vacuity Point.[9] The last two points are located on the back of the ear. Treatment may be applied to one or both ears, daily or every other day, for 15-30 minutes each time. Each point should be stimulated every five minutes during needle retention. Five to 10 sessions is considered one course of treatment, with 3-5 days rest in between courses.

To clear heat and drain fire, enrich yin and engender fluids when dry heat has damaged fluids, use Pancreas, Pancreas Gland Point, Endocrine, Lung, Stomach, and Thirst Point. To nourish yin and clear heat, downbear fire and engender fluids when stomach dryness has damaged yin and yin vacuity with exuberant fire is present, use Pancreas, Pancreas Gland Point, Stomach, Hunger Point, and Brain Point. To enrich kidney yin and secure the essence, boost the qi and secure the lower burner, warm the kidney and transform the qi when there is kidney yin vacuity depletion, vacuity cold in the lower source, or yin and yang dual vacuity, use Pancreas, Pancreas Gland Point, Endocrine, Kidney, Urinary Bladder, Liver, *Shen Men*, Thirst Point, *Shen Bao*, Vacuity Point.

TUINA

In order to nourish yin and clear heat, use one finger Zen pushing technique (*yi zhi chan tui fa*) at *Yi Shu* (M-BW-12) for 15 minutes. Then use pressing (*an*) and rubbing (*rou*) techniques for three minutes each at *Yi Shu* and *San Yin Jiao* (Sp 6). Follow this by pressing and rubbing *Gan Shu* (Bl 18), *Dan Shu* (Bl 19), and *Shen Shu* (Bl 23) for one minute each. Then use rolling (*gun*) technique on both sides of the back along the bladder channel for five minutes, treating *Yi Shu* with especially heavy pressure and rolling all the way down to the *Ba Liao* (Bl 31-34). Next, chafe (*ca*) or rub the governing vessel, and finish by using one finger Zen pushing method at *Yong Quan* (Ki 1).

FOOT ZONE MASSAGE

Chinese foot reflexology may be done at Pineal Body, Kidney, Pancreas, Bladder, and Lower Body Lymphatic areas. Another slightly different protocol consists of massaging Pancreas, Pineal Body, Stomach, Kidney, Adrenal, Lung, and Bladder.

While internally administered Chinese medicinals are the main treatment modality for diabetes within Chinese medicine, acupuncture and other externally applied techniques can be useful as adjunctive therapies, especially during initial treatment when patient and practitioner are trying to bring this condition under control using every means at their disposal. In addition, self-moxibustion, self-tuina, and self foot zone massage may be useful home therapies used by the patient on a daily basis to prevent and treat diabetic complications. However, for these externally applied therapies to be significantly effective, regular daily application over a prolonged period of time is typically required.

ENDNOTES:

[1] Yang Lian-de, quoted in *Zhong Guo Dang Dai Zhen Jiu Ming Jia Yi An (Contemporary Chinese National Acupuncture & Moxibustion Famous Masters Case Histories)*, compiled by Wang Xue-tai & Liu Guan-jun, Jilin Science & Technology Publishing Co., Changchun, 1991, p. 362
[2] Xiao Shao-qing, *Zhong Guo Zhen Jiu Chu Fang Xue (A Study of Chinese Acupuncture & Moxibustion Prescription-writing)*, Ningxia People's Publishing Co., Yinchuan, 1986, p. 275-276
[3] Yang Lian-de, *op. cit.*, p. 362
[4] Li Yong-zhi & Meng Fan-yi, *Xiao Ke (Wasting & Thirsting)*, Chinese National Chinese Medicine & Medicinals Publishing Co., Beijing, 1995, p. 121
[5] Cheng Can-ruo, quoted in *Zhong Guo Dang Dai Zhen Jiu Ming Jia Yi An (Contemporary Chinese National Acupuncture & Moxibustion Famous Masters Case Histories)*, compiled by Wang Xue-tai & Liu Guan-jun, Jilin Science & Technology Publishing Co., Changchun, 1991, p. 636
[6] *Ibid.*, p. 636
[7] Wang Jin-tao, "The Treatment of 18 Cases of Diabetes with *Song Zhen* Method of *Tui Na*," *Shan Dong Zhong Yi Za Zhi (Shandong Journal of Chinese Medicine)*, #11, 1999, p. 502
[8] Li Yi, *Zhi Zhen Zhi Bai Bing (The Finger-needle Treatment of Hundreds of Diseases)*, New Era Publishing Co., Beijing, 1997, p. 101
[9] Chen Kang-mei & Gao Xiao-lan, *Er Xue Zhi Bai Bing (The Treatment of Hundreds of Diseases with Ear Acupuncture)*, People's Army Medical Press, Beijing, 1995, p. 277-279

7

DIET & DIABETES

Diet is perhaps the single most important factor in determining the control of diabetes.[1] No matter how many hypoglycemic tablets are swallowed, insulin is injected, or even Chinese medicinals are taken, without adherence to a healthy diet, it is difficult to master diabetes. The good news is that one-third of all patients with diabetes succeed in controlling their blood glucose through dietary modifications in 6-12 weeks.[2] Although this is a book specifically about the Chinese medical treatment of diabetes mellitus, diabetes is a complex condition which commonly requires a combination of modern Western and traditional Chinese treatment. We believe this is also the case when it comes to diabetes and dietary therapy. It is our experience as clinicians working in a Western milieu that the best results come from blending the disease specificity of Western medicine with the time-tested holistic wisdom of Chinese medicine. In addition, many of the foods traditionally eaten in China by those with diabetes either are not widely available in the West or are not to the modern Western palate or lifestyle. Therefore, this chapter on diabetes and diet is divided into two parts. The first part discusses the current Western medical view on dietary therapy for this condition. Much of the information in this section comes from WebMD™ Health.[3] Other sources are cited in the endnotes. The second part of this chapter then presents traditional Chinese teachings on diet and diabetes.

WESTERN DIETARY THERAPY FOR DM

Both type 1 and 2 diabetes share the central feature of elevated blood sugar levels due to absolute or relative insufficiencies of insulin. After meals, food is digested in the stomach and intestines. Carbohydrates are broken down into sugar molecules, of which glucose is one, and proteins are digested into their constituents, amino acids. Glucose and amino acids are then absorbed directly into the bloodstream, and blood sugar levels rise. Normally, this signals the beta cells of the pancreas to secrete insulin, which pours into the bloodstream. Insulin, in turn, enables glucose and amino acids to enter cells—especially the muscle cells—where, along with other hormones, it directs whether these nutrients will be burned for energy or stored for future use. As blood sugar falls to premeal levels, the pancreas reduces the production of insulin, and the body uses its stored energy until the next meal provides additional nutrients. In type 1 diabetes, the beta cells in the pancreas that produce insulin are gradually destroyed. Eventually, insulin deficiency is absolute. Without insulin to move glucose into the cells, blood sugar levels become excessively high, a condition known as hyperglycemia. The sugar, which the body cannot use without insulin, spills over into the urine and is lost. Therefore, type 1 patients become dependent on exogenously administered insulin for survival. In this case, dietary control focuses on balancing food intake with insulin intake and energy expenditure from physical exertion.

Most type 2 diabetes patients produce variable or even normal amounts of insulin but are insulin resistant. This means they have abnormalities in liver and muscle cells that block the action of insulin, and many type 2 diabetes patients are incapable of secreting enough insulin to overcome this resistance. In this latter case, it is likely that there is an additional defect in insulin secretion by the beta cells. In addition, obesity is common in type 2 diabetes patients, and this condition appears to be related to insulin resistance. Thus the primary dietary goal for overweight type 2 patients is weight loss and maintenance.

As we have seen, people with both types of diabetes are at

risk for a number of medical complications, including heart and kidney disease. Therefore, dietary requirements for diabetes must also take these disorders into consideration.

GENERAL GOALS OF A DIABETES DIET

It used to be that people thought there was a "diabetes diet." However, in the spring of 1994, the American Diabetes Association (ADA) issued new dietary guidelines giving people with diabetes more latitude in their choices of foods.[4] At this time, there is no single diet that meets all the needs of everyone with diabetes. In fact, there is currently quite a bit of controversy in the world of diet and diabetes. Nevertheless, there are some constants. All people with diabetes should aim for healthy lipid levels and control of blood pressure. People with type 1 diabetes and those with type 2 diabetes on insulin or oral antidiabetic agents must focus on controlling blood glucose levels by coordinating calorie intake with medication or insulin administration, exercise, and other variables. Adequate calories must be maintained for normal growth in children, for increased needs during pregnancy, and after illness. For those who are overweight, suffer from type 2 diabetes, and are not taking medication, both weight loss and blood sugar control are important. A reasonable weight is usually defined as what is achievable and sustainable, rather than one that is culturally defined as desirable or ideal. Even a 10-15 pound weight loss for those who are obese can significantly help in controlling blood glucose.[5] And, according to most authorities, the general rules for healthy eating apply to everyone: limit fats (particularly saturated fats and trans-fatty acids), protein, and cholesterol, and consume plenty of fiber and fresh vegetables.

MONITORING

In patients being treated with insulin or insulin-producing or sensitizing drugs, it is important to monitor blood glucose levels carefully to avoid hypoglycemia. Patients should aim for premeal glucose levels of 80-120mg/dL for adults and teens, 100-200mg/dL for children under 12, and bedtime levels of 100-140mg/dL. Current intensive treatment for type 1 diabetes to tightly control blood sugar levels usually requires four or more daily blood sugar tests. Blood glucose levels are generally more stable in type 2 diabetes than in type 1. Therefore, experts usually recommend measuring blood levels only 1-2 times per day. Other tests are needed periodically to determine potential complications of diabetes, such as hypertension and nephropathy. Such tests may also indicate whether current diet plans are helping the patient and whether

changes should be made. For instance, glycosylated hemoglobin (HbA1C) is usually measured quarterly. Levels of 11-12% of glycosylated hemoglobin indicate poor control of carbohydrates. High levels of proteinuria (micro- and macroalbuminuria) is prognosticative of deteriorating renal function and the need to lower protein intake.[6]

PREVENTING HYPOGLYCEMIA (A.K.A. INSULIN SHOCK)

For prevention of long-term complications of diabetes, experts are now recommending that both type 1 and type 2 patients should aim at keeping blood glucose levels as close to normal as possible. This is referred to as "tight control." Such intensive insulin treatment increases the risk of hypoglycemia, which occurs when blood glucose is extremely low (below 60 mg/dL). Diabetes patients should always carry hard candy, fruit juice, or sugar packets, and family and friends should be aware of the symptoms of hypoglycemia. If the patient is helpless, they should be administered 3-5 pieces of hard candy, 2-3 packets of sugar, or half a cup (i.e., four ounces) of fruit juice. If there is inadequate response within 15 minutes, additional oral sugar should be provided or the patient should receive emergency medical treatment, including the intravenous administration of glucose. Family members and friends can also learn to inject glucagon, a hormone which, unlike insulin, raises blood glucose.

TIMING OF MEALS

While people with and without diabetes should eat the same kind of generally healthy diet, one major difference is that people with diabetes should eat approximately the same amount of food at the same time each day. People with diabetes should also space meals throughout the day instead of eating large meals once or twice per day. This can help a person avoid extremely high or low blood glucose levels.[7] The timing of meals is particularly important for people taking insulin. The types and amounts of food as well as meal and snack times should be carefully determined so that blood glucose levels are properly regulated. In general, people with type 1 diabetes should eat about 30 minutes after taking an insulin injection. Three meals should be eaten each day at regular intervals, about 4-5 hours apart. Snacks are often needed at midmorning and midafternoon, but they should be included as part of the total daily calorie requirements. One study of type 2 patients has also reported that large dinners raise fasting blood glucose levels the next morning, which may adversely affect some patients.

GUIDELINES FOR MAJOR FOOD COMPONENTS IN A DIABETES DIET

CARBOHYDRATES

Compared to fats and protein, carbohydrates have the greatest impact on blood sugar, but different carbohydrates have different effects. Carbohydrates are either complex (as in starches) or simple (as in fruits and sugars). One gram of carbohydrates equals four calories. The current recommendation by the American Diabetes Association is that carbohydrates should provide between 50-60% of daily caloric intake. However, recently, this high carbohydrate/low fat diet has come under scrutiny. Those with type 2 diabetes who tend to be overweight and insulin-resistant overproduce glucose after eating carbohydrates. This, in turn, requires more insulin to process this glucose. This then leads to appetite stimulation and production of fat. Therefore, some patients with diabetes may have problems with cholesterol and triglyceride levels when carbohydrates constitute over 50% of the diet. If triglycerides are high, carbohydrates should be reduced to 45%.

In all cases, complex carbohydrates found in whole grains and vegetables are preferred over those found in starches—such as pastas, white-flour products, and potatoes. (Patients with diabetes should consume no [or avoid] vegetables that grow underground due to their high content of amylose.) In one study, substituting special starch-free bread for normal bread resulted in a significant decline in blood glucose and hemoglobin A1 in those with type 2 diabetes. However, no difference appears to exist between complex carbohydrates and simple sugars in their ability to raise blood glucose levels. Nevertheless, this does not mean that those with diabetes should increase their sugar intake. Rather, it indicates that people with diabetes can add more fresh fruit to their diets than previously thought. Fresh fruits have a number of significant health benefits. Sugar from fruit (fructose) produces a slower increase in glucose than sucrose (table sugar). Sugar itself adds calories and increases blood glucose levels quickly, but it provides no nutrients. One study also found that sugar was a risk factor for heart disease, possibly because sugar produces very low density lipoproteins and triglycerides which are atherogenic. People with diabetes should avoid products listing more than five grams of sugar per serving. If specific amounts are not listed, patients should avoid products with sugar listed as one of the first four ingredients on the label.

PROTEIN

Proteins should provide 12-20% of calories. One gram of protein contains four calories. Studies are showing that reducing proteins in the diet helps slow the progression of kidney disease in both those with diabetes and those without. Some experts recommend that anyone with diabetes other than pregnant women should restrict protein to approximately 0.4 grams for every pound of their ideal body weight—about 10% of daily calories. However, it should be noted that, although rare, a severely low protein/low salt diet coupled with high fluid intake increases the risk for hyponatremia, a condition that can cause fatigue, confusion, and, in extreme cases, can be life-threatening. Protein is commonly recommended as part of a bedtime snack to maintain normal blood sugar levels during the night, although studies are mixed over whether it adds any protective benefits against night-time hypoglycemia. If it does, only small amounts (14 grams) may be needed to stabilize blood glucose levels. For heart protection, one 1999 study suggests that it does not matter if one choose fish, poultry, beef, or pork as long as the meat is lean. (Saturated fat in meat is the primary danger to the heart.) Fish is still probably the best source of protein for people with diabetes, however. In one study, fish protein protected rats on high-fat diets against insulin resistance, while plant protein had no effect.

FATS & OILS

All fats found in foods are made up of a mixture of three chemical building blocks: monounsaturated, polyunsaturated, and saturated fatty acids. Oils and fats are nearly always mixtures of all three fatty acids, but one type usually predominates. For example, although coconut oil is mostly saturated, it also contains small amounts of monounsaturated and polyunsaturated fatty acids. There are also three important chemical subgroups of polyunsaturated fats: omega-3, omega-6, and omega-9 fatty acids. In addition, there are trans-fatty acids. These are not naturally occurring fats but are products of food processing. However, one gram of fat is equal to nine calories, whether it is saturated or unsaturated, and one teaspoon of oil, butter, or other fats equals about five grams of fat.

Although there is much controversy on the effects of fat on health, virtually all experts strongly advise limiting intake of saturated fats (found in animal products) and trans-fatty acids (found in commercial baked goods and fast foods), which produce unhealthy cholesterol and lipid levels. However, monounsaturated and polyunsaturated fatty acids may have health benefits even though no guidelines yet exist on how much or how little of these to eat. Some experts recommend maintaining a relatively high intake of monounsaturated and polyunsaturated fats (about 32% of calorie intake), with saturated fats representing no more than 8%. Others believe that a very trim diet, 20% fat with as little as 4% saturated fat, is ideal. Still others recommend fat intake somewhere in between these extremes. Nevertheless, in all cases, the health dangers of a diet high in saturated or trans-fatty fat should not be underestimated, and all fats, both good ones and bad, add the same calories. Also of note, one study indicates that, although dietary cholesterol itself does not appear to increase the risk for heart disease in most people, people with diabetes, especially type 2 diabetes, may be an exception. Therefore, until more research is done, people with type 2 diabetes should probably consider avoiding eating eggs or other high-cholesterol foods, such as shrimp, more than once a week.

HARMFUL FATS. Reducing consumption of saturated fats and trans-fatty acids is the first essential step in managing cholesterol levels through diet. Saturated fats are found predominantly in animal products, including meat and dairy products. Saturated fats in the diet increase blood cholesterol levels. The so-called tropical oils—palm, coconut, and cocoa butter—are also high in saturated fats. However, evidence is lacking about these oils' effects on the heart. The countries with the highest palm-oil intake, Costa Rica and Malaysia, also have much lower heart disease rates and cholesterol levels than Western nations. Trans-fatty acids are also dangerous for the heart, and in addition, they may pose a risk for certain cancers. They are created by adding a hydrogen molecule to polyunsaturated or monounsaturated oils (called hydrogenation) during a process aimed at stabilizing oils to prevent them from becoming rancid and to keep them solid at room temperature. These partially hydrogenated fats both increase LDL cholesterol and reduce HDL cholesterol levels. One study of 80,000 nurses reported that women whose total fat consumption was 46% of total caloric intake had no greater risk in general for a heart attack than did those for whom fat represented 30% of calories consumed. However, women whose diets were high in trans-fatty acids had a 53% increased risk for heart attack compared to those who consumed the least of those fats. Hydrogenated fats are used in stick margarine and in many fast foods and baked goods, including most commercially produced white breads. When purchasing these foods, people with diabetes should avoid those with labels that include "partially hydrogenated" oils and understand such products may contain trans-fatty acids even if they claim to be low- or no-cholesterol or are made from unsaturated oils. Liquid margarine is not hydrogenated and is recommended, as is margarine labeled "trans-fatty acid free."

BENEFICIAL FATS & OILS. Some fat, especially from polyunsaturated and monounsaturated fats, is essential for health and is critical for healthy development in children. Polyunsaturated fats are found in safflower, sunflower, corn, cottonseed oils, and fish, while monounsaturated fats are mostly present in olive, canola, and peanut oils and in most nuts. Many studies have indicated that monounsaturated fats help to maintain healthy HDL levels and some have reported that polyunsaturated fats reduced HDL levels. It is not clear, as of this writing, that monounsaturated fat has a significant advantage over polyunsaturated fats on cholesterol levels, although monounsaturated fats may have other advantages, including antioxidant, anti-blood-clotting, and anti-inflammatory properties.

To help clarify matters, researchers are focusing on smaller building blocks called essential fatty acids (EFAs) contained in polyunsaturated oils (omega-3 and omega-6 fatty acids) and monounsaturated oils (omega-9 fatty acid). Omega-3 EFA in fish oil significantly lowers (almost 30%) triglycerides in patients with diabetes. However, omega-3 EFA may cause a slight rise in LDL and may worsen blood glucose control.[8] Omega-6 EFA improves nerve blood flow, nerve conduction, and helps prevent neuropathy in both type 1 and 2 diabetes.[9]

SOURCES OF ESSENTIAL FATTY ACIDS

- **Omega-3 polyunsaturated fatty acids:**

  They are further categorized as alpha-linolenic acid (sources include canola oil, soybeans, flaxseed, olive oil, many nuts and seeds), and docosahexaenoic and eicosapentaenoic acids (sources are oily fish and breast milk). Studies have indicated that vegetable oils containing alpha-linolenic acids reduce triglycerides and are heart protective, although fish oils, which contain docosahexaenoic and eicosapentaenoic acids, do not have much effect. Fish itself, however, has other substances that appear to have many benefits.

- **Omega-6 polyunsaturated fatty acids:**

  Further categorized as linoleic, or linolic, acid. (Sources are flaxseed, corn, soybean, and canola oil.)

- **Omega-9 monounsaturated fatty acids:**

  Categorized as oleic acid. (Sources are olive, canola, and peanut oil and avocado.)

Studies have found greater protection against heart disease from omega-6 oils than omega-3, but omega-6 is also associated with increased production of compounds called eicosanoids which enhance tumor growth in animals. Both omega-3 and omega-9 fatty acids contain chemicals that block these eicosanoids. Some researchers believe that our current Western diet now contains an unhealthy ratio of 10:1 of omega-6 to omega-3 fatty acids. (Omega-6 fatty acids are contained in many oils used for making hydrogenated fats.) This seems to suggest that the bottom line is to try to obtain a better balance of fatty acids without consuming too many calories. A number of studies indicate that, in a healthy balance, all of these fatty acids are essential to life.

Fiber

Fiber is an important dietary component in the fight for healthy cholesterol balance and is found in vegetables, fruits, and whole grains. Fiber cannot be digested by humans but passes through the intestines, drawing water with it, and is eliminated as part of fecal content. Recent studies on both men and women have reported that diets rich in fiber from whole grains reduce the risk for type 2 diabetes. Fiber is also good for the heart. High fiber diets (up to 55 grams per day) help improve cholesterol levels, control weight, and improve blood glucose and insulin levels. However, the average American eats considerably less fiber than this per day.[10] Fiber also helps prevent certain cancers and many intestinal problems. A diet rich in fiber also tends to "displace" the consumption of other, unhealthy foods with high fat content.[11]

For weight loss, insoluble fiber, found in wheat bran, whole grains, seeds, and fruit and vegetable peels, is most effective. However, soluble fiber, found in dried beans, oat bran, barley, apples, citrus fruits, and potatoes, has important benefits for the heart, particularly for lowering blood cholesterol levels. People who increase their levels of soluble fiber should also increase water and fluid intake.

Specifically healthful whole grains, fruits & vegetables

The best sources of dietary fiber, soluble or insoluble, are obtained from whole grains, particularly oats, nuts, legumes, fruits, and vegetables. Such foods also provide many other health benefits. For example, one study has reported that oat-rich diets reduced blood pressure and cholesterol levels significantly better than wheat-rich diets. In one study of 22,000 male physicians, those who ate nuts had the lowest rate of heart disease. Other studies indicate that nuts improve cholesterol levels and may even inhibit tumor growth. These benefits may derive from a fatty compound called alpha-linolenic acid and from other plant chemicals. Unfortunately, nuts are also high in calories. Pectin, a type of fiber found in apples, grapefruits, and oranges, may also protect against heart disease. Deeply colored green, red, and yellow fruits and vegetables are rich in important antioxidant vitamins and other phytochemicals. Spinach, chicory, sorrel, Swiss chard, dandelion, and turnip greens are high in vitamins and contain no fat. In general, the darker the color of the vegetable, the more vitamins it has. Cruciferous vegetables, such as broccoli, cabbage, bok choy, Brussel sprouts, cauliflower, and kale are also rich in vitamins and high in antioxidants. Isoflavones found in soybeans, tofu, tempeh, and soy milk deserves special mention. Soy products seem to have major benefits for older people and those with type 2 diabetes. Some studies have found that eating 20-25 grams a day (about 5-6 ounces of firm tofu) helps maintain healthy cholesterol levels and may also lower the risk for kidney disease and certain cancers.[12]

Sodium

Although salt does not raise blood glucose, it can raise blood pressure. Since hypertension and diabetes commonly coexist, people with diabetes should limit salt intake, particularly if they also have hypertension. A major on-going study of salt intake has found evidence that diets high in salt accelerate hypertension as people age. People who are most likely to be salt-sensitive are generally overweight, older, African American, and those who have low levels of renin, a hormone that prevents reduction of blood pressure. In addition to helping to reduce blood pressure, salt restriction enhances the benefits of certain antihypertensive drugs by reducing potassium loss. One study showed that diets with very low salt intake helped protect against kidney disease in patients who were also taking calcium-blocker drugs for high blood pressure. Possibly even more important, another study has found that salt restriction reduced levels of protein in the urine of diabetic rats. Albuminuria is an early indicator of kidney damage. About 75% of consumption of sodium and salt in Europe and the U.S. comes from commercially processed foods. However, yet another study has found an increased rate of heart attacks in people with very restrictive low salt diets. This suggests that some sodium may be needed to protect the heart. Therefore, eliminating all salt from the diet is probably not the best idea.

ALCOHOL

Alcohol contains almost as many calories per gram as fat.[13] While it was once thought that people with diabetes should totally abstain from alcohol, it is now thought that small amounts of alcohol can be included in the diets of those with DM as long as blood glucose is under good control. In fact, drinking wine appears to have some health benefits if used in moderation (*i.e.*, 1-2 glasses per day). However, in those taking insulin or sulfonylureas, alcohol may cause a hypoglycemic reaction. This is especially the case in those with hypoglycemic unawareness. To make matters worse, the symptoms of hypoglycemia (specifically, neuroglycopenia) and the symptoms of alcohol intoxication are similar: thick-tongued speech, shaking, staggering walk, mental confusion, etc.[14] Likewise, drinking alcohol on an empty stomach may also cause low blood sugar. Therefore, people with diabetes should only drink alcohol with food.

Patients with other health problems may be asked to abstain from alcohol. These include pancreatitis, high triglyceride levels, gastric problems, neuropathy, nephropathy, and certain types of heart disease (*i.e.*, cardiomyopathies). Pregnant women or those at risk for alcohol abuse should not drink alcohol.

CAFFEINE

A review of life-time records of male medical students found that by age 60, 19% of noncoffee drinkers had high blood pressure as compared to 25% of coffee drinkers that were hypertensive. Caffeine may have greater effect in people who already have elevated blood pressure. Drinking coffee increases excretion of calcium which, in turn, may increase the risk for high blood pressure. Therefore, anyone who drinks coffee should maintain an adequate calcium intake. Studies have indicated that unfiltered coffee may increase levels of LDL cholesterol and alanine-aminotransferase, an indicator of liver damage. Filtered coffee poses no such risks.

SPECIFIC DIET METHODS FOR THOSE WITH DIABETES

Anyone with diabetes needs some diet plan. One 18 month study of people with type 2 diabetes found no difference between a high carbohydrate/high fiber diet, a low fat diet, and a weight management diet. All groups, however, experienced lower glycosylated hemoglobin levels and lower LDL cholesterol levels. There were no changes in HDL cholesterol or triglycerides. The researchers concluded that the positive benefits of the diets derived not from the specific regimens but because the people in the study were attentive and focused. In other words, any diet works if patients work at it. Choosing a healthy diet and then making the effort to stick to it appear to be the primary requirements for successful control of blood glucose levels.

Several dietary methods are available for controlling blood sugar levels. The simplest method is to follow the Food Guide Pyramid, recommended by the U.S. Department of Agriculture for everyone. Some experts believe this may be sufficient for many people with diabetes. More intricate dietary methods are available for control of blood sugar. They can be effective, but they are also complex and many patients become discouraged using them. The most common method for controlling blood sugar is the use of The Diabetic Exchange Lists designed by the American Diabetes and American Dietetic Associations. More sophisticated methods include counting carbohydrate grams and adjusting them according to blood glucose levels and tabulating the total available glucose (TAG) derived from foods that are eaten. Counting calories is usually the basis for weight loss. If one of these methods works in controlling glucose levels, there is no reason to choose another. Each of them can be effective. However, because controlling diabetes is an individual affair, we believe that everyone with this condition should receive help from a dietary professional in selecting the best method for them. For instance, a person with type 2 diabetes who is overweight and insulin-resistant may need to have a different carbohydrate/protein balance than a thin person with type 1 diabetes in danger of kidney disease.

WEIGHT CONTROL

Weight control is an especially important part of the management of type 2 diabetes since extra body fat makes it difficult for people with type 2 diabetes to make and use their own insulin. It is estimated that 80-90% of type 2 DM patients are obese.[15] The benefits to health from weight loss are highest with the first pounds lost, and losing only 10% of body weight can control progression of type 2 diabetes. Such weight loss can be gradual—for instance, one pound per week. The first step is to calculate the daily caloric need for maintaining a healthy weight. This is typically 12-15 calories for each pound of ideal body weight. However, this varies depending on gender, age, and whether a person is active or sedentary. As a rough rule of thumb, one pound of fat equals about 3,500 calories. Therefore, one can typically lose one pound per week by reducing daily caloric intake by about 500 calories. Naturally, the more severe the daily calorie restriction, the faster the weight loss.

Some studies suggest that replacing foods high in fats and sugars with low fat, complex carbohydrates, such as fruits, vegetables, and whole grains, may be more effective for weight control than calorie counting. In a one-year study, those on low fat diets lost three times as much weight as those on standard low calorie diets. However, very low fat diets (15% or less of daily calories) may actually increase triglycerides and reduce HDL cholesterol levels, and such changes are risk factors for heart disease. Many people who reduce their fat intake may also not consume enough of the basic nutrients, including vitamins A and E, folic acid, calcium, iron, and zinc, and they often increase their intake of carbohydrates. People on low fat diets should consume a high variety of foods and take a multivitamin if appropriate. Simply switching to low fat or skimmed milk may help people achieve the recommended dietary goal of 30% or fewer calories from fat and also help provide calcium. Some dietary fat is essential. Such fats should be derived from nontropical plant oils and fish. All healthy diets should also be high in fiber, which studies are increasingly reporting to be an important weight-loss factor.

When trying to lose weight, however, meals should not be skipped and particularly for those who are on insulin. Skipping meals can upset the balance between food intake and insulin and can also lead to weight gain if extra food is needed too often to offset low blood sugar levels.

EATING DISORDERS & DIABETES

Up to 1/3 of young women with type 1 diabetes have eating disorders that prompt them to underdose insulin to lose weight. This is a very hazardous practice. Healthy eating habits along with good insulin control are essential in managing this complex disease. In addition, people with diabetes and eating disorders, such as anorexia nervosa and bulimia, are likely to have more episodes of ketoacidosis and hypoglycemia and their glycosylated hemoglobin levels tend to be higher.[16] Because their blood glucose is not under very good control, the risk for diabetes complications, such as neuropathy, is also much greater.

FOOD GUIDE PYRAMID & THE MEDITERRANEAN DIET

The Food Guide Pyramid contains the U.S. Department of Agriculture's general nutritional guidelines for everyone. While this pyramid is a great step forward from the four basic food groups of the 1950s and 60s, it still has some problems. Therefore, some nutritional experts have recommended modifying it to adapt to the so-called Mediterranean diet. A recent study of heart attack patients found that those on the Mediterranean diet had a 76% lower risk of major adverse cardiovascular events, including subsequent heart attacks, unstable angina, and stroke, compared to those on a normal diet. Although this study does not constitute proof for the superiority of the Mediterranean diet, it does lend additional support to that possibility. Research indicates that it is not a single food but the spectrum of foods in this diet that is responsible for whatever benefits are associated with it. The table below indicates the differences between the Food Guide Pyramid and the Mediterranean diet. Of some concern to those with diabetes with the Mediterranean diet are added calories from the high intake of olive oil, reduced iron levels, and possible lack of calcium from fewer dairy products. Experts recommend that those who choose the Mediterranean diet should use only olive oil (no margarine or butter even on bread) to avoid excess fat. They should cook in iron pans and eat foods that contain iron

---

Standard Pyramid Diet

- Groups all saturated and monounsaturated fats and oils together and recommends using them sparingly

- Recommends 2-3 daily servings of dairy products and 2-3 daily services of meat, nuts, legumes, or beans

- Vegetables: 3-5 daily servings
  Fruits: 2-4 servings (Does not specifically recommend fresh or frozen)

- Defines carbohydrates only as breads and other starchy foods and recommends 6-11 servings per day

---

Mediterranean Diet

- Advises olive oil daily in moderation
  Avoids saturated fats

- Recommends red meat only a few times a month
  Avoids high fat dairy products

- Recommends fresh fruits and vegetables and higher amounts of nuts, legumes, and beans than with the pyramid diet

- Recommends high fiber whole grains (e.g., couscous, polenta, bulgur) and potatoes

- Daily glass or two of wine

and those rich in vitamin C, which boosts iron intake. They may also need supplemental calcium. In addition, the recommended intake of wine may be problematic for some people with diabetes and for anyone who is pregnant or abuses alcohol. In addition, all people with diabetes who have indications of kidney damage should restrict protein below the intake of the general population.

DIABETIC EXCHANGE LISTS

The diabetic exchanges are six different lists of foods grouped according to similar calorie, carbohydrate, protein, and fat content. These are starch/bread, meat, vegetables, fruit, milk, and fat. The objective of the exchange lists is to maintain the proper balance of carbohydrates, proteins, and fats throughout the day. The exchange lists can be obtained by calling or writing the American Diabetes Association.

In developing a menu, patients must first establish their individual dietary requirements, particularly the optimal number of daily calories and the proportion of carbohydrates, fats, and protein. This should normally been done with their physician or a professional nutritionist. A person is allowed a certain number of exchange choices from each food list per day. The amount and type of these exchanges are based on a number of factors, including the daily exercise program, timing of insulin injections, and whether or not the individual needs to lose weight or reduce cholesterol or blood pressure levels. The exchange lists should then be used to set up menus for each day that fulfill these requirements. Foods can be substituted for each other within an exchange list but not between lists even if they have the same calorie count. In all lists, except in the fruit list, choices can be doubled or tripled to supply a serving of certain foods (*e.g.*, three starch choices equal 1 1/2 cups of hot cereal or three meat choices equal a three ounce hamburger). On these exchange lists, some foods are "free." These contain less than 20 calories per serving and can be eaten in any amount spread throughout the day unless a serving size is specified. The following are the categories given on the exchange lists:

STARCHES & BREAD. Each exchange under starches and bread contains about 15 grams of carbohydrates, three grams of protein, and a trace of fat, for a total of 80 calories. A general rule is that 1/2 cup of cooked cereal, grain, or pasta equals one exchange, and one ounce of a bread product is one serving.

MEAT & CHEESE. The exchange groups for meat and cheese are categorized by lean meat and low fat substi-

tutes, medium fat meat and substitutes, and high fat. High fat exchanges should be used at a maximum of three times a week. Fat should be removed before cooking. Exchange sizes on the meat list are generally one ounce and based on cooked meats (three ounces of cooked meat equals four ounces of raw meat).

VEGETABLES. Exchanges for vegetables are 1/2 cup cooked, one cup raw, and 1/2 cup juice. Each group contains five grams of carbohydrates, two grams of protein, and 2-3 grams of fiber. Vegetables can be fresh or frozen. Canned vegetables are less desirable because they are often high in sodium. Vegetables should be cooked by steaming without added fat.

FRUITS & SUGAR. Sugars are now included within the total carbohydrate count in the ADA exchange lists. Still, sugars should not be more than 10% of daily carbohydrates. Each exchange contains about 15 grams of carbohydrates, for a total of 60 calories.

MILK & SUBSTITUTES. The milk and milk substitutes list is categorized by a fat content similar to the meat list. A milk exchange is usually one cup or eight ounces. For those who are on weight-loss or low cholesterol diets, the skim and very low fat milk lists should be followed and the whole milk group should be avoided. Others should use the whole milk list very sparingly. All people with diabetes should avoid artificially sweetened milks.

FATS. A fat exchange is usually one teaspoon, but it may vary. People, of course, should avoid saturated and trans-fatty acids and choose polyunsaturated or monounsaturated fats instead.

Number of exchanges per day for different calorie levels					
Calories	**1200**	**1500**	**1800**	**2000**	**2200**
Starch/bread	5	8	10	11	13
Meat	4	5	7	8	8
Vegetable	2	3	3	4	4
Fruit	3	3	3	3	3
Milk	2	2	2	2	2
Fat	3	3	3	4	5

CARBOHYDRATE COUNTING & BLOOD GLUCOSE CONTROL

Carbohydrates have the greatest impact on blood sugar of all nutrients, with fats and protein playing only minor roles. If all other dietary methods fail, carbohydrate counting may be beneficial, but it is very complex and typically requires the collaboration of a physician. This technique relies on knowing the number of carbohydrate grams needed during the day, how to calculate these from food, and how rapidly different foods increase blood glucose levels. To implement this dietary method, multiple blood glucose readings are taken over a few days to determine the patient's daily insulin requirements for keeping blood sugar balanced. A special calculation is then made for the number of carbohydrate grams that are covered by that daily insulin dose. The next step is to find the number of carbohydrates in foods so that the right amount can be eaten to balance this amount of insulin. Commercial foods are labeled with carbohydrate amounts and, for

The glycemic index of some commonly eaten foods

Breads

Pumpernickel	49
Rye	64
White	69
Whole wheat	72

Grains

Barley	22
Brown rice	66
Sweet corn	58
White rice	72

Beans

Baked	43
Chickpeas	36
Kidney	33
Red lentils	27
Soy	14

Milk products

Ice cream	38
Milk	34
Yogurt	38

Cereals

All Bran®	54
Corn flakes	83
Swiss muesli	60
Oatmeal	53
Puffed rice	90
Shredded Wheat®	70

Pasta

Macaroni	46
Spaghetti	38
Spaghetti, protein enriched	28

Fruits

Apple	38
Banana	61
Orange	43
Orange juice	49
Strawberries	32

Potatoes

Instant mashed	86
Mashed	72
New	58
Sweet	50
White	87
Yams	54

Snacks

Corn chips	72
Oatmeal cookies	57
Potato chips	56

Sugars

Fructose	22
Honey	91
Refined sugar	64

other foods, a number of books are available that provide the percentage of carbohydrates to the total nutrients.

In general, one gram of carbohydrate raises blood glucose by three points in people who weigh 200 pounds, four points for those weighing 150 pounds, and five points for those who weigh 100 pounds. Patients must choose not only the appropriate amount of carbohydrates needed to raise glucose levels, but they must also know which carbohydrate-containing foods will raise blood sugar within a desired time frame. For instance, foods with "fast" carbohydrates may be needed for sudden blood sugar drops shortly before a meal, while foods with "slow" carbohydrates may be useful for long periods of exercise. To determine fast and slow carbohydrates, a glycemic index of foods has been developed. This glycemic index is an indicator of how quickly specific foods affect blood glucose (see table). The index is based on a scale of 1-100. For example, a glucose tablet equals 100 and has the most rapid effect. When taken for hypoglycemia, it can bring relief in 10-15 minutes. Some studies have shown that diets high in foods that have a low glycemic index improve blood sugar, cholesterol, and triglyceride levels and may even reduce the risk for kidney disease. It should be noted that numbers attributed to each food are not additive. In other words, adding All Bran® cereal with a glycemic index number of 49 to a banana with an index of 61 does not equal 110. However, the combination of carbohydrates with fats or protein do change that carbohydrate's impact on blood glucose. For instance, a baked potato has a very high index of 87, but, when a fat, such as butter, is added, the impact slows down and the glycemic index of the combined foods is considerably less than the potato alone.

The glycemic index is not meant as a complete dietary guide, since it does not provide nutritional guidelines for all foods. The U.S.D.A. Food Pyramid, the Mediterranean diet, or exchange lists should still serve as the basis for meal planning. This index is simply an indication of how the metabolism will respond to carbohydrates eaten. That being said, it is true that low glycemic index numbers are often associated with whole grains and other beneficial complex carbohydrates. One study tracked the glycemic indices for the traditional foods of Pima Indians: corn, lima beans, white and yellow teparies, mesquite, and acorns. These foods had a very low index, and experts believe they had protected this genetically susceptible population from the high incidence of type 2 diabetes the Pimas are experiencing now. This current high incidence is most likely from the high fat, simple carbohydrate heavy modern Western diet.

LOW CARBOHYDRATE DIETS

There are currently two low carbohydrate diets which are currently popular and are responsible for a great deal of the debate on diet and diabetes. These are the Atkins Diet created by Dr. Robert C. Atkins and the Zone Diet created by Dr. Barry Sears. Dr. Atkins recommends a diet composed of only 25% carbohydrates. Typically this equals about 20 grams of carbohydrates per day. Studies have shown that a 25% carbohydrate diet may be beneficial in type 2 diabetes patients who have failed drug therapy. High fat/low carbohydrate diets have improved blood glucose and lipid levels in those with type 2 diabetes, and a low carbohydrate diet has decreased blood glucose in healthy men.[17] However, such low carbohydrate diets increase the risk of ketoacidosis.

The two main principles of the Zone Diet are: 1) ensure that the body receives an adequate supply of low fat protein at each meal, and 2) eat proteins, fats, and fiber-rich vegetables and fruits in a ratio for which the body is genetically programmed.[18] According to Dr. Sears and his followers, by consuming the proper ratio of low density carbohydrates to fat to protein based on their genetically determine constitution, an individual can control his or her insulin production with amazing results. Low density carbohydrates are vegetables and fruits, while high density carbohydrates include both refined and unrefined grains and beans, including breads and pasta. As the proponents of the Zone Diet point out, even complex carbohydrates tend to have high glycemic indices, and both high and low density carbohydrates will cause an upward spike in blood glucose levels if too many are eaten in combination with proteins and fat depending on one's genetic predisposition.[19] In general, the Zone Diet recommends most Americans eat a diet composed of 30% fat, 30% protein, and 40% carbohydrates. This is definitely less carbohydrates than the ADA currently recommends, and the basic tenet of the Zone Diet vis à vis diabetes is to eat meals that have a low glycemic index. Some of the other basic guidelines of the Zone Diet include always eating within one hour after waking, eating a minimum of three meals and two snacks per day, eating a combination of low fat protein plus carbohydrates and fats at every meal and snack, and drinking eight 8-ounce glasses of water per day. For women, each meal should contain three ounces of protein, while men should eat four ounces of protein per meal. Further, less than 25% of all carbohydrates in any given meal or snack should come from high density carbohydrates such as grains, breads, pasta, beans, and potatoes.[20]

Dr. Charles R Attwood, MD, in an article titled, "Debunking the 'Zone Diet,'" tells the following story:

> Anne, an old friend of mine, walked up to Barry Sears at the Tom Landry Sports Medicine and Research Center in Dallas. She complained that the program outlined in his book, *Enter The Zone*—more lean meat, egg whites, poultry and fish, while limiting many grains, vegetables, and fruits—just didn't work for her. She didn't feel good, and her performance level (swimming) had declined. Anne was now back on her vegetables, fruits, and whole grains.
>
> "Stay with what works best," he said...[21]

We believe that Dr. Sears response was both common sense and very much in line with traditional Chinese medical dietary wisdom. Although certain aspects of the Zone Diet may be controversial, the fact that proponents recognize that proper diet depends on each individual's unique constitution is an important insight that is all too often overlooked by Western medicine.[22] All too often, Western physicians, nutritionists, and governmental bodies, such as the U.S.D.A., the A.D.A., and Drs. Pritikin, Atkins, *et al.*, promote one-size-fits-all, supposedly universal diets. However, everyone is not the same, and what will promote internal balance and good health in one person may cause imbalance and disease in another. It is one of the core wisdoms of Chinese medicine that each patient should receive individualized treatment, including dietary therapy, based on his or her own personal pattern of disharmony.

VITAMINS & MINERALS

According to the American Dietetic Association,

> The best nutritional strategy for promoting optimal health and reducing the risk of chronic disease is to obtain adequate nutrients from a wide variety of foods. [However,] vitamin and mineral supplementation is appropriate when well-accepted, peer-reviewed, scientific evidence shows safety and effectiveness.[23]

That being said, a 1993 *Newsweek* poll found that approximately seven out of 10 Americans used supplements at least occasionally.[24] Due to changes in diet, escalating levels of stress, degradation of agricultural soils, changes in agricultural and food manufacturing and marketing processes, and increases in environmental toxins, dietary

sources of and human needs for vitamins and minerals may be changing. As Heidi-Lee Robertson writes:

> During the last two decades... there have been tremendous advances in this field and a growing body of strong evidence which suggests that while the old daily dietary allowances are fine for warding off acute deficiencies, higher intakes of specific nutrients can promote optimal health and prevent chronic disease. This is a particularly important new concept in view of the increasing numbers of elderly in the world's population both in developing and industrialised countries, as well as the increasing cost of health care globally. Intensive research in the micronutrient field is being aimed at reducing the prevalence of micronutrient deficiencies, the so called "hidden hunger," thereby deriving some well documented reductions in morbidity and mortality in infants, children and young mothers.[25]

Micronutrient research has shown that supplementation with certain vitamins and minerals can either treat or prevent diabetes and its complications. Since vitamin supplementation is commonly practiced by Chinese medical practitioners in the People's Republic of China (as evidenced by its inclusion in the treatment plans of many published Chinese medical studies) as well as by professional practitioners of acupuncture and Chinese medicine in the West, we feel it appropriate to say a few things about the most important supplemental micronutrients in the prevention and treatment of this condition.

CHROMIUM

Chromium is a heavy metal. Studies have shown that doses of supplemental chromium at levels of 200mcg BID improve insulin senstivity and reduce blood glucose in type 2 diabetes as well as have beneficial effects on glycosylated hemoglobin and cholesterol levels.[26] However, like all heavy metals, chromium is nephrotoxic at excessive levels. Chromium bound to polynicotinate or picolinate is better than colloidal chromium for human supplementation.

ALPHA LIPOIC ACID

Alpha lipoic acid improves glucose utilization in the muscles and improves glucose sensitivity. It has been shown to reduce glucose levels in those with type 2 diabetes. It also regenerates other antioxidants and reduces oxidative stress on the nerves. Doses up to 800mg per day are typically used for the prevention of diabetic neuropathy.[27]

CoQ$_{10}$

CoQ$_{10}$ has been shown to improve insulin secretory response in those with diabetes with mitochrondrial DNA mutuation or so-called maternally inherited insulin-dependent diabetes mellitus (MIDDM). Its antioxidant effects may prevent various of the degenerative complication of diabetes and improve cardiac health.[28] CoQ$_{10}$ is produced within the body. However, its synthesis declines with age. Supplementation is usually 100-150mg per day.

VITAMIN E

Vitamin E improves blood glucose tolerance and insulin sensitivity and may also prevent the onset of diabetes. In addition, it prevents the oxidation of LDL cholesterol, thereby reducing the risk of heart disease. It also prevents inflammation of the blood vessels. Hence it may also help prevent other vascular complications of diabetes.[29] Dosage ranges are 800-1200IU per day.

FLAVONOIDS

Flavonoid antioxidants, such as quercetin, rutin, and other plant polyphenols, protect human lymphocystes against oxidative damage. They have known benefits in cataracts and other complications of oxidative damage in diabetes, such as coronary artery disease.[30] Natural sources of flavonoids include onions and tea.

VITAMIN B$_{12}$

Clinical studies have shown that supplementation with vitamin B$_{12}$ is effective in preventing peripheral neuropathy and may benefit those with retinopathy.[31] Doses range from 3-40mg per day.

VITAMIN B$_3$

Vitamin B$_3$ improves insulin production by preventing oxidative damage to the pancreas from activated immune cells in those with type 1 diabetes.[32]

VITAMIN B$_6$

Vitamin B$_6$ has been shown to prevent peripheral neuropathy and it may also prevent gestational diabetes. It prevents glycosylation of proteins and may, therefore, help prevent other complications of diabetes.[33] The usual dose is 100-200mg per day.

ZINC

Zinc is essential for normal function of many enzymes in the body and for protection against oxidation. People with diabetes commonly have a zinc deficiency.[34] Dosage range for zinc is usually 25-30mg per day. Do not take more than 50mg per day.

BIOTIN

Biotin is a cofactor in carbohydrate metabolism which has been shown to improve glucose metabolism in those with type 2 diabetes. It also prevents nerve damage.[35]

CARNITINE

Carnitine is an amino acid which increases insulin senstivity in those with type 2 diabetes via improved fat metabolism. It also helps prevent diabetic cardiomyopathy, neuropathy, and cataracts. A carnitine deficiency is common in those with diabetes.[36]

VANADIUM

Vanadium is another heavy metal which is not naturally occurring in foods. However, studies have found that supplementation with vanadium improves blood glucose control in those with type 2 diabetes. In one single-blind, placebo-controlled study, there was a 20% reduction in blood glucose and a slight reduction in hepatic insulin resistance.[37]

Based on the above research, the main supplemental micronutrients for controlling blood glucose levels include chromium, alpha lipoic acid, zinc, biotin, and vanadium. The main eye and nerve protection micronutrients are alpha lipoic acid, CoQ$_{10}$, and vitamins E, B$_3$, B$_6$, and B$_{12}$. The main micronutrients for controlling cholesterol and blood lipids are vitamins E, B$_6$, and B$_{12}$.

CHINESE DIETARY THERAPY

Chinese dietary therapy is an integral part of Chinese medicine. In general, Chinese dietary therapy is divided into two broad categories: 1) prevention of disease and maintenance of good health, and 2) the remedial treatment of disease. Under the remedial treatment of disease, there are four subdivisions: 1) matching meals with pattern discrimination; 2) protecting and nourishing the spleen and stomach; 3) careful harmonization of the five flavors; and 4) careful observation of food prohibitions.

1. MATCHING MEALS WITH PATTERN DISCRIMINATION

Treating primarily based on each patient's personal Chinese medical pattern discrimination is the hallmark of standard professional Chinese medicine. As we have seen above, the root pattern of diabetes is a qi and yin dual vacuity with dryness and heat. Therefore, the treatment principles for this root pattern are to boost the qi and nourish yin, moisten dryness (or engender fluids) and clear heat.

A. BOOSTING THE QI

Boosting the qi means to supplement the qi by fortifying the spleen. The spleen is the latter heaven source of the engenderment and transformation of the qi. All foods boost the qi at least somewhat since qi is made out of the finest essence of foods and liquids. However, it is specifically the sweet flavor within food that Chinese medical theory posits as being directly responsible for supplementing the qi. Consequently, it is not surprising that almost all foods contain at least some sweet flavor. This includes grains and legumes, fruits and vegetables, and meat and dairy products. In theory, the sweeter a food is, the more it boosts the qi—*in theory*. The problem is that the sweet flavor not only boosts the qi, it also engenders fluids. If more fluids are engendered than the spleen can move and transform, these will collect and transform into damp evils. Since the spleen is averse to dampness, these damp evils may damage the spleen, and, since the spleen is the viscus which controls the engenderment and transformation of qi, anything which damages the spleen will lead to spleen vacuity. Therefore, one cannot simply eat sweet-flavored foods in order to boost the qi. In fact, it is usually overeating sugars and sweets which has gotten the patient with diabetes into the situation they are in.

As stated above, almost all foods have some sweetness inherent in them. When we eat intensely sweet foods, we typically feel a rush of qi followed by fatigue, *i.e.*, the sugar blues. The subsequent fatigue or let-down after eating sugars and sweets in those with reactive hypoglycemia is a symptom of spleen qi vacuity. Therefore, like so much else in Chinese medicine, the key is moderation. In other words, one should eat things that are only moderately sweet and/or eat intensely sweet foods only sparingly.

B. NOURISHING YIN

All foods are composed of varying amounts of qi and *wei* or flavor. Qi is the clearest part of the clear part of food which, when transformed and dispersed, becomes the qi in the body. Flavor, as used in this technical context, does not mean the five flavors. Rather, it refers to the clear part of the turbid from which yin is engendered and transformed. The qi part of food is light and clear, while the flavor part of food is thick and relatively turbid. Flavor nourishes and enriches yin, blood, and essence. However, because it is turbid, it is more difficult to digest. Overeating foods which are relatively high flavor (also called thick-flavored foods in Chinese medicine) may cause accumulation of dampness and turbidity and damage the spleen. Foods which are high in flavor and, therefore, nourish yin primarily include animal products, such as meat, eggs, and milk products. These are extremely "nutritious" in that they nourish yin. But they are also difficult to digest and may damage the spleen and internally engender dampness and turbidity.

Therefore, just as when trying to boost the qi with food, one must proceed with moderation when trying to nourish yin with food. Animal products are usually high in fats and oils, being the main source of saturated fats, and most people with diabetes already have a history of overeating fats and oils. While, theoretically, those with a yin vacuity should eat more thick-flavored, fatty foods, such as turtle, duck, shellfish, beef, butter, and milk, in actual fact, most people with diabetes actually should eat less of these foods. As we know, yin when extreme transforms into yang. Fats and oils are not only extremely sweet in Chinese medicine, they are also warm or hot. This means fatty oily foods easily transform not only dampness but heat. In fact, a great deal of the heat so typical of diabetes was originally engendered from overeating thick-flavored, oily, fatty, rich foods which transformed internal heat.

C. MOISTENING DRYNESS

Foods which moisten dryness tend to be sweet and cool. In terms of commonly eaten foods, this mostly means fruits. Therefore, patients with diabetes accompanied by oral dryness and thirst are counseled to add more fresh fruits to their diets. However, since these fruits are intensely sweet, one has to be careful not to overconsume such sweet fruits. In particular, in the West, this means avoiding or only making sparing use of fruit juices. Fruit juices concentrate the sweetness of several pieces of fruit in a single glass or serving. As we have seen above, the glycemic index of a food is affected by the total constituents of that food, and the fiber in whole fruits helps to slow down the glycemic effect of fresh fruits. Fruit juices lack this mitigating fiber. Therefore, eating whole fresh fruits is better for one's health in terms of diabetes than drinking lots of fruit juices.

Similarly, milk and dairy products such as yogurt moisten dryness. However, people with diabetes need to be careful not to overconsume such dairy products. As we have seen above, it may have actually been overconsumption of diary products when young which subsequently leads to type 1 and maybe even type 2 diabetes.

D. CLEARING HEAT

Every food is assigned a nature in Chinese medicine. Nature in Chinese dietary therapy actually means a food's temperature. This is the effect the food has on yang heat within the body. Thus foods whose natures are cool or cold can clear evil heat. While most grains, legumes, and meats are neutral or warm in nature, there are a number of fruits and vegetables and a few grains and legumes which are cool or cold. Cool or cold vegetables include spinach, lettuce, celery, broccoli, cabbage, radish, eggplant, potato, asparagus, purslane, mushrooms, and water chestnuts. Cool or cold fruits include the summer melons, such as cucumbers, cantaloupes, watermelons, apples, pears, mulberries, mango, kiwi fruit, and grapefruit. Wheat is a cool grain as are millet, Job's tears barley, and buckwheat, and mung beans are a cool legume. In general, the hotter or more yang hyperactive a patient is, the more of these cool and cold foods they should add to their daily diet.

2. PROTECTING & NOURISHING THE SPLEEN & STOMACH

Protecting the spleen and stomach is the limiting factor for all of the above treatment principles. As we have seen, overeating sweet and/or yin-nourishing foods may damage the spleen by engendering dampness and turbidity internally, and this includes fluid-engendering, dryness-moistening foods. Similarly, overeating cool and cold foods may damage the spleen, since the spleen and stomach's functions of transforming and dispersing are nothing other than the functions of their yang qi. If one eats too many cool and cold foods, one runs the risk of clearing and draining too much yang qi from the spleen and stomach, thus damaging the spleen. Since the spleen and stomach are the latter heaven root of engenderment and transformation of all qi and blood in the body, such damage can only work against the person with diabetes.

Therefore, eating foods which theoretically restore balance to the body based on the patient's pattern discrimination must always be balanced with the necessity of protecting and promoting the function of the spleen and stomach. This is primarily achieved by adhering to what Chinese medicine calls the clear, bland diet. This means a diet which is composed of lots of fruits and vegetables, lots of whole grains and legumes, including various types of soybean products, some nuts and seeds, and only a little bit of animal products. In addition, anything very sweet, very acrid, bitter, sour, salty, or made through fermentation, such as alcohol, vinegar, cheese, or bread, should be eaten sparingly. Most food should be cooked and/or chewed thoroughly in order to help its transformation and dispersion, its separation into clear and turbid.

Basically, one must always balance eating for one's pattern discrimination and the imbalance it describes and protecting and promoting the spleen and stomach. Chinese medicine's fundamental vision of health and disease, as laid down in the *Nei Jing (Inner Classic)*, is based on the Confucian Doctrine of the Mean—every thing in moderation. The spleen and stomach are the earth phase who are located in the center and whose nature is moderation. Ultimately, this means that every patient's diet must be adjusted individually based on sex, age, natural endowment (or constitution), and activity, and the climate in which they live.

3. CAREFUL HARMONIZATION OF THE FIVE FLAVORS

Harmonization of the five flavors primarily means not overeating any one flavor. One should eat widely and not stick with only a few foods eaten over and over again day after day. It is especially important not to become addicted to specific flavors, such as sweet, salty, or acrid/spicy. Overeating sweet damages the spleen and engenders dampness. Overeating salt damages the kidneys (and heart), while overeating acrid, spicy foods engenders internal heat and damages and consumes yin.

4. CAREFUL OBSERVATION OF FOOD PROHIBITIONS

In general, food prohibitions mean not eating any foods which will aggravate the patient's condition in terms of their pattern discrimination. In other words, if a person suffers from yin vacuity and fluid dryness, then one should not eat or only eat sparingly foods which are hot, acrid, and windy natured, such as hot spices like cayenne and peppermint. In addition, certain foods are prohibited in the case of certain Chinese diseases. For instance, spinach and honey are prohibited to patients with diarrhea and involuntary seminal emission due to these foods' slippery, glossy, i.e., sliding, nature. Similarly, patients with skin diseases are forbidden fa wu or "emitting substances." Emitting substances are foods which Chinese doctors have recognized to cause (allergic) skin rashes, such as chicken, shellfish, and peanuts. Food prohibitions also mean not eating certain foods when taking certain Chinese medicinals. For instance, one is not supposed to eat radishes or drink tea when taking Radix Panacis Ginseng (Ren Shen). Such food prohibitions must be decided upon in terms of each individual patient, their main symptoms, and any Chinese medicinals they may be taking.

CHINESE DIETARY RECIPES FOR DIABETES

Beyond the above general guidelines, the Chinese dietary literature is filled with formulas or recipes for specific dishes for those with diabetes. Many of these dishes contain foods that are not commonly available in the West, and many others are simply not to most Westerners palates or lifestyle. However, below are a selection of typical Chinese diabetes recipes which may be beneficial to some Westerners.

TRICHOSANTHES ROOT CONGEE

INGREDIENTS: Radix Trichosanthis Kirlowii (Tian Hua Fen), 30g, rice (brown or white depending on preference and the strength of the patient's spleen), 50g

FUNCTIONS & INDICATIONS: Clears heat and engenders fluids; treats dryness and heat with damaged fluids due to wasting and thirsting

METHOD OF PREPARATION & ADMINISTRATION: Soak the Tian Hua Fen in water for two hours. Then add 200ml of water and decoct down to 100ml. Remove the dregs and reserve the liquid. Add 400ml of water to the rice plus the reserved medicinal liquid and cook into porridge. Eat 2-3 times per day.

SPINACH CONGEE

INGREDIENTS: Spinach, 250g, Endothelium Corneum Gigeriae Galli (Ji Nei Jin), 10g, rice, 50g

FUNCTIONS & INDICATIONS: Stops thirst, moistens dryness, and nourishes the stomach; treats wasting and thirsting

METHOD OF PREPARATION & ADMINISTRATION: Wash the spinach and cut into pieces. Add water and cook with the Ji Nei Jin for 30-40 minutes. The add the rice and make into porridge. Eat two times per day.

RADISH CONGEE

INGREDIENTS: Daikon radish, five whole ones, rice, 250g

FUNCTIONS & INDICATIONS: Clears heat and disperses food, rectifies the qi and transforms phlegm; treats wasting and thirsting with dry mouth, polyuria, and obesity

METHOD OF PREPARATION & ADMINISTRATION: Cut up the radishes and boil in water. When soft, press out the juice and cook the rice into porridge in the resulting liquid. Eat freely.

REHMANNIA CONGEE

INGREDIENTS: Uncooked Radix Rehmanniae (Sheng Di), 50g, Semen Zizyphi Spinosae (Suan Zao Ren), 30g, rice, 100g

FUNCTIONS & INDICATIONS: Enriches the liver and boosts the heart, clears heat and quiets the spirit; treats damage to yin fluids with vexatious heat and thirst, dry stools, and insomnia

METHOD OF PREPARATION & ADMINISTRATION: First decoct the Sheng Di and Suan Zao Ren in water, reserving the medicinal liquid. Then cook the rice into porridge in this liquid. Eat freely.

WATERMELON SEED CONGEE

INGREDIENTS: Watermelon seeds, 50g, rice, 30g

FUNCTIONS & INDICATIONS: Clears heat and nourishes the stomach, engenders fluids and stops thirst; treats vexatious thirst due to damage to fluids by heat

METHOD OF PREPARATION & ADMINISTRATION: Decoct the watermelon seeds in water and cook the rice into porridge in the resulting medicinal liquid. Eat freely.

ASPARAGUS CONGEE

INGREDIENTS: Tuber Asparagi Cochinensis (Tian Men Dong), 30g, rice, 50g

FUNCTIONS & INDICATIONS: Supplements the kidneys and enriches yin, nourishes the stomach and engenders fluids

METHOD OF PREPARATION & ADMINISTRATION: Decoct the *Tian Men Dong* in water and use this medicinal liquid to cook the rice into porridge. Eat freely.

CLAM PUREE

INGREDIENTS: Fresh clams, a suitable amount

FUNCTIONS & INDICATIONS: Supplements the liver and kidneys at the same time as it seeps dampness and transforms phlegm; treats lung dryness with damaged fluids and yin insufficiency wasting and thirsting

METHOD OF PREPARATION & ADMINISTRATION: Mash the flesh of fresh clams and boil in water till cooked. Take warm several times per day.

CORN SILK TEA

INGREDIENTS: Corn silk (Stigma Zeae Maydis, *Yu Mi Xu*), 30g, water, 1500ml

FUNCTIONS & INDICATIONS: Clears heat and downbears yang by disinhibiting dampness; treats diabetes complicated by hypertension due to yang hyperactivity

METHOD OF PREPARATION & ADMINISTRATION: Decoct the corn silks in water down to 700ml. Remove the dregs and drink 350ml per time, two times per day.

PIG PANCREAS SOUP

INGREDIENTS: Pig pancreas, one piece, Semen Coicis Lachyrma-jobi (*Yi Yi Ren*), 30g, Radix Astragali Membranacei (*Huang Qi*), 60g, Radix Dioscoreae Oppositae (*Shan Yao*), 120g

FUNCTIONS & INDICATIONS: Supplements the spleen and kidneys; treats middle and lower wasting and thirsting

METHOD PREPARATION & ADMINISTRATION: Cook the pig pancreas with the Chinese medicinals into soup, remove the two roots, and eat.

SCHISANDRA HARD-BOILED EGGS

INGREDIENTS: Chicken eggs, 2-4 pieces, Fructus Schisandrae Chinensis (*Wu Wei Zi*), 30-50g

FUNCTIONS & INDICATIONS: Supplements the kidneys and secures and astringes; treats lower wasting with insecurity of the kidney qi

METHOD OF PREPARATION & ADMINISTRATION: Hard boil the eggs in water in which the *Wu Wei Zi* are also decocted and then eat the eggs.

PUMPKIN & BLACK BEAN SOUP

INGREDIENTS: Skinned pumpkin pieces and black beans, a suitable amount of each

FUNCTIONS & INDICATIONS: Clears heat and supplements the center at the same time as supplementing the kidneys; treats middle and lower wasting and thirsting

METHOD OF PREPARATION & ADMINISTRATION: Cook the pumpkin and black beans into soup with water, adding a little salt or soy sauce to taste. Eat freely. In general, eat more pumpkin and other winter squash which all, when ripe, clear heat at the same time as supplementing the center.

For more information on Chinese dietary therapy and the Chinese medical descriptions of 200 commonly eaten foods, see Bob Flaws's *The Tao of Healthy Eating* also available from Blue Poppy Press.

CONCLUSION

According to Cao Hui-fen, whether one uses Western or Chinese dietary therapy, the goals of dietary therapy in those with diabetes mellitus are to:

1. Strive to keep blood glucose values within normal ranges

2. Maintain all blood lipids within normal ranges

3. Maintain the caloric intake proper to the body weight of the patient according to the patient's condition or stage of growth and whether the patient is a child, pregnant, or a nursing mother

4. Avoid emergencies in daily dietary needs and the complications of chronic illness

5. Provide not only for the diabetic's bodily needs, but also provide support for the patient's environment and lifestyle as appropriate[38]

If one can achieve these goals through dietary control and regulation, then the patient's benefit will be served no matter what the theoretical approach.

ENDNOTES:

[1] www.westondiabetes.org.uk/diet.htm

[2] www.uic.edu/depts/mcfp/geriatric/endocrine/sld008.htm

[3] http://my.webmd.com/contents/dmk/dmk_article_40029.htm

[4] www.lifeclinic.com/focus/diabetes/diet.asp

[5] www.uic.edu, op. cit.

[6] www.cdfnb.org/diabetes/diet/diet1.htm

[7] www.niddk.nih.gov/health/diabetes/pubs/niddm/diet.htm

[8] www.altdiabetes.com/Summary/Omega3EFA.htm

[9] www.altdiabetes.com/Summary/Omega6EFA.htm

[10] www.niddk.nih.gov/diabetes/diet, op cit.

[11] www.westondiabetes.org.uk, op. cit.

[12] www.soyfoods.com/symposium/ScientificProgram.html

[13] American Diabetes Association, *Complete Guide to Diabetes*, Bantam Books, NY, 1999, p. 242

[14] http://icanv.com/dec/nofr/d5.htm

[15] http://umm.drkoop.com/conditions/ency/article/002440.htm

[16] American Diabetes Association, *op. cit.*, p. 258

[17] www.altdiabetes.com/LowCarb.htm

[18] www.zoneperfect.com/Outline.htm

[19] www.getzoned.com.au/Diabetes_main.htm

[20] www.drsears.com/site/Tools/Hints/HintsHome.ns

[21] www.vegsource.com/attwood/zone.htm

[22] Another Western medical diet based on genetic predisposition is Dr. Peter D'Adamo's *Eat Right 4 Your Type*. These are four different diets based on the four blood types: A, B, AB, and O. These diets are then further refined in terms of Caucasian, African, or Asian ancestry and whether the person is a "secretor" or not. A secretor is defined as a person who secretes their blood type antigens into their body fluids, including their saliva. According to Dr. D'Adamo, many metabolic traits, including carbohydrate tolerance, are linked to secretor status. For more information on this method of genetically based dietary therapy, see www.dadamo.com/napham/LR4YT2.htm.

[23] www.eatright.org/asupple.htm

[24] *Ibid.*

[25] www.saspen.com/jcn/feb99/reflect.htm

[26] www.altdiabetes.com/Summary/Chromium.htm

[27] www.altdiabetes.com/Summary/LipoicAcid.htm

[28] www.altdiabetes.com/Summary/CoQ10.htm

[29] www.altdiabetes.com/Summary/VitE.htm

[30] www.altdiabetes.com/Summary/Flavonoids.htm

[31] www.altdiabetes.com/Summary/VitB12.htm

[32] www.altdiabetes.com/Summary/VitB3.htm

[33] www.altdiabetes/Summary/VitB6.htm

[34] www.altdiabetes/Summary/Zinc.htm

[35] www.altdiabetes/Summary/Biotin.htm

[36] www.altdiabetes.com/Summary/Carnitine.htm

[37] www.altdiabetes.com/Summary/Vanadium.htm

[38] Cao Hui-fen, "Diabetic Dietary Therapy," *Yun Nan Zhong Yi Zhong Yao Za Zhi* (*Yunnan Journal of Chinese Medicine & Medicinals*), #4, 1996, p. 66-67

8

EXERCISE & DIABETES

Regular exercise is important for the management of both types 1 and 2 diabetes. Physical activity improves the status of diabetes patients by transporting glucose to the muscles, improving circulation, and increasing insulin receptors.[1] Specific effects of moderate sustained exercise in patients with either type 1 or 2 diabetes include:

1. Lowering of blood glucose levels during and after exercise
2. Improvement of insulin sensitivity
3. Lowering of basal and postprandial insulin concentrations
4. Lowering of glycosylated hemoglobin levels
5. Decreased triglyceride levels
6. Increased high density lipids, the so-called good cholesterol
7. Improvement in mild to moderate hypertension
8. Burning of more calories, therefore increased fat loss
9. Conditioning of the cardiovascular system
10. Increased strength and flexibility
11. Improvement of attitude, sense of well-being, and quality of life
12. Reduced psychological stress [2,3]

However, there are several risks associated with exercise for those with diabetes. The following are some of the risks of exercise for patients with diabetes:

1. Hypoglycemia if diabetes is being treated with insulin or oral hypoglycemic agents
2. Hyperglycemia after very strenuous exercise
3. Hyperglycemia and ketosis in insulin-deficient patients

4. Precipitation or exacerbation of cardiovascular disease
5. Worsening of the long-term complications of diabetes, such as retinopathy, nephropathy, and both peripheral and autonomic neuropathy[4]

These risks do not mean that people with diabetes should not exercise. In medicine, one always must assess the risks of any therapy in an individual patient and then compare those risks to the potential benefits. In order to assess these risks, it is now being advised that diabetes patients over 35 years of age not already involved in regular physical activity receive a physical examination and stress test before starting an exercise plan. This examination should include:

LEVEL OF GLYCEMIC CONTROL
CARDIOVASCULAR EXAM
    BLOOD PRESSURE
    PERIPHERAL PULSES
    BRUITS
    BLOOD LIPIDS
    ECG AT REST AND DURING ACTIVITY FOR THOSE
        WITH KNOWN CARDIOVASCULAR DISEASE
NEUROLOGICAL EVALUATION
EYE EXAM BY AN OPHTHALMOLOGIST OR CERTIFIED OPTOMETRIST

According to the American Diabetes Association and the American College of Sports Medicine (ACSM), aerobic exercise is generally deemed the best for diabetes sufferers. Walking, jogging, biking, swimming, and aerobic dances are all examples of potential aerobic exercise. The definition of aerobic exercise is any physical activity which raises the heart rate at least 50% above its resting rate and keeps it at the new rate for a continuous 20 minutes.[5]

Therefore, depending on a person's cardiovascular condition, different physical activities at different levels of intensity may or may not be aerobic for a given individual. However, even moderate regular exercise can help lower blood glucose by increasing tissue sensitivity to insulin. In fact, studies of older people who engage in regular moderate aerobic exercise (*e.g.*, brisk walking or biking) lower their risk for diabetes even if they do not lose weight.

ADA & ACSM EXERCISE GUIDELINES FOR THOSE WITH DIABETES

Type: Aerobic
Frequency: 3-5 times per week
Duration: 20-60 minutes
Intensity: 50-74% of maximal aerobic capacity
Safety precautions:
    Warm up/cool down
    Careful selection of exercise type
       & intensity
    Patient education
    Proper footwear
    Avoid exercise in extreme heat or cold
    Inspect feet daily after exercise
    Blood glucose monitoring
       pre-/post-exercise
    Treatment of hypoglycemia
    Maintain adequate hydration
Increasing adherence:
    Make exercising enjoyable
    Convenient location
    Positive feedback from medical
       personnel & family

To see how a particular patient responds to exercise, a trial period of 6-12 weeks should be conducted, beginning, for instance, with 20-30 minutes of brisk walking three times per week. Depending on the patient's response to this regime, exercise may be increased from there as necessary or desirable. However, many people with diabetes will need to begin with only five minutes of activity. In that case, duration should be increased by no more than 1-2 minutes per week. Then, after the desired duration of activity has been attained, the intensity of the exercise may be increased based on fitness. In some cases, for instance in those whose pulmonary function is poor or who have peripheral vascular disease, patients may not be able to reach their desired exercise durations. In that case, one may build up to three exercise sessions per day each lasting only 5-10 minutes per session.

SPECIAL PRECAUTIONS FOR THOSE TAKING INSULIN & ANTIDIABETIC MEDICATIONS

Patients who are taking antidiabetic medications and particularly insulin should take special precautions before embarking on a workout program. The drastic changes in insulin sensitivity that occur during and after exercise require patients being treated with insulin to adjust their insulin therapy or nutritional intake in order to prevent hypoglycemia. For instance, insulin-dependent athletes may need to decrease insulin doses or take in more carbohydrates, especially in the form of pre-exercise snacks (skim milk is particularly helpful). Therefore, patients with diabetes should monitor their glucose levels carefully before, during, and after workouts. One should delay exercise if blood glucose is over 250mg/dL or under 100 mg/dL. To avoid hypoglycemia, patients with diabetes should inject insulin in sites away from the muscles they use the most during exercise.

Unlike patients treated with insulin, problems in glucose regulation do not usually occur, other than occasional hypoglycemia, with those being treated with oral antidiabetic medications and diet. In those being treated with diet alone, supplemental feedings before, during, or after exercise are unnecessary except when exercise is unusually vigorous or prolonged.

WEIGHT TRAINING & DIABETES

Although most people, including those with diabetes, benefit from including some weight or strength training in their overall exercise regime (for instance 2-3 times per week), weight training may cause problems in those with retinopathy and/or hypertension. People with retinopathy should avoid activities that involve holding one's breath or in which the head drops below the level of the waist. For those with hypertension, their blood pressure should be checked during any weight training or other activity that involves significant arm movements to insure that such activities do not elevate the blood pressure too much. If one has uncontrolled hypertension and one lifts weights, he or she should be sure to exhale during the hardest part of each exercise and inhale during the easiest part so that excessive upward changes in blood pressure are less likely to occur.

STRETCHING & DIABETES

In general, people tend to become less flexible as they age. In addition, peripheral neuropathy tends to shorten muscles. Therefore, stretching is often a desirable part of an overall exercise regime for those with diabetes. Stretching can be done on a daily basis, and is usually easier in the evening than in the morning. Stretches should be held for approximately 30 seconds each with no bouncing. Bob Anderson's classic, *Stretching*, is an excellent guide to flexibility training.[6]

PROPER HYDRATION

Adequate fluid is essential for persons with hyperglycemia since the body loses fluids in an effort to rid itself of the additional, unwanted blood glucose. In addition, people with diabetes tend to be older, and the thirst mechanism weakens as we age. This means that thirst generally does not occur in older persons until they are actually dehydrated. Therefore, patients with diabetes typically need to make a conscious effort to drink sufficient fluids. Since thirst is not a reliable guide to the body's fluid needs in older persons, weight loss can help create guidelines for water consumption. One pound of weight loss after exercise should be replaced with two cups of water or other calorie-free, caffeine-free beverage. Other guidelines for fluid intake and exercise for persons with diabetes include drinking 1-2 eight ounce glasses of water before exercise and drinking 1/2 cup of water every 10-15 minutes during exercise. Sports drinks may be helpful for people with type 1 diabetes to help maintain blood glucose levels if exercise lasts over one hour.

QIGONG

Qigong is a fairly modern Chinese term which is a catch-all for many different kinds of self-massage, exercise, and meditation. The *qi* in qigong refers to the qi of Chinese medicine. *Gong* means to work, discipline, or train. Thus qigong means to train one's qi. In general, qigong is divided into still qigong (*jing qi gong*) and stirring or active qigong (*dong qi gong*). In addition, most qigong, whether still or stirring involves some sort of patterning of the breath. Typically, there will also be some sort of visualization of the movement of qi to and through the body coordinated with any physical movements and respiration. For instance, *tai ji quan* may be seen as a type of stirring or active qigong. As early as the Jin dynasty (265-420 CE), Chao Yuan-fang described the use of qigong in the treatment of wasting and thirsting or diabetes in his *Zhu Bing Yuan Hou Lun (Treatise on the Origins & Symptoms of Various Diseases)*. More recently, tests conducted by the Physiology Section of the No. 1 Shanghai Medical University showed that qigong can quickly decrease blood glucose and enhance glucose metabolism.[7] At the Shandong College of Chinese Medicine, another study of 31 middle-aged and elderly patients with diabetes found that qigong had beneficial effects on blood glucose levels, insulin levels, microcirculation, and immunity.[8] And Gao Yan-bin devotes 30 pages to qigong in his book on Chinese medicine and diabetes. Therefore, Western patients may want to consider adding qigong to their self-care regime. In general, qigong can be safely done while taking Western antidiabetic medications and complements acupuncture and internally administered Chinese medicinals.

However, for best results, qigong should be learned from a trained and experienced teacher who can adjust one's qigong regime for each individual. As an example of the importance of a live teacher, Ken Cohen, the famous American teacher of qigong, points out that, although qigong generally promotes slow, rhythmic, abdominal breathing, chest breathing and a quicker respiratory rate may be necessary biologic adjustments for those with diseases, such as hypoglycemia, diabetes, and kidney failure, characterized by acidosis. "If hyperventilation is needed to correct a serious underlying disturbance, then to interfere with it is to court disaster."[9] In other words, just as with all other aspects of Chinese medical treatment, an individualized qigong exercise plan is necessary based on a combination of the patient's pattern discrimination and their disease diagnosis. Therefore, we have chosen not to include specific qigong exercises in this book. Nevertheless, we do endorse and recommend the use of qigong for patients with diabetes.

ENDNOTES:

[1] www.uic.edu/depts/mcfp/geriatric/endocrine/sld009.htm
[2] American Diabetes Association, *Complete Guide to Diabetes*, Bantam Books, New York, 1999, p. 268
[3] www.diabetes-midon.org/exercise.htm
[4] *Ibid.*
[5] Heart rate is not always a good indicator of exercise intensity. For example, if a patient is on beta-blockers, their heart rate will not increase as expected. Also, autonomic neuropathy may prevent the heart rate from increasing as usual during exercise.
[6] Anderson, Bob, *Stretching*, 20th edition, Shelter Publications, Bolinas, CA, 2000
[7] Chen Jin-ding, The *Treatment of Diabetes with Traditional Chinese Medicine*, trans. by Sun Ying-kui & Zhou Shu-hui, Shandong Science & Technology Press, Jinan, 1994, p. 203
[8] Jing Yu-zhong et al., "Observations on the Effects of 31 Cases of Diabetes Treated with 'Return the Spring Gong'," *Proceedings of the Second World Conference for Academic Exchange on Medical Qigong*, Bejing, 1993, p. 135
[9] Cohen, Kenneth S., *The Way of Qigong: The Art and Science of Chinese Energy Healing*, Balantine Books, NY, 1997, p. 120

9

THE TREATMENT OF DIABETES BASED ON PATTERN DISCRIMINATION

Different Chinese authors favor slightly different systems of pattern discrimination when it comes to the Chinese medical treatment of diabetes mellitus. The following patterns are those we find most common in Western patients with DM. However, these patterns only form the armature or skeleton for the Chinese medical treatment of this condition. Since individual patients vary widely and most present with complicated combinations of patterns, the treatment protocols given below must typically be modified with additions and subtractions in real life. The case histories presented below help exemplify the real-life treatment of this condition by senior practitioners.

1. SPLEEN VACUITY-LIVER DEPRESSION PATTERN

MAIN SYMPTOMS: Elevated blood glucose but no marked polydipsia, polyphagia, or polyuria, fatigue, lack of strength, psychoemotional tension, vexation, and agitation, chest oppression, abdominal distention, reduced appetite, possible blurred vision, dry, rough eyes, bilateral rib-side aching and pain, a fat, enlarged tongue with teeth-marks on its edges and white fur, and a soggy, bowstring pulse[1]

TREATMENT PRINCIPLES: Fortify the spleen and supplement the qi, course the liver and resolve depression

RX: *Xiao Yao San Jia Jian* (Rambling Powder with Additions & Subtractions)

INGREDIENTS: Rhizoma Polygonati (*Huang Jing*) and Radix Albus Paeoniae Lactiflorae (*Bai Shao*), 20g each, Caulis Polygoni Multiflori (*Ye Jiao Teng*), Radix Bupleuri (*Chai Hu*), Radix Codonopsitis Pilosulae (*Dang Shen*), Radix Angelicae Sinensis (*Dang Gui*), Rhizoma Atractylodis Macrocephalae (*Bai Zhu*), and Sclerotium

Poriae Cocos (*Fu Ling*), 9g each, and mix-fried Radix Glycyrrhizae (*Gan Cao*), 6g

FORMULA ANALYSIS: *Chai Hu* courses the liver and rectifies the qi, while *Bai Shao, Dang Gui,* and *Ye Jiao Teng* nourish the blood and, thereby, emolliate the liver. *Dang Shen, Bai Zhu, Fu Ling,* and mix-fried *Gan Cao* fortify the spleen and supplement the qi. *Huang Jing* fortifies the spleen and supplements the qi at the same time as it empirically treats wasting and thirsting disease.

ADDITIONS & SUBTRACTIONS: If liver depression has transformed heat which has damaged stomach fluids, add 12 grams each of Radix Scutellariae Baicalensis (*Huang Qin*) and Tuber Ophiopogonis Japonici (*Mai Men Dong*). If there is polydipsia or polyphagia, add 30 grams of uncooked Gypsum Fibrosum (*Shi Gao*) and 9-15 grams of Rhizoma Anemarrhenae Aspheloidis (*Zhi Mu*). If the eyes are dry and rough, add nine grams each of Flos Chrysanthemi Morifolii (*Ju Hua*) and Fructus Lycii Chinensis (*Gou Qi Zi*). If fatigue and lack of strength are marked, add 15-30 grams of Radix Astragali Membranacei (*Huang Qi*). If spleen vacuity has led to damp accumulation, add nine grams of Rhizoma Pinelliae Ternatae (*Ban Xia*). If there is chest oppression and rib-side pain, add nine grams of Tuber Curcumae (*Yu Jin*). If there is abdominal distention, add nine grams each of Rhizoma Cyperi Rotundi (*Xiang Fu*) and Radix Auklandiae Lappae (*Mu Xiang*). If there is numbness, aching, and pain, add 15-30 grams of Radix Salviae Miltiorrhizae (*Dan Shen*), 15 grams of Radix Rubrus Paeoniae Lactiflorae (*Chi Shao*), and nine grams of Semen Pruni Persicae (*Tao Ren*). If there is polyuria, add nine grams each of Ootheca Mantidis (*Sang Piao Xiao*) and Fructus Schisandrae Chinensis (*Wu Wei Zi*). If there is dizziness, head distention, headache, and/or hypertension, add 15 grams of Spica Prunellae Vulgaris (*Xia Ku Cao*), 12 grams of Concha Haliotidis (*Shi Jue Ming*), and nine grams of Flos Chrysanthemi Morifolii (*Ju Hua*).

ACUPUNCTURE & MOXIBUSTION: *Tai Chong* (Liv 3), *He Gu* (LI 4), *San Yin Jiao* (Sp 6), *Zu San Li* (St 36), *Pi Shu* (Bl 20)

FORMULA ANALYSIS: Draining *Tai Chong* and *He Gu* courses the liver and rectifies the qi, while supplementing *Zu San Li* and *Pi Shu* fortifies the spleen and supplements the qi. Even supplementing-even draining *San Yin Jiao* both courses the liver and fortifies the spleen.

ADDITIONS & SUBTRACTIONS: For abdominal distention, add draining *Qi Hai* (CV 6) and *Tian Shu* (St 25). For rib-side pain, add draining *Zu Lin Qi* (GB 41) and *Zhang Men* (Liv 13). For chest oppression, add draining *Dan Zhong* (CV 17) and *Nei Guan* (Per 6). For depression transforming heat in the liver, add draining *Xing Jian* (Liv 2). For depression transforming heat in the stomach, add draining *Nei Ting* (St 44) and use even supplementing-even draining at *Zu San Li*. For dizziness, head distention, headache, and hypertension, add draining *Qu Chi* (LI 11) and *Feng Chi* (GB 20).

2. SPLEEN VACUITY WITH DAMP ENCUMBRANCE PATTERN

MAIN SYMPTOMS: Elevated blood glucose but no marked polydipsia, polyphagia, or polyuria, fatigue, lack of strength, heavy-headedness, heavy limbs, a bland, tasteless feeling in the mouth, chest oppression, possible nausea and vomiting, abdominal distention, loose stools, a fat, enlarged tongue with teeth-marks on its edges and slimy, white fur, and a soggy, moderate (*i.e.*, relaxed or slightly slow) pulse

TREATMENT PRINCIPLES: Fortify the spleen and eliminate dampness

RX: *Shen Ling Bai Zhu San Jia Wei* (Ginseng, Poria & Atractylodes Powder with Added Flavors)

INGREDIENTS: Semen Coicis Lachyrma-jobi (*Yi Yi Ren*) and Rhizoma Polygonati (*Huang Jing*), 20g each, Semen Nelumbinis Nuciferae (*Lian Zi*) and Radix Dioscoreae Oppositae (*Shan Yao*), 15g each, Semen Dolichoris Lablab (*Bai Bian Dou*), 12g, Rhizoma Atractylodis Macrocephalae (*Bai Zhu*) and Sclerotium Poriae Cocos (*Fu Ling*), 9g each, Radix Panacis Ginseng (*Ren Shen*) and Radix Platycodi Grandiflori (*Jie Geng*), 6-9g each, Fructus Amomi (*Sha Ren*) and mix-fried Radix Glycyrrhizae (*Gan Cao*), 3-6g each

FORMULA ANALYSIS: *Ren Shen*, *Huang Jing*, *Shan Yao*, *Bai Zhu*, *Fu Ling*, *Gan Cao*, and *Yi Yi Ren* fortify the spleen and boost the qi at the same time as they dry, transform, and seep dampness. In addition, *Huang Jing* empirically treats wasting and thirsting. *Lian Zi* and *Bai Bian Dou* supplement the spleen and stop diarrhea, while *Sha Ren* rectifies the qi and dries dampness and *Jie Geng* upbears the clear.

ADDITIONS & SUBTRACTIONS: For diabetes mellitus with marked fatigue, one can delete *Huang Jing* and add 15 grams of Radix Astragali Membranacei (*Huang Qi*) and nine grams each of Fructus Schisandrae Chinensis (*Wu Wei Zi*) and Endothelium Corneum Gigeriae Galli (*Ji Nei Jin*). For qi stagnation, add 3-6 grams of Pericarpium Citri Reticulatae (*Chen Pi*). For fluid insufficiency characterized by marked oral dryness and thirst, add 9-15 grams of Radix Puerariae (*Ge Gen*).

ACUPUNCTURE & MOXIBUSTION: *Zu San Li* (St 36), *Shang Qiu* (Sp 5), *San Yin Jiao* (Sp 6), *Pi Shu* (Bl 20), *Wei Shu* (Bl 21)

FORMULA ANALYSIS: Even supplementing-even draining *Zu San Li*, *Shang Qiu*, *San Yin Jiao*, *Pi Shu*, and *Wei Shu* fortifies the spleen at the same time as it eliminates dampness.

ADDITIONS & SUBTRACTIONS: For abdominal distention and/or diarrhea, add even supplementing-even draining *Zhong Wan* (CV 12), *Tian Shu* (St 25), and *Da Chang Shu* (Bl 25). For chest oppression, nausea, and vomiting, add draining *Dan Zhong* (CV 17) and *Nei Guan* (Per 6).

3. SPLEEN VACUITY WITH STASIS & STAGNATION PATTERN

MAIN SYMPTOMS: Elevated blood glucose but no marked polydipsia, polyphagia, or polyuria, bodily emaciation, fatigue, lack of strength, dry, scaly skin, a dry mouth with scanty fluids, loose stools, frothy, bubbly urination, a dark red tongue and/or static spots or macules, and a deep, fine, choppy pulse

TREATMENT PRINCIPLES: Fortify the spleen and boost the qi, quicken the blood and transform stasis

RX: *Shuang Jie Jiang Tang Jing San Hao* (Doubly Resolving Lower the Sugar Essence No. 3)

INGREDIENTS: Radix Astragali Membranacei (*Huang Qi*), 15-30g, Rhizoma Polygonati (*Huang Jing*) and Radix Salviae Miltiorrhizae (*Dan Shen*), 20g each, Radix Et

Rhizoma Polygoni Cuspidati (*Hu Zhang*) and Caulis Polygoni Multiflori (*Ye Jiao Teng*), 15g each, and Radix Panacis Ginseng (*Ren Shen*), Cortex Radicis Moutan (*Dan Pi*), and Herba Lycopi Lucidi (*Ze Lan*), 9g each

FORMULA ANALYSIS: *Huang Qi, Huang Jing,* and *Ren Shen* fortify the spleen and boost the qi. *Dan Shen, Hu Zhang, Dan Pi,* and *Ze Lan* quicken the blood and transform stasis. *Ye Jiao Teng* nourishes the blood and stops itching. Its inclusion in this formula is based on the fact that static blood hinders the engenderment of new or fresh blood. Hence blood stasis is typically accompanied by an element of blood vacuity as evidenced by the dry, scaly skin. Further, *Huang Jing* not only boosts the qi but enriches yin and engenders fluids, and blood and fluids share a common source. This explains why blood stasis is commonly accompanied by oral dryness.

ADDITIONS & SUBTRACTIONS: For even greater spleen supplementation, add nine grams each of Rhizoma Atractylodis Macrocephalae (*Bai Zhu*) and Sclerotium Poriae Cocos (*Fu Ling*). If there is diarrhea, add 12-15 grams each of Radix Dioscoreae Oppositae (*Shan Yao*) and Semen Dolichoris Lablab (*Bai Bian Dou*).

ACUPUNCTURE & MOXIBUSTION: *Zu San Li* (St 36), *San Yin Jiao* (Sp 6), *He Gu* (LI 4), *Xue Hai* (Sp 10), *Ge Shu* (Bl 17), *Pi Shu* (Bl 20)

FORMULA ANALYSIS: Supplementing *Zu San Li* and *Pi Shu* fortifies the spleen and supplements or boosts the qi. Even supplementing-even draining *San Yin Jiao* and draining *He Gu* and *Xue Hai* quickens the blood and transforms stasis. Supplementing *Ge Shu* nourishes the blood.

ADDITIONS & SUBTRACTIONS: If there is oral dryness, add supplementing *Jia Che* (St 6), *Di Cang* (St 4), and *Cheng Jiang* (CV 24). If there are loose stools, add supplementing *Zhong Wan* (CV 12), *Tian Shu* (St 25), *Wei Shu* (Bl 21), and *Da Chang Shu* (Bl 25).

4. DAMP HEAT BREWING & STAGNATING PATTERN

MAIN SYMPTOMS: Obesity, dry mouth and throat, oral thirst, commonly a bitter taste in the mouth, possible bad breath, fatigue, dry, bound stools, urinary frequency, urgency, and astringency, possible burning pain, dark, possibly scanty, yellow urine or white, turbid urine, chest oppression, abdominal distention, possible loose stools or constipation, pruritus, a fat, enlarged tongue with slimy, white or dry, yellow tongue fur, and a slippery or soggy, rapid pulse

NOTE: This pattern describes enduring damp heat which is in the act of damaging the spleen qi and yin fluids. However, there are, as yet no pronounced symptoms of either spleen qi vacuity or true yin vacuity.

TREATMENT PRINCIPLES: Arouse the spleen and transform turbidity, clear heat and eliminate dampness

RX: *Gan Lu Xiao Du Yin Jia Wei* (Sweet Dew Disperse Toxins Drink with Added Flavors)

INGREDIENTS: Rhizoma Belamcandae Chinensis (*She Gan*), 18g, Talcum (*Hua Shi*), 15g, Fructus Cardamomi (*Bai Dou Kou*), Herba Agastachis Seu Pogostemi (*Huo Xiang*), Herba Artemisiae Capillaris (*Yin Chen Hao*), Radix Scutellariae Baicalensis (*Huang Qin*), Bulbus Fritillariae Thunbergii (*Zhe Bei Mu*), Fructus Forsythiae Suspensae (*Lian Qiao*), and Rhizoma Anemarrhenae Aspheloidis (*Zhi Mu*), 9g each, Radix Et Rhizoma Rhei (*Da Huang*), 6-9g, Caulis Akebiae (*Mu Tong*) and Herba Menthae Haplocalycis (*Bo He*), 6g each, and Rhizoma Acori Graminei (*Shi Chang Pu*), 4.5g

FORMULA ANALYSIS: *Yin Chen Hao, Hua Shi, Mu Tong,* and *Huang Qin* all clear heat and eliminate dampness. *Bai Dou Kou* and *Huo Xiang* aromatically transform dampness and arouse the spleen, while *Shi Chang Pu* and *Zhe Bei Mu* transform damp turbidity. *Lian Qio, Bo He,* and *Da Huang* clear heat. In addition, *Bo He* combined with *Yin Chen Hao* courses the liver and rectifies the qi. *Zhi Mu* enriches yin and drains fire, while *She Gan* clears heat from the lungs at the same time as it helps transform phlegm, dampness, and turbidity.

ADDITIONS & SUBTRACTIONS: If there is no constipation, either reduce the dosage of or delete *Da Huang*. If there is spleen qi vacuity, add 6-9 grams of Radix Panacis Ginseng (*Ren Shen*). If there is liver depression, add nine grams of Radix Bupleuri (*Chai Hu*). For marked strangury, add nine grams each of Folium Pyrrosiae (*Shi Wei*) and Herba Dianthi (*Qu Mai*).

ACUPUNCTURE & MOXIBUSTION: *Yin Ling Quan* (Sp 9), *Lou Gu* (Sp 7), *San Yin Jiao* (Sp 6)

FORMULA ANALYSIS: This group of points is called the Three Emperors. This is a special combination of the Dong family for diabetes mellitus. Draining *Yin Ling Quan* and *Lou Gu* clears heat and eliminates dampness. Even supplementing-even draining *San Yin Jiao* drains dampness from the spleen at the same time as it fortifies the spleen and nourishes and enriches the liver and kidneys.

ADDITIONS & SUBTRACTIONS: For abdominal distention, add *Zhong Wan* (CV 12). For chest oppression, add *Dan Zhong* (CV 17). For dry, bound stools, add *Nei Ting* (St 44), *Tian Shu* (St 25), and *Da Chang Shu* (Bl 25). For concomitant liver depression, add *Tai Chong* (Liv 3) and *He Gu* (LI 4).

5. YIN FLUID DEPLETION & VACUITY PATTERN

MAIN SYMPTOMS: Dry mouth and throat, exuberant, effulgent desire for food, dry, bound stools, weight gain or obesity, decreased physical strength and energy, a red tongue with yellow fur or white fur with scanty fluids, and a deep, bowstring pulse

TREATMENT PRINCIPLES: Supplement the kidneys and boost the stomach, enrich yin and engender fluids

RX: *Zeng Ye Tang Jia Wei* (Increase Humors Decoction with Added Flavors)

INGREDIENTS: Uncooked Radix Rehmanniae (*Sheng Di*), Radix Trichosanthis Kirlowii (*Tian Hua Fen*), and Radix Scrophulariae Ningpoensis (*Xuan Shen*), 30g each, Radix Glehniae Littoralis (*Sha Shen*), 15g, and Tuber Ophiopogonis Japonici (*Mai Men Dong*) and Radix Puerariae (*Ge Gen*), 12g each

FORMULA ANALYSIS: All the medicinals in this formula engender fluids and enrich yin. In addition, *Sheng Di, Xuan Shen,* and *Mai Men Dong* clear vacuity heat, while *Ge Gen* upbears fluids and thus stops thirst.

ADDITIONS & SUBTRACTIONS: For exuberant and effulgent desire to eat, add 30 grams each of cooked Radix Rehmanniae (*Shu Di*) and Rhizoma Polygonati Odorati (*Yu Zhu*). For dry, bound stools, add 6-9 grams of uncooked Radix Et Rhizoma Rhei (*Da Huang*) and nine grams of Fructus Immaturus Citri Aurantii (*Zhi Shi*). If there is simultaneous tension, agitation, and easy anger with a red tongue, yellow fur, and a bowstring pulse indicating yin vacuity with liver depression, add 15 grams of Radix Albus Paeoniae Lactiflorae (*Bai Shao*) and nine grams each of Radix Bupleuri (*Chai Hu*), Fructus Citri Aurantii (*Zhi Ke*), and Fructus Immaturus Citri Aurantii (*Zhi Shi*) in order to enrich yin and emolliate the liver, course the liver and rectify the qi. If there is simultaneous dizziness and vertigo, poor sleep, and a tendency to high blood pressure indicat-

ing yin vacuity with yang hyperactivity, add 15 grams of Radix Cyathulae (*Chuan Niu Xi*) and 30 grams each of Concha Margaritiferae (*Zhen Zhu Mu*) and uncooked Concha Haliotidis (*Shi Jue Ming*) to abduct heat and move it downward, enrich yin and subdue yang. If the patient is obese with a tendency to high cholesterol and a red tongue with thick, yellow fur, indicating damp heat obstructing and stagnating, add 30 grams each of Herba Artemisiae Capillaris (*Yin Chen Hao*) and Semen Coicis Lachrymajobi (*Yi Yi Ren*), 15 grams each of Rhizoma Alismatis (*Ze Xie*) and Radix Et Rhizoma Polygoni Cuspidati (*Hu Zhang*), and nine grams each of Radix Bupleuri (*Chai Hu*) and Radix Scutellariae Baicalensis (*Huang Qin*) to clear heat and disinhibit dampness.

If liver depression with depressive heat is predominant and yin vacuity is less pronounced, use *Dan Zhi Xiao Yao San Jia Jian* (Moutan & Gardenia Rambling Powder with Additions & Subtractions): Cortex Radicis Lycii Chinensis (*Di Gu Pi*), 30g, Flos Albizziae Julibrissinis (*He Huan Hua*), 15g, Radix Dioscoreae Oppositae (*Shan Yao*), 12g, Radix Angelicae Sinensis (*Dang Gui*), Radix Albus Paeoniae Lactiflorae (*Bai Shao*), Radix Bupleuri (*Chai Hu*), Sclerotium Poriae Cocos (*Fu Ling*), Rhizoma Cyperi Rotundi (*Xiang Fu*), Cortex Radicis Moutan (*Dan Pi*), Fructus Gardeniae Jasminoidis (*Zhi Zi*), Fructus Lycii Chinensis (*Gou Qi Zi*), Herba Artemisiae Capillaris (*Yin Chen Hao*), and Flos Chrysanthemi Morifolii (*Ju Hua*), 9g each, and Rhizoma Alismatis (*Ze Xie*), 6g.

ACUPUNCTURE & MOXIBUSTION: *Ge Shu* (Bl 17), *Pi Shu* (Bl 20), *Yi Shu* (M-BW-12), *Shen Shu* (Bl 23), *Zu San Li* (St 36), *Qu Chi* (LI 11), *Tai Xi* (Ki 3)

FORMULA ANALYSIS: Supplementing *Pi Shu* and even supplementing-even draining *Zu San Li* supplements the latter heaven source of qi and blood engenderment and transformation, while draining *Qu Chi* and even supplementing-even draining *Zu San Li* clears heat. Supplementing *Ge Shu, Shen Shu,* and *Tai Xi* supplements the kidneys and nourishes yin. Supplementing *Yi Shu* helps supplement the spleen at the same time as it empirically treats diabetes.

ADDITIONS & SUBTRACTIONS: If there is vexatious thirst, add *Fei Shu* (Bl 13) and *Cheng Jiang* (CV 24). If there is polyphagia and easy hunger with dry, bound stools, add *Wei Shu* (Bl 21) and *Feng Long* (St 40). If there is polyuria and night sweats, add *Fu Liu* (Ki 7) and *Guan Yuan* (CV 4). If there is diarrhea and fatigue, add *Yin Ling Quan* (Sp 9) and *Shang Ju Xu* (St 37). If there is liver depression, add *Tai Chong* (Liv 3) and *He Gu* (LI 4).

6. YIN VACUITY WITH HEAT EXUBERANCE PATTERN

MAIN SYMPTOMS: Vexatious thirst, polydipsia, polyphagia, easy hunger, bad breath, toothache, frequent, profuse, yellow-colored urination, dry, bound stools, a red tongue with scanty fluids and dry, yellow or no fur, and a fine rapid, or slippery, rapid pulse

NOTE: The difference between this and the preceding pattern is that the signs and symptoms of stomach heat are more marked. In fact, some authors call this pattern spleen-stomach dryness and heat.

TREATMENT PRINCIPLES: Supplement the kidneys and enrich yin, clear heat from the stomach and intestines

RX: *Zeng Ye Tang* (Increase Humors Decoction) plus *Bu Hu Tang* (White Tiger Decoction) plus *Xiao Ke Tang* (Disperse Thirst Decoction) with additions and subtractions

INGREDIENTS: Uncooked Radix Rehmanniae (*Sheng Di*), uncooked Gypsum Fibrosum (*Shi Gao*), and Radix Scrophulariae Ningpoensis (*Xuan Shen*), 30g each, Radix Puerariae (*Ge Gen*), 15g, Tuber Ophiopogonis Japonici (*Mai Men Dong*) and Rhizoma Anemarrhenae Aspheloidis (*Zhi Mu*), 12g each, and Radix Trichosanthis Kirlowii (*Tian Hua Fen*), Rhizoma Coptidis Chinensis (*Huang Lian*), and Fructus Immaturus Citri Aurantii (*Zhi Shi*), 9g each

FORMULA ANALYSIS: *Sheng Di, Xuan Shen,* and *Mai Men Dong* enrich yin and engender fluids. *Shi Gao, Zhi Mu, Tian Hua Fen,* and *Huang Lian* clear heat and eliminate dryness, and *Zhi Shi* rectifies the qi and frees the flow of the qi mechanism.

ADDITIONS & SUBTRACTIONS: If lung-stomach dryness and heat have damaged and consumed both qi and yin, add six grams of Radix Panacis Ginseng (*Ren Shen*). If there is yang ming heat exuberance causing constipation, add 6-9 grams of Radix Et Rhizoma Rhei (*Da Huang*) and 3-6 grams of Mirabilitum (*Mang Xiao*). If there is concomitant liver depression, see the additions and subtractions for pattern #2 above.

ACUPUNCTURE & MOXIBUSTION: Same as pattern #2 plus *Nei Ting* (St 44) and *Zhao Hai* (Ki 6).

FORMULA ANALYSIS: Draining *Nei Ting* clears heat from

the yang ming. Supplementing *Zhao Hai* enriches yin and engenders fluids.

ADDITIONS & SUBTRACTIONS: If there is constipation, add draining *Zhi Gou* (TB 6) and even supplementing-even draining *Tian Shu* (St 25) and *Da Chang Shu* (Bl 25). If there is concomitant qi vacuity, add supplementing *Pi Shu* (Bl 20) and even supplementing-even draining *Zu San Li* (St 36).

7. LUNG HEAT & FLUID DAMAGE PATTERN

MAIN SYMPTOMS: Dry mouth, dry throat, dry nose, a predilection for drinking, frequent urination, a cough with scanty phlegm or a dry cough with no phlegm, red tongue edges and tip with scanty fur and lack of fluids, and a floating, large or floating, fine pulse in the right inch position

TREATMENT PRINCIPLES: Clear the lungs and moisten dryness, nourish yin and engender fluids

RX: *Sha Shen Mai Men Dong Tang Jia Wei* (Glehnia & Ophiopogon Decoction with Added Flavors)

INGREDIENTS: Radix Glehniae Littoralis (*Sha Shen*) and Tuber Ophiopogonis Japonici (*Mai Men Dong*), 15g each, Rhizoma Phragmitis Communis (*Lu Gen*), 12g, Rhizoma Polygonati Odorati (*Yu Zhu*), Folium Mori Albi (*Sang Ye*), Radix Trichoanthis Kirlowii (*Tian Hua Fen*), and Semen Dolichoris Lablab (*Bai Bian Dou*), 9g each, and uncooked Radix Glycyrrhizae (*Gan Cao*), 3-6g

FORMULA ANALYSIS: *Sha Shen, Mai Men Dong, Tian Hua Fen, Yu Zhu,* and *Lu Gen* all engender fluids and moisten dryness especially in the stomach and lungs. *Sang Ye* clears heat from the liver and lungs. *Bai Bian Dou* fortifies the spleen and transforms dampness without damaging yin fluids, while uncooked *Gan Cao* clears heat at the same time as it harmonizes all the other medicinals in the formula.

ADDITIONS & SUBTRACTIONS: If there is concomitant liver depression qi stagnation, add nine grams each of Fructus Meliae Toosendan (*Chuan Lian Zi*) and Radix Albus Paeoniae Lactiflorae (*Bai Shao*).

ACUPUNCTURE & MOXIBUSTION: *Lie Que* (Lu 7), *Zhao Hai* (Ki 6), *Zhong Fu* (Lu 1), *Fei Shu* (Bl 13)

FORMULA ANALYSIS: Even supplementing-even draining *Lie Que* and supplementing *Zhao Hai* clears heat from the lungs at the same time as it engenders fluids and moistens dryness. Similarly, even supplementing-even draining *Zhong Fu* and *Fei Shu* clears heat from the lungs as it simultaneously moistens dryness.

ADDITIONS & SUBTRACTIONS: For more marked lung heat, add draining *Chi Ze* (Lu 5). For oral dryness and thirst, add even supplementing-even draining *Di Cang* (St 4), *Jia Che* (St 6), and *Cheng Jiang* (CV 23). For dry nose, add even supplementing-even draining *Ying Xiang* (LI 20). For cough, add even supplementing-even draining *Dan Zhong* (CV 17).

8. LIVER YIN INSUFFICIENCY PATTERN

MAIN SYMPTOMS: Polydipsia, polyuria, dry, scratchy eyes, dizziness, vertigo, tight sinews, muscular cramps, especially in the calves at night, blurred vision, night-blindness, pale, brittle nails, itching, possible numbness of the extremities, rib-side pain, and a pale tongue with a possible red tip and thin, white or scanty, dryish yellow fur, and a fine, bowstring pulse

TREATMENT PRINCIPLES: Enrich water and clear the liver

RX: *Qi Ju Di Huang Wan* (Lycium & Chrysanthemum Rehmannia Pills) plus *Yi Guan Jian* (One Link Decoction) with added flavors

INGREDIENTS: Uncooked Radix Rehmanniae (*Sheng Di*), 15g, Radix Glehniae Littoralis (*Sha Shen*) and Tuber Ophiopogonis Japonici (*Mai Men Dong*), 12g each Radix Dioscoreae Oppositae (*Shan Yao*), Fructus Corni Officinalis (*Shan Zhu Yu*), Sclerotium Poriae Cocos (*Fu Ling*), Rhizoma Alismatis (*Ze Xie*), Cortex Radicis Moutan (*Dan Pi*), Fructus Lycii Chinensis (*Gou Qi Zi*), Flos Chrysanthemi Morifolii (*Ju Hua*), Radix Angelicae Sinensis (*Dang Gui*), and Radix Albus Paeoniae Lactiflorae (*Bai Shao*), 9g each and Fructus Meliae Toosendan (*Chuan Lian Zi*), 6g

FORMULA ANALYSIS: *Sheng Di, Sha Shen, Mai Men Dong, Shan Zhu Yu, Dang Gui, Bai Shao,* and *Gou Qi Zi* all nourish liver blood and enrich kidney yin. *Dang Gui* and *Dan Pi* quicken the blood. *Shan Yao* fortifies the latter heaven spleen at the same time as it supplements the former heaven kidneys. *Ju Hua* clears the liver and brightens the eyes, while *Chuan Lian Zi* courses and clears the liver. *Fu Ling* helps *Shan Yao* fortify the spleen at the same time as it helps *Ze Xie* seep dampness and lead yang back down into the yin track.

ADDITIONS & SUBTRACTIONS: For a bitter taste in the mouth with oral dryness, add 3-6 grams of Rhizoma Coptidis Chinensis (*Huang Lian*). If there is constipation, add 9-12 grams of Semen Trichosanthis Kirlowii (*Gua Lou Ren*). If there are night sweats, add nine grams of Cortex Radicis Lycii Chinensis (*Di Gu Pi*). If there is vexatious heat and thirst, add 15-25 grams uncooked Gypsum Fibrosum (*Shi Gao*) and 9-12 grams of Rhizoma Anemarrhenae Aspheloidis (*Zhi Mu*).

ACUPUNCTURE & MOXIBUSTION: *Ge Shu* (Bl 17), *Gan Shu* (Bl 18), *Shen Shu* (Bl 23), *Qu Quan* (Liv 8), *Tai Xi* (Ki 3), *San Yin Jiao* (Sp 6)

FORMULA ANALYSIS: Supplementing *Ge Shu, Gan Shu, Qu Quan,* and *San Yin Jiao* nourishes liver blood, while supplementing *Shen Shu, Tai Xi,* and *San Yin Jiao* enriches kidney water.

ADDITIONS & SUBTRACTIONS: For blurred vision and night-blindness, add supplementing *Tai Yang* (M-HN-9) and *Jing Ming* (Bl 1). For dizziness and vertigo, add even supplementing-even draining *Feng Chi* (GB 20), *Tai Yang* (M-HN-9), and *Yin Tang* (M-HN-3). For heat in the liver, add *Tai Chong* (Liv 3) and *Xing Jian* (Liv 2). Needle *Tai Chong* through to *Xing Jian* and use even supplementing-even draining technique. For rib-side pain, add even supplementing-even draining *Zhang Men* (Liv 13) and *Qi Men* (Liv 14).

9. HEART YIN INSUFFICIENCY PATTERN

MAIN SYMPTOMS: Polydipsia, polyphagia, polyuria, heart palpitations, insomnia, profuse dreams, a red tongue tip with scanty fur, and a surging pulse in the inch position

TREATMENT PRINCIPLES: Enrich yin and nourish fluids, calm the heart and quiet the spirit

RX: *Tian Wang Bu Xin Dan Jia Jian* (Heavenly Emperor Supplement the Heart Elixir with Additions & Subtractions)

INGREDIENTS: Uncooked Radix Rehmanniae (*Sheng Di*), Radix Scrophulariae Ningpoensis (*Xuan Shen*), and Radix Salviae Miltiorrhizae (*Dan Shen*), 15g each, Tuber Ophiopogonis Japonici (*Mai Men Dong*), Tuber Asparagi Cochinensis (*Tian Men Dong*), Semen Zizyphi Spinosae (*Suan Zao Ren*), and Semen Biotae Orientalis (*Bai Zi Ren*), 12g each, Radix Angelicae Sinensis (*Dang Gui*), Sclerotium Pararadicis Poriae Cocos (*Fu Shen*), Radix Polygalae Tenuifoliae (*Yuan Zhi*), and Fructus Schisandrae

Chinensis (*Wu Wei Zi*), 9g each, and Radix Platycodi Grandiflori (*Jie Geng*) and Radix Panacis Ginseng (*Ren Shen*), 6g each

FORMULA ANALYSIS: *Sheng Di, Xuan Shen, Mai Men Dong, Wu Wei Zi,* and *Tian Men Dong* all enrich yin and nourish fluids. *Dan Shen* and *Dang Gui* nourish and quicken the heart blood. *Suan Zao Ren* and *Bai Zi Ren* nourish heart blood and quiet the heart spirit. *Yuan Zhi, Fu Shen,* and *Ren Shen* construct and quiet the heart spirit, and *Jie Geng* acts as the messenger leading the other medicinals specifically to the region of the chest.

ADDITIONS & SUBTRACTIONS: For severe heart palpitations and insomnia, add 12-15 grams of Caulis Polygoni Multiflori (*Ye Jiao Teng*) and 9-12 grams of Arillus Euphoriae Longanae (*Long Yan Rou*). For severe dry mouth and thirst, add 9-12 grams of Herba Dendrobii (*Shi Hu*). For sores on the tip of the tongue, add 3-6 grams of Rhizoma Coptidis Chinensis (*Huang Lian*) and 1.5-6 grams of Plumula Nelumbinis Nuciferae (*Lian Zi Xin*).

ACUPUNCTURE & MOXIBUSTION: *Jue Yin Shu* (Bl 14), *Xin Shu* (Bl 15), *Dan Zhong* (CV 17), *Shen Men* (Ht 7), *Nei Guan* (Per 6), *Tai Xi* (Ki 3), *San Yin Jiao* (Sp 6)

FORMULA ANALYSIS: Supplementing *Tai Xi* and *San Yin Jiao* enriches yin and nourishes fluids. Even supplementing-even draining *Jue Yin Shu, Xin Shu, Dan Zhong, Nei Guan,* and *Shen Men* supplements and clears the heart and quiets the spirit.

ADDITIONS & SUBTRACTIONS: If there is severe insomnia, add draining *Bai Hui* (GV 20) and *Feng Chi* (GB 20). If there is concomitant liver depression, add draining *Tai Chong* (Liv 3).

10. QI & YIN DUAL VACUITY PATTERN

MAIN SYMPTOMS: Polydipsia, polyphagia, and polyuria may not be marked. Instead, there is dry mouth and throat, lassitude of the spirit, fatigue, shortness of breath, low back and knee soreness and limpness, dry, bound stools, possible concomitant heart palpitations, spontaneous perspiration, dizziness, tinnitus, numbness or pain of the extremities, blurred vision, a fat tongue with teeth-marks on its edges and white fur, and a deep, fine pulse.

TREATMENT PRINCIPLES: Fortify the spleen and boost the qi, supplement the kidneys and nourish yin

RX: *Sheng Mai San* (Engender the Pulse Powder) plus *Zeng Ye Tang* (Increase Humors Decoction) with added flavors

INGREDIENTS: Uncooked Radix Rehmanniae (*Sheng Di*) and uncooked Radix Astragali Membranacei (*Huang Qi*), 30g each, Rhizoma Polygonati (*Huang Jing*), Radix Pseudostellariae Heterophyllae (*Tai Zi Shen*), Radix Scrophulariae Ningpoensis (*Xuan Shen*), Radix Puerariae (*Ge Gen*), Radix Trichosanthis Kirlowii (*Tian Hua Fen*), and Radix Dioscoreae Oppositae (*Shan Yao*), 15g each, Tuber Ophiopogonis Japonici (*Mai Men Dong*), 12g, and Fructus Corni Officinalis (*Shan Zhu Yu*) and Fructus Schisandrae Chinensis (*Wu Wei Zi*), 9g each

FORMULA ANALYSIS: *Sheng Di, Mai Men Dong, Ge Gen, Xuan Shen,* and *Tian Hua Fen* enrich yin and engender fluids. *Huang Qi, Shan Yao, Shan Zhu Yu,* and *Tai Zi Shen* boost the qi, and *Huang Jing* and *Wu Wei Zi* simultaneously supplement the qi and yin.

ADDITIONS & SUBTRACTIONS: If there is mainly qi vacuity with heart palpitations, spontaneous perspiration, shortness of breath, and lack of strength, increase the dose of *Huang Qi* and add nine grams of Radix Panacis Ginseng (*Ren Shen*) or 15-30 grams of Radix Codonopsitis Pilosulae (*Dang Shen*). If there is a dry mouth, dry stools, and a red tongue with scanty fluids due to predominant yin damage, increased the dose of *Sheng Di, Xuan Shen,* and *Tian Hua Fen* and add 15 grams each of Radix Glehniae Littoralis (*Sha Shen*) and Herba Dendrobii (*Shi Hu*). If there is fire effulgence, add 30 grams of uncooked Gypsum Fibrosum (*Shi Gao*) and 9-12 grams of Rhizoma Anemarrhenae Aspheloidis (*Zhi Mu*). If there is low back and knee soreness and limpness and numbness or pain of the extremities due to liver blood-kidney yin vacuity with malnourishment of the sinews, add 30 grams of Fructus Chaenomelis Lagenariae (*Mu Gua*), 15 grams each of Rhizoma Cibotii Barometsis (*Gou Ji*) and Radix Achyranthis Bidentatae (*Niu Xi*), and 12 grams of Lumbricus (*Di Long*) to strengthen the low back and supplement the kidneys, soothe the sinews and free the flow of the network vessels.

If there is exhaustion and fatigue as well as lack of strength of the four limbs, decreased appetite, loose stools, a fat tongue with white fur, and a deep, fine, forceless pulse due to spleen qi vacuity weakness, first use *Shen Ling Bai Zhu San* (Ginseng, Poria & Atractylodes Powder) to fortify the spleen and boost the qi: Semen Coicis Lachyrma-jobi (*Yi Yi Ren*), 30g, Semen Nelumbinis

Nuciferae (*Lian Zi*), Radix Dioscoreae Oppositae (*Shan Yao*), and Semen Dolichoris Lablab (*Bai Bian Dou*), 15g each, Radix Panacis Ginseng (*Ren Shen*), Rhizoma Atractylodis Macrocephalae (*Bai Zhu*), and Sclerotium Poriae Cocos (*Fu Ling*), 9g each, and Fructus Amomi (*Sha Ren*), Radix Platycodi Grandiflori (*Jie Geng*), and mix-fried Radix Glycyrrhizae (*Gan Cao*), 6g each.

ACUPUNCTURE & MOXIBUSTION: *Zhong Wan* (CV 12), *Qi Hai* (CV 6), *Zu San Li* (St 36), *Pi Shu* (Bl 20), *Shen Shu* (Bl 23), *Di Ji* (Sp 8), *San Yin Jiao* (Sp 6)

FORMULA ANALYSIS: Supplementing *Zhong Wan*, *Qi Hai*, *Zu San Li*, and *Di Ji* fortifies the spleen and boosts the qi, while supplementing *Shen Shu* and *San Yin Jiao* supplements the kidneys and nourishes yin.

ADDITIONS & SUBTRACTIONS: If there is simultaneous phlegm dampness obstructing internally, add draining *Feng Long* (St 40) and drain *Zhong Wan*.

11. QI & YIN DUAL VACUITY WITH SIMULTANEOUS BLOOD STASIS PATTERN

MAIN SYMPTOMS: Polydipsia, polyphagia, and polyuria may not be marked. Instead, there is dry mouth, lack of strength, heart palpitations, shortness of breath, dizziness, tinnitus, low back and knee soreness and limpness, numbness and/or pain of the extremities, blurred vision, chest oppression, chest pain, possible bilateral lower limb edema, possible windstroke and hemiplegia, abnormalities in blood flow, increased blood platelet aggregation, a fat, dark, possible purplish tongue and/or static macules and spots, dark, tortuous, distended sublingual veins, and a deep, fine pulse.

TREATMENT PRINCIPLES: Fortify the spleen and boost the qi, supplement the kidneys and nourish yin, quicken the blood and transform stasis

RX: *Yi Qi Yang Yin Huo Xue Tang* (Boost the Qi, Nourish Yin & Quicken the Blood Decoction)

INGREDIENTS: Radix Scrophulariae Ningpoensis (*Xuan Shen*), Radix Salviae Miltiorrhizae (*Dan Shen*), Rhizoma Polygonati (*Huang Jing*), uncooked Radix Astragali Membranacei (*Huang Qi*), and Radix Trichosanthis Kirlowii (*Tian Hua Fen*), 30g each, uncooked Radix Rehmanniae (*Sheng Di*), 20g, Radix Pseudostellariae Heterophyllae (*Tai Zi Shen*) and Radix Puerariae (*Ge Gen*), 15g each, Tuber Ophiopogonis Japonici (*Mai Men Dong*), 12g, Fructus Schisandrae Chinensis (*Wu Wei Zi*),

Radix Angelicae Sinensis (*Dang Gui*), Semen Pruni Persicae (*Tao Ren*), and Fructus Immaturus Citri Aurantii (*Zhi Shi*), 9g each, and uncooked Radix Et Rhizoma Rhei (*Da Huang*), 6-10g

FORMULA ANALYSIS: *Sheng Di*, *Xuan Shen*, *Tian Hua Fen*, *Wu Wei Zi*, *Mai Men Dong*, and *Ge Gen* nourish yin and engender fluids, while *Huang Qi*, *Huang Jing*, and *Tai Zi Shen* fortify the spleen and supplement the qi. *Dang Gui* nourishes and quickens the blood, while *Dan Shen* quickens and nourishes the blood. *Zhi Shi* rectifies the qi, and *Da Huang* clears heat from the yang ming and frees the flow of the stools.

ADDITIONS & SUBTRACTIONS: If there is high blood pressure, add 30 grams of Concha Margaritiferae (*Zhen Zhu Mu*), 15 grams each of Ramulus Uncariae Cum Uncis (*Gou Teng*) and Radix Cyathulae (*Chuan Niu Xi*), and six grams of Rhizoma Gastrodia Elatae (*Tian Ma*). If there is peripheral neuropathy with numbness and/or pain of the extremities, add 15 grams each of Rhizoma Cibotii Barometis (*Gou Ji*), Radix Cyathulae (*Chuan Niu Xi*), and Fructus Chaenomelis Lagenariae (*Mu Gua*) and nine grams each of Radix Gentianae Macrophyllae (*Qin Jiao*), Buthus Martensis (*Quan Xie*), and Scolopendra Subspinipes (*Wu Gong*). If there is retinopathy with seepage of blood into the fundus, add 12 grams of Thallus Algae (*Kun Bu*), nine grams each of Scapus Et Inflorescentia Eriocaulonis Buergeriani (*Gu Jing Cao*) and Semen Celosiae Argenteae (*Qing Xiang Zi*), and two grams of Radix Pseudoginseng (*San Qi*) swallowed with the decocted liquid. If there is phlegm heat causing acute cerebrovascular disease, add 30 grams of Fructus Trichosanthis Kirlowii (*Gua Lou*) and nine grams of bile-processed Rhizoma Arisaematis (*Dan Nan Xing*) in order to transform phlegm and free the flow of the brain bowel.

If qi stagnation and blood stasis are predominant, yin vacuity is less pronounced, and there is no qi vacuity, use the following unnamed formula: Herba Leonuri Heterophylli (*Yi Mu Cao*) and Radix Salviae Miltiorrhizae (*Dan Shen*), 30g each, Radix Rubrus Paeoniae Lactiflorae (*Chi Shao*), Radix Puerariae (*Ge Gen*), uncooked Radix Rehmanniae (*Sheng Di*), and cooked Radix Rehmanniae (*Shu Di*), 15g each, and Radix Auklandiae Lappae (*Mu Xiang*), Radix Angelicae Sinensis (*Dang Gui*), and Radix Ligustici Wallichii (*Chuan Xiong*), 9g each

ACUPUNCTURE & MOXIBUSTION: Same as pattern #4 above plus *Ge Shu* (Bl 17) and *Xue Hai* (Sp 10).

FORMULA ANALYSIS: Draining *Xue Hai* and even supplementing-even draining *Ge Shu* quickens the blood and dispels stasis.

12. YIN & YANG DUAL VACUITY PATTERN

MAIN SYMPTOMS: Pronounced low back and knee soreness and limpness, shortness of breath, lack of strength, a dry mouth with a desire for lots of drinks, fear of cold, chilled limbs, possible facial or lower leg edema, decreased appetite, loose stools or alternating diarrhea and constipation, turbid urine, a somber yellow, darkish facial complexion, withered auricles, loose teeth, impotence, a pale but dark tongue with white, dry fur, and a deep, fine, forceless pulse

TREATMENT PRINCIPLES: Foster yin and warm yang, supplement the kidneys and quicken the blood

RX: *Jin Gui Shen Qi Wan* (*Golden Cabinet* Kidney Qi Pills) plus *Shui Lu Er Xian Dan* (Water & Land Two Immortals Elixir) with additions and subtractions

INGREDIENTS: Radix Salviae Miltiorrhizae (*Dan Shen*), 30g, Radix Puerariae (*Ge Gen*), cooked Radix Rehmanniae (*Shu Di*), Radix Dioscoreae Oppositae (*Shan Yao*), Rhizoma Alismatis (*Ze Xie*), Sclerotium Poriae Cocos (*Fu Ling*), Sclerotium Polypori Umbellati (*Zhu Ling*), Semen Euryalis Ferocis (*Qian Shi*), and Fructus Rosae Laevigatae (*Jin Ying Zi*), 15g each, Fructus Corni Officinalis (*Shan Zhu Yu*), 12g, and Ramulus Cinnamomi Cassiae (*Gui Zhi*) and Radix Lateralis Praeparatus Aconiti Carmichaeli (*Fu Zi*), 6g each

FORMULA ANALYSIS: *Shu Di* supplemnents the kidneys and enriches yin, while *Gui Zhi* and *Fu Zi* supplement the kidneys and warm yang. *Shan Zhu Yu, Jin Ying Zi,* and *Qian Shi* supplement the kidneys and astringe the qi. *Shan Yao* and *Fu Ling* fortify the spleen and supplement the qi, while *Fu Ling, Zhu Ling,* and *Ze Xie* seep and disinhibit dampness. *Dan Shen* quickens and nourishes the blood.

ADDITIONS & SUBTRACTIONS: If there is yin vacuity with fire effulgence, add nine grams each of Rhizoma Anemarrhenae Aspheloidis (*Zhi Mu*) and Cortex Phellodendri (*Huang Bai*). If there is kidney qi not securing, increase the dosages of *Qian Shi* and *Jin Ying Zi* and add 15 grams of Fructus Alpiniae Oxyphyllae (*Yi Zhi Ren*) and nine grams of Fructus Rubi Chingii (*Fu Pen Zi*) to secure the kidneys and stop slippage. If there is concomitant liver depression and damp obstruction with frequent, urgent urination and lower abdominal falling and distention, add 15 grams each of Semen Citri Reticulatae (*Ju*

He) and Folium Pyrrosiae (*Shi Wei*), and nine grams each of Radix Bupleuri (*Chai Hu*), Fructus Citri Aurantii (*Zhi Ke*), Fructus Immaturus Citri Aurantii (*Zhi Shi*), and Semen Lichi Chinensis (*Li Zhi He*) to course and disinhibit the qi mechanism, free the flow and disinhibit urination. If spleen yang is depleted and vacuous with scanty appetite and loose stools or diarrhea, add 20-30 grams of Semen Lachryam-jobi (*Yi Yi Ren*), 15 grams of Semen Dolichoris Lablab (*Bai Bian Dou*), and 9-12 grams each of Rhizoma Atractylodis Macrocephalae (*Bai Zhu*) and Radix Codonopsitis Pilosulae (*Dang Shen*). If qi and blood, and yin and yang are all vacuous with lassitude of the spirit, lack of strength, fear of cold, chilled limbs, and pale lips, nails, and tongue, add 18 grams of Radix Astragali Membranacei (*Huang Qi*), 12 grams of Fructus Lycii Chinensis (*Gou Qi Zi*), and nine grams each of Radix Angelicae Sinensis (*Dang Gui*) and Gelatinum Cornu Cervi (*Lu Jiao Jiao*) to boost the qi and nourish the blood.

If there is heart-kidney yang decline with chest oppression, heart palpitations, if severe, inability to lie down, more severe edema, and scanty urination, use *Sheng Mai San* (Engender the Pulse Powder) plus *Wu Ling San* (Five [Ingredients] Poria Powder) with added flavors: uncooked Radix Astragali Membranacei (*Huang Qi*), 18g, Fructus Schisandrae Chinensis (*Wu Wei Zi*), Sclerotium Poriae Cocos (*Fu Ling*), Sclerotium Polypori Umbellati (*Zhu Ling*), and Rhizoma Alismatis (*Ze Xie*), 15g each, Rhizoma Atractylodis Macrocephalae (*Bai Zhu*) and Tuber Ophiopogonis Japonici (*Mai Men Dong*), 12g each, Radix Panacis Gisneng (*Ren Shen*), Ramulus Cinnamomi Cassiae (*Gui Zhi*), and Semen Lepidii Descurainiae (*Ting Li Zi*), 9g each, and Fructus Zizyphi Jujubae (*Da Zao*), 5-7 pieces.

If there is spleen-kidney decline and vanquishment with phlegm dampness obstructing the center and turbid evils collected internally, a somber white facial complexion, superficial edema, epigastric glomus and oppression, torpid intake, nausea, dry, bound stools, and thick, slimy tongue fur, use *Huang Lian Wen Dan Tang Jia Wei* (Coptis Warm the Gallbladder Decoction with Added Flavors) in order to transform phlegm and harmonize the stomach, free the flow of the bowels and downbear turbidity: Rhizoma Pinelliae Ternatae (*Ban Xia*) and Sclerotium Poriae Cocos (*Fu Ling*), 12g each, Pericarpium Citri Reticulatae (*Chen Pi*), Fructus Immaturus Citri Aurantii (*Zhi Shi*), Caulis Bambusae In Taeniis (*Zhu Ru*), and wine stir-fried Radix Et Rhizoma Rhei (*Da Huang*), 9g each, Rhizoma Coptidis Chinensis (*Huang Lian*), 3-6g, Radix Glycyrrhizae (*Gan Cao*), 1-3g, and Fructus Zizyphi

Jujubae (*Da Zao*), 3-5 pieces. If the stools are not constipated, remove or reduce *Da Huang*. If there is phlegm heat complicated by blood stasis causing either peripheral neuropathy or cerebral vascular disease, add nine grams each of Lumbricus (*Di Long*), Bombyx Batryticatus (*Jiang Can*), Zaocys Dhumnades (*Wu Shao She*), and/or Spina Gleditschiae Chinensis (*Zao Jiao Ci*).

ACUPUNCTURE & MOXIBUSTION: *Qi Hai* (CV 6), *Guan Yuan* (CV 4), *Zhong Wan* (CV 12), *Zu San Li* (St 36), *Pi Shu* (Bl 20), *Shen Shu* (Bl 23), *San Yin Jiao* (Sp 6)

FORMULA ANALYSIS: Supplementing *Zhong Wan*, *Zu San Li*, and *Pi Shu* fortifies the spleen, the latter heaven root of qi and blood engenderment and transformation. Supplementing *San Yin Jiao* and moxaing *Qi Hai*, *Guan Yuan*, and *Shen Shu* supplements the kidneys and invigorates yang.

ADDITIONS & SUBTRACTIONS: For marked liver depression qi stagnation, add draining *Tai Chong* (Liv 3) and *He Gu* (LI 4). For concomitant dampness and turbidity, add draining *Shang Qiu* (Sp 5) and *Feng Long* (St 40) and even supplementing-even draining *Zhong Wan*. If yang vacuity is marked, add moxibustion at *Ming Men* (GV 4). If there is spleen yang vacuity, add moxibustion at *Pi Shu* and *Wei Shu* (Bl 21). If there are heart palpitations, add even supplementing-even draining *Nei Guan* (Per 6) and *Shen Men* (Ht 7). If there is severe edema and scanty urination, add draining *Yin Ling Quan* (Sp 9) and *Zhong Ji* (CV 3) and use even supplementing-even draining at *Guan Yuan*. If there is concomitant blood stasis, add draining *Xue Hai* (Sp 10).

ABSTRACTS OF REPRESENTATIVE CHINESE RESEARCH:

Peng Geng-ru & Zhao Lin, "A Clincial Audit of the Treatment of 92 Cases of Type II Diabetes with *Xiao Ke Tang* (Wasting & Thirsting Decoction) & Glyburide," *Hu Nan Zhong Yi Za Zhi* (*Hunan Journal of Chinese Medicine*), #2, 2002, p. 17-18: Of the 92 patients in the treatment group, 59 were male and 33 were female. These patients ranged in age from 39-61 years, with a median age of 53.18 ± 7.16 years. The shortest course of disease among these patients was half a year, the longest was 15 years, and median duration was 4.95 ± 3.79 years. There was also a comparison group of 76 patients, among whom 42 were male and 43 were female. These patients ranged in age from 42-60 years, with a median age of 50.27 ± 8.12 years. The shortest course of disease in this group was one year, the longest was 13 years, and the median duration was 4.58 ± 2.74 years. Therefore, there was no significant

statistical difference in these two groups in terms of sex, age, or disease course. All the patients has a fasting glucose level equal to or higher than 7.8mmol/L and non-fasting blood glucose level of 11.1mmol/L or more. All were given an oral glucose tolerance test (OGTT) and all were diagnosed with type 2 diabetes mellitus.

The treatment group received the following Chinese medicinals: Semen Fagopyri Esculenti (*Qiao Mai*), 18g, Radix Trichosanthis Kirlowii (*Tian Hua Fen*) and Radix Codonopsitis Pilosulae (*Dang Shen*), 15g each, Radix Astragali Membranacei (*Huang Qi*), 12g, and Fructus Schisandrae Chinensis (*Wu Wei Zi*), Radix Salviae Miltiorrhizae (*Dan Shen*), and Semen Dolichoris Lablab (*Bai Bian Dou*), 10g each. One *ji* of these medicinals was decocted in water and administered orally per day. In addition, both groups were administered 2.5-5mg of glyburide each time, two times per day. Both regimes were continued for 12 weeks.

Marked effect was defined as fasting blood glucose (FBG) lowered to 7.2mmol/L or a reduction by 30%. Postprandial blood glucose (PPBG) was reduced to 8.25mmol/L or a reduction by 30%. In addition, clinical symptoms either disappeared or were markedly decreased. Some effect meant that FBG was lowered to 8.25mmol/L or reduced 10-29%, PBG was 9.9mmol/L or reduced 10-29%, and clinical symptoms markedly improved. No effect meant that there was no change in FBG or PBG or a reduction of less than 10% and no obvious improvement in clinical symptoms. Based on these criteria, 51 patients (55.4%) in the treatment group were judged to have experienced a marked effect, 32 (34.8%) got some effect, and nine (9.8%) got no effect, for a total amelioration rate of 90.2%. In the comparison group, 28 (36.8%) got a marked effect, 25 (32.9%) got some effect, and 23 (30.3%) got no effect, for a total amelioration rate of 69.7%. In addition, there was an overall 20% better result in terms of improvements in fatigue, lack of strength, oral thirst, polyuria, polyphagia, and tongue signs in the treatment group than in the comparison group. Therefore, this study suggests that Chinese medicinals and glyburide are more effective than glyburide alone for the treatment of type 2 diabetes. In addition, the authors state there were no side effects with the Chinese medicinals.

Su Ping-mao & Zhang Guo-xia, "A Summary of the Treatment of 57 Cases of Diabetic Dawn Phenomenon with Master Lei's *Su Xiang Hua Zuo Fang* (Penetratingly Aromatic Transforming Turbidity Formula)," *Hu Nan Zhong Yi Za Zhi* (*Hunan Journal of Chinese Medicine*), #2, 2001, p. 16-17: A certain percentage of diabetic patients manifest symptoms of elevated blood glucose between 5-7

AM. This is referred to as diabetic dawn phenomenon. In this study, there were a total of 89 patients, 40 of whom were seen as out-patients and 49 of whom were in-patients. All received dietary and exercise therapy and all received one or more types of oral hypoglycemic agents. In addition, all had a body mass index (BMI) between 26.4-28.0kg/m. The treatment group was comprised of 57 patients, 30 men and 27 women, 39-61 years of age, with an average age of 47 years. Their disease course had lasted from 1-6 years, with an average duration of four years. From 2-3 AM, their blood glucose was 4.0-6.0mmol/L, with an average of 5.6mmol/L. From 7-8 AM, fasting blood glucose was 9.0-12.0mmol/L, with an average of 10.9mmol/L. Urine glucose was 0.5-2.0g/24hrs, with an average of 0.8g/24hrs. In the comparison group, there were 19 men and 13 women 40-62 years of age, with average age of 49 years. Their course of disease ran between 1-7 years, with an average course of five years. Two to 3 AM blood glucose, 7-8 AM fasting blood glucose, and urine glucose was essentially the same as the treatment group. Thus there was no significant statistical difference in terms of age, sex, disease duration, BMI, blood glucose, or urine glucose. Diagnostic criteria for type 2 diabetes was based on the criteria of the American Diabetes Association. The Chinese medical pattern discrimination of phlegm dampness was based on national standards for Chinese medicine and diabetes and included chest and ductal glomus and oppression, torpid intake, nausea, obesity, bodily encumbrance and fatigue, head distention, and heavy limbs.

The treatment group received the following Chinese medicinals in addition to their usual oral hypoglycemic agents: Radix Salviae Miltiorrhizae (*Dan Shen*), 30g, Herba Agastachis Seu Pogostemi (*Hua Xiang*), Herba Eupatorii Fortunei (*Pei Lan*), Radix Scutellariae Baicalensis (*Huang Qin*), and Ramulus Euonymi Alati (*Gui Jian Yu*), 15g each, and Rhizoma Pinelliae Ternatae (*Ban Xia*), Pericarpium Citri Reticulatae (*Chen Pi*), Cortex Magnoliae Officinalis (*Hou Po*), Pericarpium Arecae Catechu (*Da Fu Pi*), and Folium Nelumbinis Nuciferae (*Ou Ye*), 10g each. One *ji* of these medicinals was decocted in water and administered per day. The comparison group received 500mg of dimethyldiguanide between 3-4 AM in addition to their usual oral hypoglycemic agents, and both groups were re-examined after one week.

In terms of outcomes criteria, a good effect meant that fasting blood glucose between 7-8 AM was 4.4-6.1mmol/L. An ordinary effect was defined as a fasting blood glucose between 7-8 AM of 6.2-7.0mmol/L, and a poor effect was a fasting blood glucose between 7-8 AM higher than

7.0mmol/L. Based on these criteria, 30 patients (52.6%) in the treatment group were considered to have gotten a good effect, 18 (31.6%) got an ordinary effect, and nine (15.8%) got no effect, for a total effectiveness rate of 84.2%. In the comparison group, 16 (50.0%) got a good effect, 10 (31.3%) got an ordinary effect, and 6 (18.8%) got no effect, for a total effectiveness rate of 81.3%. Although there was no significant statistical difference in outcomes between these two groups, the treatment group did not have to be wakened in the middle of the night for administration of dimethyldiguanide and, therefore, slept more and better.

Zhou Jun-huai, "The Integrated Chinese-Western Medical Treatment of 50 Cases of Type II Diabetes," *Hu Nan Zhong Yi Za Zhi (Hunan Journal of Chinese Medicine)*, #2, 2001, p. 44: Patients in this study were all diagnosed with type 2 diabetes according to 1985 WHO criteria. In the treatment group, there were 50 patients made up of 32 men and 18 women from 39-75 years of age, with an average age of 51.8 years. Their disease course had lasted from two months to eight years. Six cases controlled their condition through diet alone, while the other 44 used sulfonylurea-type oral hypoglycemic agents. There were also 50 patients in the comparison group – 28 men and 22 women aged 41-77, with an average age of 53.7 years. Their course of disease had lasted four months to nine years. Four controlled their condition through diet alone and the rest used sulfonylurea-type oral hypoglycemics.

Treatment for those in the so-called treatment group consisted of the following Chinese medicinals on top of their standard treatment: uncooked Radix Astragali Membranacei (*Huang Qi*), 40g, Radix Trichosanthis Kirlowii (*Tian Hua Fen*), Radix Salviae Miltiorrhizae (*Dan Shen*), and Rhizoma Alismatis (*Ze Xie*), 20g each, Radix Albus Paeoniae Lactiflorae (*Bai Shao*), Tuber Ophiopogonis Japonici (*Mai Men Dong*), and Radix Dioscoreae Oppositae (*Shan Yao*), 15g each, and Rhizoma Polygonati Odorati (*Yu Zhu*), Fructus Schisandrae Chinensis (*Wu Wei Zi*), and Herba Dendrobii (*Shi Hu*), 10g each. One *ji* of these medicinals was decocted in water and administered per day continuously for two months. Additions and subtractions to the above were made on the basis of differences in symptoms. In the comparison group, besides their standard therapy, patients received 0.25mg of dimethyldiguanide each time, three times per day for two months.

Marked effect meant that FBG was less than 6.0mmol/L and PPBG was less than 8.0mmol/L. Ordinary effect meant a FBG more than 6.0mmol/L and less than 7.8mmol/L and a PPBG more than 8.0mmol/L and less than 10.0mmol/L. Poor effect meant a FBG more than 7.8mmol/L and a PPBG more than 10.0mmol/L. Based on these criteria, 40 patients (80%) in the treatment group got a marked effect, eight (16%) got an ordinary effect, and two (4%) got a poor effect in terms of FBG. In terms of PPBG, 40 (80%) got a marked effect, nine (18%) got an ordinary effect, and one (2%) got a poor effect. In the comparison group, in terms of FBG, 20 (40%) got a marked effect, five (10%) got an ordinary effect, and five (10%) got a poor effect. In terms of PPBG, 14 (28%) got a marked effect, 26 (52%) got an ordinary effect, and 10 (20%) got a poor effect. These outcomes suggest that Chinese medicinals combined with sulfonylurea-type hypoglycemic agents are more effective for the treatment of type 2 diabetes than dimethyldiguanide and sulfony-lurea-type oral hypoglycemic agents alone.

Wu Chen *et al.*, "A Clinical Analysis of the Influence of Acupuncture on Blood Glucose & Blood Lipids in Patients with Diabetes," *He Nan Zhong Yi (Henan Chinese Medicine)*, #1, 2001, p. 42-43: There were 26 type 2 diabetes patients in this study, including 12 men and 14 women. Two were less than 40 years old, 11 were 41-50, eight were 51-65, and five were over 65, with an average age of 56.5 years. Four cases had developed diabetes within the year, 14 had had diabetes for 1-5 years, six, for 6-10 years, and two for more than 10 years, with an average disease course of 4.46 years. Nine cases exhibited the pattern of yin vacuity with dryness and heat, seven exhibited qi and yin dual vacuity, six exhibited blood stasis with heat exuberance, and four exhibited yin and yang dual vacuity.

The main points consisted of: *Yi Shu* (M-BW-12), *Pi Shu* (Bl 20), *Shen Shu* (Bl 23), *San Jiao Shu* (Bl 22), *Qu Chi* (LI 11), *Zhi Gou* (TB 6), *Zu San Li* (St 36), *San Yin Jiao* (Sp 6), and *Tai Xi* (Ki 3). If there was yin vacuity with dryness and heat, *Tai Yuan* (Lu 9) and *Nei Ting* (St 44) were added. If there was qi and yin dual vacuity, *Qi Hai Shu* (Bl 24) and *Guan Yuan* (CV 4) were added. If there was blood stasis with heat exuberance, *He Gu* (LI 4) and *Ge Shu* (Bl 17) were added. If there was yin and yang dual vacuity, *Qi Hai* (CV 6) and *Ming Men* (GV 4) were added. After obtaining the qi, even supplementing-even draining hand technique was used and the needles were retained for 30-60 minutes each treatment. Two to three treatments were given per week, with 10 treatments equaling one course. A rest of 3-5 days was given between successive courses.

In terms of outcomes, a marked effect was defined as basic disappearance of symptoms, FBG less than 7.2mmol/L, and PPBG less than 8.33mmol/L or a 30% reduction in blood sugar. Cholesterol was less than 5.96mmol/L, and triglycerides were less than 1.47mmol/L. Some effect

meant that there was marked improvement in symptoms, FBG was less than 8.33mmol/L, PPBG was less than 10.0mmol/L or blood glucose was reduced 10-29%, cholesterol was less than 6.48mmol/L, and triglycerides were less than 1.70mmol/L. No effect meant that reductions in blood glucose and blood lipids did not meet the above criteria. Based on these criteria, 11 patients got a marked effect, 12 got some effect, and only three got no effect, for a total amelioration rate of 88.46%.

Su Yu-dian & Niu Tong-zhou, "Experiences in the Treatment of Diabetes with Rhizoma Atractylodis (*Cang Zhu*)," *Zhong Yi Za Zhi (Journal of Chinese Medicine)*, #9, 1998, p. 573: Twenty type 2 diabetes patients were treated in this study, 12 of whom were men and eight, women. These patients ranged in age from 30-61 years old. One case had had diabetes less than half a year, 10 cases had had diabetes from 1/2-3 years, eight cases had had diabetes from 3-6 years, and one case had had diabetes for more than seven years. Eight cases had a mild degree condition, six had a medium degree condition, and six had a heavy or serious degree condition. Twelve cases had previously used Western oral hypoglycemic medicines, seven had used both Western and Chinese medicines, and one case used insulin.

All the patients in this study were administered *Jin Shui Xiang Sheng Yin* (Metal & Water Mutually Engendering Drink): Rhizoma Atractylodis (*Cang Zhu*), 15g, and Radix Astragali Membranacei (*Huang Qi*), Radix Glehniae Littoralis (*Sha Shen*), Tuber Asparagi Cochinensis (*Tian Men Dong*), Tuber Ophiopogonis Japonici (*Mai Men Dong*), Radix Scrophulariae Ningpoensis (*Xuan Shen*), uncooked Radix Rehmanniae (*Sheng Di*), Radix Dioscoreae Oppositae (*Shan Yao*), Fructus Corni Officinalis (*Shan Zhu Yu*), and Fructus Schisandrae Chinensis (*Wu Wei Zi*), 10g each. One *ji* of these medicinals was decocted in water and administered orally per day, and one month equaled one course of treatment. If patients had concomitant blood stasis, Radix Salviae Miltiorrhizae (*Dan Shen*), Fructus Crataegi (*Shan Zha*), Semen Pruni Persicae (*Tao Ren*), and Flos Carthami Tinctorii (*Hong Hua*) were added. If there was concomitant glaucoma, sparrow blindness, or deafness, the above formula was combined with *Qi Hu Di Huang Wan Jia Jian* (Lycium & Chrysanthemum Rehmannia Pills with Additions & Subtractions). If there were ulcers or abscesses, it was combined with *Wu Wei Xiao Du Yin* (Five Flavors Disperse Toxins Drink). If ulcers and sores had produced pus, it was combined with *Huang Qi Liu Yi Tang* (Astragalus Six [to] One Decoction). Using this protocol, 10 cases were judged cured, seven improved, and three got no effect, for an 85% total amelioration rate.

Lin Zhi-gang, "A Study of the Efficacy of Treating Type II Diabetes with Integrated Acupuncture & Medicinals," *Fu Jian Zhong Yi Yao (Fujian Chinese Medicine & Medicinals)*, #2, 2000, p. 19-20: There were 70 patients in this study, all of whom had been diagnosed with type 2 diabetes and whose blood glucose was poorly controlled by Western hypoglycemic agents. Forty of these patients were men and 30 were women. Their ages ranged from 31-80 years, and their disease duration ranged from six months to 32 years. Thirty-five of these patients were treated with Chinese herbs and the other 35 were treated with Chinese herbs and acupuncture. Fasting and one, two, and three hour postprandial blood glucose was similar in both these groups before treatment, and patients continued to take their insulin or oral hypoglycemics during this study.

These patients were further divided into three patterns. Those with yin vacuity in the herb group received the following Chinese medicinals: uncooked Radix Astragali Membranacei (*Huang Qi*), 30g, Radix Trichosanthis Kirlowii (*Tian Hua Fen*), Radix Scrophulariae Ningpoensis (*Xuan Shen*), Radix Puerariae (*Ge Gen*), and Radix Dioscoreae Oppositae (*Shan Yao*), 20g each, Radix Pseudostellariae Heterophyllae (*Tai Zi Shen*) and uncooked Radix Rehmanniae (*Sheng Di*), 15g each, Rhizoma Coptidis Chinensis (*Huang Lian*), 10g, and Cortex Radicis Moutan (*Dan Pi*), 6g. One *ji* was decocted in water and administered per day. Those in the combined therapy group with this pattern also were treated once each day with acupuncture at *San Yin Jiao* (Sp 6) for 20 minutes each time.

Those in the qi and yin dual vacuity group received the following medicinals: uncooked Radix Astragali Membranacei (*Huang Qi*), 30g, Radix Codonopsitis Pilosulae (*Dang Shen*), Radix Glehniae Littoralis (*Sha Shen*), and Radix Puerariae (*Ge Gen*), 20g each, and Radix Disocoreae Oppositae (*Shan Yao*), 15g. Those in the combined therapy group with this pattern were also needled daily at *San Yin Jiao* (Sp 6) and *Zu San Li* (St 36) for 20 minutes each time.

Those in the yin and yang dual vacuity group received the following medicinals: uncooked Radix Astragali Membranacei (*Huang Qi*), 30g, uncooked Radix Rehmanniae (*Sheng Di*), Radix Puerariae (*Ge Gen*), Fructus Lycii Chinensis (*Gou Qi Zi*), and Carapax Amydae Chinensis (*Bie Jia*), 20g each, Fructus Corni Officinalis (*Shan Zhu Yu*), Radix Dioscoreae Oppositae (*Shan Yao*), Semen Cuscutae Chinensis (*Tu Si Zi*), and Plastrum Testudinis (*Gui Ban*), 15g each, and Herba Epimedii (*Xian Ling Pi*), 12g. Those in the combined therapy group were also needled once per day at *San Yin Jiao* (Sp 6) and *Zu San*

Li (St 36) and moxaed with a moxa roll for 20 minutes each time, two times per day at *Yong Quan* (Ki 1).

Thirty days after initiating this protocol, a marked effect was defined as FBG less than 6.11mmol/L, two hour PPBG less than 11.1mmol/L or FBG and PPBG less than before treatment by more than 5.0mmol/L. Some effect meant that FBG was 6.11-7.8mmol/L, two hour PPBG was 11.1-15.0mmol/L, or both FBG and PPBG had been lowered between 3-5mmol/L. No effect meant that FBG was more than 7.8mmol/L, two hour PPBG was more than 15mmol/L, or both FBG and PPBG had decreased less than 3mmol/L. Based on these criteria, 15 patients in the Chinese medicinals group only got a marked effect, 12 got some effect, and eight got no effect for a total amelioration rate of 77.1%. In the combined therapy group, 29 got a marked effect, five got some effect, and only one got no effect, for a total amelioration rate of 97.1%.

Li Guang-ping, "The Treatment of 30 Cases of Sulfonylurea-type Hypoglycemic Medicine Subsequent Loss of Effectiveness with Integrated Chinese-Western Medicine," *Fu Jian Zhong Yi Yao (Fujian Chinese Medicine & Medicinals)*, #6, 2000, p. 13-14: Thirty patients were treated in this study. All had been taking sulfonylurea-type hypoglycemic drugs which had been effective for one year but which had then become ineffective. Fasting blood glucose in all these patients was equal or more than 10mmol/L, and glycosylated hemoglobin was equal or more than 9.5%. Among these 30 patients, there were 14 males and 16 females. Eighteen were taking oral glyburide and 12 were taking gliclazide. The median age was 55.8 ± 3.4 years, and the median duration of DM was 6.5 ± 0.9 years. All had varying degrees of fatigue and lack of strength in the four limbs.

In terms of treatment, on top of their Western hypoglycemic medications, all the patients in this study were administered the following Chinese medicinals: Radix Astragali Membranacei (*Huang Qi*), Radix Dioscoreae Oppositae (*Shan Yao*), Rhizoma Polygonati (*Huang Jing*), and Radix Pseudostellariae Heterophyllae (*Tai Zi Shen*), 30g each, Rhizoma Atractylodis Macrocephalae (*Bai Zhu*), Sclerotium Poriae Cocos (*Fu Ling*), Endoethelium Corneum Gigeriae Galli (*Ji Nei Jin*), and Radix Angelicae Sinensis (*Dang Gui*), 15g each, Radix Platycodi Grandiflori (*Jie Geng*), 10g, and uncooked pork pancreas, 1/3 of a whole one. One *ji* of these medicinals were decocted in water per day and administered orally in three divided doses for eight weeks.

In terms of treatment outcomes, FBG went from a median 12.78 ± 2.1mmol/L before treatment to 8.2 ± 1.34mmol/L after treatment. Two hour PPBG went from a median 20.8 ± 3.28mmol/L before treatment to 12.5 ± 3.2mmol/L after treatment. Glycosylated hemoglobin went from a median of 12.8 ± 1.2mmol/L before treatment to 8.8 ± 0.9mmol/L after treatment. Total cholesterol went from a median 5.89 ± 0.37 before treatment to 5.98 ± 0.26mmol/L after treatment. Triglycerides went from a median 1.96 ± 0.32 before treatment to 1.63 ± 0.65mmol/L after treatment.

Zhou Jun-huai, "The Integrated Chinese-Western Medical Treatment of 50 Cases of Type II Diabetes," *Hu Nan Zhong Yi Za Zhi (Hunan Journal of Chinese Medicine)*, #2, 2001, p. 44: Altogether, there were 100 patients in this study, all of whom had been diagnosed with type 2 diabetes by 1985 WHO criteria. These patients were evenly divided into a treatment and a comparison group. In the treatment group, there were 32 males and 18 females aged 39-75 years, with an average age of 51.8 years. Their course of disease had lasted from two months to eight years. Six patients were able to control their blood sugar by dietary restrictions alone. The other 44 used sulfonylurea-type medications. In the comparison group, there were 28 males and 22 females aged 41-77 years, with an average age of 53.7 years. These patients' course of disease had lasted from four months to nine years. Four of these patients were able to control their blood sugar through diet alone, while the other 46 used suflonylurea-type medications.

In terms of treatment, those in the comparison group were also administered 0.25mg of dimethylbiguanide three times per day. Those in the treatment group were given the same Western medical treatment as the comparison group plus the following self-composed Chinese medicinal formula: uncooked Radix Astragali Membranacei (*Huang Qi*), 40g, Radix Salviae Miltiorrhizae (*Dan Shen*), Rhizoma Alismatis (*Ze Xie*), and Radix Trichosanthis Kirlowii (*Tian Hua Fen*), 20g each, Tuber Ophiopogonis Japonici (*Mai Men Dong*), Radix Dioscoreae Oppositae (*Shan Yao*), and Radix Panacis Ginseng (*Ren Shen*), 15g each, and Fructus Schisandrae Chinensis (*Wu Wei Zi*) and Herba Dendrobii (*Shi Hu*), 10g each. One *ji* of these medicinals was decocted in water and administered per day continuously for two months. Suitable additions and subtractions were made based on the clinical signs and symptoms.

Marked effect was defined as FBG less than 6.0mmol/L and PPBG less than 8.0mmol/L. Typical effect was defined as FBG more than 6.0mmol/L and less than 7.8mmol/L and PPBG more than 8.0mmol/L and less than 10.0mmol/L. Relatively poor effect was defined as FBG more than 7.8mmol/L and PPBG more than 10.0mmol/L. Based on these criteria, 40 cases (80%) of the patients in

the treatment group were judged to have gotten a marked effect, eight (16%) got a typical effect, and two (4%) got a poor effect in terms of FBG. In terms of PPBG, 40 cases (80%) in the treatment group got a marked effect, nine (18%) got a typical effect, and one (2%) got a poor effect. In the comparison group, in terms of FBG, 20 (40%) got a marked effect, 25 (50%) got a typical effect, and five (10%) got a poor effect. In terms of PPBG, 14 (28%) got a marked effect, 26 (52%) got a typical effect, and 10 (20%) got a poor effect. According to the author, this study suggests that dimethylbiguanide is more effective for lowering blood glucose when administered with Chinese medicinals.

Wang Jun-hua & Wang Cheng-cui, "The Treatment of 30 Cases of Type II Diabetes with Integrated Chinese-Western Medicine," *Shan Xi Zhong Yi (Shanxi Chinese Medicine)*, #2, 2001, p. 25-26: There were 60 patients altogether in this study, all of whom were diagnosed with type 2 diabetes according to 1985 WHO criteria. These 60 patients were divided into two groups, a treatment group which received both Chinese and Western medicine and a comparison group which received only Western medicine. There were 13 men and 17 women in the treatment group aged 41-70, with an average age of 58. These patients had had diabetes for 2-18 years, with an average disease duration of six years. In the comparison group, there were 14 men and 16 women aged 40-60, with an average age of 53 years. They had been ill from eight months to 18 years, with an average disease course of 5.6 years. Hence there was no marked statistical difference between these two groups in terms of age, sex, or disease duration.

Patients in the treatment group received the following Chinese medicinals: Radix Dioscoreae Oppositae (*Shan Yao*), 30g, Rhizoma Coptidis Chinensis (*Huang Lian*), uncooked Radix Rehmanniae (*Sheng Di*), Radix Astragali Membranacei (*Huang Qi*), and Semen Coicis Lachryma-jobi (*Yi Yi Ren*), 15g each, and Radix Puerariae (*Ge Gen*), Radix Trichosanthis Kirlowii (*Tian Hua Fen*), Rhizoma Atractylodis (*Cang Zhu*), Sclerotium Poriae Cocos (*Fu Ling*), and Pericarpium Citri Reticulatae (*Chen Pi*), 12g each. If there was torpid intake, Rhizoma Atractylodis Macrocephalae (*Bai Zhu*) and Endothelium Corneum Gigeriae Galli (*Ji Nei Jin*) to fortify the spleen and disperse food. If there was abdominal distention, Fructus Citri Aurantii (*Zhi Ke*) and Semen Raphani Sativi (*Lai Fu Zi*) were added to rectify the qi and disperse distention. If there was blood stasis, Radix Salviae Miltiorrhizae (*Dan Shen*) was added to quicken the blood and transform stasis. If there was fever, Flos Lonicerae Japonicae (*Jin Yin Hua*) and Fructus Forsythiae Suspensae (*Lian Qiao*) were added to clear heat and resolve toxins. And if there were either epistaxis or bleeding gums, Radix Pseudoginseng (*San Qi*) and Radix Rubiae Cordifoliae (*Qian Cao Gen*) were added to stop bleeding. One *ji* of these medicinals was decocted in water and administered per day in two or three divided doses. In addition, all patients in both the treatment and comparison groups received glyburide. If FBG was 7.8-11.9mmol/L, the dose of glyburide was 2.5mg per day. If FBG was equal to or more than 12.0mmol/L, the dose was 2.5mg BID. If there were other concomitant conditions, those conditions also received standard Western medical treatment. Both groups underwent treatment for four weeks.

Marked effect was defined as disappearance or basic disappearance of clinical symptoms, FBG less than 7.2mmol/L, and two hour PPBG less than 8.3mmol/L. Improvement was defined as decrease in symptoms, FBG less than 8.3mmol/L, and two hour PPBG less than 10.0mmol/L. No effect meant that there was no obvious improvement in symptoms and blood glucose did not meet the above requirements. Based on these criteria, eight cases in the treatment group got a marked effect, 13 got some effect, and nine got no effect, for a total amelioration rate of 70.0%. In the comparison group, three cases got a marked effect, seven got some effect, and 20 got no effect, for a total amelioration rate of 33.3%. Therefore, there was a significant difference in outcomes between these two groups suggesting that glyburide is more effective when combined with individually prescribed Chinese medicinals.

Qing Zhao-qian, "A Survey of the Treatment of 60 Cases of Type II Diabetes with *Shen Qi Yu Xiao Tang* (Ginseng & Astragalus Cure Wasting Decoction – Plus a Comparison with 30 Cases Treated with Gliclazide," *Zhe Jiang Zhong Yi Za Zhi* (*Zhejiang Journal of Chinese Medicine*), #5, 2001, p. 190-191: All 90 patients in this study were diagnosed with type 2 DM according to 1985 WHO criteria. Further, all were diagnosed as exhibiting the pattern of qi and yin dual vacuity. Fifty-two of these patients were in-patients and 38 were out-patients. In the treatment group of 60 patients, 27 were male and 33 were female, aged 38-72, with a median age of 58.27 ± 8.42 years and a disease course of 0.5-19 years, with a median disease duration of 11.15 ± 2.56 years. Twenty-nine cases had accompanying high cholesterol, 26 had hypertension, 34 had coronary heart disease, 20 had fatty livers, nine had retinopathy, eight had peripheral neuropathy, and six had nephropathy. Among the 30 patients in the so-called comparison group, there were 12 males and 18 females aged 39-73, with a median age of 57.33 ± 7.59 years and a disease course of 0.5-18 years, with a median duration of 10.29 ± 2.37 years. In this group, 14 cases had accompanying

hyperlipidemia, 12 had hypertension, 16 had coronary heart disease, nine had fatty livers, six had retinopathy, five had peripheral neuropathy, and two had kidney disease. Therefore, there was no marked statistical difference in age, sex, disease course, or accompanying conditions between these two groups.

The treatment group were given the following Chinese medicinals: Radix Astragali Membranacei (*Huang Qi*), 30g, Radix Pseudostellariae Heterophyllae (*Tai Zi Shen*), and Radix Dioscoreae Oppositae (*Shan Yao*), 20g each, Radix Glehniae Littoralis (*Sha Shen*), Radix Scrophulariae Ningpoensis (*Xuan Shen*), Rhizoma Polygonati (*Huang Jing*), and uncooked Radix Rehmanniae (*Sheng Di*), 15g each, Rhizoma Polygonati Odorati (*Yu Zhu*), 12g, Radix Panacis Ginseng (*Ren Shen*) and Fructus Corni Officinalis (*Shan Zhu Yu*), 10g each, and Fructus Schisandrae Chinensis (*Wu Wei Zi*), 6g. One *ji* of these medicinals was decocted in water and administered per day. One month equaled one course of treatment, and, typically, patients underwent three courses before evaluation. In the comparison group, patients were administered 80mg of gliclazide TID. After three weeks of this regime, patients' dosages were adjusted up or down as necessary to a maximum of 240mg per day. As in the treatment group, one month equaled one course of treatment, and patients typically underwent three courses of treatment before evaluation.

Marked effect was defined as basic disappearance or marked reduction of symptoms, FBG less than 7.2mmol/L or decreased by 30%, and PPBG less than 8.3mmol/L or decreased by 30%. Some effect meant that there was marked improvement in symptoms, FBG was less than 8.3mmol/L, and PPBG was less than 10.0mmol/L or reduced by more than 10%. No effect meant that there were no obvious improvements in symptoms and no lowering of FBG or PPBG. Based on these criteria, in the treatment group, 24 cases (40%) were judged to have experienced a marked effect, 33 (55%) got some effect, and three cases (5%) got no effect, for a total amelioration rate of 95%. In the comparison group, 12 cases (40%) got a marked effect, 11 cases (36.7%) got some effect, and seven cases (23.3%) got no effect, for a total amelioration rate of 76.7%. Therefore, there was a marked statistical difference in the outcomes of these two groups. In addition, median reductions in fasting and postprandial blood glucose were markedly greater in the treatment group as opposed to the comparison group.

Chen Jian-fei, "A Hemorrheological Study on the Effect of Acupuncture in Treating Diabetes Mellitus," *Journal of Traditional Chinese Medicine*, #2, 1987, p. 95-100: For four years, the author performed rheological studies on 20 patients with diabetes. Of this group, eight were male and 12 were female. Their ages ranged from 16-82 years old. Their course of disease ranged from two months to 23 years, with nine cases having suffered for over five years. Seventeen cases were non-insulin dependent and three cases were insulin-dependent. The median FBG was 240.5 ±18.05 mg/dL. The patients were divided into two groups. The acupuncture only group consisted solely of type 2 patients, and the acupuncture plus drug group was comprised of both type 1 and 2 patients with insufficient insulin secretion. This second group received insulin or oral hypoglycemic drugs in addition to acupuncture treatment if, after one course of treatment, they did not have any marked blood glucose reduction. Two groups of acupuncture points were used. The ruling points were *Zu San Li* (St 36), *Pi Shu* (Bl 20), and *Ge Shu* (Bl 17). The additional points, applied according to the patients' patterns, were *Fei Shu* (Bl 13), *Wei Shu* (Bl 21), *Shen Shu* (Bl 23), *Zhong Wan* (CV 12), *Qu Chi* (LI 11), *Feng Long* (St 40), *Fu Liu* (Ki 7), *Yin Ling Quan* (Sp 9), *Di Ji* (Sp 8), and/or *San Yin Jiao* (Sp 6).

Blood tests for viscosity were taken before and after acupuncture, with improved results in both treatment groups (P < 0.001-0.01). The acupuncture plus drug group experienced better results than the acupuncture only group, with total amelioration rates of 77.1% and 94% respectively. In addition, the hematocrit, sedimentation rate, and sedimentation rate equation K values were all markedly reduced after acupuncture treatment. These rates were 78.6%, 85.7%, and 71.4% respectively. The acupuncture plus drug group also experienced reductions in fibrinogen and prothrombin levels after acupuncture. The average blood sugar level of patients in the acupuncture group was 227.9 mg/dL before treatment and 138.9 mg/dL after treatment. Of the 14 patients in that group, seven experienced marked improvement, three experienced some improvement, and one got no results. The six patients in the acupuncture plus drug group had an average blood glucose level of 322.5 mg/dL before treatment and 157.3 mg/dL after treatment. In this group, there were two cases who experienced marked improvement, three cases who got some improvement, and one case which got no results. The acupuncture treatment group had a higher amelioration rate than the acupuncture plus drug group (93% and 86% respectively). Both groups also had lowered levels of cholesterol and triglycerides. The average cholesterol of the patients was 204.7 mg/dL, and the average triglyceride was 161.2 mg/dL before treatment. After treatment, the average cholesterol level dropped by 41.7 mg/dL and triglyceride dropped as much as 49.4 mg/dL.

Lin Yun-gui *et al.*, "Treatment of Diabetes with Moxibustion," *Journal of Traditional Chinese Medicine*, #1, 1987, p. 12-14: A group of 13 patients with diabetes with blood sugar levels above 150 mg/dL were treated with moxibustion. All the patients had high blood sugar levels even though they regulated their diets and took oral medications (one of the patients also took insulin in addition to oral medication). There were seven men in the study and six women. One was between 31-39 years of age, five were between 40-49 years of age, and seven were between 50-59 years of age. The duration of illness was two years for one patient, 3-5 years for six patients, and over six years for one patient. Before moxibustion treatment, the blood sugar levels ranged between 150-250 mg/dL, with an average of 175 mg/dL.

Moxa cones were used (1.5cm in diameter and 2cm long) supported on fresh ginger slices (2cm in diameter and 3-4mm thick). The acupuncture points were grouped and used alternately, with nine additional points applied according to the patients' patterns. Ten to 30 moxa cones were used on each point, with treatment every other day, each treatment lasting over three hours. Each course of treatment was composed of 25 sessions. The acupuncture points were grouped as follows and used alternately:

1. *Zu San Li* (St 36), *Zhong Wan* (CV 12)
2. *Ming Men* (GV 4), *Shen Zhu* (GV 12), *Pi Shu* (Bl 20)
3. *Qi Hai* (CV 6), *Guan Men* (St 22)
4. *Ji Zhong* (GV 6), *Shen Shu* (Bl 23)
5. *Hua Gai* (CV 20), *Liang Men* (St 21)
6. *Da Zhui* (GV 14), *Gan Shu* (Bl 18)
7. *Xing Jian* (Liv 2), *Zhong Ji* (CV 3), *Fu Ai* (Sp 16)
8. *Fei Shu* (Bl 13), *Ge Shu* (Bl 17), *Shen Shu* (Bl 23)

For upper wasting with polydipsia, *Jin Jin & Yu Ye* (M-HN-20, acupuncture), *Nei Guan* (Per 6), *Yu Ji* (Lu 10), and *Shao Fu* (Ht 8) were added. For middle wasting, *Pi Shu* (Bl 20) and *Da Du* (Sp 2) were added. For lower wasting with polyuria, *Ran Gu* (Ki 2) and *Yong Quan* (Ki 1) were added. Fasting blood sugar tests were performed daily, and all oral medications and insulin were discontinued during this moxibustion study. At the end of one course of treatment the average blood sugar level was 138 mg/dL. After the second course of treatment, the average blood sugar level was 130 mg/dL.

Li Yi, "The Treatment of 26 Cases of Diabetes Using the Methods of Boosting the Qi, Nourishing Yin & Quickening the Blood," *Yun Nan Zhong Yi Zhong Yao Za Zhi (Yunnan Journal of Chinese Medicine & Medicinals)*, #1, 1997, p. 12: The fasting blood glucose for most of the patients in this study was more than 7.8 mmol/L, and the urine glucose test was positive. Of the group, six patients were male, and 20 were female. The youngest was 38 years old, and the oldest was 68, with an average age of 53 years. The shortest duration of illness was six months; the longest was eight years.

The prescription consisted of: uncooked Radix Rehmanniae (*Sheng Di*), Radix Dioscoreae Oppositae (*Shan Yao*), Radix Astragali Membrancei (*Huang Qi*), and Cortex Ziziphi (*Huai Zao Pi*), 30g each, Rhizoma Atractylodis (*Cang Zhu*), Radix Scrophulariae Ningpoensis (*Xuan Shen*), Rhizoma Polygonati (*Huang Jing*), and Rhizoma Polygonati Odorati (*Yu Zhu*), 20g each, Radix Salviae Miltiorrhizae (*Dan Shen*), Herba Dendrobii (*Shi Hu*), and Rhizoma Anemarrhenae Aspheloidis (*Zhi Mu*), 15g each, and Fructus Gardeniae Jasminoidis (*Zhi Zi*) and Endothelium Corneum Gigeriae Galli (*Ji Nei Jin*), 12g each. For dry mouth and extreme thirst, Radix Trichosanthis Kirlowii (*Tian Hua Fen*) and Fructus Pruni Mume (*Wu Mei*) were added. For lower burner damp heat and genital itching, Cortex Phellodendri (*Huang Bai*) was added. For copious, clear urination, Ootheca Mantidis (*Sang Piao Xiao*) and Fructus Schisandrae Chinensis (*Wu Wei Zi*) were added. For shortness of breath and disinclination to speak, Radix Pseudostellariae (*Tai Zi Shen*) and Radix Panacis Qinquefolii (*Xi Yang Shen*) were added. For low back and lower limb aching and limpness, Cortex Eucommiae Ulmoidis (*Du Zhong*) was added. If there was unclear vision, then Scapus Et Inflorescentia Eriocaulonis Buergeriani (*Gu Jing Cao*) was added. If there was insomnia and profuse dreams, then Semen Zizyphi Spinosae (*Suan Zao Ren*) and Caulis Polygoni Multiflori (*Ye Jiao Teng*) were added. One *ji* was administered per day, and two weeks constituted one course of treatment. In addition, patients were counseled on controlling the amount of food eaten and avoiding acrid, peppery, greasy, and sweet foods.

Patients were considered recovered if the FBG was less than 6.7mmol/L, urine glucose was negative, and the symptoms disappeared. Patients were considered to have had gotten a good effect if the FBG was less than 9.4mmol/L, urine glucose was negative, and the symptoms had improved. Patients were considered to have gotten no effect if the FBG was more than 9.4mmol/L, urine glucose was positive, and the clinical symptoms were only slightly better. Based on these criteria, eight cases were considered recovered (30.77%), 15 cases were considered to have gotten a good effect (57.69%), and three cases were considered to have gotten no effect (11.53%), for a total amelioration rate of 88.64%. The shortest course of treatment was two weeks, and the longest was six weeks. The average treatment time was four weeks.

Luo Shan, "The Treatment of Diabetes Using the Methods of Boosting the Qi, Enriching Yin & Draining Fire," *Hu Bei Zhong Yi Za Zhi (Hubei Journal of Chinese Medicine)*, #3, 1998, p. 41-42: Among the 50 patients in this study, 31 were male and 19 were female. Two patients were 20 years of age or younger, 38 patients were between 21-60 years of age, and 10 patients were older than 60 years of age. For 24 patients, the duration of illness was under a year; for 22 patients, the duration was 1-5 years; and for four patients, the duration of illness was more than five years. For 11 patients, FBG was 6.1-10.08mmol/L; for 23 patients, FBG was 10.09-12.32mmol/L; and for 16 patients, FBG was higher than 12.32mmol/L. The urine glucose test was (++) for four patients, (+++) for 17 patients, and (++++) for 29 patients. Eight patients also had cardiovascular disease, nine had cerebrovascular disease, two had pulmonary tuberculosis, 14 had urinary infections, five patients had boils, six had biliary infections, seven had peripheral neuritis, and seven had visual disturbances.

The basic prescription consisted of: uncooked Radix Astragali Membrancei (*Huang Qi*), Radix Dioscoreae Oppositae (*Shan Yao*), and Radix Trichosanthis Kirlowii (*Tian Hua Fen*), 30g each, Fructus Corni Officinalis (*Shan Zhu Yu*), 20g, Rhizoma Atractylodis Macrocephalae (*Bai Zhu*), uncooked Radix Rehmanniae (*Sheng Di*), Radix Scrophulariae Ningpoensis (*Xuan Shen*), Cortex Radicis Moutan (*Dan Pi*), Tuber Ophiopogonis Japonici (*Mai Men Dong*), and Fructus Schisandrae Chinensis (*Wu Wei Zi*), 15g each, and Radix Panacis Qinquefolii (*Xi Yang Shen*) (or Radix Pseudostellariae Heterophyllae [*Tai Zi Shen*]), 10g. For vexatious thirst with desire for liquids and profuse urination, a red tongue with thin fur, rapid pulse, and other marked heat signs, Gypsum Fibrosum (*Shi Gao*), Rhizoma Anemarrhenae Aspheloidis (*Zhi Mu*), and Rhizoma Coptidis Chinensis (*Huang Lian*) were added. For ravenous hunger, cooked Radix Rehmanniae (*Shu Di*) was added. For frequent, profuse, and clear urination and a very weak cubit pulse suggesting vacuity cold, Cortex Cinnamomi Cassiae (*Rou Gui*), Radix Lateralis Praeparatus Aconiti Carmichaeli (*Fu Zi*), Radix Morindae Officinalia (*Ba Ji Tian*), and Ootheca Mantidis (*Sang Piao Xiao*) were added. For profuse sweating, Os Draconis (*Long Gu*) and Concha Ostreae (*Mu Li*) were added. When angina or coronary heart disease was present, Fructus Trichosanthis Kirlowii (*Quan Gua Lou*), Radix Pseudoginseng (*San Qi*), and Radix Salviae Miltiorrhizae (*Dan Shen*) were added. In addition, any infections, peripheral neuritis, and/or visual disturbances were treated with appropriate medicinals. One *ji* was administered per day on an empty stomach, and 20 days constituted one course of treatment. The routine use of Western drugs to reduce glucose levels in the blood and urine was continued until the glucose levels dropped, at which time the drugs were discontinued. Using this protocol, 19 patients recovered, 30 had some improvement, and one got no result.

REPRESENTATIVE CASE HISTORIES:

CASE 1[2]

The patient was an adult male of unspecified age who was first examined on Jun. 2, 1975. The man's desire for food had increased and he rapidly hungered. If he did not eat, his stomach clamored and he had borborygmus. His mouth was dry with a desire to drink. His symptoms were consistent with upper thirsting and middle wasting. The patient's tongue was red with thin fur, and his pulse was small and slippery. The man was diagnosed as suffering from diabetes, and his patterns were categorized as stomach bowel blazing heat with spleen movement loss of normalcy. Therefore, the treatment principles were to nourish the stomach and clear heat, supplement the spleen and rectify the qi. The following medicinals were prescribed based on these principles: uncooked Gypsum Fibrosum (*Shi Gao*), 15g, uncooked Radix Rehmanniae (*Sheng Di*), 12g, Radix Codonopsitis Pilosulae (*Dang Shen*), stir-fried Rhizoma Atractylodis Macrocephalae (*Bai Zhu*), Sclerotium Poriae Cocos (*Fu Ling*), Folium Lophatheri Gracilis (*Dan Zhu Ye*), processed Rhizoma Cyperi Rotundi (*Xiang Fu*), Rhizoma Anemarrhenae Aspheloidis (*Zhi Mu*), and uncooked Semen Coicis Lachryma-jobi (*Yi Yi Ren*), 9g each, and Radix Puerariae (*Ge Gen*) and Radix Auklandiae Lappae (*Mu Xiang*), 4.5g each.

The second examination occurred on Jun. 9. After taking the above medicinals, the man's dry mouth had decreased and his clamoring stomach and rapid hungering were also less. However, he still had abdominal distention and borborygmus, his pulse was still small and slippery, and his tongue was still red with thin fur. In addition, its center was fissured and cracked. Therefore, the treatment principles were changed to clear stomach heat and nourish fluids and humors, for which the formula was: uncooked Gypsum Fibrosum (*Shi Gao*), 15g, Rhizoma Anemarrhenae Aspheloidis (*Zhi Mu*), Radix Codonopsitis Pilosulae (*Dang Shen*), Sclerotium Poriae Cocos (*Fu Ling*), uncooked Radix Rehmanniae (*Sheng Di*), Folium Lophatheri Gracilis (*Dan Zhu Ye*), uncooked Semen Coicis Lachryma-jobi (*Yi Yi Ren*), and processed Rhizoma Cyperi Rotundi (*Xiang Fu*), 9g each, and Radix Puerariae (*Ge Gen*) and Radix Auklandiae Lappae (*Mu Xiang*), 4.5g each.

The third examination occurred on Jun. 16. At this point, the abdominal distention and borborygmus had receded and the clamoring stomach and rapid hungering had disappeared. Oral dryness was better, but there was a sensation of dizziness and head distention. The root of the patient's tongue had slimy fur, the central fissures had receded, and his pulse was still small and slippery. This suggested that the stomach heat had been eliminated. Therefore, the patient was administered spleen-supplementing, stomach-nourishing ingredients to secure and consolidate the treatment effects: Radix Codonopsitis Pilosulae (*Dang Shen*), stir-fried Rhizoma Atractylodis Macrocephalae (*Bai Zhu*), Sclerotium Poriae Cocos (*Fu Ling*), Rhizoma Anemarrhenae Aspheloidis (*Zhi Mu*), and uncooked and cooked Semen Germinatus Oryzae Sativae (*Gu Ya*), 9g each, and stir-fried Fructus Citri Aurantii (*Zhi Ke*), Radix Puerariae (*Ge Gen*), and mix-fried Radix Glycyrrhizae (*Gan Cao*), 3g.

CASE 2[3]

The patient was a 57 year-old agricultural worker who was first examined on Sept. 16, 1981. For the previous four years, the man had had polydipsia and polyuria and had been diagnosed at a local hospital as suffering from diabetes. The patient had been treated with both Chinese and Western medicines and the severity of his condition had decreased. However, six months before, the disease had recurred and his symptoms had increased. His mouth was dry with a desire to drink. In fact, he drank 5000ml per day. His urination had also increased to 4000ml per day. This was accompanied by a decrease in appetite, fatigue, lack of strength, emission of chill on both lower limbs, a sensation of bodily heat, easy perspiration on movement, and occasional spasms within his penis. The patient's blood pressure was 110/70, and his pulse rate was 76 BPM. Respiration was 18 times per minute, and body temperature was 36.8°C. Blood glucose was 234mg/dL, and urine glucose was (+++). The man's tongue was pale with white fur, and his pulse was deep, fine, and weak.

Based on the above signs and symptoms, this patient's pattern was categorized as kidney qi vacuity with loss of regulation of water and fire and ministerial fire flaming upward, brewing and binding in the center. Therefore, the man was prescribed *Jin Gui Shen Qi Wan Jia Jian* (*Golden Cabinet* Kidney Qi Pills with Additions & Subtractions): cooked Radix Rehmanniae (*Shu Di*), 18g, Radix Polygoni Multiflori (*He Shou Wu*) and Radix Dioscoreae Oppositae (*Shan Yao*), 12g each, Sclerotium Poriae Cocos (*Fu Ling*), Cortex Radicis Moutan (*Dan Pi*), Rhizoma Alismatis (*Ze*

Xie), and Fructus Schisandrae Chinensis (Wu Wei Zi), 10g each, and Ramulus Cinnamomi Cassiae (Gui Zhi), 6g.

After taking six ji of the above formula, the man's drinking and urinating was cut in half. Therefore, he was represcribed 30 ji of the same formula plus Radix Morindae Officinalis (Ba Ji Tian), Herba Epimedii (Xian Ling Pi), Semen Trigonellae Foeni-graeci (Hu Lu Ba), and Fructus Foeniculi Vulgaris (Xiao Hui Xiang), after which, the patient's drinking and urinating were normal. the man's psyche improved, his fear of cold disappeared, his blood glucose dropped to 94.7mg/dL, and his urine glucose turned negative. The same formula was continued in order to secure and consolidate the treatment effect until the patient was discharged from the hospital on Nov. 4 of the same year. On follow-up some time later, there had been no recurrence.

CASE 3[4]

The patient was a 59 year-old female who was first examined on May 16, 1979. Three months previous, the patient's mouth had become dry and thirsty and she had begun drinking more water. This was then accompanied by frequent, excessive urination. Gradually, she had become fatigued and had lost her strength. Other signs and symptoms included spontaneous perspiration, night sweats, shortness of breath, emaciation. The woman's doctor had increased her treatment for pulmonary tuberculosis, but this had not had any effect on the above symptoms. Therefore, she was sent to Dr. Du for examination. In addition to the above, Dr. Du found a low, faint voice, scanty appetite, lack of taste, a pale tongue with white fur, and a fine pulse which was weak at both cubits. X-rays did not show any abnormalities. Blood glucose was 346mg/dL, and urine glucose was (+++). Therefore, the woman was diagnosed with diabetes.

Based on her signs and symptoms, Dr. Du discriminated this patient's pattern as lung-spleen qi vacuity with kidney yang insufficiency. Therefore, based on the treatment principles of supplementing the kidney source, fortifying and moving spleen earth, and supplementing and boosting the lung qi, she was prescribed the following Chinese medicinals: Radix Dioscoreae Oppositae (Shan Yao), Semen Astragali Complanati (Sha Yuan Zi), and Fructus Rosae Laevigatae (Jin Ying Zi), 15g each, Sclerotium Poriae Cocos (Fu Ling), Fructus Lycii Chinensis (Gou Qi Zi), and Radix Puerariae (Ge Gen), 12g each, uncooked Radix Rehmanniae (Sheng Di), cooked Radix Rehmanniae (Shu Di), Rhizoma Alismatis (Ze Xie), Cortex Radicis Moutan (Dan Pi), Fructus Corni Officinalis (Shan Zhu Yu), Tuber

Ophiopogonis Japonici (Mai Men Dong), and Fructus Immaturus Citri Aurantii (Zhi Shi), 9g each, and Radix Lateralis Praeparatus Aconiti Carmichaeli (Fu Zi) and Ramulus Cinnamomi Cassiae (Gui Zhi), 6g each.

On the second examination which occurred on June 19, the woman had taken 17 ji of the above medicinals and her polydipsia and polyuria had markedly decreased. Her sweating had also decreased and her psyche had improved. Her pulse had become bowstring and fine, while her tongue was pale red with thin, yellow fur. Urine glucose was (++). Therefore, 15 grams of Rhizoma Polygonati (Huang Jing) and nine grams of Radix Trichosanthis Kirlowii (Tian Hua Fen) were added to the original formula.

On Jul. 20, the woman was seen for the third time by Dr. Du. Over the intervening time, all the patient's symptoms had gradually improved. However, she was still short of breath and had a dry mouth. Blood glucose was 300mg/dL, and urine glucose was (+-++). Therefore 10 grams each of cooked Radix Rehmanniae (Shu Di) and uncooked Radix Rehmanniae (Sheng Di) were added to the above formula as well as three grams of Radix Panacis Ginseng (Ren Shen) and 1.5 grams of Rhizoma Coptidis Chinensis (Huang Lian). At the same time, the Dan Pi and Mai Men Dong were removed. In mid-December, the woman was seen for the fourth time, and all her symptoms had been eliminated. Her blood glucose was 123mg/dL, and urine glucose was (-). The patient stopped taking the medicinals for two months and, when re-examined, there had been no recurrence. She was instructed on proper dietary therapy. Ten years later on follow-up there had still been no recurrence.

CASE 4[5]

The patient was a 66 year-old male who was first examined on August 7, 1985. The man complained of chest pain and dizziness. He had already been diagnosed with coronary artery disease and high blood pressure for 10 years. Over the last half year, the man's lower limbs had become numb and he had developed oral thirst and rapid hungering. The patient's blood glucose was 267mg/dL and urine glucose was (+++). The patient was placed on Western hypoglycemic medications which were effective. However, when the man stopped taking these, his blood sugar increased again. The man was addicted to alcohol and fatty, salty foods. His body was robust and his upper abdomen was potbellied. His lips were purple and dark and he had extremely foul breath. There was oral thirst and a desire to drink, increased intake of grains, and constipation. His urine was yellow but its amount was not excessive. The man's tongue was red and fissured in the center with scanty fur. His pulse was fine, rapid, bow-string, and slippery.

Based on these signs and symptoms, the patient's pattern was discriminated as central fire blazing and exuberant with stomach yin depletion and consumption and heat stasis in the blood network vessels. The treatment principles were to enrich and moisten dry earth, clear and discharge evil fire, cool the blood and free the flow of the network vessels. Therefore, he was prescribed the following medicinals: Radix Trichosanthis Kirlowii (*Tian Hua Fen*), fresh Rhizoma Imperatae Cylindricae (*Bai Mao Gen*), and Rhizoma Phragmitis Communis (*Lu Gen*), 60g each, uncooked Gypsum Fibrosum (*Shi Gao*), 50g, uncooked Radix Rehmanniae (*Sheng Di*), Radix Scrophulariae Ningpoensis (*Xuan Shen*), Herba Lycopi Lucidi (*Ze Lan*), and Semen Trichosanthis Kirlowii (*Gua Lou Ren*), 30g each, and Cortex Radicis Moutan (*Dan Pi*) and Radix Pseudostellariae Heterophyllae (*Tai Zi Shen*), 10g each.

After taking the above medicinals continuously for half a month, all the patient's symptoms greatly decreased. Therefore, he was prescribed the same formula minus *Shi Gao, Gua Lou Ren*, and *Dan Pi* and with *Tian Hua Fen, Bai Mao Gen*, and *Lu Gen* reduced to 30 grams each. In addition, 30 grams of Radix Dioscoreae Oppositae (*Shan Yao*) were added. This prescription was administered for three months, after which the patient's blood glucose was normal and his urine glucose was negative. The man was counseled on his alcohol consumption, was forbidden sweets and fats, and recommended to control his intake of carbohydrates at the same time as increasing his intake of vegetables and bean products.

CASE 5[6]

The patient was a 46 year old male who habitually ate fatty, sweet foods. During the previous three years, due to excessive taxation and fatigue and emotional discomfort, the man had come to feel a lack of strength in his body and limbs accompanied by vexatious thirst and a predilection for drinking, frequent, numerous, excessive urination, a sweet, bitter taste and slimy feeling in his mouth, constant hunger, occasional abdominal glomus and fullness, borborygmus, constipation, emaciation, low back and knee soreness and limpness, tinnitus, rough eyes, heart palpitations, insomnia, a low, faint voice, aversion to wind, and generalized pruritus. The patient's tongue fur was thick, slimy, and whitish yellow. His pulse was slippery and fine. Urine glucose was (++++), urine ketones (++), and blood glucose was 18.68mmol/L (336.6mg/dL). The diagnosis was

diabetes mellitus, and the man's patterns were categorized as heat above and vacuity below with simultaneous damp heat depression and obstruction. Therefore, treatment was to clear the upper and supplement the lower, seep dampness and discharge heat. The medicinals prescribed consisted of: uncooked Gypsum Fibrosum (*Shi Gao*), 30g, Radix Dioscoreae Oppositae (*Shan Yao*), 20g, Radix Codonopsitis Pilosulae (*Dang Shen*), Radix Astragali Membranacei (*Huang Qi*), Herba Artemisiae Capillaris (*Yin Chen Hao*), and Fructus Rosae Laevigatae (*Jin Ying Zi*), 15g each, Caulis Bambusae In Taeniis (*Zhu Ru*), Sclerotium Poriae Cocos (*Fu Ling*), and Fructus Corni Officinalis (*Shan Zhu Yu*), 12g each, and Rhizoma Anemarrhenae Aspheloidis (*Zhi Mu*), Tuber Asparagi Cochinensis (*Tian Men Dong*), and Fructus Kochiae Scopariae (*Di Fu Zi*), 9g each. One *ji* of these medicinals was decocted in water and administered per day.

After taking the above formula as an in-patient for two months, urine glucose and ketones had turned negative, blood glucose was 7.6mmol/L (137mg/dL), and all his symptoms had disappeared. Therefore, the following medicinals were made into pills: uncooked Radix Rehmanniae (*Sheng Di*), cooked Radix Rehmanniae (*Shu Di*), Fructus Corni Officinalis (*Shan Zhu Yu*), and Radix Dioscoreae Oppositae (*Shan Yao*), 40g each, Sclerotium Poriae Cocos (*Fu Ling*), Cortex Radicis Moutan (*Dan Pi*), Radix Codonopsitis Pilosulae (*Dang Shen*), Cornu Degelatinum Cervi (*Lu Jiao Shuang*), and Tuber Ophiopogonis Japonici (*Mai Men Dong*), 30g each, and Fructus Schisandrae Chinensis (*Wu Wei Zi*), 20g. These medicinals were ground into powder and made into pills with water. The patient took five grams of these each time, two times per day in order to secure and consolidate the treatment effect. On follow-up after one year, there had been no recurrence of disease.

CASE 6[7]

The patient was a 35 year old female who complained of oral thirst, excessive hunger, dizziness, head distention, heart vexation, easy anger, stomach duct glomus and fullness, and genital itching for three years. She had been previously diagnosed with diabetes and vaginitis for which she had been prescribed *Xiao Ke Wan* (Wasting & Thirsting Pills), *Gan Lu Xiao Ke Wan* (Sweet Dew Wasting & Thirsting Pills), insulin, and gliclazide with unremarkable effects. She had also been prescribed fluid-engendering, thirst-stopping, yin-nourishing ingredients without effect. Recently, the woman's eyesight had become blurred, and this was what brought her to Zhu Jin-zhong who found that her pulse was soggy and moderate (*i.e.*, relaxed or slightly slow) and her tongue had slightly slimy, white fur. Zhu categorized this woman's patterns as upper dryness and lower cold with damp depression untransformed and liver wood not spreading. Dr. Zhu thought that the previous attempts to enrich this woman's yin had strengthened dampness and caused detriment to her yang. Therefore, he prescribed *Chai Hu Gui Zhi Gan Jiang Tang Jia Jian* (Bupleurum, Cinnamon Twig & Dry Ginger Decoction with Additions & Subtractions): Radix Scrophulariae Ningpoensis (*Xuan Shen*) and Radix Trichosanthis Kirlowii (*Tian Hua Fen*), 15g each, Radix Bupleuri (*Chai Hu*), Ramulus Cinnamomi Cassiae (*Gui Zhi*), Radix Scutellariae Baicalensis (*Huang Qin*), and Concha Ostreae (*Mu Li*), 10g each, and Radix Glycyrrhizae (*Gan Cao*), 6g. After taking 15 *ji* of this formula, the patient's oral thirst and genital itching greatly decreased, her psyche improved, and her urine glucose went from (++++) to (+). Therefore, another 15 *ji* were administered, after which her genital itching disappeared, her urine glucose was (±), and all her symptoms were eliminated.

CASE 7[8]

The patient was a 70 year old female who had been diagnosed with diabetes at 50 years of age. This woman had had recurrent urinary tract infections since she was 40 and lower limb paralysis, aching, and pain for the past 20 years. In the past two years, oral thirst with a desire to drink, fatigue, lack of strength, frequent urination, urinary pain, and lower limb aching, pain, and paralysis had all gotten worse. In fact, the woman's urination had become so frequent, she was incontinent. In addition, there was severe lower limb edema, and, if she drank many fluids, this would lead to vomiting. Her lower limb pain was worse at night, and she urinated so frequently, she found it difficult to go to sleep. The patient was also vexed, agitated, and restless. She had taken a number of Western medications, none of which had been markedly effective. At the time of examination, the woman's tongue had slimy, yellow fur and her pulse was vacuous, bowstring, slippery, and rapid. Based on these signs and symptoms, Dr. Zhu categorized this patient's patterns as qi and yin dual vacuity with phlegm and dampness depressed and stagnating and depression transforming fire. Therefore, the treatment principles were to supplement the qi and nourish yin, eliminate dampness and drain fire, for which he prescribed *Qi Mai Di Huang Tang Jia Jian* (Astragalus Ophiopogon & Rehmannia Decoction with Additions & Subtractions): Radix Astragali Membranacei (*Huang Qi*) and uncooked Radix Rehmanniae (*Sheng Di*), 15g each, Radix Panacis Ginseng (*Ren Shen*), Tuber Ophiopogonis Japonici (*Mai Men Dong*), Fructus Schisandrae Chinensis (*Wu Wei Zi*), Rhizoma Atractylodis (*Cang Zhu*), Sclerotium Poriae

Cocos (*Fu Ling*), Rhizoma Alismatis (*Ze Xie*), Massa Medica Fermentata (*Shen Qu*), and Cortex Radicis Moutan (*Dan Pi*), 10g each, Radix Angelicae Sinensis (*Dang Gui*), 6g, and Folium Perillae Frutescentis (*Zi Su Ye*), 3g. After taking 20 *ji* of this formula, the woman's eating and drinking and psyche improved and her aching and pain, paralysis, frequent urination, and urinary pain decreased. Therefore, the above formula was made into pills, each pill weighing nine grams. The woman then took one pill each time, three times per day for two years, at the end of which time, all her urinary frequency and pain and edema had disappeared and her lower limb paralysis and aching and pain had mostly disappeared.

CASE 8[9]

The patient was a 52 year old male. During the past three years, the patient was commonly hungry and thirsty. In addition, he experienced frequent urination and loss of weight. The man said that he habitually ate rich, fatty foods and drank alcohol. Fasting blood glucose was 150mg/dL and two hour PPBG was 180mg/dL. Fasting urine glucose was (+) and, postprandial, it was (+++). The patient was diagnosed with diabetes mellitus and was started on tolbutamide. When the man took this medication, his symptoms abated, but, if he stopped this medication, they recurred. Therefore, he decided to try acupuncture. In terms of his Chinese medical signs and symptoms, the man presented with lassitude of the spirit, a lusterless facial complexion, and a low, weak voice, oral thirst, polydipsia, frequent urination, nocturia, thin, slimy, yellow tongue fur, and a bowstring, vacuous pulse.

Based on these signs and symptoms, the man's patterns were categorized as stomach heat, lung-kidney yin vacuity, and kidney qi not securing and astringing. Therefore, the treatment principles were to nourish the yin of the lungs and kidneys and regulate and rectify the spleen and stomach. The points selected included: *Shen Shu* (Bl 23), *Yi Shu* (M-BW-22), *San Yin Jiao* (Sp 6), and *Yu Ji* (Lu 10). These points were needled once per day with even supplementing-even draining technique and were retained for 30 minutes each treatment. During this course of treatment, the patient was requested to suspend his oral hypoglycemic medications and to abstain from rich foods and alcohol. After five treatments, the oral thirst had abated and water intake was reduced by half. Urination was reduced to 3-4 times per day and once during the night. Excessive hunger was also somewhat decreased.

Therefore, in order to increase the supplementation of the lungs and kidneys, supplementing *Tai Xi* (Ki 3) and *Fei Shu* (Bl 13) were added to the above formula. After five more treatments, the excessive hunger, thirst, and urination continued to gradually improve. The tongue fur became white and moist, and the pulse turned bowstring and moderate (*i.e.*, relaxed or slightly slow). This indicated that kidney qi and yin had been restored. Thus two more points were added to the above prescription—*Qi Hai* (CV 6) and *Zu San Li* (St 36)—needled with even supplementing-even draining technique in order to clear heat from the stomach. After needling, a plum blossom needle was used to tap the *Hua Tuo Jia Ji* (B-BW-35) from T11-L5. After 15 treatments with this modified protocol, the patient's psyche had improved and the three polys, *i.e.*, polydipsia, polyphagia, and polyuria, were completely relieved. Fasting blood glucose was now 130mg/dL, and two hour PPBG was 170mg/dL. Urine glucose was negative.

In order to secure and consolidate the above treatment effects, the following points were selected: *Shen Shu* (Bl 23), *Yi Shu* (M-BW-22), *Pi Shu* (Bl 20), *Zhong Ji* (CV 3), *Zu San Li* (St 36), *San Yin Jiao* (Sp 6), and *Yang Ling Quan* (GB 34). Three to four of these points were chosen each time, and needling was administered every other day. After the needles were withdrawn, the *Hua Tuo Jia Ji* points were needled with a plum blossom needle as described above. After two more months of treatment, all the patient's symptoms had completely disappeared, fasting blood glucose was 100mmol/L, and urine glu cose was negative. On follow-up after six months, there had been no recurrence.

CASE 9[10]

The patient was a 56 year old male cadre who was diagnosed with diabetes in March 1979. The man had been treated but without marked effect. He still had vexatious thirst, polydipsia, a dry mouth, lack of strength in his four limbs, and frequent, profuse urination. However, his bowel movements were normal. Fasting blood glucose was 453mg/dL, urine glucose was (+++), and ketones were negative. His tongue was pale with thick, slimy, white fur, and his pulse was deep and forceless.

Based on the above signs and symptoms, the man's pattern was discriminated as qi and yin dual vacuity upper wasting. Therefore, the treatment principles were to enrich yin and supplement the qi, clear heat and engender fluids, assisted by fortifying the spleen and eliminating dampness. The points chosen were: *Yang Ling Quan* (GB 34) and *Zhi Gou* (TB 6) to course the liver, rectify the qi, and disinhibit dampness, and *Guan Yuan* (CV 4) and *Dai Mai* (GB 26) to supplement the kidneys. In addition, the man was also prescribed the following Chinese medicinals: Gypsum Fibrosum (*Shi Gao*), Radix Astragali Membranacei (*Huang Qi*), uncooked Radix Discoreae Oppositae (*Shan Yao*), Fructus Pruni Mume (*Wu Mei*), Herba Artemisiae Capillaris (*Yin Chen Hao*), and Radix Trichosanthis Kirlowii (*Tian Hua Fen*), 50g each, Rhizoma Alismatis (*Ze Xie*), 40g, and Rhizoma Anemarrhenae Aspheloidis (*Zhi Mu*), 20g. One *ji* of these were decocted in water per day and administered in three divided doses. After taking 100 *ji* of this formula and receiving 50 acupuncture treatments, the patient's fasting blood glucose was 89mg/dL, his fasting urine glucose was negative, and so was his two hour postprandial urine glucose.

CASE 10[11]

The patient was a 45 year old male cadre who was diagnosed with diabetes on Dec. 6, 1979. This man had previously been treated with Chinese medicinals without apparent effect. His signs and symptoms included dry mouth, vexatious thirst, abdominal distention, fatigue, lack of strength, constipation, bodily emaciation, a red tongue tip and slimy, white fur, and a deep, slippery pulse. Fasting blood glucose was 240mg/dL, and urine glucose was (++). Based on these signs and symptoms, the man's pattern was categorized as lung dryness and spleen dampness. The treatment principles were to clear heat and engender fluids, fortify the spleen and disinhibit dampness. The points selected for these purposes consisted of: *Shen Men* (Ht 7), *Fu Liu* (Ki 7), and *Yin Ling Quan* (Sp 9). The Chinese herbal prescription consisted of: Radix Trichosanthis Kirlowii (*Tian Hua Fen*) and uncooked Radix Dioscoreae Oppositae (*Shan Yao*), 100g each, Gypsum Fibrosum (*Shi Gao*) and Semen Coicis Lachrymajobi (*Yi Yi Ren*), 50g each, Radix Astragali Membranacei (*Huang Qi*), 30g, Rhizoma Coptidis Chinensis (*Huang Lian*), 20g, and Rhizoma Anemarrhenae Aspheloidis (*Zhi Mu*), 15g. One *ji* of these medicinals was decocted in water per day and administered orally in three divided doses.

After taking four *ji* of the above medicinals, the dry mouth, vexatious thirst, abdominal distention, fatigue, and lack of strength were all decreased. The tip of the tongue was pale and the tongue fur was now thin and white, while the patient's pulse was deep, bowstring, and fine. Therefore, 15 grams of Rhizoma Cyperi Rotundi (*Xiang Fu*) was added to the previous formula and another four *ji* were administered. Now all the patient's symptoms were greatly decreased. The patient was given another 60 *ji* of this basic formula with additions and subtractions and he received 30 acupuncture treatments, after which his FBG was 98mg/dL and his urine glucose was negative.

CASE 11[12]

The patient was a 63 year old female agricultural worker who was first examined on Jan. 4, 1997. The woman had been diagnosed with diabetes for more than a year, and previous medication had lowered her fasting blood glucose to 7.2mmol/L. The woman was continuously taking 15mg of gliclazide, but she still had oral thirst and polyuria which her Western medication was not able to control. Each day, this woman would drink 4000ml of fluids, then she would have polyuria which was especially severe at night. In addition, her low back was sore, her gums were swollen, she was fearful of chill, her psyche was dull and listless, her tongue was pale with thin, white fur, and her pulse was soft.

Based on these signs and symptoms, the woman's pattern was discriminated as kidney yang insufficiency failing to steam and vaporize fluids, causing thirst above, and kidney qi insufficiency failing to secure and contain, causing frequent urination below. For this, the patient was prescribed Zhang Zhong-jing's *Shen Qi Wan Jia Wei* (Kidney Qi Pills with Added Flavors): cooked Radix Rehmanniae (*Shu Di*) and Radix Dioscoreae Oppositae (*Shan Yao*), 30g each, Fructus Corni Officinalis (*Shan Zhu Yu*), Sclerotium Poriae Cocos (*Fu Ling*), and Rhizoma Alismatis (*Ze Xie*), 15g each, Cortex Radicis Moutan (*Dan Pi*), Ootheca Mantidis (*Sang Piao Xiao*), Radix Trichosanthis Kirlowii (*Tian Hua Fen*), and Fructus Alpiniae Oxyphyllae (*Yi Zhi Ren*), 10g each, Radix Lateralis Praeparatus Aconiti Carmichaeli (*Fu Zi*) and Radix Linderae Strychnifoliae (*Wu Yao*), 6g each, and Cortex Cinnamomi Cassiae (*Rou Gui*), 3g. After taking 10 *ji* of this formula, the woman's oral thirst was improved, however, her urination was still frequent. Therefore, 30 grams each of calcined Os Draconis (*Long Gu*) and Concha Ostreae (*Mu Li*) were added and 10 more *ji* were administered. At this point, both the thirst and urination were basically controlled. Therefore, she was given *Shen Qi Wan* in pill form in order to secure and consolidate the treatment effects.

CASE 12[13]

The patient was a 50 year old female who had been diagnosed with diabetes for two years. Because long-term Western medical treatment had had little effect, she looked hopefully to Chinese medicine. The symptoms seen were vexatious thirst with profuse urination, low back and leg aching and weakness, lassitude of the spirit, lack of strength, dizziness, blurred vision, difficult bowel movements, and, with each passing day, increasingly noticeable emaciation. Her tongue was red with thin fur, and her pulse was fine with a weak cubit position. Her FBG was 9.8mmol/L.

Accordingly, the patient's pattern discrimination was enduring dryness and heat with liver and kidney qi and yin both damaged. The treatment principles were to enrich and supplement the liver and kidneys, boost the qi and enrich yin, and clear heat and moisten dryness. The prescription consisted of: Radix Astragali Membranacei (*Huang Qi*), 30g, Radix Codonopsitis Pilosulae (*Dang Shen*), 30g, Radix Puerariae (*Ge Gen*), 15g, Radix Anemarrhenae Asphodeloidis (*Zhi Mu*), 9g, Cortex Radicis Lycii Chinensis (*Di Gu Pi*), 15g, Radix Trichosanthis Kirlowii (*Tian Hua Fen*), 15g, uncooked Radix Rehmanniae (*Sheng Di*), 15g, Radix Scrophulariae Ningpoensis (*Xuan Shen*), 15g, Tuber Ophiopogonis Japonici (*Mai Dong*), 12g, Fructus Schisandrae Chinensis (*Wu Wei Zi*), 6g, Fructus Lycii Chinensis (*Gou Qi Zi*), 12g, Radix Dioscoreae Oppositae (*Shan Yao*), 15g, Fructus Corni Officinalis (*Shan Zhu Yu*), 12g, and uncooked Radix Polygoni Multiflori (*He Shou Wu*), 12g. After taking these medicinals for two weeks, the patient's signs and symptoms were markedly alleviated, and, one month later, her blood glucose had dropped to 6.9mmol/L. Regulating treatment was continued, and, on follow-up three months later, her blood glucose was essentially normal.

CASE 13[14]

The patient was a 62 year old female who had a history of hypertension and hypercholesterolemia for the past eight years. Two weeks before she came in, she suddenly developed hemiplegia and was diagnosed with a brain infarction and diabetes. She had already had Western medical emergency treatment. At the time of examination, her spirit was completely withered and weak, her limbs on the left side were paralyzed, and she had numbness and tingling in her limbs, dizziness, and a dry mouth. Night-time urination was frequent and copious. Her tongue was enlarged and dark with thin, slimy fur. Her pulse was deep and fine. Her blood pressure was 20/12kPa, and her blood glucose was 11.8mmol/L.

Based on the above signs and symptoms, the patient's pattern discrimination was liver-kidney qi and yin dual depletion with phlegm stasis obstructing and impeding the channels and network vessels. The treatment principles were to enrich and nourish liver and kidney qi and yin, transform phlegm, quicken the blood, and free the flow of the network vessels. The prescription consisted of: Radix Astragali Membranacei (*Huang Qi*), 30g, Radix Angelicae Sinensis (*Dang Gui*), 12g, Radix Ligustici Wallichii (*Chuan Xiong*), 9g, Hirudo Seu Whitmania (*Shui Zhi*), 9g, Lumbricus (*Di Long*), 12g, uncooked Radix Rehmanniae (*Sheng Di*), 15g, Radix Scrophulariae Ningpoensis (*Xuan Shen*), 15g, Radix Puerariae (*Ge Gen*),

30g, Rhizoma Atractylodis (*Cang Zhu*), 9g, Rhizoma Gastrodiae Elatae (*Tian Ma*), 9g, Ramulus Uncariae Cum Uncis (*Gou Teng*), 18g added at the end, Rhizoma Acori Graminei (*Chang Pu*), 9g, Rhizoma Alismatis (*Ze Xie*), 30g, and Herba Lycopi Lucidi (*Ze Lan*), 15g. This formula was administered for two months with various additions and subtractions, at which time the function of the limbs and body on the left side was gradually restored and the other symptoms also showed evidence of amelioration. Blood pressure and blood glucose became stabilized and normal.

Case 14[15]

The patient was a 62 year old male who had a history of diabetes for eight years. However, his blood glucose remained elevated and was not decreasing. In order to lower it, he was given Western medicines combined with insulin treatment. The patient was obese, and he constantly had a bitter taste in his mouth and bad breath, while his gums were swollen and painful. He had thirst with a desire for fluids but did not drink much water. He was hungry, yet ate scantily. His stools were sloppy and stagnant, his urine was yellow and scanty, and he was dizzy and fatigued. His tongue was deviated and red with teethmarks on its edges and thick, slimy, yellow fur. His pulse was soggy and slippery. His FBG was 9.1mmol/L.

Based on the preceding signs and symptoms, this patient's pattern discrimination was prolonged wasting and thirsting with spleen qi suffering detriment. This had resulted in a breakdown of movement and transformation. Thus dampness and heat had congested and become exuberant, with fullness of the triple burner. Consequently, the treatment principles were to clear and transform dampness and heat, supplement the spleen and engender fluids. The prescription consisted of: Rhizoma Atractylodis (*Cang Zhu*), 12g, Rhizoma Atractylodis Macrocephalae (*Bai Zhu*), 12g, Rhizoma Coptidis Chinensis (*Huang Lian*), 3g, Radix Scutellariae Baicalensis (*Huang Qin*), 15g, uncooked Semen Coicis Lachryma-jobi (*Yi Yi Ren*), 30g, *Liu Yi San* (Six to One Powder), 30g wrapped, Radix Astragali Membranaei (*Huang Qi*), 30g, Radix Codonopsitis Pilosulae (*Dang Shen*), 15g, Radix Dioscoreae Oppositae (*Shan Yao*), 15g, Radix Trichosanthis Kirlowii (*Tian Hua Fen*), 15g, Herba Dendrobii (*Shi Hu*), 15g, Radix Puerariae (*Ge Gen*), 15g, Radix Scrophulariae Ningpoensis (*Xuan Shen*), 10g, and Fructus Cardamomi (*Bai Kou Ren*), 3g. One week after taking these medicinals, all the patient's symptoms were somewhat improved. Therefore, the previous formula was modified, with *Cang Zhu* being used at up to 30 grams. The patient was treated for two months. Eventually these Chinese medicinals enabled the dampness and heat to be cleared and the condition to be entire-ly eliminated. On re-examination, the patient's blood glucose was 6.0mmol/L. Later, his insulin use was discontinued, and his use of Western hypoglycemic medicines was less than before treatment. On follow-up a half year later, the patient's condition had basically stabilized.

Case 15[16]

The patient was a 41 year old female who had been diagnosed with diabetes for over four years. Previously, she had taken oral herbal prescriptions one after another to lower her blood glucose levels and harmonize the center, but all with no good results. Therefore, she came to the Chinese author's clinic for treatment. Her symptoms were thirst, hunger, profuse urination, emaciation, extreme exhaustion, vexation and agitation, dry stools, and numbness and lack of strength in her lower limbs. The tongue body was red, and the fur was thin, white, and dry. The pulse was fine and rapid. The blood glucose was 16mmol/L, the urine glucose was (++++), and urine ketones were (++).

Based on the preceding signs and symptoms, the Chinese medical pattern discrimination was lung and stomach exuberant heat. The basic prescription consisted of: uncooked Radix Astragali Membranacei (*Huang Qi*), Radix Dioscoreae Oppositae (*Shan Yao*), and Radix Trichosanthis Kirlowii (*Tian Hua Fen*), 30g each, Fructus Corni Officinalis (*Shan Zhu Yu*), 20g, Rhizoma Atractylodis Macrocephalae (*Bai Zhu*), uncooked Radix Rehmanniae (*Sheng Di*), Radix Scrophulariae Ningpoensis (*Xuan Shen*), Cortex Radicis Moutan (*Dan Pi*), Tuber Ophiopogonis Japonici (*Mai Men Dong*), and Fructus Schisandrae Chinensis (*Wu Wei Zi*), 15g each, and Radix Panacis Qinquefolii (*Xi Yang Shen*), 10g. In addition, Gypsum Fibrisum (*Shi Gao*), Rhizoma Anemarrhenae Aspheloidis (*Zhi Mu*), and Rhizoma Coptidis Chinensis (*Huang Lian*) were added to the basic formula. Ten consecutive *ji* were prescribed, and, after that, all the patient's symptoms were alleviated and there was no thirst, no red tongue, and no dry stools. However, the profuse sweating continued. Therefore, *Shi Gao* and *Zhi Mu* were subtracted, and Os Draconis (*Long Gu*) and Concha Ostreae (*Mu Li*) were added. Another 10 *ji* were prescribed, after which the patient recovered. Her blood glucose was 5.8 mmol/L and the urine glucose was negative. Then *Liu Wei Di Huang Wan* (Six Flavors Rehmannia Pills) and *Shen Ling Bai Zhu San* (Ginseng, Poria & Atractylodes Powder) were prescribed as a follow-up course of treatment. One year later, there had been no recurrence of this illness.

Case 16[17]

The patient was a 52 year old male cadre who was first

examined in April 1987 and whose main symptoms were oral thirst, polydipsia, easy hungering, polyuria, and bodily emaciation which had lasted three years. The patient had been previously diagnosed with type 2 DM. His FBG at that time was 15.54mmol/L (280mg/dL), and his urine glucose was (+++). The man had been treated at a local hospital with glyburide and Chinese medicinals but without very marked treatment effects. Fasting blood glucose had become 9.99-13.32mmol/L (180-240mg/dL), but he had developed retinal vessel sclerosis. At the time Dr. Yang first saw this patient, he had a dry mouth with desire to drink, polyphagia, night-time polyuria (4-5 urinations per night), incessant spontaneous perspiration, tidal heat, lack of strength, dry stools, and blurred vision. In addition, his tongue was red with scanty fur, and his pulse was fine, rapid, and forceless. Fasting blood glucose was 11.6mmol/L (210mg/dL) and urine glucose was (+++).

Based on these signs and symptoms, the man's Chinese medical pattern was categorized as qi and yin dual vacuity, and the treatment principles were to boost the qi and nourish yin. Therefore, Dr. Yang needled *Fei Shu* (Bl 13), *Yi Shu* (M-BW-12), *Pi Shu* (Bl 20), *Shen Shu* (Bl 23), *Tai Yuan* (Lu 9), *Tai Bai* (Sp 3), and *Tai Xi* (Ki 3). The back transport points were needled with supplementing technique and not needle retention. The source points were needled with supplementing technique and 15 minute retention. This treatment was given once every other day, and, after 12 treatments, the patient's condition had markedly improved. The polydipsia and polyphagia had basically disappeared and the night-time urinations had decreased. The man's vision had improved, FBG was 7.9mmol/L (143mg/L), and urine glucose was (+). However, he still suffered from incessant spontaneous perspiration. Therefore, *Tai Xi* was removed and draining *He Gu* (LI 4) and supplementing *Fu Liu* (Ki 7) was added. After another course of treatment, all the symptoms had disappeared, the patient's psyche had improved, his FBG was 5.3mmol/L (96mg/L), and urine glucose was negative. Yet another course of treatment was given in order to secure and consolidate the treatment effect. On follow-up two years later, the patient's FBG was 6.2mmol/L (113mg/L) and his urine glucose was still negative.

CASE 17[18]

The patient was a 46 year old female who had suffered from oral thirst and frequent urination for three months. In addition, there was lassitude of the spirit, lack of strength in her extremities, emaciation, a tendency to hunger, and continuous pruritus. Her FBG was 13.3mmol/L (240mg/dL), urine glucose was (++), and urine ketones were negative. Therefore, the woman was diagnosed with diabetes and administered oral hypoglycemic medications. Unfortunately, although her symptoms improved, there was dizziness and nausea, and, thus, the patient stopped these medications and came to Dr. Chen for acupuncture. At the time Dr. Chen examined this woman, her blood pressure was 140/70mmHg, her tongue was pale with thin, yellow, turbid fur, her pulse was slippery, fine, and rapid, and she weighed 51kg.

Based on these signs and symptoms, the woman's Chinese medical pattern was categorized as kidney yin vacuity, and the treatment principles were to enrich yin and moisten the lungs, clear the stomach and downbear fire. The points Dr. Chen chose were *Tai Xi* (Ki 3) and *Guan Yuan* (CV 4) combined with *Yu Ji* (Lu 10) and *Zu San Li* (St 36). *Tai Xi* and *Guan Yuan* were needled with supplementing technique, and *Yu Ji* and *Zu San Li* were needled with draining technique. After obtaining the qi, the needles were retained for 20 minutes.

At the second examination, the patient reported that her fatigue and vexatious thirst had both improved after the acupuncture. However, she was still hungry and still had frequent urination. Her tongue and pulse were the same as before. Therefore, Dr. Chen needled the same points as before plus the Kidney ear point on the right side in order to more strongly secure the root and support the righteous, and on the third examination, the patient reported her lassitude of the spirit had improved yet again and that the symptoms of the three wastings had decreased. In addition, her night-time urinations had gone from 5-6 per night to 2-3. Her tongue was now pale with thin fur, and her pulse was slippery and fine. This meant that her kidney yin had obtained supplementation and that dryness and fire had been somewhat leveled. Therefore, draining *Kong Zui* (Lu 6) and *Yin Ling Quan* (Sp 9) and supplementing *Shen Shu* (Bl 23) were added to the original treatment. In addition, Dr. Chen needled the left Kidney ear point instead of the right.

On the fourth examination, the patient said that all her symptoms had gradually decreased and that her body weight had been increasing daily. Her tongue was pale with thin fur, and her pulse was now simply fine. Therefore, her kidney qi was judged to have recuperated and dryness and fire had gradually receded. Thus Dr. Chen needled *Yu Ji* (Lu 10) and *Zhong Wan* (CV 12) with draining technique and *Guan Yuan* (CV 4) with supplementing, and he did not needle any ear points. Instead, he used a plum blossom needle to needle the bladder channel on the upper and lower back in order to course and free the flow of the channel and network vessel qi and blood and to regulate and harmonize yin and yang.

On the fifth examination, the patient's affect had become crisp and clear and her sallow yellow facial complexion had gradually receded. Her voice and speech were clear and distinct, and her walk was strong and healthy. The pruritus had markedly decreased. However, the woman still had a hungry sensation and still urinated 4-6 times per day. Her tongue and pulse were the same as before. Therefore, Dr. Chen chose to needle her with the original method, and, by the sixth examination, the patient's facial complexion was now red and moist and she reported that she felt strong and healthy overall. She was still slightly hungry and sometimes slightly thirsty, but her skin no longer itched. Her body weight had increased to 54kg, her tongue was pale red with thin, white fur, and her pulse was fine and moderate. Fasting blood glucose was 8.3mmol/L (150mg/dL), and urine glucose was negative.

For the next three weeks, the patient was treated with regulating therapy because her righteous qi had not yet completely recovered. Therefore, she was mainly needled at *Fei Shu* (Bl 13), *Kong Zui* (Lu 6), *Zu San Li* (St 36), and *San Yin Jiao* (Sp 6). Auxiliary points included *Ming Men* (GV 4), *Shen Shu* (Bl 23), *Guan Yuan* (CV 4), *Zhong Ji* (CV 3), and *Tai Xi* (Ki 3). The woman was also instructed to warm moxa the conception vessel below her navel and *Zu San Li* for 30 minutes each time, two times each day. After these three weeks, the woman was able to walk five miles each day without discomfort, she had no thirst, and her eating was normal. Her skin no longer itched, and her blood and urine examinations were both normal. She had gained yet another two kilos of body weight, her tongue was pale red, her tongue fur was thin and moist, and her pulse was moderate. Therefore, she was judged cured and the acupuncture was stopped. On follow-up after six months, everything was still normal.

REMARKS:

1. The Chinese medical pattern discrimination and treatment of type 1 (IDDM) and type 2 (NIDDM) are the same. For instance, Guo Zhen-qiu, in *Zhong Yi Er Ke Xue* (*A Study of Chinese Medical Pediatrics*), describes the treatment of "pediatric diabetes." In this discussion, he says that most cases of pediatric diabetes are insulin–dependent diabetes. Having said that, he then goes on to give the same basic patterns as are typically given in Chinese *nei ke* or internal medicine texts, *i.e.*, lung heat transforming dryness, stomach heat burning fluids, yin vacuity-fire effulgence, yin vacuity-yang hyperactivity, and yin detriment reaching yang with kidney qi not securing. However, although acupuncture and Chinese medicine can rarely cure type 1 diabetes, they can cure type 2 diabetes as long as the disease had not progressed too far and acupuncture and Chinese medicinal therapy is supported by proper diet and lifestyle. Chinese medicine has been shown to control the symptoms of type 1 DM. It typically does not control the actual sugar levels in the blood.

2. Diabetes mellitus is a progressive disease, and Lu Renhe, as reported by Chen Jin-ding, has a three stage classification system which describes the commonly seen patterns at different stages in the progression of this condition. This staging system is a useful adjunct to the pattern discrimination given above.

STAGE I: YIN VACUITY

This describes the first stage of this disease when the patient still has a strong physique and is full of energy and vigor. However, endurance is typically lowered, there is a red tongue with yellow fur, and only mild hyperglycemia and hyperlipidemia. Urine glucose is absent, but there often is concomitant hypertension. This stage usually manifests either of two patterns:

A. Yin vacuity with ascendant liver yang hyperactivity

B. Ascendant liver yang hyperactivity due to yin vacuity

The difference between these two patterns is that the relative importances of yin vacuity and yang hyperactivity are reversed. In the first case, the treatment principles are to nourish yin and emolliate the liver, while, in the second case, the principles are to nourish yin and subdue yang.

STAGE II: HEAT TRANSMISSION

This stage describes the progressive condition where yang hyperactivity has given rise to outright heat. Patients are typically averse to heat and like cold and commonly exhibit polydipsia, polyphagia, polyuria, fatigue, emaciation, and elevated blood and urine glucose. Lu Ren-he subdivides this stage into four patterns:

A. Accumulated heat in the yang ming, for which one should clear and drain heat from the yang ming

B. Heat toxins in the lungs, for which one should clearing the lungs and resolvie toxins

C. Liver depression transforming heat, for which one should course the liver and rectify the qi, clear heat and resolve depression

D. Spleen vacuity complicated by damp heat, for which one should fortify the spleen and supplement the qi at the same time as clearing heat and eliminating dampness

STAGE III: DRYNESS & HEAT DAMAGING QI & YIN WITH NON-FREE FLOW OF THE CHANNELS & NETWORK VESSELS

In this stage, the condition has progressed even further and patients typically present with one or more of the complications of DM. General signs and symptoms include dry mouth and tongue, low back and knee soreness and limpness, aching and pain of the extremities, fatigue, a dark red tongue, and elevated blood and urine glucose. Lu Ren-he subdivides this stage into six patterns:

A. Dryness & heat damaging the qi & yin (meaning the spleen and kidneys respectively), for which one should supplement the qi, nourish yin, and moisten dryness

B. Malnourishment of the channels & network vessels due to dryness & heat damaging the qi & yin, for which one should mainly move the qi and quicken the blood, disinhibit the channels and free the flow of the network vessels. (This pattern mostly describes peripheral neuropathy.)

C. Dryness & heat damaging the lungs & spleen, for which one should fortify the spleen and supplement the qi, clear heat and moisten the lungs

D. Dryness & heat damaging the heart & spleen, for which one should supplement the kidneys and boost the qi at the same time as treating the heart and spleen

E. Dryness & heat damaging the qi & yin with stagnation of the middle burner, for which one should supplement the qi and nourish yin, clear heat and harmonize the middle burner

F. Dryness & heat damaging the qi & yin with liver depression & blood stasis, for which one should supplement the qi and yin at the same time as coursing the liver and rectifying the qi, quickening the blood and dispelling stasis

While we agree in general with Lu's three stages of DM, we would like to point out that, in many patients, liver depression transforming heat, liver depression and spleen vacuity, and/or spleen vacuity and damp heat may precede yin vacuity and yang hyperactivity, in fact being the mechanisms whereby yin is damaged and yang becomes hyperactive. For instance, it is Prof. Lu Jing-zhong's opinion that spleen vacuity is responsible for the origin and development of DM. In particular, Prof. Lu feels that, while the patient is still asymptomatic, the principles of fortifying and moving or transporting the middle and rectifying the spleen should be the main ones.[19] Similarly, Wu Shen-tao is of the opinion that the symptoms of insulin resistance (which often precedes DM), such as vexation and oppression, a bitter taste in the mouth, a torpid intake, and constipation, are shao yang channel symptoms.

According to Li Yong-zhi and Meng Fan-yi, lung-stomach dryness and heat damaging fluids is the pattern that accounts for most DM patients in the first five years of their disease course. From years 5-10, lung-kidney yin vacuity or qi and yin dual vacuity are the main patterns. After 10 years of suffering from diabetes, they say that qi and yin dual vacuity and yin and yang dual vacuity are the main patterns. However, they also say that, after five years, most cases are complicated by blood stasis.

3. Also according to Li and Meng, it is possible to correlate the progression of patterns in this disease with certain Western laboratory examinations.

A. Patients presenting with lung stomach dryness and heat damaging fluids usually have normal or only slightly elevated levels of serum insulin. Patients with lung-kidney yin vacuity have lower than normal serum insulin levels, while qi and yin dual vacuity patients have even lower insulin levels, and those with yin and yang dual vacuity have very low insulin levels.

B. Patients with dryness and heat damaging fluids tend to have lower amounts of blood glucose and blood lipids and less glycosylated hemoglobin, while those with qi and yin dual vacuity have higher amounts of blood glucose and lipids and more glycosylated hemoglobin.

C. In women with DM, the ratio between estradiol (E_2) and testosterone (T) is lower than that in normal women, and, as the disease progresses from kidney yin vacuity, to kidney qi vacuity, to kidney yin and yang dual vacuity, this ratio gradually gets lower and lower.

D. Serum glucocorticoid hormones in patients with diabetes tend to be higher than normal. In those presenting with yin vacuity, glucocorticoid hormones in the blood are only a little higher than normal. However, as one progresses to yin and yang dual vacuity, these hormones get even higher.

E. Circulating nucleotides also have a rough relationship with Chinese medical patterns. For instance, the cAMP/cGMP ratio tends to be normal in those with yin vacuity and dryness and heat, while it is lower than normal in those with qi and yin dual vacuity and even lower in those with yin and yang dual vacuity.

F. In patients with yin vacuity and dryness and heat, bilateral point temperature balances are roughly equal. However, in those with qi and yin dual vacuity, bilateral differences in point temperature tend to be relatively large, thus showing disturbances in the movement of the qi and blood throughout the body.

G. Sixty to seventy percent of patients with blood stasis have slower than normal blood flow, disturbances in microcirculation, higher than normal platelet aggregation, increased blood coagulation substances, and lowered erythrocyte membrane flow.

At present, the above laboratory examinations are not yet accepted as definitive standard criteria for making a Chinese medical pattern discrimination. However, they are suggestive, and it is probably only a matter of time before the outcomes of such laboratory examinations are routinely included in the pathognomonic signs of Chinese medical patterns.

4. Chen Xia-bo compared the pattern discrimination of 54 patients whose blood sugar could not be controlled by oral hypoglycemic agents to those of 67 patients whose blood sugar was satisfactorily controlled by oral hypoglycemic agents. The study group consisted of those whose blood glucose could not be adequately controlled by oral hypoglycemic agents, while the comparison group consisted of those whose blood glucose was adequately controlled by oral hypoglycemics.

RISK FACTORS FOR TYPE 2 DIABETES		
	Study group	Comparison group
Qi vacuity	66.7%	62.7%
Blood vacuity	9.3%	10.4%
Yin vacuity	88.9%	77.6%
Yang vacuity	48.2%	8.9%
Heart vacuity	27.8%	19.4%
Liver vacuity	83.3%	53.7%
Spleen (stomach) vacuity	38.9%	47.8%
Lung vacuity	11.1%	17.9%
Kidney vacuity	92.6%	56.7%
Qi stagnation	14.8%	32.8%
Blood stasis	85.2%	47.8%
Phlegm dampness	29.6%	38.8%
Damp heat	5.6%	34.3%
Dryness & heat	7.4%	62.7%

These comparisons suggest that oral hypoglycemic agents are more effective in patients with more replete heat, less blood stasis, and less liver-kidney and yang vacuities. In other words, oral hypoglycemics appear to work best in patients whose patterns are more replete and which typically correspond to the earlier stages of DM. This is corroborated by the fact that oral hypoglycemics lose their effectiveness in 5% of patients each year a person has had diabetes.

5. According to Ding Xue-ping *et al.*, among those with type 2 diabetes, concomitant damp heat or heat exuberance is associated with increased insulin resistance as well as with increased glucagon secretion abnormalities.

6. Although it is not hard to control diabetes with a combination of Chinese and Western medicines, it is difficult to stop the disease's progression once the disease has gone too far. For instance, once yin disease has reached yang, the disease has become difficult to treat and difficult to reverse. Stated another way, upper and middle wasting can be treated, but lower wasting is difficult to treat. In that case, Chinese medicine is only able to achieve certain effects. Therefore, it is important to know and recognize the signs and symptoms which are considered malign transformations (*e hua*) or malign conditions (*e hou*) of wasting and thirsting disease. These include:

A. Loss of spirit due to great damage to the qi and blood with decline and faintness of the righteous qi

B. The appearance of qi urination, *i.e.*, extreme polyuria

C. A transformation from polyphagia to inability to eat. If severe, there may even be nausea and vomiting.

D. Spirit mind abstraction, somnolence, and vexation and agitation, and any other manifestation of yang qi vacuity

In addition, stirring of wind, wind stroke, water swelling, and welling and flat abscesses are all symptoms of a worsening of the patient's condition.

Typically, complicating conditions, such as retinopathy, ateriosclerosis, neuropathy, and nephropathy, manifest 10-15 years after the initial onset of diabetes, and, commonly, these conditions take a turn for the worse 15-20 years after that initial onset. Therefore, it is important to treat this condition early on when a cure is still possible.

7. In terms of the real-life clinical practice, most Western middle-aged patients begin with varying amounts of liver depression and stomach heat. This heat may be depressive heat, damp heat, or even potentially phlegm heat. In most cases, there is also spleen qi vacuity. As enduring heat damages fluids, one first gets fluid dryness which later evolves into true yin vacuity. In this case, enduring fluid dryness of the lungs and stomach eventually reaches the kidneys. Now there is liver depression, spleen qi vacuity, and yin vacuity. As enduring liver depression and inhibition of the qi mechanism as well as dampness and heat damage the spleen more and more, this eventually causes a spleen-kidney yang dual vacuity. Now there is a qi and blood, yin and yang dual vacuity. Because the qi moves the blood and because blood and fluids flow together, qi stagnation and dampness may cause concomitant blood stasis. In addition, because phlegm is nothing other than congealed dampness, many cases of diabetes either are or eventually become complicated by phlegm. Although the above patterns and their accompanying formulas provide a general guideline for treatment, in real life, one basically has to assess the relative amounts of liver depression, heat (what kind of heat and where it is located), spleen qi vacuity, yin, blood, and fluid insufficiencies, yang vacuity, phlegm, and blood stasis and then construct a treatment plan which takes each disease mechanism into account according to their proportions in the patient's pattern discrimination. This means creating an individualized formula for each patient's personal combination of patterns. Most patients with diabetes have at least three patterns simultaneously: liver depression, some kind of evil heat, and spleen qi and/or yin fluid insufficiency. The older the patient or the longer the patient has had diabetes, the more additional patterns they will typically display.

Because most cases of diabetes are complicated by a number of symptoms or conditions, Ding Xue-ping gives the following generic modifications which can be added to various formulas for diabetes. For heart palpitations, add 30 grams each of Radix Pseudostellariae Heterophyllae (Tai Zi Shen) and Concha Margaritiferae (Zhen Zhu Mu), 18 grams of Dens Draconis (Long Chi), nine grams of Rhizoma Polygoni Odorati (Yu Zhu), and three grams of Rhizoma Nardostachytis (Gan Song). For chest impediment categorized as phlegm and stasis, add 12 grams of Radix Salviae Miltiorrhizae (Dan Shen), nine grams each of Fructus Trichosanthis Kirlowii (Gua Lou) and Bulbus Allii (Cong Bai), six grams of Flos Carthami Tinctorii (Hong Hua), and three grams of Ramulus Cinnamomi Cassiae (Gui Zhi). For hemiplegia and aphasia, add 12 grams of Eupolyphaga Seu Opisthoplatia (Tu Bei Chong), nine grams each of Tuber Curcumae (Yu Jin) and Hirudo Seu Whitmania (Shui Zhi), six grams of Concretio Silicea Bambusae (Tian Zhu Huang), and 4.5 grams of Buthus Martensis (Quan Xie). For headache and dizziness due to hypertension, add 30 grams

of Dens Draconis (Long Chi), 18 grams each of Concha Margaritiferae (Zhen Zhu Mu) and Concha Haliotidis (Shi Jue Ming), and 0.6 grams of Cornu Caprae (Shan Yang Jiao), powdered and swallowed with the decoction. For numbness and piercing pain of the extremities due to peripheral neuropathy, add nine grams of Bombyx Batryticatus (Jiang Can), six grams of Lumbricus (Di Long), and 4.5 grams of Buthus Martensis (Quan Xie). For retinopathy, add 30 grams of Radix Salviae Miltiorrhizae (Dan Shen), 18 grams of Concha Haliotidis (Shi Jue Ming), and 15 grams each of Spica Prunellae Vulgaris (Xia Ku Cao) and Herba Lycopi Lucidi (Ze Lan). For nausea and vomiting, add nine grams of Endothelium Corneum Gigeriae Galli (Ji Nei Jin), six grams of Folium Perillae Frutescentis (Zi Su Ye), and three grams of Rhizoma Coptidis Chinensis (Huang Lian). For diarrhea, add nine grams each of Fructus Psoraleae Corylifoliae (Bu Gu Zhi) and Semen Myristicae Fragrantis (Rou Dou Kou). For constipation, add 12 grams of Herba Cistanchis Deserticolae (Rou Cong Rong) and nine grams of Radix Angelicae Sinensis (Dang Gui). For edema, add 30 grams of Radix Stephaniae Tetrandrae (Han Fang Ji) and 15 grams each of Herba Lycopi Lucidi (Ze Lan) and Herba Leonuri Heterophylli (Yi Mu Cao). For vaginal pruritus or strangury, add 30 grams each of Radix Et Rhizoma Polygoni Cuspidati (Hu Zhang), Herba Oldenlandiae Diffusae Cum Radice (Bai Hua She She Cao), and Rhizoma Smilacis Galbrae (Tu Fu Ling), 15 grams of Fructus Kochiae Scopariae (Di Fu Zi), and nine grams of Herba Pyrrosiae (Shi Wei). If there is simultaneous external contraction with fever and sore throat, add 12 grams of Radix Lithopsermi Seu Arnebiae (Zi Cao), nine grams each of Fructus Arctii Lappae (Niu Bang Zi) and Folium Daqingye (Da Qing Ye), and three grams of Fructificatio Lasiospherae Seu Calvatiae (Ma Bo). If aversion to cold is marked, add 12 grams each of Folium Perillae Frutescentis (Zi Su Ye) and Semen Praeparatum Sojae (Dan Dou Chi). If there is cough with yellow phlegm, add 30 grams each of Semen Benincase Hispidae (Dong Gua Zi) and Herba Houttuyniae Cordatae Cum Radice (Yu Xing Cao) and 12 grams each of Pulvis Indigonis (Qing Dai) and Folium Eriobotryae Japonicae (Pi Pa Ye). If there are sores, add 30 grams each of Herba Oldenlandiae Diffusae Cum Radice (Bai Hua She She Cao) and Rhizoma Smilacis Glabrae (Tu Fu Ling) and 15 grams of Radix Cynanchi Baiwei (Bai Wei).[20]

8. According to modern Western medicine, the incidence of diabetes is closely related to emotional factors. In one published study, 48% of patients with diabetes suffer from some form of emotional dysphoria. In another study, it is estimated that 76% of diabetes patients are type A personalities. Type A persons have strong ambitions, are compulsive workers, and are easily agitated and/or angered.[21] This helps underscore the importance of treating the liver, through coursing and resolving as well as nourishing and emolliating, when treating DM with Chinese medicine.

9. Because most cases of diabetes involve qi and yin vacuities with either replete or vacuity heat, the main Chinese medicinals for the treatment of diabetes are: Radix Panacis Ginseng (*Ren Shen*), Radix Codonopsitis Pilosulae (*Dang Shen*), Radix Astragali Membranacei (*Huang Qi*), Radix Dioscoreae Oppositae (*Shan Yao*), Fructus Schisandrae Chinensis (*Wu Wei Zi*), Rhizoma Polygonati (*Huang Jing*), Fructus Lycii Chinensis (*Gou Qi Zi*), cooked Radix Rehmanniae (*Shu Di*), uncooked Radix Rehmanniae (*Sheng Di*), Radix Scrophulariae Ningpoensis (*Xuan Shen*), Radix Trichosanthis Kirlowii (*Tian Hua Fen*), Tuber Ophiopogonis Japonici (*Mai Men Dong*), Tuber Asparagi Cochinensis (*Tian Men Dong*), Gypsum Fibrosum (*Shi Gao*), Rhizoma Anemarrhenae Aspheloidis (*Zhi Mu*), and Radix Salviae Miltiorrhizae (*Dan Shen*). Most Chinese medicinal formulas for the treatment of diabetes include a selection of several of the foregoing medicinals depending on the patient's pattern(s).

In the same vein, the following medicinals have all been shown to have hypoglycemic effects. Therefore, most formulas for diabetes contain a number of these medicinals.

MEDICINALS WHICH CLEAR HEAT: Bombyx Batryticatus (*Jiang Can*), Cortex Phellodendri (*Huang Bai*), Cortex Radicis Lycii Chinensis (*Di Gu Pi*), Folium Mori Albi (*Sang Ye*), Radix Et Rhizoma Polygoni Cuspidati (*Hu Zhang*), Radix Puerariae (*Ge Gen*), Radix Scrophulariae Ningpoensis (*Xuan Shen*), Radix Trichosanthis Kirlowii (*Tian Hua Fen*), Rhizoma Anemarrhenae Asphodeloidis (*Zhi Mu*)

MEDICINALS WHICH SUPPLEMENT: Cortex Radicis Acanthopanacis Gracilistylis (*Wu Jia Pi*), Fructus Corni Officinalis (*Shan Zhu Yu*), Fructus Lycii Chinensis (*Gou Qi Zi*), Herba Epimedii (*Xian Ling Pi*), Radix Astragali Membranacei (*Huang Qi*), Radix Dioscoreae Oppositae (*Shan Yao*), Radix Panacis Ginseng (*Ren Shen*), Radix Polygoni Multiflori (*He Shou Wu*), uncooked Radix Rehmanniae (*Sheng Di*), cooked Radix Rehmanniae (*Shu Di*), Rhizoma Atractylodis Macrocephalae (*Bai Zhu*), Rhizoma Polygonati (*Huang Jing*), Rhizoma Polygonati Odorati (*Yu Zhu*), Tuber Ophiopogonis Japonici (*Mai Men Dong*)

MEDICINALS WHICH DISINHIBIT OR DRY DAMPNESS: Fructus Xanthii Sibirici (*Cang Er Zi*), Rhizoma Alismatis (*Ze Xie*), Rhizoma Atractylodis (*Cang Zhu*), Sclerotium Poriae Cocos (*Fu Ling*), Stylus Zeae Maydis (*Yu Mi Xu*)

OTHER MEDICINALS: Fructus Germinatus Hordei Vulgaris (*Mai Ya*), Fructus Schisandrae Chinensis (*Wu Wei Zi*), Herba Agrimoniae Pilosae (*Xian He Cao*), Semen Litchi Sinensis (*Li Zhi He*)

10. One theory of Chinese medicine holds, "Wasting and thirsting has dryness without dampness." However, in clinic one often sees concurrent damp heat evils and especially in those where long-term control of blood glucose is not good. The spleen is responsible for lingering damp heat. The spleen rules the latter heaven, and, during the course of wasting and thirsting, qi and yin are both necessarily consumed. If the spleen qi suffers vacuity detriment, on the one hand, movement and transformation have no power, while, on the other, yin liquids lack a source. This often leads to yin vacuity dryness and heat becoming extreme. Long-standing spleen vacuity loss of movement causes damp evils to encumber and obstruct. Thus heat transforms, and dampness and heat become mutually locked. If severe, this may lead to the brewing of toxins and the transformation of stasis.

When treating this situation with medicinals, one cannot only address the root yin vacuity of wasting and thirsting. However, the method of transforming dampness is prohibited since it might aggravate the disease mechanism of yin vacuity dryness. Yet, one can also not simply address the spleen vacuity. In that case, the single or self-same flavor that supplements the qi would also result in sweetly and warmly strengthening heat and thus aggravating dry heat's damage of yin. In this case, the methods of clearing and transforming dampness and heat should be combined with supplementing the spleen and engendering fluids. Of the damp-transforming medicinals, the chief one chosen in the treatment of diabetes is Rhizoma Atractylodis (*Cang Zhu*). It is outstandingly successful in moving the spleen, constraining the essence, and lowering glucose levels.

11. Zhao Jie believes that spleen yin vacuity is an important pattern of this condition. However, after considering Zhao's arguments, we don't think spleen yin vacuity is that useful a pattern in the treatment of this condition. The symptoms that Zhao posits for spleen yin vacuity include decreased food intake, a dry mouth but no desire to drink, abdominal distention, vexation and fullness, constipation, a dry tongue with scanty fluids, and a fine, rapid pulse. To us, these signs and symptoms add up to nothing other than stomach heat and dryness with a minor element of spleen qi vacuity. Zhao goes on to say that he believes there are three degrees or subpatterns of spleen yin vacuity. These are simple spleen yin vacuity (for which he recommends Radix Puerariae, *Ge Gen*,

Radix Trichosanthis Kirlowii, *Tian Hua Fen*, Cortex Radicis Lycii Chinensis, *Di Gu Pi*, Semen Praeparatus Sojae, *Dan Dou Chi*, Rhizoma Anemarrhenae Asphodeloidis, *Zhi Mu*, Radix Glehniae Littoralis, *Sha Shen*, Tuber Ophiopogonis Japonici, *Mai Men Dong*, Semen Plantaginis, *Che Qian Zi*, Radix Dioscoreae Oppositae, *Shan Yao*, Semen Dolichoris Lablab, *Bai Bian Dou*, and Semen Coicis Lachyrma-jobi, *Yi Yi Ren*), qi and yin dual vacuity, possibly complicated by damp obstruction, and spleen qi falling downward. The pattern of qi and yin dual vacuity has been dealt with above. The symptoms Zhao attributes to spleen qi falling downward are polyuria and sweet-flavored urine. However, Zhao does not offer any specific advice for treating these.

12. Because most diabetes begins, at least in part, due to faulty diet, dietary therapy *must* play a part in the patient's overall treatment plan. For more on this issue, please see Chapter 7 on diet and diabetes.

ENDNOTES:

[1] Bowstring is our preferred translation for *xian mai* or what Wiseman and Feng Ye translate as string-like.

[2] Zhang Hong-xiang, as anthologized in the Shanghai Municipal Department of Health's *Shang Hai Lao Zhong Yi Jiang Yan Xuan Bian (A Selected Compilation of Shanghai Old Chinese Doctors Experiences)*, Shanghai Science & Technology Publishing Co., Shanghai, 1984, p. 168-169

[3] Guo Wei, as anthologized in Shi Yu-guang & Dan Shu-jian's *Xiao Ke Zhuan Zhi (Wasting & Thirsting Expertise)*, Chinese Medicine Ancient Books Publishing Co., 1997, p. 69-70

[4] Du Yu-mao, as anthologized in Shi Yu-guang & Dan Shu-jian, *op. cit.*, p. 82-83

[5] Hu Qiao-cheng, as anthologized in Shi Yu-guang & Dan Shu-jian, *op. cit.*, p. 98-99

[6] Zhao Jin-duo, as anthologized in Dan Shu-jian & Chen Zi-hua's *Xiao Ke Juan (The Wasting & Thirsting Book)*, Chinese National Chinese Medicine & Medicinals Publishing Co., Beijing, 1999, p. 225-226

[7] Zhu Jin-zhong, as anthologized in Dan Shu-jian & Chen Zi-hua, *op. cit.*, p. 204

[8] *Ibid.*, p. 206

[9] Chen Ji-rui & Wang, Nissi, *Acupuncture Case Histories from China*, Eastland Press, Seattle, 1988, p. 90-92

[10] Xiao Shao-qing, *Zhong Guo Zhen Jiu Chu Fang Xue (A Study of Chinese Acupuncture & Moxibustion Prescription-writing)*, Ningxia People's Publishing Co., Yinchuan, 1986, p. 275-276

[11] *Ibid.*, p. 276

[12] Shen Zhao-xiong, "Raising the Borders of [Zhang] Zhong-jing's Formulas for the Treatment of Wasting & Thirsting," *Jiang Su Zhong Yi (Jiangsu Chinese Medicine)*, #5, 1999, p. 30

[13] Xiao Yan-qian, "Important Examples in the Discrimination & Treatment of Diabetes," *Shang Hai Zhong Yi Yao Za Zhi (Shanghai Journal of Chinese Medicine & Medicinals)*, #9, 1997, p. 14-15

[14] *Ibid.*

[15] *Ibid.*

[16] Luo Shan, "The Treatment of Diabetes Using the Method of Boosting the Qi, Enriching Yin, & Draining Fire," *Hu Bei Zhong Yi Za Zhi (Hubei Journal of Traditional Chinese Medicine)*, #3, 1998, p. 41-42

[17] Yang Lian-de, as anthologized in *Zhong Guo Dang Dai Zhen Jiu Ming Jia Yi An (Contemporary Chinese National Acupuncture & Moxibustion Famous Masters' Case Histories)*, compiled by Wang Xue-tai & Liu Guan-jun, Jilin Science & Technology Publishing Co., Changchun, 1991, p. 361

[18] Chen Quan-xin, as anthologized in *Zhong Guo Dang Dai Zhen Jiu Ming Jia Yi An (Contemporary Chinese National Acupuncture & Moxibustion Famous Masters' Case Histories)*, compiled by Wang Xue-tai & Liu Guan-jun, Jilin Science & Technology Press, Changchun, 1991, p. 441-442

[19] Du Ting-hai & Lu Xiao-hong, "Prof. Lu Jing-zhong's Experiences in the Pattern Discrimination & Treatment of Asymptomatic Diabetes," *Xin Zhong Yi (New Chinese Medicine)*, #7, 2001, p. 11

[20] Xia Cheng-dong, "Plucking the Essentials of Professor Ding Xue-ping's Experiences in the Treatment of Diabetes," *Xin Zhong Yi (New Chinese Medicine)*, #2, 2001, p. 17

[21] Lu Ren-he, *Tang Niao Bing Ji Qi Bing Fa Zheng Zhong Xi Yi Zhen Zhi Xue (The Onset of Diabetes and Its Diagnosis & Treatment by Chinese & Western Medicine)*, People's Health & Hygiene Press, Beijing, 1997, p. 47

10

GESTATIONAL DIABETES

Gestational diabetes mellitus (GDM) is defined as any degree of glucose intolerance with onset or first recognition during pregnancy.[1] This definition is applicable whether or not insulin is used for treatment and whether or not the condition persists after pregnancy. It does not exclude the possibility that an unrecognized glucose intolerance may have antedated or begun concomitantly with pregnancy. Three to five percent of all pregnant women in the United States are diagnosed as having gestational diabetes resulting in approximately 185,000 cases per year.[2] The actual prevalence of GDM may be as high as 14% of all pregnancies depending on the population studied and the diagnostic tests employed.[3] Gestational diabetes usually develops because of a faulty physical interaction between the mother and baby. During the second trimester, somewhere between 24-28 weeks, the placenta begins producing many hormones. One of these hormones may block the action of insulin in the mother, thus creating insulin resistance. If the mother cannot produce enough extra insulin to overcome this resistance, her blood sugar will rise. The mother's high blood sugar then stimulates the baby to make more insulin and move more sugar into his or her cells, causing him or her to gain extra weight. If left unregulated, these changes can have serious harmful effects on both the mother and child.

While any woman may develop gestational diabetes, some of the risk factors are a previous diagnosis of GDM, severe physical or emotional stress if prone to GDM, obesity, a family history of diabetes, a history of miscarriage, having previously given birth to a very large infant (i.e., greater than nine pounds), stillbirth, or a child with a birth defect, or having too much amniotic fluid (polyhydraminos). Women over 25 years of age are also at greater risk than those under 25.[4] Western medical screening for GDM is routinely performed (unless otherwise indicated) between weeks 24-28 of gestation in women meeting one or more of the following criteria:

1. Twenty-five years of age or older
2. Less than 25 years of age and obese (i.e., 20% or more over desired body weight or a body mass index (BMI) equal to or over $27kg/m^2$
3. A family history of diabetes in a first degree relative
4. Member of an ethnic/racial group with a high prevalence of diabetes, e.g., Hispanic American, Native American, Asian American, African American, or Pacific Islander.

Such screening tests consist of a 50g oral glucose load followed by plasma glucose determination one hour later. A value equal to or greater than 140mg/dL (7.8mmol/L) one hour after a 50g load indicates the need for a full diagnostic 100g three hour oral glucose tolerance test (OGTT) performed in the fasting state. A Western medical diagnosis of gestational diabetes is made if two or more of the following blood sugar levels are higher than the following criteria:

1. Fasting blood glucose > 105mg/dL
2. One hour blood glucose > 190mg/dL
3. Two hour blood glucose > 165mg/dL
4. Three hours blood glucose > 145mg/dL

The Western medical treatment of gestational diabetes consists of immediate dietary modification in order to regulate blood sugar levels. If dietary modification alone is not able to control blood glucose, insulin injections may be necessary. In order to determine blood glucose levels, women with GDM must self-monitor their blood glucose up to four times per day as well as test for ketones in their urine 1-2 times per week. For some women, exercising, such as walking after meals or at specific times of the day, helps to keep blood sugars in better control.[5]

Risks to the mother if GDM is not controlled include the possibility of delivery by Ceasarean section due to the baby's large size or the development of toxemia (a.k.a. eclampsia), increased urinary tract infections, and development of pregnancy induced high blood pressure. About 5% of women with GDM develop toxemia during pregnancy.[6] Approximately 40% of women diagnosed with GDM develop type 2 diabetes later in life.[7] In one large study, more than half of all women with GDM developed overt type 2 diabetes within 15 years of pregnancy.[8] The risks to the infant include macrosomia (i.e., a large, fat baby), shoulder dystocia, neonatal hypoglycemia, increased risk for obesity and diabetes, prolonged neonatal jaundice, low blood calcemia, and respiratory distress syndrome. In the majority of cases, GDM disappears automatically after delivery.

CHINESE MEDICAL DISEASE CATEGORIZATION: The traditional Chinese disease categories which correspond to gestational diabetes or its complications include *ren shen fan re*, vexatious heat during pregnancy, *ren shen fan ke*, vexatious thirst during pregnancy, *ren shen xuan yun*, dizziness and vertigo during pregnancy, *ren shen tou zhang tong*, head distention and pain during pregnancy, *ren shen xian zheng*, epilepsy during pregnancy, *ren shen xiao bian lin tong*, urinary strangury and pain during pregnancy, and *ren shen duo niao*, polyuria during pregnancy.

CHINESE DISEASE MECHANISMS: During pregnancy, yin, essence, blood, and fluids are transported downward to the uterus in order to foster and nourish the fetus. If, due to natural endowment insufficiency or habitual bodily yin vacuity, this may leave yin and blood within the mother's body depleted and vacuous. Thus yin vacuity may engender heat internally, and this heat may further damage and consume yin fluids, leading to the easy engenderment of wasting and thirsting disease. It is also possible for habitual depression to cause the liver to lose its spreading. Because the fetus already obstructs the mother's qi mechanism as it grows in size towards the end of the pregnancy, qi stagnation often becomes more severe during the last trimester, and enduring or aggravated depression may transform fire which may also damage and consume yin fluids. Further, habitual addiction to sweets and fats may also cause accumulation of heat brewing internally. If, during the later half of pregnancy when yin and blood tend to become vacuous and insuffi-

cient and yang qi tends to become exuberant, such exuberant yang qi may join with these heat evils, thus exacerbating each other. Hence, there is yin vacuity with heat exuberance which is also able to give rise to wasting and thirsting disease.

TREATMENT BASED ON PATTERN DISCRIMINATION:

1. YIN VACUITY WITH HEAT EXUBERANCE PATTERN

MAIN SYMPTOMS: Dry mouth and parched throat, vexatious thirst, polydipsia, frequent, numerous, excessive urination, polyphagia, rapid hungering, dry, bound stools, a red tongue with scanty fluids, and a slippery, rapid pulse

TREATMENT PRINCIPLES: Enrich yin and clear heat

RX: *Zeng Ye Tang* (Increase Humors Decoction) plus *Bai Hu Tang* (White Tiger Decoction) with additions and subtractions

INGREDIENTS: Uncooked Gypsum Fibrosum (*Shi Gao*), 20g, uncooked Radix Rehmanniae (*Sheng Di*) and Radix Scrophulariae Ningpoensis (*Xuan Shen*), 15g each, Radix Glehniae Littoralis (*Sha Shen*) and Tuber Ophiopogonis Japonici (*Mai Men Dong*), 12g each, and Rhizoma Anemarrhenae Aspheloidis (*Zhi Mu*) and Radix Scutellariae Baicalensis (*Huang Qin*), 9g each

FORMULA ANALYSIS: *Sheng Di, Xuan Shen, Sha Shen* and *Mai Men Dong* enrich yin and increase humors. *Huang Qin, Shi Gao,* and *Zhi Mu* clear heat and engender fluids.

ADDITIONS & SUBTRACTIONS: If there are dry, bound stools, one can increase the doses of *Sheng Di* and *Xuan Shen* in order to enrich yin and increase humors, moisten the intestines and free the flow of the stools. If there is simultaneous obstruction and stagnation of the qi mechanism with chest and rib-side distention and oppression, add nine grams each of Pericarpium Citri Reticulatae Viride (*Qing Pi*), Fructus Meliae Toosendan (*Chuan Lian Zi*), and Fructus Citri Aurantii (*Zhi Ke*) to course the liver and rectify the qi. If oral thirst is severe, add nine grams each of Herba Dendrobii (*Shi Hu*), Rhizoma Phragmitis Communis (*Lu Gen*), and Fructus Pruni Mume (*Wu Mei*) to engender fluids and stop thirst.

ACUPUNCTURE & MOXIBUSTION: *Tai Xi* (Ki 3), *Zhao Hai* (Ki 6), *Nei Ting* (St 44)

FORMULA ANALYSIS: Supplementing *Tai Xi* and *Zhao*

Hai supplements the kidneys and enriches yin. Draining *Nei Ting* clears heat.

ADDITIONS & SUBTRACTIONS: If oral thirst is severe, add supplementing *Cheng Jiang* (CV 24) and *Lie Que* (Lu 7). If there is concomitant liver depression qi stagnation, add draining *Tai Chong* (Liv 3).

2. QI & YIN VACUITY PATTERN

MAIN SYMPTOMS: Shortness of breath, lack of strength, dry mouth and a desire to drink, dry, bound stools, frequent, numerous, excessive urination, a fat tongue with white fur, and a deep, fine, slippery pulse

TREATMENT PRINCIPLES: Boost the qi and nourish yin

RX: *Sheng Mai San* (Engender the Pulse Powder) plus *Zeng Ye Tang* (Increase Humors Decoction) with additions and subtractions

INGREDIENTS: Rhizoma Polygonati (*Huang Jing*), 20g, Radix Pseudostellariae Heterophyllae (*Tai Zi Shen*), Radix Glehniae Littoralis (*Sha Shen*), uncooked Radix Rehmanniae (*Sheng Di*), and Radix Scrophulariae Ningpoensis (*Xuan Shen*), 15g each, Tuber Ophiopogonis Japonici (*Mai Men Dong*) and Tuber Asparagi Cochinensis (*Tian Men Dong*), 12g each, and Fructus Schisandrae Chinensis (*Wu Wei Zi*), Fructus Lycii Chinensis (*Wu Wei Zi*), and Fructus Corni Officinalis (*Shan Zhu Yu*), 9g each

FORMULA ANALYSIS: *Tai Zi Shen* and *Huang Jing* boost the qi and nourish yin. *Sheng Di, Xuan Shen, Mai Men Dong, Tian Men Dong, Sha Shen,* and *Wu Wei Zi* enrich yin and engender fluids. *Shan Zhu Yu* and *Gou Qi Zi* enrich and supplement the liver and kidneys.

ADDITIONS & SUBTRACTIONS: If there is lassitude of the spirit, lack of strength, and other such obvious qi vacuity symptoms, add 15-30 grams of Radix Astragali Membranacei (*Huang Qi*) and 9-15 grams of Radix Codonopositis Pilosulae (*Dang Shen*). If there is dry mouth and polydipsia due to yin vacuity and internal heat, add nine grams each of Rhizoma Anemarrhenae Aspheloidis (*Zhi Mu*), Fructus Pruni Mume (*Wu Mei*), and Herba Dendrobii (*Shi Hu*) to clear heat, enrich yin, and engender fluids. If there is dizziness or vertigo due to liver-kidney yin vacuity, add 9-15 grams each of Flos Chrysanthemi Morifolii (*Ju Hua*) and Ramulus Uncariae Cum Uncis (*Gou Teng*). If there is polyphagia and rapid hungering, add 12 grams each of cooked Radix Rehmanniae (*Shu Di*) and Rhizoma Polygonati Odorati (*Yu Zhu*).

ACUPUNCTURE & MOXIBUSTION: *Tai Xi* (Ki 3), *Zu San Li* (St 36), *Pi Shu* (Bl 20), *Shen Shu* (Bl 23)

FORMULA ANALYSIS: Supplementing *Zu San Li* and *Pi Shu* supplements the spleen and boosts the qi. Supplementing *Tai Xi* and *Shen Shu* supplements the kidneys and enriches yin.

ADDITIONS & SUBTRACTIONS: If there is dry mouth and polydipsia, add supplementing *Cheng Jiang* (CV 24), *Zhao Hai* (Ki 6), and *Lie Que* (Lu 7). If there is liver-kidney yin vacuity, add supplementing *Qu Quan* (Liv 8), *Ge Shu* (Bl 17), and *Gan Shu* (Bl 18). If there is polyphagia and rapid hungering, add draining *Nei Ting* (St 44) and use even supplementing-even draining technique at *Zu San Li*.

3. LIVER-KIDNEY YIN VACUITY PATTERN

MAIN SYMPTOMS: Low back and knee soreness and limpness, frequent, numerous, excessive urination which is possibly turbid like rice-washing water, dry mouth and a desire to drink, dizziness or vertigo, a red tongue with scanty fluids, and a deep, fine, slippery pulse

TREATMENT PRINCIPLES: Enrich and supplement the liver and kidneys

RX: *Liu Wei Di Huang Wan* (Six Flavors Rehmannia Pills)

INGREDIENTS: Radix Dioscoreae Oppositae (*Shan Yao*), 15g, cooked Radix Rehmanniae (*Shu Di*), 12g, and Fructus Corni Officinalis (*Shan Zhu Yu*), Sclerotium Poriae Cocos (*Fu Ling*), Rhizoma Alismatis (*Ze Xie*), and Cortex Radicis Moutan (*Dan Pi*), 9g each

FORMULA ANALYSIS: *Shu Di* enriches the kidneys and fosters the essence. It is the ruling medicinal in this formula. *Shu Di* is assisted by *Shan Zhu Yu* which nourishes the liver and kidneys and boosts the essence. *Shan Yao* supplements spleen yin and gathers the finest essence. *Fu Ling* blandly seeps dampness from the spleen. It also assists *Shan Yao* to boost the spleen. *Ze Xie* clears and discharges kidney fire as well as protects from *Shu Di*'s enriching sliminess. *Dan Pi* clears and discharges liver fire. It also helps control *Shan Zhu Yu*'s warmth in addition to quickening the blood and transforming stasis.

ADDITIONS & SUBTRACTIONS: If there is yin vacuity with fire effulgence, add nine grams each of Rhizoma Anemarrhenae Aspheloidis (*Zhi Mu*) and Cortex Phellodendri (*Huang Bai*) to enrich yin and downbear fire. If there is yin vacuity and yang hyperactivity with dizziness and vertigo, one can add 12 grams each of Tuber Ophiopogonis Japonici (*Mai Men Dong*) and Plastrum Testudinis (*Gui Ban*) and nine grams each of Flos Chrysanthemi Morifolii (*Ju Hua*) and Ramulus Uncariae Cum Uncis (*Gou Teng*) to enrich yin and level the liver. If there is bilateral lower leg edema, low back soreness, and turbid urine, add nine grams each of Radix Dipsaci (*Xu Duan*), Semen Cuscutae Chinensis (*Tu Si Zi*), Sclerotium Polypori Umbellati (*Zhu Ling*), and Cortex Radicis Mori Albi (*Sang Bai Pi*) to supplement the kidneys and quiet the fetus, disinhibit water and disperse swelling.

ACUPUNCTURE & MOXIBUSTION: *Tai Xi* (Ki 3), *Qu Quan* (Liv 8), *Ge Shu* (Bl 17), *Gan Shu* (Bl 18), *Shen Shu* (Bl 23)

FORMULA ANALYSIS: Supplementing *Tai Xi* and *Shen Shu* supplements the kidneys and enriches yin. Supplementing *Qu Quan*, *Ge Shu*, and *Gan Shu* supplements the liver and nourishes the blood.

ADDITIONS & SUBTRACTIONS: If there is yin vacuity with yang hyperactivity, add draining *Bai Hui* (GV 20), *Feng Chi* (Bl 20), and *Yin Tang* (M-HN-3) and replace *Qu Quan* with even supplementing-even draining *Tai Chong* (Liv 3). If there is high blood pressure, omit *Qu Quan* and add draining *Qu Chi* (LI 11) and *Feng Chi* (GB 20) and even supplementing-even draining *Tai Chong* and *Zu San Li* (St 36). If there is lower limb edema and turbid urine (meaning obvious proteinemia), add draining *Yin Ling Quan* (Sp 9) and *Zhong Ji* (CV 3).

REPRESENTATIVE CASE HISTORIES:

CASE 1[9]

The patient was a 28 year old female who was first examined on Oct. 8, 1989. She was two months pregnant with anorexia, nausea, vomiting, and dysphoria. Recently, the woman had begun vomiting immediately after eating. Other symptoms included fatigue, lack of strength, and somnolence. Urine ketones were (++), urine sugar was (++++), blood sugar was 6.5mmol/L, blood pressure was 18/10kPa, and there was coffee-like mucus in her vomitus. The patient was so weak that she had to be supported by others when brought into the clinic. She was emaciated and was disinclined to speak since this further exhausted her. The woman reported she had been constipated for half a year, often had a feverish sensation, was thirsty, and that her urine was dark and scanty. Her tongue was red

and dry with thin, yellow fur, and her pulse was fine and rapid. The patient's mother had a history of diabetes.

Based on the above signs and symptoms, the patient's pattern was categorized as liver-stomach disharmony with gallbladder heat and dry blood damaging the network vessels, and qi and yin dual vacuity. Therefore, the treatment principles were to rectify the liver and boost the qi, engender fluids and stop vomiting. The prescription written included: Radix Scrophulariae Ningpoensis (*Xuan Shen*), 18g, Caulis Perillae Frutescentis (*Zi Su Geng*), Radix Codonopsitis Pilosulae (*Dang Shen*), and Pericarpium Trichosanthis Kirlowii (*Gua Lou Pi*), 15g each, and Radix Bupleuri (*Chai Hu*), stir-fried Radix Scutellariae Baicalensis (*Huang Qin*), Rhizoma Coptidis Chinensis (*Huang Lian*), Fructus Evodiae Rutecarpae (*Wu Zhu Yu*), Caulis Bambusae In Taeniis (*Zhu Ru*), and Rhizoma Pinelliae Ternatae (*Ban Xia*), 6g each. These medicinals were decocted in water and administered internally.

After two *ji* of the above formula, the patient had one bowel movement and the number of times she vomited was reduced. Her spirit improved and the amount of urine decreased. However, the woman was still dizzy and nauseated and had a red tongue with thin fur and a fine, bowstring, slippery, but forceless pulse. Urine sugar was (++) and the ketones in her urine had become negative. Therefore, the following modification of the above formula was prescribed: Radix Codonopsitis Pilosulae (*Dang Shen*) and Radix Scrophulariae Ningpoensis (*Xuan Shen*), 15g each, uncooked Radix Rehmanniae (*Sheng Di*) and Ramulus Loranthi Seu Visci (*Sang Ji Sheng*), 12g each, Tuber Ophiopogonis Japonici (*Mai Men Dong*), Sclerotium Poriae Cocos (*Fu Ling*), and Caulis Perillae Frutescentis (*Zi Su Geng*), 10g each, Caulis Bambusae In Taeniis (*Zhu Ru*), 9g, Rhizoma Coptidis Chinensis (*Huang Lian*) and stir-fried Radix Scutellariae Baicalensis (*Huang Qin*), 6g each, and Radix Glycyrrhizae (*Gan Cao*), 3g.

After three *ji* of this formula, the patient's bowels were freely flowing and vomiting occurred only occasionally. She still had nausea in the mornings, and her urine sugar was (+). Her blood sugar was not tested. In order to secure and consolidate the treatment effect, the woman was prescribed *Xiang Sha Liu Jun Zi Wan* (Auklandia & Amomum Six Gentlemen Pills) for three days with the intention to fortify the spleen and supplement the qi, harmonize the stomach and secure the fetus. The woman was also recommended to check her blood sugar occasionally to check for any changes in her diabetes.

REMARKS:

1. While the above three patterns may be the main ones in gestational diabetes, these three root patterns may be complicated by a number of other commonly seen disease mechanisms, especially phlegm dampness, depressive or phlegm heat, liver depression qi stagnation, and blood stasis. Therefore, it is likely that the above formulas will have to be modified with additions and subtractions.

2. As part of their basic education, all acupuncturists learn that certain acupuncture points are forbidden during pregnancy. However, what many Western acupuncturists do not understand is that these prohibitions are not absolute. Such acupuncture points are forbidden during pregnancy only if *unwarranted*. When the patient's condition—either their pattern or their symptoms—indicates their use, then they can and even should be used unless another point or points will work equally as well. In general, it is not easy to initiate labor at full term with acupuncture, let alone causing an accidental abortion with acupuncture. For instance, in the case of pre-eclampsia, acupuncture should definitely be used as a first aid treatment to lower the blood pressure and prevent seizures, and typically one or more points used in such a treatment are otherwise contraindicated during pregnancy.

ENDNOTES:

[1] Metzger, B.E., "Proceedings of the Third International Workshop-Conference on Gestational Diabates Mellitus," 1991, p. 201
[2] www.amoc.org/gesdiab.htm
[3] www.diabetes.org/diabetescare/supplement198/s60.htm
[4] www.nichd.nih.gov/publications/pubs/gest1.htm
[5] www.diabetes.ca/about_diabetes/gestational.htm
[6] www.nichd.nih.gov/publications/pubs/gest2.htm
[7] www.amoc.org, op. cit.
[8] www.nichd.nih.gov/publications/pubs/gest2.htm
[9] Chen Jin-ding, *The Treatment of Diabetes with Traditional Chinese Medicine*, trans. by Sun Ying-kui & Zhou Shu-hui, Shandong Science & Technology Press, Jinan, 1994, p. 141-143

11

HEPATOGENIC DIABETES

Secondary hepatic parenchymal damage diabetes refers to diabetes mellitus secondary to typically chronic liver disease. This condition is also called hepatogenic diabetes. Chronic liver disease causes decreased glucose tolerance in 50-80% of cases and diabetes in 15-30% of cases. In addition, many oral hypoglycemic agents may cause damage to the liver, and, while injected insulin is not injurious to the liver, it is difficult to adjust the dose. Therefore, injection of insulin commonly results in hypoglycemia which does not benefit the recuperation of the liver.

TREATMENT BASED ON PATTERN DISCRIMINATION:

1. LIVER DEPRESSION & DAMP HEAT PATTERN

MAIN SYMPTOMS: Torpid intake but no severe emaciation, abdominal distention, lack of strength, rib-side distention and pain, if severe, possible yellowing of the body and eyes which is fresh and bright in color, thirst not leading to drinking or possible thirst with a desire to drink but not actually drinking, short, yellow urination but not profuse urination, a bitter taste in the mouth, a red tongue with slimy, yellow fur, and a soggy, rapid or bowstring, rapid pulse

NOTE: This pattern is mostly seen in those with chronic active hepatitis and diabetes mellitus.

TREATMENT PRINCIPLES: Clear the liver and discharge heat, disinhibit dampness and move or transport the spleen

RX: *Qing Gan Jiang Tang Tang* (Clear the Liver & Lower Sugar Decoction)

INGREDIENTS: Herba Artemisiae Capillaris (*Yin Chen Hao*) and Herba Taraxaci Mongolici Cum Radice (*Pu Gong Ying*), 30g each, Gypsum Fibrosum (*Shi Gao*), 20g, Radix Scutellariae Baicalensis (*Huang Qin*), Rhizoma Coptidis Chinensis (*Huang Lian*), Fructus Forsythiae Suspensae (*Lian Qiao*), Radix Bupleuri (*Chai Hu*), Herba Agastachis Seu Pogostemi (*Huo Xiang*), Radix Et Rhizoma Polygoni Cuspidati (*Hu Zhang*), Tuber Curcumae (*Yu Jin*), uncooked Fructus Gardeniae Jasminoidis (*Zhi Zi*), stir-fried Rhizoma Atractylodis Macrocephalae (*Bai Zhu*), Semen Coicis Lachryma-jobi (*Yi Yi Ren*), and uncooked Radix Glycyrrhizae (*Gan Cao*), 10g each, and Fructus Cardamomi (*Bai Dou Kou*), 6g

FORMULA ANALYSIS: *Yin Chen Hao, Pu Gong Ying, Shi Gao, Huang Qin, Huang Lian, Hu Zhang, Zhi Zi,* and *Lian Qiao* clear heat and eliminate dampness from the liver-gallbladder. *Chai Hu* and *Yu Jin* course the liver and resolve depression. *Huo Xiang, Bai Zhu, Yi Yi Ren,* and *Bai Dou Kou* arouse the spleen and dry and disinhibit dampness. Uncooked *Gan Cao* both clears heat and resolves toxins and harmonizes all the other medicinals in this formula.

ADDITIONS & SUBTRACTIONS: If torpid intake and scanty appetite are marked, add 15 grams of stir-fried Fructus Germinatus Hordei Vulgaris (*Mai Ya*) and nine grams of Endothelium Corneum Gigeriae Galli (*Ji Nei Jin*). If there is ductal glomus and nausea, add nine grams each of Rhizoma Pinelliae Ternatae (*Ban Xia*) and Rhizoma Acori Graminei (*Shi Chang Pu*).

ACUPUNCTURE & MOXIBUSTION: *Tai Chong* (Liv 3), *Xing Jian* (Liv 2), *Yang Ling Quan* (GB 34), *Yin Ling Quan* (Sp 9)

FORMULA ANALYSIS: Needling *Tai Chong* through to

Xing Jian and needling *Yang Ling Quan* through to *Yin Ling Quan*, both with draining technique, courses the liver and resolves depression, clears heat and disinhibits dampness.

ADDITIONS & SUBTRACTIONS: If torpid intake and scanty appetite are marked, add draining *Zhong Wan* (CV 12) and *Zu San Li* (St 36). If there is ductal glomus and nausea, add draining *Zhong Wan* (CV 12), *Nei Guan* (Per 6), and *Zu San Li* (St 36). If there is jaundice, add draining *Zhi Yang* (GV 9). If spleen vacuity is pronounced, use even supplementing-even draining at *Zu San Li* and add supplementing *Pi Shu* (Bl 20) and *Wei Shu* (Bl 21).

2. LIVER QI DEPRESSION & STAGNATION PATTERN

MAIN SYMPTOMS: Absence of jaundice, rib-side distention and pain, chest oppression and a tendency to sighing, easy anger, fatigue, lack of strength, ductal and abdominal distention and fullness, torpid intake, scanty appetite, dry, hard, irregular stools, no thirst or thirst but no polydipsia, clear, long urination, spider nevi, liver palms, a liverish facial expression, a normal or dark tongue with thin, dry, white fur, and a fine, bowstring pulse. In this case, FBG is normal or only slightly high, but PPBG is markedly elevated.

NOTE: This pattern is mostly seen in those with chronic hepatitis or those with liver cirrhosis accompanied by diabetes. In actual fact, it is a liver wood-spleen-stomach-earth disharmony pattern, not just a liver pattern regardless of its name as the following treatment principles and plan show.

TREATMENT PRINCIPLES: Course the liver and rectify the qi, fortify the spleen and harmonize the stomach

RX: *Shu Gan Jiang Tang Tang* (Course the Liver & Lower Sugar Decoction)

INGREDIENTS: Radix Puerariae (*Ge Gen*) and Radix Trichosanthis Kirlowii (*Tian Hua Fen*), 30g each, Radix Astragali Membranacei (*Huang Qi*) and processed Rhizoma Atractylodis (*Cang Zhu*), 20g each, Radix Bupleuri (*Chai Hu*), Fructus Citri Aurantii (*Zhi Ke*), Rhizoma Cyperi Rotundi (*Xiang Fu*), Radix Angelicae Sinensis (*Dang Gui*), stir-fried Rhizoma Atractylodis Macrocephalae (*Bai Zhu*), and stir-fried Radix Albus Paeoniae Lactiflorae (*Bai Shao*), 10g each, and uncooked Radix Glycyrrhizae (*Gan Cao*), 6g

FORMULA ANALYSIS: *Ge Gen* and *Tian Hua Fen* engen-

der fluids and moisten dryness. *Chai Hu, Xiang Fu,* and *Zhi Ke* course the liver and rectify the qi. *Dang Gui* and *Bai Shao* nourish the blood and emolliate the liver. *Huang Qi, Cang Zhu,* and *Bai Zhu* fortify the spleen, and uncooked *Gan Cao* harmonizes all the other medicinals in this formula.

ADDITIONS & SUBTRACTIONS: If there is short, reddish urination, add 15 grams each of Herba Artemisiae Capillaris (*Yin Chen Hao*) and Talcum (*Hua Shi*). If there are liver palms or spider nevi, add 15 grams each of Cortex Radicis Moutan (*Dan Pi*) and uncooked Radix Rehmanniae (*Sheng Di*). If there are loose stools, add 15 grams each of Radix Dioscoreae Oppositae (*Shan Yao*) and Semn Coicis Lachryma-jobi (*Yi Yi Ren*).

ACUPUNCTURE & MOXIBUSTION: *Tai Chong* (Liv 3), *He Gu* (LI 4), *Zu San Li* (St 36), *San Yin Jiao* (Sp 6)

FORMULA ANALYSIS: Draining *Tai Chong* and *He Gu* courses the liver and rectifies the qi. Supplementing *Zu San Li* and *San Yin Jiao* fortifies the spleen and boosts the qi.

ADDITIONS & SUBTRACTIONS: If there is concomitant damp heat, add draining *Yin Ling Quan* and use even supplementing-even draining at *San Yin Jiao*. If there is short, reddish urination, also drain *Zhong Ji* (CV 3). If there is concomitant blood stasis, add draining *Xue Hai* (Sp 10) and use even supplementing-even draining at *San Yin Jiao*. If spleen vacuity is marked, add supplementing *Pi Shu* (Bl 20) and *Wei Shu* (Bl 21). If liver blood vacuity is marked, add supplementing *Ge Shu* (Bl 17) and even supplementing-even draining *Gan Shu* (Bl 18).

3. LIVER-KIDNEY YIN VACUITY PATTERN

MAIN SYMPTOMS: Emaciation, vexatious heat in the five hearts, epistaxis, bleeding gums, hypochondral glomus and lumps (*i.e.,* hepatosplenomegaly), abdominal distention, torpid intake and poor appetite or polyphagia and rapid hungering, constipation, polyuria, dry lips, dry mouth with a desire to drink, a red tongue with peeled fur and lack of fluids, and a bowstring, fine, rapid pulse. In addition, one mostly sees liver palms, spider nevi, and, if severe, jaundice and ascites.

NOTE: This pattern is mostly seen in those with chronic hepatitis or liver cirrhosis and diabetes with a relatively long disease course.

TREATMENT PRINCIPLES: Emolliate and nourish, clear and discharge, enrich and supplement the liver and kidneys

RX: *Yang Gan Jiang Tang Tang* (Nourish the Liver & Lower Sugar Decoction)

INGREDIENTS: Tuber Asparagi Cochinensis (*Tian Men Dong*), Tuber Ophiopogonis Japonici (*Mai Men Dong*), and Radix Trichosanthis Kirlowii (*Tian Hua Fen*), 30g each, uncooked Radix Rehmanniae (*Sheng Di*), 25g, Radix Polygoni Multiflori (*He Shou Wu*), Rhizoma Polygonati Odorati (*Yu Zhu*), and processed Rhizoma Polygonati (*Huang Jing*), 15g each Rhizoma Anemarrhenae Aspheloidis (*Zhi Mu*), Fructus Lycii Chinensis (*Gou Qi Zi*), Radix Scrophulariae Ningpoensis (*Xuan Shen*), Cortex Radicis Lycii Chinensis (*Di Gu Pi*), and Cortex Radicis Moutan (*Dan Pi*), 10g each, and uncooked Radix Glycyrrhizae (*Gan Cao*), 6g

FORMULA ANALYSIS: *Tian Men Dong, Mai Men Dong, Tian Hua Fen, Huang Jing,* and *Yu Zhu* engender fluids and moisten dryness. *Xuan Shen, Dan Pi, Di Gu Pi,* and *Zhi Mu* clear heat and cool the blood. *He Shou Wu* and *Gou Qi Zi* nourish the liver and supplement the kidneys. Uncooked *Gan Cao* clears heat at the same time as it harmonizes all the other medicinals in this formula.

ADDITIONS & SUBTRACTIONS: If there are bleeding gums or epistaxis, add 15 grams each of Herba Artemisiae Apiaceae (*Qing Hao*) and Radix Gentianae Macrocphyllae (*Qin Jiao*). If there is ascites, add 15 grams each of Semen Plantaginis (*Che Qian Zi*), Sclerotium Polypori Umbellati (*Zhu Ling*), and stir-fried Radix Dioscoreae Oppositae (*Shan Yao*). If there is hypochondral glomus or lumps, add 15 grams each of Carapax Amydae Sinensis (*Bie Jia*) and Rhizoma Sparganii (*San Leng*) and nine grams of Pericarpium Citri Reticulatae Viride (*Qing Pi*).

ACUPUNCTURE & MOXIBUSTION: *Tai Chong* (Liv 3), *Tai Xi* (Ki 3), *San Yin Jiao* (Sp 6), *Ge Shu* (Bl 17), *Gan Shu* (Bl 18), *Shen Shu* (Bl 23)

FORMULA ANALYSIS: Supplementing *Tai Chong, San Yin Jiao, Ge Shu,* and *Gan Shu* nourishes the blood and emolliates the liver. Supplementing *Tai Xi, San Yin Jiao,* and *Shen Shu* enriches yin and supplements the kidneys.

ADDITIONS & SUBTRACTIONS: To clear heat from the blood, add draining *Xue Hai* (Sp 10) and *Qu Chi* (LI 11). To clear heat from the stomach, add draining *Nei Ting* (St 44). To treat hypochondral glomus and lumps, draining *Xue Hai* (Sp 10), *Zhang Men* (Liv 13), and *Qi Men* (Liv 14). For upper abdominal distention, add draining *Zhong Wan* (CV 12). For lower abdominal distention, add draining *Qi Hai* (CV 6) and *Tian Shu* (St 25). For constipation, add *Zhi Gou* (TB 6), *Zhao Hai* (Ki 6), *Nei Ting* (St 44), *Tian Shu* (St 25), and *Da Chang Shu* (Bl 25).

ABSTRACTS OF REPRESENTATIVE CHINESE RESEARCH:

Wei Su-xia, "The Treatment of 40 Cases of Hepatogenic Diabetes Via the Liver," *Si Chuan Zhong Yi (Sichuan Chinese Medicine)*, #10, 1999, p. 16-17: Among the 40 patients in this study, there were 28 men and 12 women aged 30-71 years old. Thirty-three patients had chronic hepatitis, six had cirrhosis, and one had liver cancer. Diagnostic criteria included a history of chronic hepatitis, abnormal liver function, the three polys, FBG equal to or more than 7.0mmol/L, and two hour PPBG equal to or more than 11mmol/L. Patients were discriminated and treated according to the three patterns and Chinese herbal formulas presented above. One *ji* of these medicinals was decocted in water and administered per day in two divided doses. One month equaled one course of treatment, and treatment efficacy was judged after two such courses.

Marked effect meant that the clinical symptoms disappeared, FBG was less than 6.66mmol/L, PPBG was less than 8.3mmol/L, and urine glucose was negative. Some effect was defined as a marked improvement in clinical symptoms, FBG less than 6.66mmol/L, PPBG less than 10mmol/L, and urine glucose negative. No effect meant that these criteria were not met. Based on these criteria, 26 patients were deemed to have gotten a marked effect, 11 patients got some effect, and three patients got no effect. Thus the total amelioration rate was 92%.

Zhu Yong-juan, "Clinical Observation of 100 Cases of Type II Hepatogenic Diabetes," *Shang Hai Zhong Yi Yao Za Zhi (Shanghai Journal of Chinese Medicine & Medicinals)*, #7, 1999, p. 19-20: In this study, there were 46 men and 54 women. The youngest was 30 years of age, and the oldest was 82 years of age. The average age was 56 years. The shortest duration of disease was one year and the longest duration was 17 years. The average duration of disease was four years. There were 14 cases of liver and kidney disease, 46 cases of itching skin, 68 cases of vision problems, and 24 cases of neuropathy. Nine cases had a fasting blood glucose between 7.7-9.6mmol/L; 27 cases had a fasting blood glucose between 9.7-11.5mmol/L; 32 cases had a fasting blood glucose between 11.6-13.4mmol/L; 28 cases had a fasting blood glucose between 13.5-15.3mmol/L; and four cases had a fasting blood glucose between 15.4-17.2mmol/L. The average fasting blood glucose was 12.54mmol/L. Postprandial blood glucose levels ranged from 11.3-23.8mmol/L, with an average of 17.43mmol/L.

Coursing the liver and regulating the qi were the primary treatment principles. The formula consisted of: Semen Litchi Chinensis (*Li Zhi He*), 20g, Radix Astragali (*Huang Qi*), 15g, Sclerotium Poriae Cocos (*Fu Ling*), Herba Portulacae Oleraceae (*Ma Chi Xian*), and Lignum Suberalatum Euonymi (*Gui Jian Yu*), 12g each, Radix Albus Paeoniae Lactiflorae (*Bai Shao Yao*), Radix Angelicae Sinensis (*Dang Gui*), Radix Bupleuri (*Chai Hu*), Radix Ligustici Wallichii (*Chuan Xiong*), Rhizoma Atractylodis Macrocephalae (*Bai Zhu*), and Radix Puerariae (*Ge Gen*), 9g each, and Folium Nelumbinis Nuciferae (*He Ye*), 6g. For liver depression-spleen vacuity, six grams of Radix Panacis Ginseng (*Ren Shen*) and as much as 30 grams of Radix Astragali Membrancei (*Huang Qi*) were added. For liver depression transforming into fire, six grams of Fructus Gardeniae Jasminoidis (*Shan Zhi*) and nine grams of Cortex Radicis Moutan (*Dan Pi*) were added. If depressive heat had damaged yin, 15 grams of Cortex Radicis Lycii Chinensis (*Di Gu Pi*) together with *Liu Wei Di Huang Wan Jia Jian* (Six Flavors Rehmannia Pills with Additions & Subtractions) were added. For severe thirst, 12 grams of Rhizoma Phragmitis Communis (*Lu Gen*) were added. For blood stasis, 15 grams of Radix Salviae Miltiorrhizae (*Dan Shen*) and 12 grams of Semen Pruni Persicae (*Tao Ren*) were added. For yang vacuity edematous swelling or albuminuria, *Fu Gui Ba Wei Wan* (Aconite & Cinnamon Eight Flavors Pills) were added. For numbness and aching pain in the arms and legs, 30 grams of Ramulus Mori Albi (*Sang Zhi*) were added. For dimness of vision, 15 grams of Fructus Tribuli Terrestris (*Bai Ji Li*), 12 grams of Concha Haliotidis (*Shi Jue Ming*), and nine grams of Flos Chrysanthemi Morifolii (*Ju Hua*) were added. For skin itching, 10 grams each of Fructus Kochiae Scopariae (*Di Fu Zi*) and Radix Sophorae Flavescentis (*Ku Shen*) were added. If the flesh was festering (with infection), *Jin Huang San* (Golden Yellow Powder) was used as an external wash. One *ji* of the above medicinals were decocted in water each day for 30 days, with one month equaling one course of treatment. The duration of treatment was four months.

If symptoms were alleviated, the fasting blood glucose was lower than 6.1mmol/L, and glycosuria was (±), then the results were considered very good. If symptoms were alleviated, the fasting blood glucose was lowered by 1.5-2.0mmol/L, and the glycosuria was (+ - ++), then the results were considered moderately good. If there was no change in the symptoms and the blood glucose and glycosuria were not lowered, then there were no results. Of the 100 patients in this study, 40 had very good results, 51 had moderately good results, and nine had no results, for a total amelioration rate of 91%. After four months of treatment, the fasting blood glucose levels ranged from 5.8-15.8mmol/L and the average was 10.4mmol/L. Postprandial blood glucose levels ranged from 9.7-21.2mmol/L, with an average of 13.49mmol/L.

REPRESENTATIVE CASE HISTORIES:

CASE 1[1]

The patient was a 37 year old male who was first examined on Feb. 10, 1996. The patient had a history of chronic hepatitis B for three years. In 1994, he had been diagnosed as also suffering from diabetes due to polydipsia, polyuria, an FBG of 9.1mmol/L, and a two hour PPBG of 15mmol/L. The patient had previously been treated with *Xiao Ke Wan* (Wasting & Thirsting Pills) and Chinese medicinals to clear heat and nourish yin. However, control of blood glucose was not satisfactory (two hour PPBG 14-14mmol/L). The patient's facial complexion was dark and stagnant and he had chest oppression, heart vexation, fatigue, lack of strength, abdominal distention, loose, noncrisp stools 2-3 times per day, turbid, yellow urine with lots of frothy bubbles, a dry mouth with a sticky, slimy feeling, thirst but no polydipsia, a red tongue with thick, slimy, yellow fur, and a bowstring, slippery, rapid pulse. FBG was 8.4mmol/L, one hour PPBG was 14.2mmol/L, two hour PPBG was 17mmol/L, fasting C-peptides were 2.78ng/ml, one hour postprandial C-peptides were 4.9ng/ml, and two hour postprandial C-peptides were 5.7ng/ml. HBsAg and HBeAg were both positive as was antibodies to HBc.

Based on the above signs and symptoms, this patient's Chinese medical patterns were categorized as liver depression and damp heat. Therefore he was treated with *Shu Gan Jiang Tang Tang* (Course the Liver & Lower Sugar Decoction): Radix Puerariae (*Ge Gen*) and Radix Trichosanthis Kirlowii (*Tian Hua Fen*), 30g each, Radix Astragali Membranacei (*Huang Qi*) and processed Rhizoma Atractylodis (*Cang Zhu*), 20g each, Radix Bupleuri (*Chai Hu*), Fructus Citri Aurantii (*Zhi Ke*), Rhizoma Cyperi Rotundi (*Xiang Fu*), Radix Angelicae Sinensis (*Dang Gui*), stir-fried Rhizoma Atractylodis Macrocephalae (*Bai Zhu*), and stir-fried Radix Albus Paeoniae Lactiflorae (*Bai Shao*), 10g each, and uncooked Radix Glycyrrhizae (*Gan Cao*), 6g. After taking 15 *ji* of this formula, the oral thirst was gone. After one whole course of treatment, the chest oppression, heart vexation, ductal distention, and loose stools all also had disappeared. His urination was clear and long, and his tongue had become pale red with thin, white fur. Fasting blood glucose was 6.6mmol/L, two hour PPBG was 9.1mmol/L, and liver function had returned to normal. On follow-up after two years, blood and urine glucose were within normal parameters.

CASE 2[2]

The patient was a 62 year old male worker who was first examined on Mar. 10, 1973. In 1964, this patient had had icteric hepatitis. He had been treated in a hospital and had improved. However, in 1973, he developed secondary liver cirrhosis. At the same time, diabetes manifested with oral thirst and polyuria. In addition, there was devitalized eating, fatigue, lack of strength, lancinating rib-side pain, ductal and abdominal distention, slightly loose, noncrisp stools, and a purplish red tongue with slimy, yellow fur and teeth-marks on its edges. Further, there was hepato-splenomegaly, urine glucose was (+++), FBG was 280mg/dL, and liver function was abnormal.

Based on these signs and symptoms, the patient's Chinese medical patterns were categorized as enduring damp heat causing liver blood stasis and obstruction and loss of spleen's movement with qi and yin dual vacuity. Therefore, the treatment principles were to clear heat and transform dampness, regulate and rectify the liver and spleen, boost the qi and nourish yin. Based on these principles, the following Chinese medicinals were prescribed: Radix Astragali Membranacei (Huang Qi), Radix Codonopsitis Pilosulae (Dang Shen), Radix Salviae Miltiorrhizae (Dan Shen), Radix Trichosanthis Kirlowii (Tian Hua Fen), Herba Dendrobii (Shi Hu), Fructus Ligustri Lucidi (Nu Zhen Zi), and Herba Oldenlandiae Diffusae Cum Radice (Bai Hua She She Cao), 15g each, and Radix Rubrus Paeoniae Lactiflorae (Chi Shao), Radix Albus Paeoniae Lactiflorae (Bai Shao), Cortex Phellodendri (Huang Bai), Pericarpium Citri Reticulatae (Chen Pi), Fructus Schisandrae Chinensis (Wu Wei Zi), Rhizoma Atractylodis (Cang Zhu), and Radix Scrophulariae Ningpoensis (Xuan Shen), 10g each.

After taking nine ji of these medicinals, the patient's oral thirst and polyuria were slightly decreased and his stools were more crisp. However, they could still be loose sometimes. Hence, Dr. Wan rewrote the patient's prescription as follows: Radix Astragali Membranacei (Huang Qi), Radix Dioscoreae Oppositae (Shan Yao), Radix Salviae Miltiorrhizae (Dan Shen), and Herba Oldenlandiae Diffusae Cum Radice (Bai Hua She She Cao), 30g each, Radix Trichosanthis Kirlowii (Tian Hua Fen), Herba Dendrobii (Shi Hu), and Herba Leonuri Heterophylli (Yi Mu Cao), 15g each, and Rhizoma Atractylodis (Cang Zhu), Radix Scrophulariae Ningpoensis (Xuan Shen), Radix Rubrus Paeoniae Lactiflorae (Chi Shao), Fructus Schisandrae Chinensis (Wu Wei Zi), and Herba Patriniae Heterophyllae Cum Radice (Bai Jiang Cao), 10g each.

After taking 12 ji of these medicinals, the oral thirst and

polyuria completely remitted and the patient's stools were formed. Liver function had returned to normal, and FBG was 150mg/dL. Therefore, Dr. Wan added 10 grams of Semen Pruni Persicae (Tao Ren) to the original formula plus three grams of Radix Rubrus Panacis Ginseng (Hong Shen). The patient took these Chinese medicinals for another month. When he was re-examined on Jun. 2, blood glucose was normal and liver function was still normal. Afterwards, the patient took 8-10 ji of the original formula and, after 10 years, there was no recurrence.

CASE 3[3]

The patient was a 47 year old female who was first examined on Oct. 5, 1979. In 1963, this woman had suffered from acute schistosomiasis, for which she was treated and had improved. However, in 1977, her liver function became abnormal. The Western diagnosis was schistosomiasal liver cirrhosis. Then, in 1979, the patient was diagnosed with diabetes. At the time of Dr. Wan's examination, there was liver area aching and pain, fatigue, lack of strength, a dry mouth but scanty drinking, devitalized eating, dizziness, profuse dreams during sleep at night, vexation, agitation, and restlessness, sometimes loose stools and sometimes constipation, yellow urine, relatively profuse night-time urination, and sometimes early, sometimes late menstruation which was sometimes scanty and sometimes profuse and which contained a small number of blood clots. The patient's eyelids were slightly swollen, her tongue tip was red and its edges were purple with thin, yellow fur, and a bowstring, fine pulse. Both hands lacked warmth, hard lumps could be felt in the abdomen, and there was pitting edema of both lower limbs. Urine glucose was (++), FBG was 170mg/dL, and liver function was abnormal. Schistosomiasal liver cirrhosis was confirmed by ultrasound.

Based on the above signs and symptoms, this patient's Chinese medical patterns were discriminated as liver blood not flowing smoothly with loss of regularity of spleen movement, damp heat brewing and exhausting the former, kidney qi insufficiency, loss of regulation of the chong and ren, and heart spirit loss of nourishment. Therefore, the treatment principles were to clear and eliminate dampness and heat, regulate the qi and blood, supplement the spleen and kidneys, and nourish the heart spirit, for which the patient was prescribed: Radix Pseudostellariae Heterophyllae (Tai Zi Shen), Radix Dioscoreae Oppositae (Shan Yao), Caulis Polygoni Multiflori (Ye Jiao Teng), Radix Salviae Miltiorrhizae (Dan Shen), and Herba Oldenlandiae Diffusae Cum Radice (Bai Hua She She Cao), 30g each, Radix Trichosanthis Kirlowii (Tian Hua Fen), Fructus Corni Officinalis (Shan Zhu Yu),

Herba Leonuri Heterophylli (*Yi Mu Cao*), Fructus Forsythiae Suspensae (*Lian Qiao*), and Herba Dendrobii (*Shi Hu*), 15g each, and Herba Epimedii (*Xian Ling Pi*), Semen Astragali Complanati (*Sha Yuan Zi*), PlumulaNelumbinis Nuciferae (*Lian Zi Xin*), and Herba Agastachis Seu Pogostemi (*Huo Xiang*), 10g each.

After taking 30 *ji* of these medicinals, liver function and blood glucose had both returned to normal and urine glucose was negative. The patient continued to rely on the original formula for regulation and rectification. On follow-up after nine years, the liver area was comfortable, the patient's psyche was good, and there were no abnormalities in liver function or blood glucose.

REMARKS:

1. It is estimated that 1.25 million Americans are infected with HBV, 2.7 million are infected with HCV, and 70,000 are infected with HDV. Many people infected with these viruses go unrecognized for many years until their condition eventually becomes symptomatic. Because many people with chronic liver disease also have a history of alcohol abuse, not a few persons with chronic liver disease currently have or may be expected to develop diabetes. In addition, 10% of patients receiving dialysis test positive for HCV, and diabetes is a major cause of nephropathy requiring dialysis.

ENDNOTES:

[1] Wei Su-xia, "The Treatment of 40 Cases of Hepatogenic Diabetes Via the Liver," *Si Chuan Zhong Yi (Sichuan Chinese Medicine)*, #10, 1999, p. 17

[2] Wan Wen-mo, anthologized in Shi Yu-guang & Dan Shu-jian's *Xiao Ke Zhuan Zhi (Wasting & Thirsting Expertise)*, Chinese Medicine Ancient Books Publishing Co., 1997, p. 136-137

[3] *Ibid.*, p. 137-138

12

DIABETIC KETOACIDOSIS

Diabetic ketoacidosis (DKA) is a state of relative (in relation to glucagon) or absolute insulin deficiency which leads to a state of hyperglycemia with subsequent osmotic diuresis and volume depletion in turn leading to dehydration and acidosis due to ketonemia, ketonuria, and loss of bicarbonate in the urine. The most common causes of this condition are underlying infection, disruption of insulin treatment, dehydration, emotional stress, or new onset of diabetes.[1] In the U.S., DKA is primarily seen in patients with type 1 diabetes. The incidence is roughly two per every 100 years of diabetes, with approximately 3% of type 1 diabetic patients initially presenting with DKA.[2] This condition may also occur exceptionally in type 2 diabetes patients. It tends to occur in individuals younger than 19 years, i.e., the more brittle type 1 diabetic patients, but may occur in diabetic patients of any age. Diabetic ketoacidosis accounts for 14% of all hospital admissions for patients with diabetes and 16% of all diabetes-related fatalities. With modern fluid management, the overall mortality rate of DKA is about 2% per episode. However, in children under 10 years, DKA causes 70% of diabetes-related fatalities. In pregnant patients, the fetal mortality rate is as high as 30%, with this rate climbing to 60% in DKA with coma. Before the discovery of insulin in 1922, the mortality rate for all patients with DKA was 100%.[3]

In those patients with known diabetes, the precipitating factor for DKA can be identified in more than 80% of cases.[4] The most common cause, except in cases where the patient has simply missed or stopped taking their insulin, is a relative lack of insulin secondary to an increased requirement for insulin in turn due to some increased physiologic stress. Such physiologic stressors may include infection (40% of cases), especially pneumonia and urinary tract infections, myocardial infarction, cerebrovascular accident, complicated pregnancy, trauma, psychoemotional stress, and surgery. Other precipitating factors may include other endocrine disorders, alcohol consumption, and the use of certain medications, including steriods, calcium channel blockers, Pentamidine, beta-blocking agents, and Dilantin. Approximately 20-30% of cases are idiopathic.[5]

The presenting symptoms of DKA include fatigue, generalized malaise, possible altered mental status, i.e., decreased alertness, thirst, and polyuria. Depending on the duration of the symptoms, the patient may also be able to report recent weight loss. As the patient becomes increasingly ill, they may begin to vomit and complain of abdominal pain (a most reliable symptom). The physical signs of DKA can be variable. Most patients will have some degree of tachycardia, but the blood pressure is often normal. Evidence of dehydration, such as loss of skin turgor and dry mucus membranes, may be present. There may be either high fever or hypothermia, and the respiratory rate may be either normal or somewhat rapid. In addition, there is typically acetone ("fruity") breath odor.[6] Laboratory diagnosis of DKA is based on elevated blood glucose (usually above 250mg/dL), a low serum bicarbonate level (usually below 15mEq/L), an elevated anion gap (calculated), and demonstrable ketonemia.

Diabetic ketoacidosis is an acute, life-threatening condition requiring emergency care. Typically, management consists of airway maintenance, supplemental oxygen as needed, treatment for shock, rehydration via IV fluid replacement therapy, potassium replacement (at least for adults), and IV administration of insulin to treat the hyperglycemia.[7] Complications of Western medical treatment for DKA may include brain edema due to osmotic dysequilibrium between the brain and plasma when glucose is lowered too rapidly (less than 1% in adults), acute pulmonary edema, hyperkalemia, hypophosphatemia, and hypoglycemia.

CHINESE MEDICAL DISEASE CATEGORIZATION: Based on its clinical symptoms: DKA mainly corresponds to the Chinese disease categories of *tou tong*, headache, *fan ke*, vexatious thirst, *ou tu*, vomiting, *shen si huang hu*, spirit mind abstraction, and *shen zhi hun mi*, coma.

CHINESE DISEASE MECHANISMS:

The signs and symptoms of this condition are mainly due to three disease mechanisms: 1) dryness and heat binding internally consuming and damaging qi and yin, 2) qi not transforming yin with retention of turbid evils, and 3) static blood obstruction and stagnation. In real life, this dryness and heat are most commonly due to some combination of habitual bodily yang exuberance, emotional stress causing qi depression to transform fire, overeating warm, acrid foods which damage and consume yin, and overeating sweet, fluid-engendering foods which damage the spleen qi. The spleen becomes too weak to move and transform fluids which gather and collect, transforming into dampness and then into damp heat. In addition, consumption of yin vacuity due to aging may give rise to inability to control yang, with engenderment of internal heat. If dryness and heat damage fluids, there is vexatious thirst and polydipsia, dry skin and mucus membranes, dry, red tongue and lips, tachycardia, and possible emission of heat or fever. If the spleen qi becomes too vacuous and weak to move and transform fluids, not only may this give rise to damp heat, but it may also engender phlegm turbidity. If this phlegm turbidity counterflows upward and attacks the stomach, it may cause nausea and vomiting. If it ascends even further, it may confound the clear orifices, resulting in spirit mind abstraction and coma. If the spleen qi becomes too vacuous and weak to transform the finest essence of food and liquids, this may lead to weight loss and emaciation. If dryness and heat boil and cook the constructive and blood, the blood will become sticky and stagnant. This tendency towards the creation of blood stasis is also aggravated by liver depression qi stagnation failing to move the blood, spleen qi vacuity weakness failing to empower the movement of the blood, and phlegm dampness obstructing the free flow of the blood. Blood stasis in the vessels of the heart may give rise to chest oppression and heart pain. In the area of the abdomen, it may give rise to abdominal pain. Stasis obstructing the vessels of the brain may lead to loss of normalcy of brain function, and stasis obstructing the vessels of the body and extremities may give rise to hypothermia as may yin exhaustion leading to yang desertion.

TREATMENT BASED ON PATTERN DISCRIMINATION:

1. QI & YIN DUAL DAMAGE PATTERN

MAIN SYMPTOMS: Oral thirst, polydipsia, frequent urination with large volume, extreme lack of strength, heart palpitations, a red tongue with scanty fur, and a fine, rapid pulse

NOTE: This pattern is mostly seen in those with mild DKA with the main symptoms of polydipsia, polyuria, and extreme lack of strength.

TREATMENT PRINCIPLES: Boost the qi and nourish yin, clear heat and engender fluids

RX: *Sheng Mai San* (Engender the Pulse Powder) plus *Zeng Ye Tang* (Increase Fluids Decoction) with additions and subtractions

INGREDIENTS: Uncooked Radix Rehmanniae (*Sheng Di*) and Radix Scrophulariae Ningpoensis (*Xuan Shen*), 30g each, Radix Pseudostellariae Heterophyllae (*Tai Zi Shen*), Radix Glehniae Littoralis (*Sha Shen*), and uncooked Radix Astragali Membranacei (*Huang Qi*), 15g each, Tuber Ophiopogonis Japonici (*Mai Men Dong*), 12g, and Fructus Schisandrae Chinensis (*Wu Wei Zi*), Radix Trichosanthis Kirlowii (*Tian Hua Fen*), Herba Dendrobii (*Shi Hu*), Rhizoma Anemarrhenae Aspheloidis (*Zhi Mu*), Fructus Immaturus Citri Aurantii (*Zhi Shi*), and Sclerotium Poriae Cocos (*Fu Ling*), 9g each

FORMULA ANALYSIS: *Huang Qi, Tai Zi Shen,* and *Fu Ling* fortify the spleen and boost the qi. *Mai Men Dong, Sheng Di, Xuan Shen, Shi Hu,* and *Sha Shen* enrich yin and engender fluids. *Tian Hua Fen* and *Zhi Mu* clear heat and engender fluids in order to eliminate vexatious thirst. *Wu Wei Zi* constrains yin and engenders fluids, while *Zhi Shi* moves the qi in order to protect against *Sheng Di* and *Xuan Shen*'s enriching sliminess.

ADDITIONS & SUBTRACTIONS: If there is concomitant constipation, add nine grams of wine-processed Radix Et Rhizoma Rhei (*Da Huang*). If the tongue is dark red, add 12 grams each of Radix Angelicae Sinensis (*Dang Gui*), Radix Salviae Miltiorrhizae (*Dan Shen*), and Radix Rubrus Paeoniae Lactiflorae (*Chi Shao*) in order to quicken the blood and transform stasis. If there are diabetic sores with secondary infections, add 15 grams each of Herba Violae Yedoensitis Cum Radice (*Zi Hua Di*

Ding), Flos Chrysanthemi Indici (*Ye Ju Hua*), and Radix Rubrus Paeoniae Lactiflorae (*Chi Shao*). If there is infection due to toothache or peridontitis, add 15 grams eac hof Radix Achyranthis Bidentatae (*Niu Xi*) and Radix Angelicae Dahuricae (*Bai Zhi*) and add three grams of Herba Asari Cum Radice (*Xi Xin*). If there is external contraction of wind cold, add nine grams each of Radix Ledebouriellae Divaricatae (*Fang Feng*), Radix Et Rhizoma Notopterygii (*Qiang Huo*), and Folium Perillae Frutescentis (*Zi Su Ye*). If there is external contraction of wind heat, add 15 grams each of Folium Daqingye (*Da Qing Ye*) and Radix Puerariae (*Ge Gen*) and nine grams of Radix Bupleuri (*Chai Hu*). If there is concomitant urinary tract infection, add 15 grams each of Herba Violae Yedoensitis Cum Radice (*Zi Hua Di Ding*) and Rhizoma Imperatae Cylindricae (*Bai Mao Gen*) and nine grams each of Fructus Kochiae Scopariae (*Di Fu Zi*) and Cortex Phellodendri (*Huang Bai*). If there is enduring high ketonemia, add 15 grams each of Folium Daqingye (*Da Qing Ye*), Radix Isatidis Seu Baphicacanthi (*Ban Lan Gen*), and Radix Lithospermi Seu Arnebiae (*Zi Cao*), and three grams of Cortex Cinnamomi Cassiae (*Rou Gui*). If there is hyperthyroidism or enlargement of the thyroid gland, add 15 grams of Spica Prunellae Vulgaris (*Xia Ku Cao*), 12 grams each of Concha Arcae (*Wa Leng Zi*) and Concha Ostreae (*Mu Li*), and nine grams each of Bulbus Fritillariae Thunbergii (*Zhe Bei Mu*), Herba Sargassii (*Hai Zao*), Thallus Algae (*Kun Bu*), and Endothelium Corneum Gigeriae Galli (*Ji Nei Jin*).

If vexatious thirst is severe with marked lack of strength, one can use *Bai Hu Jia Ren Shen Tang Jia Jian* (White Tiger Plus Ginseng Decoction with Additions & Subtractions): uncooked Gypsum Fibrosum (*Shi Gao*), 30g, Radix Dioscoreae Oppositae (*Shan Yao*), 15g, Tuber Ophiopogonis Japonici (*Mai Men Dong*), 12g, Radix Trichosanthis Kirlowii (*Tian Hua Fen*) and Rhizoma Anemarrhenae Aspheloidis (*Zhi Mu*), 9g each, Radix Panacis Ginseng (*Ren Shen*), 6-9g, and mix-fried Radix Glycyrrhizae (*Gan Cao*), 3-6g.

ACUPUNCTURE & MOXIBUSTION: *Tai Xi* (Ki 3), *San Yin Jiao* (Sp 6), *Zu San Li* (St 36), *Nei Ting* (St 44)

FORMULA ANALYSIS: Supplementing *Tai Xi* and *San Yin Jiao* nourishes and enriches yin fluids, while supplementing *San Yin Jiao* and *Zu San Li* fortifies the spleen and boosts the qi. Draining *Nei Ting* clears heat from the yang ming.

ADDITIONS & SUBTRACTIONS: If there is concomitant blood stasis, add draining *Xue Hai* (Sp 10) and use even supplementing-even draining at *San Yin Jiao* (Sp 6). If there is emission of heat, add draining *Qu Chi* (LI 11) and *He Gu* (LI 4).

2. DRYNESS & HEAT ENTERING THE BLOOD WITH BLOOD STASIS AND RETENTION OF TURBIDITY PATTERN

MAIN SYMPTOMS: Oral thirst, polydipsia, frequent urination with large volume, bodily fatigue, lack of strength, stomach duct glomus, torpid intake, nausea with a desire to vomit, dizziness, dry, bound stools, a dark red tongue with white, slimy or yellow, slimy fur, and a bowstring, slippery pulse

NOTE: This pattern describes a more severe presentation than the preceding pattern.

TREATMENT PRINCIPLES: Clear heat and harmonize the blood, dispel dampness and transform turbidity

RX: *Huang Lian Jie Du Tang* (Coptis Resolve Toxins Decoction) plus *Zeng Ye Tang* (Increase Fluids Decoction) with additions and subtractions

INGREDIENTS: Radix Trichosanthis Kirlowii (*Tian Hua Fen*) and Radix Astragali Membranacei (*Huang Qi*), 30g each, uncooked Radix Rehmanniae (*Sheng Di*) and Radix Scrophulariae Ningpoensis (*Xuan Shen*), 20g each, Radix Dioscoreae Oppositae (*Shan Yao*), 15g, Radix Rubrus Paeoniae Lactiflorae (*Chi Shao*) and Sclerotium Poriae Cocos (*Fu Ling*), 12g each, Cortex Radicis Moutan (*Dan Pi*), Rhizoma Atractylodis (*Cang Zhu*), Herba Eupatorii Fortunei (*Pei Lan*), Fructus Immaturus Citri Aurantii (*Zhi Shi*), Radix Scutellariae Baicalensis (*Huang Qin*), and wine-processed Radix Et Rhizoma Rhei (*Da Huang*), 9g each, and Rhizoma Coptidis Chinensis (*Huang Lian*) and Fructus Gardeniae Jasminoidis (*Zhi Zi*), 6g each

FORMULA ANALYSIS: *Huang Lian*, *Huang Qin*, and *Zhi Zi* clear heat and drain fire. *Dan Pi*, *Sheng Di*, and *Chi Shao* cool and quicken the blood. *Cang Zhu*, *Pei Lan*, and *Fu Ling* penetratingly and aromatically transform turbidity. *Zhi Shi* and *Da Huang* rectify the qi, free the flow of the bowels, and drain turbidity. *Huang Qi*, *Shan Yao*, *Sheng Di*, and *Xuan Shen* boost the qi and enrich yin.

ADDITIONS & SUBTRACTIONS: If there is dizziness and headache, add 12 grams each of Ramulus Uncariae Cum Uncis (*Gou Teng*), uncooked Concha Ostreae (*Mu Li*), and Concha Margaritiferae (*Zhen Zhu Mu*) and nine grams of Flos Chrysanthemi Morifolii (*Ju Hua*). If there is blurred vision, add 12 grams of Concha Haliotidis (*Shi Jue Ming*) and nine grams each of Fructus Lycii Chinensis (*Gou Qi Zi*), Semen Celosiae Argenteae (*Qing Xiang Zi*), and Semen Leonrui Heterophylli (*Chong Wei Zi*). If there is thirst and drinking without limit, add 30 grams of uncooked Gypsum Fibrosum (*Shi Gao*) and nine grams each of Rhizoma Anemarrhenae Aspheloidis (*Zhi Mu*) and Radix Trichosanthis Kirlowii (*Tian Hua Fen*). If there is nausea and vomiting, add nine grams each of Caulis Bambusae In Taeniis (*Zhu Ru*), Rhizoma Pinelliae Ternatae (*Ban Xia*), and Pericarpium Citri Reticulatae (*Chen Pi*). If there is polyuria, add nine grams each of Semen Euryalis Ferocis (*Qian Shi*), Fructus Rosae Laevigatae (*Jin Ying Zi*), Fructus Rubi Chingii (*Fu Pen Zi*), and Semen Cuscutae Chinensis (*Tu Si Zi*). If there is chest oppression and piercing pain, add 30 grams of Radix Salviae Miltiorrhizae (*Dan Shen*) and nine grams each of Lignum Dalbergiae Odoriferae (*Jiang Xiang*), Fructus Citri Sacrodactylis (*Fo Shou*), Fructus Crataegi (*Shan Zha*), and Flos Carthami Tinctorii (*Hong Hua*). If there is sleepiness and decreased awareness, add nine grams each of Rhizoma Acori Graminei (*Shi Chang Pu*), Radix Polygalae Tenuifoliae (*Yuan Zhi*), and Tuber Curcumae (*Yu Jin*). If there is protein in the urine, double the amount of *Huang Qi* and add 30 grams of Herba Oldenlandiae Diffusae Cum Radice (*Bai Hua She She Cao*), 15 grams of Herba Leonuri Heterophylli (*Yi Mu Cao*), and nine grams of Radix Dipsaci (*Xu Duan*). If there are accompanying sores and ulcers, add 15 grams each of Flos Lonicerae Japonicae (*Jin Yin Hua*), Herba Taraxaci Mongolici Cum Radice (*Pu Gong Ying*), Herba Portulacae Oleraceae (*Ma Chi Xian*) and Herba Violae Yedoensitis Cum Radice (*Zi Hua Di Ding*).

ACUPUNCTURE & MOXIBUSTION: *Tai Xi* (Ki 3), *San Yin Jiao* (Sp 6), *Zu San Li* (St 36), *Yin Ling Quan* (Sp 9), *Nei Ting* (St 44), *Zhong Wan* (CV 12), *Tian Shu* (St 25), *Pi Shu* (Bl 20), *Da Chang Shu* (Bl 25)

FORMULA ANALYSIS: Supplementing *Tai Xi* and even supplementing *San Yin Jiao* nourishes and enriches yin fluids. Draining *Yin Ling Quan* and even supplementing-even draining *San Yin Jiao* drains and disinhibits dampness. Supplementing *Pi Shu* and even supplementing-even draining *Zu San Li* fortifies the spleen and boosts the qi. Draining *Nei Ting, Zhong Wan, Tian Shu,* and *Da Chang Shu* frees the flow of the bowels and drains heat and turbidity.

ADDITIONS & SUBTRACTIONS: If there is dizziness and headache, add draining *Xing Jian* (Liv 2), *Feng Chi* (GB20), and *Tai Yang* (M-HN-9). If there is blurred vision, add even supplementing-even draining *Jing Ming* (Bl 1), *Feng Chi* (GB 20), and *Tai Yang* (M-HN-9). If there is nausea and vomiting, add draining *Nei Guan* (Per 6). If there is chest oppression and piercing pain, add draining *Nei Guan* (Per 6), *Dan Zhong* (CV 17), *He Gu* (LI 4), and *Xue Hai* (Sp 10).

3. HEAT BLOCKING THE CLEAR ORIFICES PATTERN

MAIN SYMPTOMS: Headache, vexation and agitation, vexatious thirst leading to drinking, large, deep breaths, a fruity odor to the breath, if severe, somnolence and coma, scanty, yellow-colored urination, a crimson red tongue with possible black or brown fur and scanty fluids, and a fine, rapid pulse

NOTE: This pattern is mostly seen in heavy or serious DKA.

TREATMENT PRINCIPLES: Clear heat and open the orifices

RX: *Qing Gong Tang Jia Jian* (Clear the Palace Decoction with Additions & Subtractions)

INGREDIENTS: Uncooked Radix Rehmanniae (*Sheng Di*), 30g, Radix Scrophulariae Ningpoensis (*Xuan Shen*), Tuber Ophiopogonis Japonici (*Mai Men Dong*), and Radix Salviae Miltiorrhizae (*Dan Shen*), 15g each, Radix Panacis Quinquefolii (*Xi Yang Shen*), Tuber Asparagi Cochinensis (*Tian Men Dong*), Herba Lophatheri Gracilis (*Dan Zhu Ye*), Rhizoma Acori Graminei (*Shi Chang Pu*), Tuber Curcumae (*Yu Jin*), and Cornu Bubali (*Shui Niu Jiao*), 9g each, Fructus Schisandrae Chinensis (*Wu Wei Zi*), 6g, and Rhizoma Coptidis Chinensis (*Huang Lian*), 3g

FORMULA ANALYSIS: *Shui Niu Jiao, Huang Lian, Shi Chang Pu,* and *Yu Jin* clear heat and flush phlegm, arouse the spirit and open the orifices. *Xi Yang Shen, Sheng Di, Xuan Shen, Tian Men Dong,* and *Mai Men Dong* boost the qi and engender fluids, enrich yin and increase humors.

ADDITIONS & SUBTRACTIONS: For even better results, also take the ready-made medicine *An Gong Niu Huang Wan* (Quiet the Palace Bezoar Pills).

ACUPUNCTURE & MOXIBUSTION: *Shi Xuan* (M-UE-1)

FORMULA ANALYSIS: Pricking the *Shi Xuan* to bleed clears heat and arouses the spirit.

ADDITIONS & SUBTRACTIONS: For loss of consciousness, add draining *Ren Zhong* (GV 26) to open the orifices and arouse the brain.

4. YIN EXHAUSTION & YANG DESERTION PATTERN

MAIN SYMPTOMS: Eyes sunken in their sockets, coma, fixed eyes and torpid spirit, gaping mouth, shortness of breath, distressed rapid breathing, ashen white or cyanotic face and lips, oily perspiration, reversal chilling of the four limbs, a cyanotic tongue, and a faint pulse on the verge of expiry

NOTE: This pattern is mostly seen in those with low blood pressure, *i.e.*, shock.

TREATMENT PRINCIPLES: Boost the qi and secure desertion

RX: *Si Ni Jia Ren Shen Tang Jia Wei* (Four Counterflows Plus Ginseng Decoction with Added Flavors)

INGREDIENTS: Radix Rubrus Panacis Ginseng (*Hong Shen*), uncooked Concha Ostreae (*Mu Li*), and uncooked Os Draconis (*Long Gu*), 30g each, Tuber Ophiopogonis Japonici (*Mai Men Dong*), 15g, Radix Lateralis Praeparatus Aconiti Carmichaeli (*Fu Zi*), Fructus Schisandrae Chinensis (*Wu Wei Zi*), Fructus Corni Officinalis (*Shan Zhu Yu*), and mix-fried Radix Glycyrrhizae (*Gan Cao*), 9g each, and dry Rhizoma Zingiberis (*Gan Jiang*), 6g

FORMULA ANALYSIS: *Hong Shen* boosts the qi and secures desertion. *Fu Zi* and *Gan Jiang* rescue yang and stem counterflow. *Mai Men Dong, Wu Wei Zi, Shan Zhu Yu, Mu Li,* and *Long Gu* constrain yin and secure desertion.

ACUPUNCTURE & MOXIBUSTION: *Zu San Li* (St 36), *Guan Yuan* (CV 4)

FORMULA ANALYSIS: Moxibustion of *Zu San Li* and *Guan Yuan* boosts the qi and secures desertion.

ABSTRACTS OF REPRESENTATIVE CHINESE RESEARCH:

Qiao Yu-qiu & Xie Mao-ling, "The Treatment of 26 Cases of Diabetic Ketoacidosis with *Huang Lian Wen Dan Tang* (Coptis Warm the Gallbladder Decoction) Combined with Western Medicinals," *Zhe Jiang Zhong Yi Za Zhi* (*Zhejiang Journal of Chinese Medicine*), #3, 2000, p. 112: There were 26 patients in this study, 16 males and 10 females aged 4-76. Their main symptoms were vexatious thirst, polydipsia, nausea, vomiting, torpid intake, emacia-

tion, lack of strength, frequent, profuse urination, and poor affect. Accompanying conditions included dry skin, low blood pressure, a small difference in arterial pressure, and bradycardia. Patient's tongues were red with dry, yellow fur, and their pulses were deep, fine, rapid, and forceless.

Treatment consisted of administration of the following basic formula: uncooked Radix Rehmanniae (*Sheng Di*), Radix Dioscoreae Oppositae (*Shan Yao*), and Radix Astragali Membranacei (*Huang Qi*), 30g each, Sclerotium Poriae Cocos (*Fu Ling*), Radix Scrophulariae Ningpoensis (*Xuan Shen*), and Radix Trichosanthis Kirlowii (*Tian Hua Fen*), 15g each, and Rhizoma Coptidis Chinensis (*Huang Lian*), ginger-processed Rhizoma Pinelliae Ternatae (*Ban Xia*), Pericarpium Citri Reticulatae (*Chen Pi*), Caulis Bambusae In Taeniis (*Zhu Ru*), and Fructus Immaturus Citri Aurantii (*Zhi Shi*), 9g each. If there was abdominal pain and diarrhea, six grams of Fructus Amomi (*Sha Ren*) were added. If there was dizziness and heart palpitations, 15 grams of Tuber Ophiopogonis Japonici (*Mai Men Dong*), 12 grams of Fructus Schisandrae Chinensis (*Wu Wei Zi*), and nine grams of Rhizoma Gastrodiae Elatae (*Tian Ma*) were added. If there was fever, cough, chest oppression, and panting, 30 grams of uncooked Gypsum Fibrosum (*Shi Gao*), 15 grams of Fructus Trichosanthis Kirlowii (*Quan Gua Lou*), 12 grams of Rhizoma Anemarrhenae Aspheloidis (*Zhi Mu*), and nine grams of Semen Pruni Armeniacae (*Xing Ren*) were added. If there was coma, nine grams of Radix Panacis Quinquefolii (*Xi Yang Shen*) were added. If there was bilateral lower limb numbness or pricking pain, 30 grams each of Caulis Milletiae Seu Spatholobi (*Ji Xue Teng*), Radix Salviae Miltiorrhizae (*Dan Shen*), and Herba Pycnostelmae (*Xu Zhang Jing*), and 15 grams of Radix Ligustici Wallichii (*Chuan Xiong*) were added. One *ji* of these medicinals were decocted in water per day and administered orally. In addition, Western medicines were used to control blood glucose, antibiotics were used if there was accompanying infection, and supplemental fluids were administered to balance electrolytes.

After five days of this protocol, all these patients' clinical symptoms either markedly improved or basically disappeared. Their tongues turned moist and their pulses went from deep, fine, rapid, and forceless to deep and fine. Further administration of these Chinese medicinals with additions and subtractions was continued in order to secure and consolidate the treatment effects.

REPRESENTATIVE CASE HISTORIES:

CASE 1[8]

The patient was a 35 year old male who had been diagnosed with diabetes three years before and prescribed orally administered glyburide. When examined by Dr. Chen, the man presented with polydipsia, polyuria, emaciation, lassitude of the spirit, fatigue, disinclination to talk, numbness of the extremities, nausea, torpid intake, dry stools, a dark tongue with yellow fur and scanty fluids, and a bowstring, slippery pulse. The man's fasting blood sugar was 20.3mmol/L, urine glucose was (++++), and ketones in the urine were (++). The patient was diagnosed with diabetic ketosis, and his Chinese medical pattern was categorized as qi and yin dual vacuity with dryness and heat complicated by internal toxic heat exuberance. For this, the treatment principles were to clear heat and resolve toxins, supplement the qi and nourish yin. Therefore, the following modification of *Xiao Tong Tang* (Disperse Ketones Decoction) was prescribed: Radix Scrophulariae Ningpoensis (*Xuan Shen*), Radix Trichosanthis Kirlowii (*Tian Hua Fen*), and Radix Astragali Membranacei (*Huang Qi*), 30g each, uncooked Radix Rehmanniae (*Sheng Di*), Radix Dioscoreae Oppositae (*Shan Yao*), and Sclerotium Poriae Cocos (*Fu Ling*), 15g each, Rhizoma Atractylodis (*Cang Zhu*) and Herba Eupatorii Fortunei (*Pei Lan*), 12g each, Caulis Bambusae In Taeniis (*Zhu Ru*) and Fructus Gardeniae Jasminoidis (*Zhi Zi*), 10g each, Rhizoma Coptidis Chinensis (*Huang Lian*), 9g, and Radix Et Rhizoma Rhei (*Da Huang*) and Radix Glycyrrhizae (*Gan Cao*), 6g each. In addition, the patient was instructed to take 2.5mg of glyburide each time, three times per day.

After three *ji* of the above formula, the patient reported alleviation of the thirst, increase of strength in his lower limbs, better spirit, and one bowel movement with soft stools per day. The man's tongue and pulse were the same as before. Urine glucose was (+++) and urine ketones were (+). Therefore, 12 more *ji* were administered continuously, after which, the patient's nausea and vomiting had disappeared and his appetite had increased. At this point in time, the man was eating 250g of cereal foods per day. Fasting blood sugar was 15.7mmol/L, liver function was normal, urine glucose was (++), and urine ketones were negative. In order to consolidate the therapeutic effect, a Chinese medicinal formula for supplementing the kidneys, fortifying the spleen, and nourishing and quickening the blood was prescribed along with continuous treatment of the diabetes with glyburide. On follow-up after half a year, urine ketones were still negative.

CASE 2[9]

The patient was a 23 year old woman who had had diabetes for three years. She was thirsty and she experienced weakness in her lower back and knees. Her appetite was excessive, her urination was profuse, and she was emaciated. Her body weight had fallen from 62kg to 51kg. The woman's tongue was red, and her pulse was fine and bowstring. Her fasting blood glucose was 11.6mmol/L, urine glucose was (++), urine ketones were (+), and blood ketones were 2.2mmol/L. The patient's Chinese medical pattern was categorized as qi and yin dual vacuity, and the treatment principles were to nourish yin and boost the qi. Seventy-five grams of cooked Radix Rehmanniae (*Shu Di*), 25 grams of Radix Astragali Membranacei (*Huang Qi*), and 10 grams of Radix Panacis Ginseng (*Ren Shen*) were orally administered as a boiled decoction, one *ji* per day. In addition, the patient increased her intake of water to assist the elimination of ketones. After four days of this regime, the urine ketones were negative. Therefore, an additional six *ji* of the prescription were administered. After that, all the patient's symptoms were relieved, and, three months later, all tests remained negative.

CASE 3[10]

The patient was a 45 year old male who was first examined on Mar. 5, 1994. For a half day, the man had been drinking alcohol and eating "thick flavors," *i.e.*, rich foods. He was drinking water without limit, yet his mouth was dry and his tongue was parched. There was white, pus-like foam at the corner of his mouth. His urination was frequent and profuse and this was worse at night. In addition, he was constipated, had lack of strength in his four limbs, and increased appetite yet loss of weight. He was dizzy and had a headache, and the man's eyes and face were both red. Blood glucose was 18.5mmol/L, urine glucose was (++++), ketones were (++), cholesterol was 6.25mmol/L, and serum diacid glycerides were 9.2mmol/L. The patient's tongue was red with burnt, blackish fur in the center. His pulse was bowstring and slippery.

Based on the above signs and symptoms, this patient's Chinese medical pattern was categorized as damp heat accumulating and gathering in the stomach and intestines with yang ming dryness and heat damaging fluids. Therefore, the treatment principles were to clear heat and drain fire, nourish yin and engender fluids, moisten the intestines and free the flow of the stools. The formula used was *Ren Shen Bai Hu Tang Jia Wei* (Ginseng White Tiger Decoction with Added Flavors): uncooked Gypsum Fibrosum (*Shi Gao*), 30g, uncooked Radix Rehmanniae (*Sheng Di*), Tuber Ophiopogonis Japonici (*Mai Men Dong*), Radix Trichosanthis Kirlowii (*Tian Hua Fen*), Herba Dendrobii (*Shi Hu*), Semen Pruni (*Yu Li Ren*), and Semen Cannabis Sativae (*Huo Ma Ren*), 15g each, Rhizoma Anemarrhenae Aspheloidis (*Zhi Mu*), Radix

Salviae Miltiorrhizae (*Dan Shen*), and Cortex Radicis Moutan (*Dan Pi*), 10g each, and uncooked Radix Glycyrrhizae (*Gan Cao*) and Radix Panacis Quinquefolii (*Xi Yang Shen*), 3g each. At the same time, the patient was administered 5mg of glyburide TID.

After taking seven *ji*, the drinking of water was reduced, the man's appetite was controlled, and the headaches and red eyes had improved. However, there was still a dry mouth and exhaustion. The tongue fur had turned yellow and slimy, and the pulse was now bowstring and rapid. Urine glucose was (++++), ketones had turned negative, and blood glucose was 13.5mmol/L. Therefore, 10 grams each of uncooked Fructus Crataegi (*Shan Zha*) and Herba Eupatorii Fortunei (*Pei Lan*) were added to the above formula, and another seven *ji* were prescribed. After this, all the patient's symptoms had remitted, blood glucose was 7mmol/L, serum cholesterol was 4.1mmol/L, serum diacid glycerides were 1.66mmol/L, and urine glucose and ketones were negative. The dose of glyburide was reduced, the patient was counseled on dietary restrictions, and four weeks later, his blood glucose and lipids were still normal.

CASE 4[11]

The patient was a 34 year old female who was first examined on Feb. 15, 1990 and who had had diabetes for seven years. Due to the death of her mother, grief and exhaustion had caused a severe headache on Feb. 9. This was accompanied by generalized fatigue, stomach duct glomus and oppression, no thought of eating for two days, and nausea and vomiting which had continued up to the time of treatment. The patient's facial complexion was flushed red, she was confused, and she was somnolent. If she drank water, she vomited. However, her two excretions were free-flowing and uninhibited. The edges of her tongue were red and the fur in the center was thin, yellow, and dry. Her pulse was small and slippery. Urine glucose was (++++), urine ketones were (+), and blood glucose was 14.9mmol/L.

Based on the above signs and symptoms, the patient's patterns were categorized as qi and yin dual vacuity with chaos and counterflow of the qi mechanism. The treatment principles were to boost the qi and nourish yin, engender fluids and stop vomiting. Therefore, she was prescribed *Sheng Mai San* (Engender the Pulse Powder) plus *Xuan Fu Dai Zhe Tang* (Inula & Hematite Decoction) with additions and subtractions: Haemititum (*Dai Zhe Shi*), 25g, Radix Pseudostellariae Heterophyllae (*Tai Zi Shen*), 15g, and Tuber Ophiopogonis Japonici (*Mai Men Dong*), Fructus Schisandrae Chinensis (*Wu Wei Zi*), Flos

Inulae Racemosae (*Xuan Fu Hua*), Rhizoma Pinelliae Ternatae (*Ban Xia*), Caulis Bambusae In Taeniis (*Zhu Ru*), Rhizoma Alismatis (*Ze Xie*), Sclerotium Poriae Cocos (*Fu Ling*), Folium Lophatheri Gacilis (*Dan Zhu Ye*), and Herba Dendrobii (*Shi Hu*), 10g each. In addition, the patient was prescribed 5mg of glyburide TID.

Two days later, the woman's symptoms had markedly decreased and she was able to eat a small amount of food. She still slept excessively and dreaded stirring. Each afternoon, she still had nausea and a clamoring stomach sensation, but there was no vomiting. Her tongue fur had turned thin and white. Urine glucose was (++) and ketones had turned negative. This meant that stomach turbidity had been downborne. Therefore, six grams each of Radix Platycodi Grandiflori (*Jie Geng*) and Bulbus Fritillariae Thunbergii (*Zhe Bei Mu*) were added to the original formula to disinhibit the lungs and transform phlegm. After another three *ji*, all the patient's symptoms had improved except for fatigue and lack of strength. Urine glucose was (+), ketones were negative, and blood glucose was 11.3mmol/L. The same formula was prescribed again, and, 10 days later, without using insulin, the patient's blood glucose was 9.4mmol/L.

CASE 5[12]

The patient was a 56 year old female who was first examined on May 20, 1997. This woman's body was emaciated and her facial complexion was blackish. She had low back and knee soreness and limpness, lack of warmth in the four extremities, dread of cold and fear of chill, frequent, numerous urination, turbid urine like fat or grease, a dry mouth leading to drinking, urination each time she drank, a dry tongue and parched throat, a small, pale tongue with dry, white fur, and a deep, fine, forceless pulse. The patient had a history of diabetes and chyluria for 10 years. Her blood glucose was 11.2mmol/L, urine glucose was (+++), ketones were (+++), and chyle was (++).

Based on these signs and symptoms, the woman's pattern was discriminated as yin and yang dual vacuity, and the treatment principles were to warm yang, enrich yin, and supplement the kidneys assisted by dividing and clearing urine turbidity. Therefore, she was prescribed *Ba Wei Shen Qi Wan* (Eight Flavors Kidney Qi Pills) plus *Wu Zi Yan Zong Wan* (Five Seeds Increase Progeny Pills) with modifications: Rhizoma Dioscoreae Hypoglaucae (*Bie Xie*) and Semen Plantaginis (*Che Qian Zi*), 15g each, uncooked Radix Rehmanniae (*Sheng Di*), cooked Radix Rehmanniae (*Shu Di*), Fructus Corni Officinalis (*Shan Zhu Yu*), Radix Dioscoreae Oppositae (*Shan Yao*),

Sclerotium Poriae Cocos (*Fu Ling*), Rhizoma Alismatis (*Ze Xie*), Radix Salviae Miltiorrhizae (*Dan Shen*), Cortex Radicis Moutan (*Dan Pi*), Fructus Rubi Chingii (*Fu Pen Zi*), Fructus Schisandrae Chinensis (*Wu Wei Zi*), Semen Cuscutae Chinensis (*Tu Si Zi*), Rhizoma Polygonati (*Huang Jing*), and Radix Lateralis Praeparatus Aconiti Carmichaeli (*Fu Zi*), 10g each, and Cortex Cinnamomi Cassiae (*Rou Gui*), 2g. In addition, the patient was prescribed 5mg of glyburide TID.

After one week of this regime, the number of urinations had decreased and the urine was clear and without turbidity. In addition, the oral dryness and thirst and the dread of cold had somewhat decreased. The tongue was pale red with white fur, and the pulse was fine and forceless. Urine glucose was (++), ketones were (+), but chyle was negative. Therefore, *Rou Gui* was subtracted from the original formula and 10 grams of Fructus Pruni Mume (*Wu Mei*) were added. After seven *ji* of this formula, the dry mouth had improved, the urine was clear, night-time urination was less numerous, and low back soreness was not severe. Blood glucose was 8.8mmol/L, urine glucose was (+), and ketones and chyle were negative. At this point, *Ba Wei Shen Qi Wan* (Eight Flavors Kidney Qi Pills) were prescribed in ready-made form to prevent the recurrence of chyluria and stabilize the blood glucose.

REMARKS:

1. According to Chen Jin-ding, there are few published reports on the Chinese medical treatment of DKA. However, Chen states that, "TCM treatment is often applied clinically and can bring about rather satisfactory effects."[13] Chen also states, "Continuous use of Chinese herbs can promote earlier restoration of the strength and prevent ketone [*sic*] in the urine from occurring again, which can help stabilize the disease and regulate the dosage of the Western drugs as well as insulin."[14] Because, in a Western setting, a diagnosis of DKA is usually made in a hospital emergency room or intensive care unit, most Western practitioners of Chinese medicine have not had, up till now, opportunity to treat this condition. Recently, the Sound Shore Medical Center in New Rochelle has been allowing acupuncture interns from Mercy College to treat patients in its ICU. If this trend were to continue, this situation may change.

2. It is Bi Ya-an's experience that using a large dose of cooked Radix Rehmanniae (*Shu Di*), for instance 75 grams per day, is instrumental in reducing ketones in diabetic patients with a basic qi and yin dual vacuity pattern. In that case, *Shu Di* may be combined with such qi supplements as Radix Astragali Membranacei (*Huang Qi*) and Radix Panacis Ginseng (*Ren Shen*) as in case #2 above.

ENDNOTES:

[1] www.emedicine.com/EMERG/topic135.htm
[2] *Ibid.*
[3] *Ibid.*
[4] www.embbs.com/cr/dka/precip.htm
[5] www.emedicine.com, *op. cit.*
[6] www.vh.org/Providers/ClinRef/FPHandbook/Chapter05/11-5.htm
[7] http://family.georgetown.edu/welchjj/netscut/endocrinology/diabetic_ketoacidosis.htm
[8] Chen Jin-ding, *op. cit.*, p. 178-179
[9] Bi Ya-an, "The Treatment of Diabetic Ketosis with Cooked Radix Rehmanniae (*Shu Di*)," *Jiang Su Zhong Yi (Jiangsu Journal of Chinese Medicine)*, #1, 2000, p. 33
[10] Kang Lu-wa, "An Inquiry into the Treatment of Diabetic Ketosis," *Si Chuan Zhong Yi (Sichuan Chinese Medicine)*, #8, 1999, p. 13
[11] *Ibid.*, p. 13
[12] *Ibid.*, p. 13
[13] Chen Jin-ding, *op. cit.*, p. 172
[14] *Ibid.* p. 176

NONKETOTIC HYPEROSMOLARITY

Nonketotic hyperosmolarity (NKH) is another well-known complication of diabetes. Also referred to as hyperglycemic hyperosmolar nonketotic coma, it is most commonly seen in older patients with type 2 diabetes and results from sustained hyperglycemic diuresis with inability to compensate with increased oral fluid intake. It is characterized by severe fluid and electrolyte depletion due to osmotic diuresis produced by extreme levels of glucose in the serum. Patients with this condition may lose up to one quarter of their extracellular fluid. However, since only less than 10% of patients with this condition present in a coma, nonketotic hyperosmolarity better describes the condition which the majority of patients present. In actual fact, DKA and NKH are a continuum. At one extreme is pure DKA without significant hyperosmolarity and possibly only modest degrees of glucose elevation with marked ketosis and increased free fatty acids. At the other extreme is NKH with extreme elevations of glucose and hyperosmolarity but without significant ketosis and mildly increased free fatty acids. In the middle, there are a range of patients which present with features of both these conditions. According to Western medicine, the precipitating factors which lead to the development of NKH in patients with type 2 diabetes are similar to those that cause DKA. The single most common precipitating factor is illness and especially pneumonia. In addition, many Western medications can precipitate NKH.[1]

Nonketotic hyperosmolarity is a slowly progressive disorder, and it is not uncommon to have a 3-10 day history of increasing thirst, polyuria, and malaise. Symptoms of an underlying infection may be present, but, in other cases, there is little history. Patients usually present with signs of dehydration, such as dry mucus membranes, tachycardia, poor skin turgor, and low-grade fever. Blood pressure is usually unaffected, unless there is severe dehydration or

infection. Likewise, unless the patient has pneumonia, respiratory symptoms are usually absent because there is no acidosis. Changes in mental status, such as lethargy and disorientation are common, but frank coma is rare. Seizures may occur in up to one-fourth of patients and can be focal or generalized. In terms of laboratory examinations, serum glucose is in excess of 600mg/dL, serum osmolarity is greater than 3330mOsm/kg, ketones are either absent or minimal, arterial pH is above 7.3, and serum bicarbonate is above 20mEq/L. The Western medical treatment and complication of NKH are essentially the same as for DKA. Although cerebral edema is more common in those with NKH (due to hyperosmolarity) than those with DKA, this complication is still quite rare in nonketotic hyperosmolarity.

CHINESE MEDICAL DISEASE CATEGORIZATION: The main clinical symptoms of nonketotic hyperosmolarity correspond to the traditional Chinese disease categories of *fan ke*, vexatious thirst, *duo niao*, profuse urination, *lao juan*, taxation fatigue, *shen si huang hu*, spirit mind abstraction, *duan xian*, epilepsy, and *shen zhi hun mi*, coma.

CHINESE DISEASE MECHANISMS:

There are three main disease mechanisms at work in those with NKH. These are: 1) contraction of external evils with heat blocking the clear orifices, 2) yin fluid depletion and consumption with blood and fluid stasis and stagnation, and 3) yin detriment reaching yang with yin exhaustion and yang desertion. Either of these first two mechanisms can give rise to the third. As stated above, the basic disease mechanism of diabetes is yin fluid depletion and consumption with dryness and heat tending to exuberance. If such patients are invaded by external evils, they are all the more likely for these evils to transform heat. If this heat falls internally into the heart wrapper (or pericardium), it may block and obstruct the clear orifices. Hence the heart-brain becomes chaotic and confused and the spirit brilliance loses its function. This may produce either coma or agitation, confusion, and restlessness.

If external evils are contracted and transform heat, they may not immediately fall inward to the pericardium. In fact, in most cases, they do not. However, they may further damage and consume yin fluids, thus aggravating the basic yin fluid vacuity detriment. In addition, high temperatures with profuse perspiration, vomiting, diarrhea, insufficient drinking of liquids, or the adverse effects of a number of different medications can all also worsen a diabetic patient's underlying yin vacuity. As yin and fluids become more vacuous and insufficient, the skin and mucus membranes become drier and vexatious thirst may increase. Because the brain loses its nourishment, the spirit brilliance may not function correctly. Hence there may be spirit mind torpor and stagnation, a bland affect, and, if severe, even coma. Because the kidneys lose their nourishment, kidney function may decline. Likewise, because the intestines become dry, the stools may become dry and bound or constipated. Further, because blood and fluids share a common source and flow together, dryness and heat damaging yin fluids may lead to the movement of the blood becoming uneasy or unsmooth, and this may result in blood stasis. If static blood then obstructs the channels and vessels of the four limbs, there may be partial paralysis, while if static blood obstructs the vessels of the brain, there may be seizures.

In any of these cases, because yin and yang are mutually rooted, if yin detriment reaches yang, there may be yin exhaustion and yang desertion leading to reversal chilling of the four limbs, cyanotic lips and nails, a somber white facial complexion, weak respiration, and a faint pulse on the verge of expiry.

TREATMENT BASED ON PATTERN DISCRIMINATION:

1. YIN FLUID DEPLETION & DETRIMENT PATTERN

MAIN SYMPTOMS: Oral thirst, polyuria, fatigue, lack of strength, dry, bound stools, a bland affect, slowed reactions to stimuli, dry, red lips and tongue, dy, parched skin with lack of elasticity, and a vacuous, rapid pulse

NOTE: This pattern is mostly seen in those without or prior to coma.

TREATMENT PRINCIPLES: Enrich yin and increase fluids

RX: *Zeng Ye Tang Jia Wei* (Increase Fluids Decoction with Added Flavors)

INGREDIENTS: Uncooked Radix Rehmanniae (*Sheng Di*), Radix Scrophulariae Ningpoensis (*Xuan Shen*), and Radix Trichosanthis Kirlowii (*Tian Hua Fen*), 30g each, Radix Glehniae Littoralis (*Sha Shen*), 15g, Tuber Ophiopogonis Japonici (*Mai Men Dong*), 12g, and Radix Puerariae (*Ge Gen*), 9g

ANALYSIS OF FORMULA: *Sheng Di, Xuan Shen,* and *Mai Men Dong* enrich yin and increase fluids. They are also able to moisten the intestines and free the flow of the stools, increase water and float the boat. *Sha Shen, Ge Gen,* and *Tian Hua Fen* nourish yin and engender fluids, upbear fluids and stop thirst.

ADDITIONS & SUBTRACTIONS: If there is still constipation after taking the above medicinals, add 15 grams of Semen Trichosanthis Kirlowii (*Gua Lou*) and nine grams of wine-processed Radix Et Rhizoma Rhei (*Da Huang*). If vexatious thirst is marked, add 30 grams of uncooked Gypsum Fibrosum (*Shi Gao*) and 12 grams of Rhizoma Anemarrhenae Aspheloidis (*Zhi Mu*). If fatigue is pronounced, add 30 grams of Radix Astragali Membranacei (*Huang Qi*) and 15 grams of Radix Pseudostellariae Heterophyllae (*Tai Zi Shen*).

ACUPUNCTURE & MOXIBUSTION: *Tai Xi* (Ki 3), *San Yin Jiao* (Sp 6), *Shen Shu* (Bl 23)

FORMULA ANALYSIS: Supplementing *Tai Xi, San Yin Jiao,* and *Shen Shu* supplements the kidneys and enriches yin.

ADDITIONS & SUBTRACTIONS: If there is oral thirst and polydipsia, add draining *Nei Ting* (St 44) and supplementing *Cheng Jiang* (CV 24). If there is constipation, add supplementing *Zhao Hai* (Ki 6), draining *Zhi Gou* (TB 6), and even supplementing-even draining *Tian Shu* (St 25) and *Da Chang Shu* (Bl 25). If fatigue is marked, add supplementing *Zu San Li* (St 36) and *Pi Shu* (Bl 20).

2. HEAT BLOCKING THE CLEAR ORIFICES PATTERN

MAIN SYMPTOMS: High fever, coma, vexation and agitation, deranged speech, no speech, constipation, reddish urine, dry, cracked lips, dry, parched skin, a crimson tongue with dry, yellow fur, and a fine, slippery, rapid pulse

NOTE: This pattern mostly presents in those with a concurrent infection and coma or delirium due to high fever.

TREATMENT PRINCIPLES: Clear heat and cool the blood, arouse the spirit and open the orifices

RX: *Qing Gong Tang Jia Wei* (Clear the Palace Decoction with Added Flavors)

INGREDIENTS: Radix Salviae Miltiorrhizae (*Dan Shen*), Flos Lonicerae Japonicae (*Jin Yin Hua*), and Cornu Bubali (*Shui Niu Jiao*) taken with the decocted liquid, 30g each, Radix Scrophulariae Ningpoensis (*Xuan Shen*) and uncooked Radix Rehmanniae (*Sheng Di*), 20g each, Fructus Forsythiae Suspensae (*Lian Qiao*) and Radix Rubrus Paeoniae Lactiflorae (*Chi Shao*), 15g each, Tuber Ophiopogonis Japonici (*Mai Men Dong*), 12g, PlumulaNelumbinis Nuciferae (*Lian Zi Xin*) and wine-processed Radix Et Rhizoma Rhei (*Da Huang*), 9g each, and Rhizoma Coptidis Chinensis (*Huang Lian*), 6g

FORMULA ANALYSIS: *Sheng Di, Xuan Shen,* and *Mai Men Dong* enrich yin and clear heat. *Lian Zi Xin* and *Huang Lian* clear the heart and drain heat. *Jin Yin Hua* and *Lian Qiao* clear heat and resolve toxins. *Dan Shen* and *Chi Shao* cool and quicken the blood. Wine-processed *Da Huang* frees the flow of the bowels and drains heat.

ADDITIONS & SUBTRACTIONS: If there is coma, also administer one pill of *An Gong Niu Huang Wan* (Quiet the Palace Bezoar Pills) via nasal intubation.

ACUPUNCTURE & MOXIBUSTION: *Shi Xuan* (M-UE-1), *Ren Zhong* (GV 26)

FORMULA ANALYSIS: Bleeding *Shi Xuan* clears heat and arouses the spirit, while draining *Ren Zhong* opens the orifices and arouses the brain.

3. YIN EXHAUSTION & YANG DESERTION PATTERN

MAIN SYMPTOMS: A somber white facial complexion, lack of consciousness of human affairs, no speech, sunken eye sockets, a dry, cracked tongue, reversal chilling of the four limbs, low blood pressure, scanty urination or anuria, and a faint pulse on the verge of expiry

NOTE: This pattern is mostly seen in patients with diabetic hyperosmolar nonketotic coma with circulatory collapse.

TREATMENT PRINCIPLES: Rescue yang and stem counterflow

RX: *Si Ni Jia Ren Shen Tang Jia Wei* (Four Counterflows Plus Ginseng Decoction with Added Flavors)

INGREDIENTS: Radix Rubrus Panacis Ginseng (*Hong Shen*), 15g, Tuber Ophiopogonis Japonici (*Mai Men Dong*), 12g, Fructus Corni Officinalis (*Shan Zhu Yu*), Fructus Schisandrae Chinensis (*Wu Wei Zi*), Radix Lateralis Praeparatus Aconiti Carmichaeli (*Fu Zi*), and dry Rhizoma Zingiberis (*Gan Jiang*), 9g each, and mix-fried Radix Glycrrhizae (*Gan Cao*), 6g

FORMULA ANALYSIS: *Fu Zi* and *Gan Jiang* resuce yang and stem counterflow. *Hong Shen, Shan Zhu Yu, Mai Men Dong, Wu Wei Zi,* and mix-fried *Gan Cao* boost the qi, nourish yin, and secure desertion.

ACUPUNCTURE & MOXIBUSTION: *Su Liao* (GV 25), *Nei Guan* (Per 6), *Zu San Li* (St 36), *Xing Fen* (M-HN-23)

FORMULA ANALYSIS: Supplementing *Zu San Li* boosts the qi and stems desertion. Draining *Nei Guan* quickens the blood within the heart and opens blockage. Supplementing *Su Liao* and *Xing Fen* arouses the brain and raises the blood pressure.

REMARKS:

1. As with DKA above, this is an emergency condition typically requiring in-patient hospital care, often in an ICU. However, after emergency treatment has stabilized the patient, Chinese medicine may be used to promote faster recovery with less side effects and lower doses of Western medicines.

ENDNOTES:

[1] www.embbs.com/cr/dka/pathdia.htm

14

Diabetic Lactic Acidosis

Lactic acidosis refers to a type of high anion gap acidosis in which there is a pathological buildup of lactic acid in the body (with elevated lactate levels in excess of 5mmol/L), decreased blood pH (below 7.35), and increased lactate/pyruvate ratio. Lactate is normally generated by muscle glycolysis. Lactate levels increase when there is either tissue anoxia or impaired utilization by the liver or kidneys. Tissue anoxia (type A lactic acidosis) may be due physiologically to exercise or pathologically to shock, anemia, carbon monoxide, cyanide, cardiac failure, or pneumonia. Impaired utilization of lactate by the liver and kidneys (type B lactic acidosis) may be due to hepatic failure, alcohol, malignancy, salycylate overdose, or, in diabetic patients, due to biguanide hypoglycemic agents.[1] While not as common as diabetic ketoacidosis, lactic acidosis is a rare but serious metabolic complication that can occur due to the use of metformin (n,N-dimethylbiguanide, Glucophage). The incidence of metformin lactic acidosis is approximately 0.03 cases per 1,000 patient years. Metformin is an oral medication for controlling elevated blood glucose levels in type 2 diabetes. Lactic acidosis due to metformin use is only one-tenth as common as that due to phenformin, another biguanide hypoglycemic which has been withdrawn from the U.S. market. However, when it does occur, lactic acidosis due to metformin use is fatal in approximately 50% of cases.[2] In cases of metformin lactic acidosis, metformin plasma levels are higher than 5mcg/ml. Most reported cases have occurred primarily in elderly diabetic patients with significant renal insufficiency, including both intrinsic renal disease and renal hypoperfusion often in conjunction with multiple concomitant medical/surgical problems and multiple concomitant medications. In particular, patients with unstable or acute congestive heart failure are at increased risk for lactic acidosis. Other risk factors include trauma, severe dehydration, intravenous pyelography, arteriography, acute asthma attacks, status epilepticus, rapid ascent to high altitudes, intestinal obstruction and jejuno-ileal bypass, and impending surgery. In addition, alcohol potentiates the effects of metformin on lactate metabolism.

The symptoms of lactic acidosis are nonspecific and may be hard to distinguish from those of the underlying disease. They include malaise, shortness of breath, severe weakness, nausea, vomiting, altered consciousness (i.e., disorientation), fatigue, respiratory distress, abdominal pain, muscle aches and pains, and thirst. As the condition worsens, there may also be hypothermia, hypotension, and resistant bradyarrhythmias. Patients on metformin are routinely instructed on the symptoms of lactic acidosis as well as to inform their physician immediately if they occur.

Metformin lactic acidosis is a medical emergency requiring immediate supportive and remedial therapy in a hospital setting. A definitive Western medical diagnosis of lactic acidosis is made by laboratory tests which, in part, rule out the presence of ketonuria and ketonemia, thus distinguishing lactic acidosis from ketoacidosis. Western medical treatment consists of immediate cessation of metformin, possible intravenous sodium bicarbonate therapy, and possible hemodialysis to correct the acidosis and remove the accumulated metformin in life-threatening acidosis. Unfortunately, bicarbonate therapy seldom, if ever, improves the usual high mortality rate of severe lactic acidosis and, in certain conditions, such as lactic acidosis associated with cancer and cardiac arrest, may worsen the acidosis by depressing cardiac performance and stimulating phosphofructokinase to make more lactic acid.[3] Thus bicarbonate therapy is controversial.

CHINESE MEDICAL DISEASE CATEGORIZATION: Diabetic lactic acidosis corresponds to the traditional disease categories of *e xin*, nausea, *ou tu*, vomiting, *shen zhi huang hu*, spirit mind abstraction, *fan ke*, vexatious thirst, *qi cu*, hasty breathing, and *pi juan fa li*, fatigue and lack of strength.

CHINESE DISEASE MECHANISMS:

While the main disease mechanisms of diabetes are yin vacuity with dryness and heat, many diabetic patients develop this yin vacuity due to long-term spleen vacuity with dampness and turbidity. This dampness and turbidity may transform into damp heat which damages and consumes yin or may obstruct the free flow of yang qi, thus transforming liver depression into depressive heat. In addition, when yin fluids are bound up as evil dampness, they become unavailable to nourish and moisten the body, thus causing or aggravating yin vacuity from that perspective as well. In any case, this underlying dampness and turbidity do not go away when any of these mechanisms eventually give rise to yin vacuity with dryness and heat.

Further, because yin and yang are mutually rooted, yin disease will eventually reach yang, resulting in a dual yin and yang vacuity. If yang qi is too vacuous and weak to move and transform yin fluids, this will only add to the presence of damp, turbid evils, including phlegm. If these damp, turbid evils stagnate and obstruct the qi mechanism, upbearing and downbearing may lose their normalcy. In that case, clear yang will not be upborne, leading to headache, dizziness, and distention, while turbid yin is not downborne. Rather, it may counterflow upward to attack the stomach, resulting in nausea and vomiting. If turbid yin lodges in and stagnates between the intestines, this may lead to abdominal pain and diarrhea. If turbid yin congests and obstructs the lung qi, blocking its downward diffusion, it may result in large, excessively deep breaths. If phlegm turbidity confounds and mists the clear orifices, the spirit brilliance may lose its function. Hence there is spirit clouding, somnolence, abstraction, and a bland affect. Likewise, hypothermia may be due to yang qi vacuity and/or blockage and obstruction of the free flow of yang qi phlegm, dampness, and turbid yin.

TREATMENT BASED ON PATTERN DISCRIMINATION:

1. PHLEGM TURBIDITY CONFOUNDING & MISTING THE CLEAR ORIFICES PATTERN

MAIN SYMPTOMS: Spirit mind abstraction, mental confusion, difficulty thinking, nausea, vomiting, unclear speech, if severe, coma, slimy, white tongue fur, and a bowstring, slippery pulse

TREATMENT PRINCIPLES: Flush phlegm and open the orifices

RX: *Di Tan Tang* (Flush Phlegm Decoction)

INGREDIENTS: Processed Rhizoma Pinelliae Ternatae (*Ban Xia*), Pericarpium Citri Reticulatae (*Chen Pi*), Fructus Immaturus Citri Aurantii (*Zhi Shi*), Sclerotium Poriae Cocos (*Fu Ling*), Radix Panacis Ginseng (*Ren Shen*), Rhizoma Acori Graminei (*Shi Chang Pu*), and Caulis Bambusae In Taeniis (*Zhu Ru*), 9g each, and bile-processed Rhizoma Arisaematis (*Dan Nan Xing*) and Radix Glycyrrhizae (*Gan Cao*), 6g each

FORMULA ANALYSIS: *Ban Xia, Dan Nan Xing,* and *Chen Pi* dry dampness and transform phlegm. *Ren Shen, Fu Ling,* and *Gan Cao* fortify the spleen and boost the qi. *Zhu Ru* and *Zhi Shi* harmonize the stomach and downbear counterflow. *Shi Chang Pu* dispels phlegm and opens the orifices.

ADDITIONS & SUBTRACTIONS: For best results, this decoction should be administered with *Su He Xiang Wan* (Liquid Styrax Pills), a ready-made Chinese medicine which also dispels phlegm and opens the orifices. If nausea and vomiting are marked, add nine grams each of Herba Agastachis Seu Pogostemi (*Huo Xiang*) and Herba Eupatorii Fortunei (*Pei Lan*) to penetratingly and aromatically transform turbidity, harmonize the stomach and stop vomiting. If there is abdominal pain, add 18 grams of Radix Albus Paeoniae Lactiflorae (*Bai Shao*) and 12 grams of Rhizoma Corydalis Yanhusuo (*Yan Hu Suo*) to relax cramping and stop pain. If qi vacuity is pronounced, add 15-30 grams of Radix Astragali Membranacei (*Huang Qi*) and 15 grams of Rhizoma Polygonati (*Huang Jing*) to strengthen and increase the function of boosting the qi.

ACUPUNCTURE & MOXIBUSTION: *Feng Long* (St 40), *Zhong Wan* (CV 12), *Nei Guan* (Per 6), *Feng Chi* (GB 20)

FORMULA ANALYSIS: Draining *Feng Long* transforms phlegm, especially when combined with *Zhong Wan.* Draining *Nei Guan* harmonizes the stomach and stops vomiting when combined with *Zhong Wan.* Draining *Feng Chi* opens the orifices of the head and treats dizziness.

ADDITIONS & SUBTRACTIONS: If there is coma, add draining *Ren Zhong* (GV 26) with strong stimulation to arouse the brain and open the orifices.

2. TURBID YIN COUNTERFLOWING UPWARD PATTERN

MAIN SYMPTOMS: Dizziness, headache, nausea, vomiting, no thought for eating or drinking, chest oppression, abdominal distention, somnolence gradually evolving into coma, a fat, pale tongue with slimy, white fur, and a deep, moderate (*i.e.*, relaxed or slightly slow) pulse

TREATMENT PRINCIPLES: Harmonize the stomach and downbear counterflow

RX: *Wen Dan Tang Jia Jian* (Warm the Gallbladder Decoction with Additions & Subtractions)

INGREDIENTS: Fructus Evodiae Rutecarpae (*Wu Zhu Yu*), Pericarpium Citri Reticulatae (*Chen Pi*), processed Rhizoma Pinelliae Ternatae (*Ban Xia*), Caulis Bambusae In Taeniis (*Zhu Ru*), Sclerotium Poriae Cocos (*Fu Ling*), Herba Agastachis Seu Pogostemi (*Huo Xiang*), and Herba Eupatorii Fortunei (*Pei Lan*), 9g each, and Rhizoma Coptidis Chinensis (*Huang Lian*), 3g

FORMULA ANALYSIS: *Huo Xiang* and *Pei Lan* penetratingly and aromatically transform turbidity. *Ban Xia*, *Chen Pi*, and *Zhu Ru* harmonize the stomach, downbear counterflow, and stop vomiting. *Fu Ling* fortifies the spleen and seeps dampness. *Huang Lian* and *Wu Zhu Yu* aromatically open and bitterly downbear, harmonize the stomach and stop vomiting.

ADDITIONS & SUBTRACTIONS: For best results, this decoction should be administered with *Su He Xiang Wan* (Liquid Styrax Pills), a ready-made Chinese medicine which also flushes phlegm and opens the orifices. If dehydration is evident with dry, parched skin, add 12 grams each of uncooked Radix Rehmanniae (*Sheng Di*), Radix Scrophulariae Ningpoensis (*Xuan Shen*), and Tuber Ophiopogonis Japonici (*Mai Men Dong*) to enrich yin and increase humors. If qi vacuity is marked, add 15-30 grams of Radix Astragali Membranacei (*Huang Qi*), 15 grams of Rhizoma Polygonati (*Huang Jing*), and nine grams of Radix Panacis Ginseng (*Ren Shen*). If there is reversal chilling of the four extremities with a faint, fine pulse on the verge of expiry, add nine grams each of Radix Rubrus Panacis Ginseng (*Hong Shen*), Fructus Schisandrae Chinensis (*Wu Wei Zi*), and Tuber Ophiopogonis Japonici

(*Mai Men Dong*) and six grams each of dry Rhizoma Zingiberis (*Gan Jiang*), Radix Lateralis Praeparatus Aconiti Carmichaeli (*Fu Zi*), and mix-fried Radix Glycyrrhizae (*Gan Cao*).

ACUPUNCTURE & MOXIBUSTION: *Zu San Li* (St 36), *Feng Long* (St 40), *Zhong Wan* (CV 12), *Nei Guan* (Per 6), *Feng Chi* (GB 20)

FORMULA ANALYSIS: Even supplementing-even draining *Zu San Li* and *Zhong Wan* fortifies the spleen and supplements the qi at the same time as it harmonizes the stomach and downbears counterflow. Draining *Feng Long* transforms phlegm, especially when combined with *Zhong Wan*. Draining *Nei Guan* harmonizes the stomach and stops vomiting when combined with *Zu San Li* and *Zhong Wan*. Draining *Feng Chi* opens the orifices of the head and treats dizziness.

ADDITIONS & SUBTRACTIONS: If somnolence slips into coma, add even supplementing-even draining *Ren Zhong* (GV 26) with strong stimulation to arouse the brain and open the orifices. If there is dehydration, add supplementing *Tai Xi* (Ki 3) and *San Yin Jiao* (Sp 6) to supplement the kidneys and nourish yin. If qi vacuity is marked, add supplementing *Pi Shu* (Bl 20) and *Wei Shu* (Bl 21). If there is reversal chilling of the extremities, add moxibustion at *Guan Yuan* (CV 4) and *Qi Hai* (CV 6).

REMARKS:

1. When this condition is severe, its mortality rate is high. Therefore, it is reasonable to consider any treatment methods which may improve the survival rate. Since Chinese medicine appears to hasten recovery from diabetic ketoacidosis, it is reasonable to think that it may also help improve treatment outcomes when combined with standard Western medical care.

2. In China, Chinese medicinals are administered through nasal feeding tubes to patients who are comatose.

ENDNOTES:

[1] www.mcevoy.demon.co.uk/Medicine/Pathology/Biochem/Renal/Lactic.htm
[2] www.rxlist.com/cgi/generic/metformi_wcp.htm
[3] www.psl.msu.edu/class/442/metab_acid_Merck.htm

15

DIABETIC HYPERTENSION

Hypertension refers to abnormally elevated blood pressure, and hypertension is especially common among people with type 2 or non-insulin-dependent diabetes. According to the American Diabetes Association, nearly 60% of people with type 2 diabetes also have high blood pressure,[1] while the U.S. Center for Disease Control puts this number at closer to 65%.[2] The Western medical diagnosis of hypertension is based on measuring systolic and diastolic blood pressure using a blood pressure cuff. Since blood pressure may fluctuate, at least two blood pressure readings should be taken on separate days, and care should be taken to insure the proper sized cuff for the size of the arm. For instance, using too small a cuff on a larger than normal arm will tend to read hypertensive. The upper limit of normal blood pressure in adults is 140/90mm/Hg.

If patients have mild hypertension and no heart problems, diet and lifestyle changes may suffice if carried out with determination. Such diet and lifestyle modifications include weight loss, restricted intake of sodium, exercise, and relaxation. For more severe hypertension or for mild cases that do not respond to changes in diet and lifestyle within one year, drug treatment is usually considered necessary. Antihypertensive medications typically fall into one of five categories: diuretics, ACE inhibitors or receptor inhibitors, beta-blockers, vasodilators, and calcium channel blockers. ACE inhibitors are the first line therapy for hypertension in diabetics because of their renal and cardiovascular effects. Low doses of beta-blockers may also be given for secondary prevention. However, these should be used with caution due to their masking of hypoglycemic symptoms. ACE inhibitors block angiotensin-converting enzyme (ACE), an enzyme that indirectly causes blood vessels to constrict. ACE inhibitors include captoril, enalapil, lisinopril, and ramipril. Beta-blockers block the effects of adrenalin, thus decreasing the heart

rate and blood pressure. There are a number of beta-blockers now available, including propranol, olacebutolo, latenolol, betaxolol, cartedolol, and carvedolol.

Nearly 15% of persons with hypertension are not currently on medication, and untreated hypertensives are at great risk for developing disabling or fatal heart disease, cerebral hemorrhage or infarction, or renal failure. Hypertension is the most important risk factor predisposing a person to stroke. However, of those hypertensives on antihypertensive medication, only 27% of American adults with high blood pressure are well controlled. The rest are on medication which is not optimally controlling their blood pressure. Unfortunately, all Western antihypertensive medicines have side effects. Some of these side effects are distressing, such as loss of sex drive, urinary incontinence, cold extremities, heart arrhythmias, fatigue, constipation, and allergy symptoms. Therefore, achieving patient adherence is difficult, especially since treatment is lifelong or, at least, indefinite.

CHINESE DISEASE MECHANISMS:

There are three key disease mechanisms in diabetic hypertension. These are liver-kidney yin vacuity, ascendant liver yang hyperactivity, and phlegm turbidity obstructing the center. If, due to stress and emotional frustration and upset, liver depression transforms heat, or, due to overeating acrid, spicy, hot foods, oily, greasy, fried foods, and drinking alcohol, heat is engendered in the stomach, enduring heat may damage and consume yin fluids. In that case, yin may fail to control yang which then counterflows and floats upward, thus giving rise to vacuity heat, ascendant liver yang hyperactivity, or even internal stirring of wind. On the other hand, overeating sugar and sweets or oily, fatty foods which engender dampness internally may damage the spleen. If the spleen becomes vacuous and weak, it may fail to move and transform water fluids which may, instead, collect and transform into damp evils. If dampness endures, and especially if it is worked on by either cold or heat, it may congeal into phlegm which obstructs the free flow of qi and blood and blocks the orifices of the heart. Because liver depression may cause or aggravate spleen qi vacuity, in real life, most cases of diabetes are complicated by spleen vacuity. Further, because spleen qi vacuity may not engender and transform blood sufficiently, blood vacuity due to spleen vacuity may evolve into liver blood-kidney yin vacuity over time. If spleen qi vacuity endures, it typically evolves eventually into a spleen qi-kidney yang dual vacuity. Therefore, one can also find cases of kidney yin and yang dual vacuity hypertension.

According to Li Dong-yuan, upward stirring of ministerial fire, as in either vacuity heat flaming upward or ascendant liver yang hyperactivity, may damage the spleen. Vice versa, a strong, healthy spleen may help keep ministerial fire from stirring frenetically and counterflowing upward. Thus Li's yin fire theory helps to explain why hypertension is such a common complication of diabetes.

TREATMENT BASED ON PATTERN DISCRIMINATION:

1. ASCENDANT LIVER YANG HYPERACTIVITY

MAIN SYMPTOMS: Headache, head distention, dizziness, tinnitus, a red facial complexion and red eyes, vexation and agitation, easy anger, insomnia, profuse dreams, a dry mouth, a bitter taste in the mouth, low back and knee soreness and limpness, if severe, dizziness with a desire to lie down or pounding head pain, nausea and a desire to vomit, numbness of the extremities, possible tremors of the limbs, unclear speech, a red tongue with yellow fur, and a bowstring, slippery pulse

TREATMENT PRINCIPLES: Level the liver and subdue yang

RX: *Tian Ma Gou Teng Yin Jia Jian* (Gastrodia Uncaria Drink with Additions & Subtractions)

INGREDIENTS: Concha Margaritiferae (*Zhen Zhu Mu*) and uncooked Concha Ostreae (*Mu Li*), 30g each, Ramulus Uncariae Cum Uncis (*Gou Teng*), Concha Haiotidis (*Shi Jue Ming*), Radix Cyathulae (*Chuan Niu Xi*), and stir-fried Fructus Immaturus Sophorae Japonicae (*Huai Hua Mi*), 15g each, Cortex Eucommiae Ulmoidis (*Du Zhong*) and Fructus Tribuli Terrestris (*Bai Ji Li*), 12g

each, Rhizoma Gastrodiae Elatae (*Tian Ma*), Flos Chyrsanthemi Morifolii (*Ju Hua*), Radix Scutellariae Baicalensis (*Huang Qin*), and Fructus Gardeniae Jasminoidis (*Zhi Zi*), 9g each

FORMULA ANALYSIS: *Tian Ma* and *Gou Teng* level the liver and extinguish wind. *Shi Jue Ming, Zhen Zhu Mu*, and uncooked *Mu Li* subdue yang. *Huang Qin, Zhi Zi*, and *Ju Hua* clear the liver and drain heat. *Du Zhong, Chuan Niu Xi*, stir-fried *Huai Hua Mi*, and *Bai Ji Li* nourish and supplement the liver and kidneys and level liver yang.

ADDITIONS & SUBTRACTIONS: If liver fire tends to be exuberant, one can add nine grams each of Radix Gentianae Scabrae (*Long Dan Cao*) and Cortex Radicis Moutan (*Dan Pi*) to clear the liver and drain fire. If there is bowel repletion constipation, add 12 grams each of uncooked Radix Rehmanniae (*Sheng Di*) and Radix Scrophulariae Ningpoensis (*Xuan Shen*) and 3-9 grams of Radix Et Rhizoma Rhei (*Da Huang*) to enrich yin and increase fluids, free the flow of the bowels and drain fire. If liver yang hyperactivity is extreme enough to transform wind, add nine grams each of Cornu Caprae (*Shan Yang Jiao*) and Haemititum (*Dai Zhe Shi*) to settle the liver and extinguish wind. If there is polydipsia, add 30 grams of Radix Trichosanthis Kirlowii (*Tian Hua Fen*) and 15 grams of Rhizoma Anemarrhenae Aspheloidis (*Zhi Mu*). If there is marked polyphagia, add 3-6 grams of Rhizoma Coptidis Chinensis (*Huang Lian*) and 20 grams of Rhizoma Atractylodis (*Cang Zhu*).

ACUPUNCTURE & MOXIBUSTION: *Feng Chi* (GB 20), *Qu Chi* (LI 11), *Zu San Li* (St 36), *Xing Jian* (Liv 2), *Tai Chong* (Liv 3), *Yang Ling Quan* (GB 34), *Tai Yang* (M-HN-9)

FORMULA ANALYSIS: Needling *Tai Chong* through to *Xing Jian* with draining technique as well as draining *Yang Ling Quan, Feng Chi*, and *Tai Yang* levels the liver and subdues yang. Because the yang ming has lots of qi and lots of blood, draining *Zu San Li* and *Qu Chi* can also drain replete yang qi from the body as a whole.

ADDITIONS & SUBTRACTIONS: If there is headache and distention, add *Bai Hui* (GV 20) and *Yi Feng* (TB 17). If there is insomnia or profuse dreams, add *An Mian* (M-HN-22a & b) and *Shen Men* (Ht 7). If there is low back aching and pain, add *Shen Shu* (Ki 3) and *Yao Yan* (M-BW-24). If there is knee soreness and limpness, add *Xi Yan* (St 35, medial and lateral). If there is bowel repletion constipation, add *Zhi Gou* (TB 6), *Tian Shu* (St 25), and *Da Chang Shu* (Bl 25). If there is polydipsia, add *Lie Que* (Lu 7) and *Zhao Hai* (Ki 6). If there is polyphagia, add *Nei Ting* (St 44).

2. LIVER BLOOD-KIDNEY YIN VACUITY PATTERN

MAIN SYMPTOMS: Dizziness, tinnitus, blurred vision, dry, astringent eyes, low back and knee soreness and limpness, vexatious heat in the five hearts, dry mouth, parched throat, impaired memory, insomnia, falling hair and loose teeth, possible bilateral red cheeks, an emaciated body, frequent, scanty, dark-colored night-time urination, a red tongue with scanty fur, and a bowstring, fine pulse

TREATMENT PRINCIPLES: Supplement the liver and kidneys, nourish the blood and enrich yin

RX: *Qi Ju Di Huang Tang Jia Jian* (Lycium & Chrysanthemum Rehmannia Decoction with Additions & Subtractions)

INGREDIENTS: Radix Scrophulariae Ningpoensis (*Xuan Shen*), 15g, cooked Radix Rehmanniae (*Shu Di*), Fructus Corni Officinalis (*Shan Zhu Yu*), Radix Dioscoreae Oppositae (*Shan Yao*), Cortex Eucommiae Ulmoidis (*Du Zhong*), Radix Achyranthis Bidentatae (*Niu Xi*), Ramulus Loranthis Seu Visci (*Sang Ji Sheng*), and Radix Albus Paeoniae Lactiflorae (*Bai Shao*), 12g each, Fructus Lycii Chinensis (*Gou Qi Zi*), 9g

FORMULA ANALYSIS: *Shu Di, Shan Zhu Yu, Sang Ji Sheng, Xuan Shen, Du Zhong, Gou Qi Zi, Bai Shao,* and *Niu Xi* enrich and supplement the liver and kidneys and lead heat to move downward. *Shan Yao* supplements the kidneys and spleen, remembering that the former and latter heaven bolster and support each other. *Fu Ling* also fortifies the spleen and supplements the qi at the same time as it seeps dampness, thus leading yang downward into the yin tract. It is aided in this endeavor by *Ze Xie* which also seeps dampness and disinhibits urination. *Dan Pi* clears vacuity heat on the one hand while it quickens the blood on the other. This is based on the saying, "In enduring disease, there must be stasis." *Ju Hua* clears the liver and brightens the eyes.

ADDITIONS & SUBTRACTIONS: If dizziness is severe, add 12 grams each of Os Draconis (*Long Gu*), Concha Ostreae (*Mu Li*), Carapax Amydae Sinensis (*Bie Jia*), and/or Concha Margaritiferae (*Zhen Zhu Mu*) to subdue floating yang. For noninteraction between the heart and kidneys with more pronounced vexation and agitation, insomnia, profuse dreams, and impaired memory, add 12 grams each of Semen Biotae Orientalis (*Bai Zi Ren*), Semen Zizyphi Spinosae (*Suan Zao Ren*), and Gelatinum Corii Asini (*E Jiao*) and three grams of Rhizoma Coptidis Chinensis (*Huang Lian*). In case of severe dry mouth and parched throat, add 12 grams each of Tuber Ophiopogonis

Japonici (*Mai Men Dong*), Radix Glehniae Littoralis (*Sha Shen*), and Rhizoma Polygonati (*Huang Jing*).

If there is yin vacuity with fire effulgence, one can use *Zhi Bai Di Huang Wan Jia Wei* (Anemarrhena & Phellodendron Rehmannia Pills with Added Flavors) instead to enrich yin and drain fire, level and subdue floating yang: Spica Prunellae Vulgaris (*Xia Ku Cao*), 15g, uncooked Os Draconis (*Long Gu*), uncooked Concha Ostreae (*Mu Li*), Concha Margaritiferae (*Zhen Zhu Mu*), and cooked Radix Rehmanniae (*Shu Di*), 12g each, Radix Dioscoreae Oppositae (*Shan Yao*), Fructus Corni Officinalis (*Shan Zhu Yu*), Sclerotium Poriae Cocos (*Fu Ling*), Cortex Radicis Moutan (*Dan Pi*), Rhizoma Alismatis (*Ze Xie*), Rhizoma Anemarrhenae Aspheloidis (*Zhi Mu*), and Cortex Phellodendri (*Huang Bai*), 9g each. If there is simultaneous spleen-kidney yang vacuity, add nine grams each of Herba Cistanchis Deserticolae (*Rou Cong Rong*), Herba Epimedii (*Xian Ling Pi*), Rhizoma Curculiginis Orchioidis (*Xian Mao*), and Gelatinum Cornu Cervi (*Lu Jiao Jiao*), and 3-6 grams of Cortex Cinnamomi Cassiae (*Rou Gui*) to warm and supplement the spleen and kidneys.

ACUPUNCTURE & MOXIBUSTION: *Feng Chi* (GB 20), *Qu Chi* (LI 11), *Zu San Li* (St 36), *Tai Chong* (Liv 3), *San Yin Jiao* (Sp 6), *Tai Xi* (Ki 3)

FORMULA ANALYSIS: Supplementing *San Yin Jiao* and *Tai Xi* supplements the kidneys and enriches yin. Even supplementing-even draining *Tai Chong* supplements the liver at the same time as it subdues yang. Draining *Feng Chi, Zu San Li,* and *Qu Chi* also subdues yang and downbears counterflow.

ADDITIONS & SUBTRACTIONS: For insomnia, add *Nei Guan* (Per 6), *Shen Men* (Ht 7), and *Bai Hui* (GV 20). For dizziness and tinnitus, add *Bai Hui* (GV 20) and *Yi Geng* (TB 17). For heart palpitations, add *Nei Guan* (Per 6), *Shen Men* (Ht 7), *Dan Zhong* (CV 17), *Jue Yin Shu* (BL14), and *Xin Shu* (Bl 15). For low back aching and pain, add *Shen Shu* (Bl 23) and *Yao Yan* (M-BW-24). For dry mouth and polydipsia, add *Lie Que* (Lu 7) and *Zhao Hai* (Ki 6). For dry eyes and blurred vision, add *Guang Ming* (GB 37) and *Jing Ming* (Bl 1). For simultaneous yang vacuity, moxa *Qi Hai* (CV 6) and *Guan Yuan* (CV 4).

3. PHLEGM TURBIDITY OBSTRUCTING THE CENTER PATTERN

MAIN SYMPTOMS: Dizziness, fatigue, heavy-headedness, a bitter taste in the mouth and/or a slimy, sticking feeling, chest oppression, nausea and vomiting, bodily obesity, a fat tongue with thick, turbid, slimy, white or slimy, yellow fur, and a bowstring, slippery or soft, soggy pulse

NOTE: Although the name of this pattern does not say so, there is an element of depressive heat in the symptom-sign picture which is also addressed by the medicinal formula below. In real-life practice, phlegm turbidity mostly complicates ascendant liver yang hyperactivity, especially if the patient is obese.

TREATMENT PRINCIPLES: Clear and transform phlegm and turbidity

RX: *Huang Lian Wen Dan Tang Jia Jian* (Coptis Warm the Gallbladder Decoction with Additions & Subtractions)

INGREDIENTS: Radix Cyathulae (*Chuan Niu Xi*), 12g, Rhizoma Pinelliae Ternatae (*Ban Xia*), Pericarpium Citri Reticulatae (*Chen Pi*), Caulis Bambusae In Taeniis (*Zhu Ru*), Rhizoma Acori Graminaei (*Shi Chang Pu*), Rhizoma Gastrodiae Elatae (*Tian Ma*), and Rhizoma Alismatis (*Ze Xie*), 9g each, Rhizoma Coptidis Chinensis (*Huang Lian*) and bile-treated Rhizoma Arisaematis (*Dan Nan Xing*), 6g each

FORMULA ANALYSIS: *Ban Xia* and *Chen Pi* rectify the qi and transform phlegm. *Huang Lian* and *Dan Nan Xing* clear and transform phlegm heat. *Tian Ma* and *Shi Chang Pu* extinguish wind and open the orifices. *Ze Xie* and *Chuan Niu Xi* abduct heat and move it downward.

ADDITIONS & SUBTRACTIONS: If the tongue is purple and dark due to phlegm and stasis mutually binding, add nine grams each of Radix Salviae Miltiorrhizae (*Dan Shen*), Radix Rubrus Paeoniae Lactiflorae (*Chi Shao*), Radix Ligustici Wallichii (*Chuan Xiong*), Semen Pruni Persicae (*Tao Ren*), and Flos Carthami Tinctorii (*Hong Hua*) to quicken the blood and transform stasis. If there is simultaneous ascendant liver yang hyperactivity, add 15 grams each of Ramulus Uncariae Cum Uncis (*Gou Teng*) and Concha Margaritiferae (*Zhen Zhu Mu*) to level the liver and subdue yang. If phlegm turbidity congestion is exuberant with the sound of phlegm in the throat and unclear speech, add Concretio Siliceae Bambusae (*Tian Zhu Huang*) and Succus Bambusae (*Zhu Li*) to transform phlegm turbidity. If there is phlegm heat bowel repletion, add nine grams each of Fructus Trichosanthis Kirlowii (*Gua Lou*) and Fructus Immaturus Citri Aurantii (*Zhi Shi*), 3-9 grams of Radix Et Rhizoma Rhei (*Da Huang*), and 3-6 grams of Mirabilitum (*Mang Xiao*) to transform phlegm and free the flow of the bowels. For stomach duct distention and fullness, add six grams each of Fructus

Amomi (*Sha Ren*), Fructus Cardamomi (*Bai Dou Kou*), and Radix Auklandiae Lappae (*Mu Xiang*) to rectify the qi and aromatically transform dampness. For spleen yang vacuity diarrhea, add nine grams of Semen Myristicae Fragrantis (*Rou Dou Kou*) and 3-6 grams of dry Rhizoma Zingiberis (*Gan Jiang*). For heart palpitations with a bound or regularly intermittent pulse, add 30 grams of Semen Zizyphi Spinosae (*Suan Zao Ren*), 12 grams of Tuber Curcumae (*Yu Jin*), and nine grams of Ramulus Cinnamomi Cassiae (*Gui Zhi*) to free the flow of yang, loosen the chest, and quiet the spirit.

ACUPUNCTURE & MOXIBUSTION: *Feng Chi* (GB 20), *Qu Chi* (LI 11), *Zu San Li* (St 36), *Tai Chong* (Liv 3), *Nei Guan* (Per 6), *Feng Long* (St 40), *Yin Ling Quan* (Sp 9)

FORMULA ANALYSIS: Draining *Feng Chi*, *Qu Chi*, *Zu San Li*, and *Tai Chong* level the liver and subdue yang and are empirically known to lower the blood pressure. *Nei Guan* and *Feng Long* transform phlegm and harmonize the stomach. *Yin Ling Quan* seeps dampness, and phlegm is nothing other than congealed dampness.

ADDITIONS & SUBTRACTIONS: If there is nausea and vomiting, add *Zhong Wan* (St 36). If there is chest oppression, add *Dan Zhong* (CV 17). If there is a bitter taste in the mouth, add *Xing Jian* (Liv 2).

ABSTRACTS OF REPRESENTATIVE CHINESE RESEARCH:

Tong Jie *et al.*, "The Treatment of 122 Cases of Diabetic Hypertension with *Ping Gan Huo Xue Jiao Nang* (Calm the Liver and Quicken the Blood Capsule)," *Shan Dong Zhong Yi Za Zhi* (*Shandong Journal of Chinese Medicine*), #2, 2000, p. 78-79: The authors of this report treated 122 cases of diabetic hypertension with *Ping Gan Huo Xue Jiao Nang* (Calm the Liver & Quicken the Blood Capsules). The treatment group included 122 patients, and the comparison group included 60 patients. Of these, 104 were men, and 78 were women. Their ages ranged from 41-73 years old, and the average age was 51.6 years. The course of disease ranged from 2-14 years, with an average duration of 4.6 years. There were 68 cases of diabetic nephropathy with hypertension, 79 cases of diabetic hypertension without nephropathy, and 35 cases of diabetic arteriosclerosis with hypertension. According to the authors, diabetic hypertension presents two primary patterns: 1) liver-kidney yin vacuity pattern and 2) blood stasis with liver wind internally stirring. Therefore, *Ping Gan Huo Xue Jiao Nang* was administered to the treatment group. This formula consisted of: Bombyx Batryticatus (*Jiang Can*), 1.5 parts, Tuber Curcumae (*Yu Jin*), 1.5 parts,

Concha Haliotidis (*Shi Jue Ming*), 1 part, Ramulus Uncariae Cum Uncis (*Gou Teng*), 1 part, Radix Albus Paeoniae Lactiflorae (*Bai Shao*), 2 parts, Semen Zizyphi Spinosae (*Suan Zao Ren*), 2 parts, Fructus Schisandrae Chinensis (*Wu Wei Zi*), 3 parts, Semen Pruni Persicae (*Tao Ren*), 1 part, Radix Ligustici Wallichii (*Chuan Xiong*), 2 parts, Hirudo Seu Whitmania (*Shui Zhi*), 0.2 parts, Radix Polygoni Multiflori (*He Shou Wu*), 1.5 parts, Radix Bupleuri (*Chai Hu*), 1 part, Caulis Polygoni Multiflori (*Ye Jiao Teng*), 1 part, Cortex Albizziae Julibrissinis (*Hu Huan Pi*), 1 part, Radix Achyranthis Bidentatae (*Niu Xi*), 1.5 parts, uncooked Radix Rehmanniae (*Sheng Di*), 3 parts, and Flos Chrysanthemi Morifolii (*Ju Hua*), 1.2 parts. All these were ground into powder and encapsulated with each capsule containing 0.5g of powder. Four to six of these capsules were given three times per day after meals. The comparison group was administered nifedipine, 10-20mg orally three times per day. In the treatment group of 122 cases, 81 cases showed marked improvement, 27 cases showed some improvement, and 14 cases showed no improvement, for a total amelioration rate of 88.5%. In the comparison group of 60 cases, 41 cases showed marked improvement, 11 cases showed some improvement, and eight cases showed no improvement, for a total amelioration rate of 86.7%.

Zhang Xue-juan & Hu Ke-jie, "A Discussion of the Treatment of Diabetic Hypertension," *Hei Long Jiang Zhong Yi Yao* (*Heilongjiang Journal of Chinese Medicine & Medicinals*), #5, 1998, p. 21-22: The authors of this report treated 26 cases of diabetic hypertension. In this study, there were 17 men and nine women whose ages ranged from 51-68 years old, with an average age of 60.1 years. The course of these patients disease had lasted from 3.5-16 years. The patients were given amiloride, 5mg once per day orally upon rising in the morning, and *Niu Huang Jiang Ya Pian* (Bovine Bezoar Downbear Pressure Tablts),one pill orally two times per day. Of these 26 patients, 20 showed marked improvement, four showed some improvement, and two were without results using this protocol, and the total amelioration rate was 92.3%. The primary medicinals in *Niu Huang Jiang Ya Pian* are: Calculus Bovis (*Niu Huang*), Cornu Antelopis Saiga-tatarici (*Ling Yang Jiao*), Margarita (*Zhen Zhu*), Borneolum (*Bing Pian*), Radix Astragali Membranacei (*Huang Qi*), Tuber Curcumae (*Yu Jin*), and Radix Albus Paeoniae Lactiflorae (*Bai Shao*).

REPRESENTATIVE CASE HISTORIES:

CASE 1[3]

The patient was a 52 year old female agricultural worker who was diagnosed with diabetes and hypertension in Jun.

1985. Her main complaints were polydipsia, polyuria, and emaciation. Fasting blood glucose was 18.3mmol/L, urine glucose was (+++), and blood pressure was 27/13kPa. The patient was treated with glybenzcyclamide, *Fu Fang Jiang Ya Pian* (Compound Lower Pressure Tablets), and *Xiao Ke Wan* (Wasting & Thirsting Pills) which decreased the urine glucose temporarily. However, urine glucose rose again if she discontinued or reduced these medications. In the previous two months, the woman had begun to feel dizzy. This was accompanied by headache, vexation and agitation, heart palpitations or even tachycardia, easy anger, thirst with a desire to drink, dry, rough eyes, dry stools, frequent urination, a dark red tongue with scanty fur, and a bowstring, rapid pulse. Blood pressure was 24/13kPa.

Based on these signs and symptoms, the patient's patterns were categorized as liver-kidney yin vacuity complicated by heart yin insufficiency. The treatment principles were to nourish the kidneys and emolliate the liver, nourish yin and subdue yang, assisted by nourishing the heart and quieting the spirit. The formula prescribed consisted of: Radix Trichosanthis Kirlowii (*Tian Hua Fen*) and stir-fried Semen Zizyphi Spinosae (*Suan Zao Ren*), 30g each, uncooked Radix Rehmanniae (*Sheng Di*) and Radix Scrophulariae Ningpoensis (*Xuan Shen*), 15g each, Fructus Lycii Chinensis (*Gou Qi Zi*), Radix Dioscoreae Oppositae (*Shan Yao*), Fructus Corni Officinalis (*Shan Zhu Yu*), Tuber Ophiopogonis Japonici (*Mai Men Dong*), and Semen Biotae Orientalis (*Bai Zi Ren*), 12g each, Sclerotium Poriae Cocos (*Fu Ling*) and Rhizoma Alismatis (*Ze Xie*), 10g each, Flos Chrysanthemi Morifolii (*Ju Hua*) and Cortex Radicis Moutan (*Dan Pi*), 9g each, and Radix Glycyrrhizae (*Gan Cao*), 6g. In addition, *Xiao Ke Wan* (Wasting & Thirsting Pills), 10 pills TID, and *Xiao Ke Ping* (Wasting & Thirsting Leveler), eight tablets TID were administered. The patient was advised to stop taking the *Fu Fang Jiang Ya Pian* and to control her diet, eating only 150g of carbohydrates per day.

After taking 15 *ji* of the above formula, the patient's dry mouth was relieved, her blood pressure was 20/13kPa, and FBG was (+). However, the patient still had a bitter taste in the mouth. Therefore, 10 grams of Rhizoma Coptidis Chinensis (*Huang Lian*) was added to her formula. After 15 more *ji*, FBG was 10mmol/L, fasting urine glucose was (+), and, two hours postprandial, it was (++). Blood pressure was now 21/12kPa. While her other symptoms became less severe, the woman still had blurred vision, which was diagnosed as diabetic cataracts through ophthalmological examination. The patient was prescribed an unidentified medicine and some eye drops for external application as well as Chinese medicinals to boost the qi and supplement the kidneys, nourish yin and clear heat: Radix Astragali Membranacei (*Huang Qi*), Radix Trichosanthis Kirlowii (*Tian Hua Fen*), Radix Salviae Miltiorrhizae (*Dan Shen*), and cooked Radix Rehmanniae (*Shu Di*), 30g each, Fructus Corni Officinalis (*Shan Zhu Yu*), 20g, Radix Dioscoreae Oppositae (*Shan Yao*), Radix Albus Paeoniae Lactiflorae (*Bai Shao*), Radix Puerariae (*Ge Gen*), and Radix Scrophulariae Ningpoensis (*Xuan Shen*), 15g each, Fructus Lycii Chinensis (*Gou Qi Zi*) and Herba Dendrobii (*Shi Hu*), 12g each, Rhizoma Coptidis Chinensis (*Huang Lian*), 10g, Flos Chrysanthemi Morifolii (*Ju Hua*), 9g, and Radix Glycyrrhizae (*Gan Cao*), 6g.

The above medicinals were taken by the patient for two months or more, during which time her blood pressure remained around 20/12kPa and blood glucose remained at 7-8mmol/L. At this point, the decoction was stopped and *Xiao Ke Wan* and *Xiao Ke Ping*, eight tablets each TID, were continued as well as *Qi Ju Di Huang Wan* (Lycium & Chrysanthemum Rehmannia Pills), one pill TID, in order to secure and consolidate the treatment effects. Eventually, the woman underwent cataract surgery.

CASE 2[4]

The patient was a 62 year old female retired clerical worker who first examined on Jan. 15, 1991 and who had had diabetes for seven years. The patient's major complaints were dry mouth, thirst but little drinking, dizziness, heart palpitations, shortness of breath, chest oppression, and paroxysmal cardiac pain which radiated to her back. The woman had previously been diagnosed as suffering from diabetes, hypertension, and coronary heart disease at another hospital and had been prescribed a number of different Western hypoglycemic and antihypertensive medications as well as nitroglycerin which had not been markedly effective. On examination, the patient was found to be obese with a clear mind, dark tongue with thick, white fur, and a bowstring, slippery pulse. Her blood pressure was 22/12kPa, total cholesterol was 7.5mmol/L, triglycerides were 2.4mmol/L, blood glucose was 9.6mmol/L, urine glucose was (+++), and urine ketones were negative. In addition, ECG showed abnormalities consistent with coronary heart disease.

Based on the above signs and symptoms, the patient's Chinese medical pattern was discriminated as internal accumulation of phlegm dampness with blood stasis obstructing the network vessels. Therefore, the treatment principles were to transform phlegm and dispel obstruc-

tion, quicken the blood and stop pain. The Chinese medicinal prescription consisted of: Radix Salviae Miltiorrhizae (*Dan Shen*), 30g, Rhizoma Gastrodiae Elatae (*Tian Ma*), Fructus Trichosanthis Kirlowii (*Gua Lou*), and Sclerotium Poriae Cocos (*Fu Ling*), 15g each, Rhizoma Atractylodis Macrocephalae (*Bai Zhu*), Rhizoma Acori Graminei (*Shi Chang Pu*), Caulis Bambusae In Taeniis (*Zhu Ru*), and Radix Ligustici Wallichii (*Chuan Xiong*), 12g each, Rhizoma Pinelliae Ternatae (*Ban Xia*), 10g, Pericarpium Citri Reticulatae (*Chen Pi*) and Fructus Citri Aurantii (*Zhi Ke*), 9g each, and Radix Glycyrrhizae (*Gan Cao*), 6g. In addition, *Xiao Ke Wan* (Wasting & Thirsting Pills), 10 pills TID, and *Xiao Ke Ping* (Wasting & Thirsting Leveler), 8 tablets TID, were prescribed.

After 15 *ji* of the above formula, the dizziness and headache had been alleviated. Therefore, *Fu Fang Jiang Ya Pian* (Compound Lower Pressure Tablets) [sic] and the nitroglycerin were discontinued. Forty more *ji* of this formula with additions and subtractions were administered, and all the symptoms were markedly relieved. Blood glucose was 5.2mmol/L, total cholesterol was 4.9mmol/L, triglycerides were 0.8mmol/L, urine glucose was negative, and blood pressure was 20/10kPa. Electrocardiogram showed some improvement in the S-T segment as well. Therefore, the decocted Chinese medicinals were discontinued, although *Xiao Ke Wan* was continued at five pills BID and *Xiao Ke Ping* was continued at six tablets BID in order to secure and consolidate the treatment effects. In addition, the patient was instructed to get more exercise and control her diet to prevent aggravation of her diabetes.

CASE 3[5]

The patient was a 66 year old male office worker who had been diagnosed with diabetes three years previously. He was first examined on Mar. 5, 1990 complaining of chest oppression, shortness of breath, lassitude of the spirit, dizziness, and frequent lancinating pain in the precordial region which radiated to his left upper back and shoulder. This pain was induced by exercise and was relieved by rest or by taking *Huo Xin Dan* (Quicken the Heart Elixir). The patient did not have obvious polydipsia, polyphagia, or polyuria. The man's facial complexion was lusterless, his consciousness was clear, he had a red tongue with scanty fur, and a bowstring, fine pulse. His blood pressure was 20/14kPa, blood glucose was 9.8mmol/L, total cholesterol was 7.2mmol/L, triglycerides were 1.6mmol/L, and urine glucose was (++). Urine ketones were negative. There were also abnormalities in ECG consistent with coronary heart disease.

Based on the above signs and symptoms, the patient was diagnosed with hypertension and coronary heart disease, and his Chinese medical patterns were categorized as qi and yin dual vacuity with blood stasis obstructing the heart. Therefore, the treatment principles were to boost the qi and nourish yin assisted by quickening the blood and dispelling stasis. The Chinese medicinal prescription consisted of: Radix Salviae Miltiorrhizae (*Dan Shen*) and Radix Trichosanthis Kirlowii (*Tian Hua Fen*), 30g each, Radix Astragali Membranacei (*Huang Qi*), 20g, Radix Codonopsitis Pilosulae (*Dang Shen*), Tuber Ophiopogonis Japonici (*Mai Men Dong*), Radix Puerariae (*Ge Gen*), and Radix Glehniae Littoralis (*Sha Shen*), 15g each, Radix Ligustici Wallichii (*Chuan Xiong*) and Rhizoma Anemarrhenae Aspheloidis (*Zhi Mu*), 12g each, Fructus Schisandrae Chinensis (*Wu Wei Zi*) and Rhizoma Corydalis Yanhusuo (*Yan Hu Suo*), 9g each, and Radix Glycyrrhizae (*Gan Cao*), 6g. In addition, eight pills of *Xiao Ke Wan* (Wasting & Thirsting Pills) and one pill of *Niu Huang Jiang Ya Wan* (Bezoar Lower Pressure Pills) were administered TID.

After 30 *ji*, during which various additions and subtractions were made depending on the patient's symptoms, all the symptoms had disappeared. Blood glucose was 5.2mmol/L, total cholesterol was 5.2mmol/L, triglycerides were 1.0mmol/L, urine glucose was negative, and ECG was normal. Therefore, the man was instructed to get more exercise, control his diet, and to take *Xiao Ke Ping* (Wasting & Thirsting Leveler), six tablets BID, in order to secure and consolidate the treatment effects.

CASE 4[6]

The patient was a 41 year old female who was first examined on Mar. 21, 1983. In November of the preceding year, the patient had developed oral thirst which led to increased drinking, increasingly frequent urination, dizziness, tinnitus, and emotional dysphoria. One month later, the disease's condition worsened and the woman went to her local hospital for examination. At that point, it was found that her blood glucose was 243mg/dL, urine glucose was (++), and blood pressure was 150/110mmHg. Therefore, the patient was diagnosed with diabetes and hypertension and she was sent to another, unnamed hospital for treatment. At this hospital, the patient was prescribed the Western medicine, *Fu Fang Jiang Ya Pian* (Compound Lower Pressure Tablets), and, after being treated for two months, her symptoms remitted and she was discharged from the hospital. However, not long after, her symptoms returned. She then came to Dr. Guo for

examination and treatment. Dr. Guo found a dry tongue, oral thirst with a desire to drink, frequent, profuse urination in excess of 2000ml per day, lassitude of the spirit, shortness of breath, torpid intake, a clouded spirit and head oppression, occasional tinnitus, emission of heat from the hearts of the hands, generalized distention, and slight lower limb edema. At this point, the patient's blood glucose was 213mg/dL, urine glucose was (+), and blood pressure was 140/105mmHg. The woman's tongue was pale red with a combination of white, slimy and dry, yellow fur, and her pulse was deep, fine, soggy, and bowstring.

Based on the above signs and symptoms, the patient's patterns were discriminated as qi and yin dual vacuity with damp depression transforming dryness and yin vacuity-yang hyperactivity. Therefore, the treatment principles were to boost the qi and enrich yin, clear heat and disinhibit dampness, level the liver and downbear counterflow. The formula Dr. Guo prescribed consisted of: uncooked Radix Astragali Membranacei (*Huang Qi*), Radix Dioscoreae Oppositae (*Shan Yao*), and uncooked Semen Coicis Lachryma-jobi (*Yi Yi Ren*), 30g each, Concha Haliotidis (*Shi Jue Ming*), decocted first, Radix Trichosanthis Kirlowii (*Tian Hua Fen*), Cortex Radicis Mori Albi (*Sang Bai Pi*), Cortex Radicis Lycii Chinensis (*Di Gu Pi*), Magnetitum (*Ci Shi*), decocted first, Radix Salviae Miltiorrhizae (*Dan Shen*), Herba Dendrobii (*Shi Hu*), Fructus Ligustri Lucidi (*Nu Zhen Zi*), and Herba Ecliptae Prostratae (*Han Lian Cao*), 15g each, Tuber Ophiopogonis Japonici (*Mai Men Dong*), Tuber Apsaragi Cochinensis (*Tian Men Dong*), Pumice (*Hai Fu Shi*), and Rhizoma Atractylodis (*Cang Zhu*), 10g each, Fructus Amomi (*Sha Ren*), 5g, and Rhizoma Coptidis Chinensis (*Huang Lian*), 3g.

After taking 30 *ji* of these medicinals, the patient's affect was improved and all her symptoms had disappeared. Her blood glucose was 120mg/dL, urine glucose was negative, and blood pressure was between 130-140/90-96mmHg. Therefore, the original formula was made into pills. On May 30, 1985, all examinations were normal. Hence medicinals to boost the qi, enrich yin, and engender fluids were made into pills in order to secure and consolidate the treatment effects. While this patient was being treated with Chinese medicinals, she completely stopped taking her Western medicines, and the Chinese medicines alone were able to effect a cure.

REMARKS:

1. Acupuncture is definitely an effective modality for

treating hypertension. It can often significantly reduce systolic pressure within a matter of minutes. However, for reducing diastolic pressure, regular repeated treatments are usually required.

2. Auriculotherapy may be done either with ear needles, Semen Vaccariae Segetalis (*Wang Bu Liu Xing*), ion pellets, magnets, or press needles. For best results, needles should be retained for 1-2 hours.

A. For ascendant liver yang hyperactivity pattern: Liver, Gallbladder, Hypertension Point, Eye 1, Eye 2

B. For liver-kidney yin vacuity pattern: Kidney, Adrenal, Internal Secretion, Subcortex, Stomach

C. For phlegm turbidity obstructing the center pattern: Spleen, Stomach, Lung, Tip of the Ear

3. Although Chinese textbooks do not typically include a qi vacuity pattern of hypertension, especially in diabetes, spleen qi vacuity complicates many, if not most, cases in Western patients. In that case, formulas should be modified appropriately. However, one should avoid using Radix Panacis Ginseng (*Ren Shen*) which has a known empirical effect of raising blood pressure. Radix Codonopsitis Pilosulae (*Dang Shen*), on the other hand, has a known empirical effect of lowering blood pressure. Another commonly used qi supplement which raises blood pressure is Radix Glycyrrhizae (*Gan Cao*).

4. Exercise is also very effective for reducing blood pressure as is weight loss.

5. Biofeedback, meditation, and deep relaxation are all useful adjuncts for helping to reduce high blood pressure associated with stress.

6. Currently, there is a debate over whether the type A personality predisposes one towards developing hypertension. In one study, 78% of hypertensive patients had type A personalities as compared to only 60% of those in the normotensive group.[7] This suggests that a type A personality is a risk factor for developing hypertension. However, another study conducted and authored by Joseph E. Schwartz of the State University of New York at Stony Brook states that, "No evidence from this study supports the hypertensive personality hypothesis."[8] Those in this study with mild hypertension were no more likely to possess type A characteristics than those with normal blood pressure.

ENDNOTES:

[1] American Diabetes Association, *Complete Guide to Diabetes*, Bantam Books, NY, 1999, p. 304-5
[2] www.cdc.gov/diabetes/pubs/facts98.htm
[3] Chen Jin-ding, *The Treatment of Diabetes with Traditional Chinese Medicine*, trans. by Sun Ying-kui & Zhou Shu-hui, Shandong Science & Technology Press, Jinan, 1994, p. 160-162
[4] *Ibid.*, p. 162-164
[5] *Ibid.*, p. 164-165
[6] Guo Wei-yi, anthologized in Shi Yu-guang & Dan Shu-jian's *Xiao Ke Zhuan Zhi (Wasting & Thirsting Expertise)*, Chinese Medicine Ancient Books Publishing Co., 1997, p. 70-71
[7] www.lboro.ac.uk/departments/hu/projects/abstracts/95hb0031.htm
[8] www.obgyn.net/newsrx/general_health-Hypertension-20010212-7.asp

16

DIABETIC
HYPERLIPOPROTEINEMIA

Dyslipidemia or abnormal blood lipid profiles are quite common in diabetes, especially type 2 diabetes. In fact, half of all type 2 diabetics exhibit some form of dyslipidemia.[1] Both type 1 and type 2 diabetes increase the risk of dyslipidemia threefold in men and possibly even more in women.[2] Commonly, such blood lipid dyscrasias take the form of abnormally high levels of low density lipids (LDL cholesterol) and triglycerides and abnormally low levels of high density lipids (HDL cholesterol). Hypertriglyceridemia is the most common lipid abnormality in diabetics.[3] Since blood lipid abnormalities, obesity, and type 2 diabetes seem to go hand in hand, researchers now question whether obesity and diabetes are the cause of such blood lipid dyscrasias. For instance, 80% of diabetics with dyslipidemia are obese.[4] It is now thought that hyperinsulinemia may cause up-regulation of LDL cholesterol binding and down-regulation of HDL cholesterol binding. Diabetic hyperlipoproteinemia is usually due to some combination of genetic predisposition, endocrinopathy, and excessive dietary intake of sugar and cholesterol. Smoking and obesity are reversible risk factors. Because the incidence of coronary heart disease rises in a linear fashion with the level of serum cholesterol, this condition is seen as a precursor to coronary heart disease via atherosclerosis.

The Western medical diagnosis of this condition is based on analysis of blood lipids and proteins. The Western medical treatment of diabetic hyperlipoproteinemia involves weight loss, dietary restriction of carbohydrates and alcohol, treatment of hyperglycemia, treatment of coexisting hypertension with lipid-neutral antihypertensive agents, and administration of either niacin (in the form of niaspan) or gemfibrozil if blood lipids are not controllable by diet alone as is commonly the case in those with diabetes. The American Diabetes Association rec-ommends an LDL cholesterol level of less than 100mg/dL for all diabetics.[5]

CHINESE DISEASE MECHANISMS:

Because diabetic hyperlipoproteinemia is often asymptomatic, at least in its beginning stages, it is difficult to discuss its Chinese medical disease mechanisms. However, if we consider two aspects of this condition, we can identify at least two main mechanisms. First, hyperlipoproteinemia is very much associated with obesity, and secondly, it leads to heart disease due to atherosclerosis. In Chinese medicine, adipose tissue or fat is seen as phlegm, dampness, and turbidity, while many of the symptoms of heart disease are indications of blood stasis. Therefore, phlegm turbidity and blood stasis are two important disease mechanisms in this condition, and the presence of one often leads to the presence of the other. For instance, the qi moves the blood. Therefore, enduring qi stagnation due to liver depression may result in blood stasis. Since the qi also moves water fluids, qi depression also commonly becomes complicated by phlegm depression. In that case, phlegm and stasis bind together, and their presence further aggravates liver depression qi stagnation.

Phlegm turbidity may also be due to disturbance in the function of the main viscera that control the movement and transformation of water fluids—the spleen and kidneys. As discussed above, spleen vacuity may be due to a number of different causes and mechanisms. It may be due to overeating sweets and sugars and oily, fatty foods. It may be due to liver depression attacking the spleen via the control cycle. It may be due to too much anxiety and thinking, too little exercise, and too much fatigue. If the spleen becomes vacuous and weak, it may fail in its duty to move and transport water fluids which collect and transform into damp evils. Over time, these damp evils may then congeal into phlegm, and the presence of phlegm hinders and obstructs the free flow of qi and blood. Enduring spleen qi vacuity may evolve into kidney yang vacuity, and vacuous yang may not be able to warm and transform water fluids. Or, blood vacuity due to spleen vacuity may evolve into liver-blood-kidney yin vacuity. Since qi is transformed from yin, kidney yin vacuity always includes some element of qi vacuity. In this case, the kidney-bladder qi transformation may also be disturbed, causing a collection and accumulation of damp evils which, over time, may congeal into phlegm.

As we have discussed above, the core disease mechanisms of diabetes are a liver-spleen disharmony with some kind of heat evils and yin vacuity. While most practitioners know that enduring heat may damage and consume body fluids, thus leading eventually to a yin vacuity, dampness may also cause yin vacuity. Damp evils are transformed out of righteous fluids. If righteous fluids become bound up as dampness and, therefore, unavailable for enriching and moistening the body, this may lead to yin fluid insufficiency and dryness. This helps explain why most diabetics have a combination of damp evils with simultaneous yin vacuity or fluid dryness. If one understands this scenario, one will be better able to understand the four main patterns of diabetic hyperlipoproteinemia presented below.

TREATMENT BASED ON PATTERN DISCRIMINATION:

1. QI & YIN DUAL VACUITY WITH BLOOD STASIS PATTERN

MAIN SYMPTOMS: Fatigue, lack of strength, heart palpitations, shortness of breath, a dry mouth and parched throat, spontaneous perspiration or night sweats, numbness of the extremities or aching and pain, possible concomitant dizziness and/or chest oppression, a dark, fat tongue or possible static macules or spots and white fur, and a deep, bowstring pulse

---

NOTE: The pulse will only be deep in this case as long as there is no simultaneous heat of any kind, and heat does complicate most, if not all, cases of diabetes.

TREATMENT PRINCIPLES: Boost the qi and nourish yin, quicken the blood and transform stasis

RX: *Jiang Zhi Yi Hao Fang* (Fat-lowering Formula No. 1)

INGREDIENTS: Radix Trichosanthis Kirlowii (*Tian Hua Fen*), Radix Salviae Miltiorrhizae (*Dan Shen*), and Rhizoma Polygonati (*Huang Jing*), 30g each, Radix Pseudostellariae Heterophyllae (*Tai Zi Shen*), 15g, Tuber Ophiopogonis Japonici (*Mai Men Dong*), Radix Puerariae (*Ge Gen*), and Radix Polygoni Multiflori (*He Shou Wu*), 12g each, Fructus Schisandrae Chinensis (*Wu Wei Zi*), Radix Angelicae Sinensis (*Dang Gui*), Hirudo Seu Whitmania (*Shui Zhi*), and Semen Pruni Persicae (*Tao Ren*), 9g each

FORMULA ANALYSIS: *Huang Jing, Tai Zi Shen, Mai Men Dong, He Shou Wu,* and *Wu Wei Zi* boost the qi and nourish yin. *Ge Gen* and *Tian Hua Fen* engender fluids and stop thirst. *Dang Gui, Dan Shen, Tao Ren,* and *Shui Zhi* quicken the blood and transform stasis.

ADDITIONS & SUBTRACTIONS: If there is simultaneous numbness and pain of the extremities, add nine grams each of Rhizoma Cibotii Barometsis (*Gou Ji*), Radix Achyranthis Bidentatae (*Niu Xi*), and Fructus Chaenomleis Lagenariae (*Mu Gua*). If there is dizziness and vertigo, add 12 grams each of Radix Achyranthis Bidentatae (*Niu Xi*), Ramulus Uncariae Cum Uncis (*Gou Teng*), Concha Haliotidis (*Shi Jue Ming*), and Flos Chrysanthemi Morifolii (*Ju Hua*). If there is chest oppression, add nine grams each of Fructus Trichosanthis Kirlowii (*Gua Lou*), Bulbus Allii (*Cong Bai*), Fructus Citri Sacrodactylis (*Fo Shou*), and Lignum Dalbergiae Odoriferae (*Jiang Xiang*). If there is marked qi vacuity, add 6-9 grams of Radix Panacis Ginseng (*Ren Shen*) and 15-45 grams of Radix Astragali Membranacei (*Huang Qi*). If there is spleen vacuity with heavy dampness, add nine grams each of Rhizoma Atractylodis Macrocephalae (*Bai Zhu*) and Rhizoma Alismatis (*Ze Xie*) and 18 grams of Herba Artemisiae Capillaris (*Yin Chen Hao*). If there is constipation, add 6-9 grams of Radix Et Rhizoma Rhei (*Da Huang*) and nine grams each of Fructus Trichosanthis Kirlowii (*Gua Lou*) and Cortex Magnoliae Officinalis (*Hou Po*).

ACUPUNCTURE & MOXIBUSTION: *Zu San Li* (St 36), *Nei Guan* (Per 6), *Shen Shu* (Bl 23), *Tai Xi* (Ki 3), *San Yin Jiao* (Sp 6), *Xue Hai* (Sp 10)

FORMULA ANALYSIS: Supplementing *Zu San Li* fortifies the latter heaven to support the former heaven. In addition, it lowers fat. Draining *Nei Guan* moves the qi, lowers fat, and prevents heart disease. When combined together, *Zu San Li* and *Nei Guan* are empirically known to treat hyperlipoproteinemia. Supplementing *Shen Shu* and *Tai Xi* enriches yin and supplements the kidneys. Draining *Xue Hai* and even supplementing-even draining *San Yin Jiao* quickens the blood and transforms stasis.

ADDITIONS & SUBTRACTIONS: If there is numbness and tingling of the fingers, add even supplementing-even draining of *Ba Xie* (M-UE-22). If there is numbness of the toes, add even supplementing-even draining of *Ba Feng* (M-LE-8). If there is dizziness and vertigo, add draining *Feng Chi* (GB 20), *Yi Feng* (TB 17), and *Bai Hui* (GV 20). If there is chest oppression, add draining *Dan Zhong* (CV 17), *Jue Yin Shu* (Bl 14), and *Xin Shu* (Bl 15). If there is constipation, add draining *Zhi Gou* (TB 6), *Yang Ling Quan* (GB 34), *Tian Shu* (St 25), and *Da Chang Shu* (Bl 25). If there are loose stools or diarrhea due to spleen vacuity, add supplementing *Pi Shu* (Bl 20), *Wei Shu* (Bl 21), *Tian Shu* (St 25), and *Da Chang Shu* (Bl 25).

2. LIVER-KIDNEY INSUFFICIENCY WITH BLOOD STASIS PATTERN

MAIN SYMPTOMS: Low back and knee soreness and limpness, dizziness, tinnitus, impaired memory, insomnia, blurred vision, rough, dry eyes, bilateral lower limb numbness or soreness, limpness, and lack of strength, a tendency to dry stools, a dark red tongue with scanty fluids, and a deep, bowstring pulse

TREATMENT PRINCIPLES: Supplement and enrich the liver and kidneys, quicken the blood and transform stasis

RX: *Jiang Zhi Er Hao Fang* (Fat-lowering Formula No. 2)

INGREDIENTS: Radix Salviae Miltiorrhizae (*Dan Shen*) and Rhizoma Polygonati (*Huang Jing*), 30g each, Fructus Crataegi (*Shan Zha*), 20g, Ramulus Loranthi Seu Visci (*Sang Ji Sheng*), 15g, Fructus Corni Officinalis (*Shan Zhu Yu*), Radix Polygoni Multiflori (*He Shou Wu*), Semen Cassiae Torae (*Jue Ming Zi*), and Rhizoma Alismatis (*Ze Xie*), 12g each, Fructus Mori Albi (*Sang Shen*), Fructus Lycii Chinensis (*Gou Qi Zi*), Flos Chrysanthemi Morifolii (*Ju Hua*), and Semen Glycinis Hispidae (*Hei Dou*), 9g each

FORMULA ANALYSIS: *Shan Zhu Yu, Gou Qi Zi, He Shou Wu, Sang Shen,* and *Hei Dou* supplement and enrich the liver and kidneys. *Ju Hua* and *Jue Ming Zi* clear the liver and brighten the eyes. *Dan Shen* and *Shan Zha* quicken the blood and transform stasis. *Huang Jing* boosts the qi and supplements the kidneys, and *Ze Xie* disinhibits dampness and downbears turbidity.

ADDITIONS & SUBTRACTIONS: If there is a concomitant kidney yang insufficiency with fear of cold and chilled limbs, add nine grams each of Herba Epimedii (*Yin Yang Huo*), Semen Euryalis Ferocis (*Qian Shi*), and Fructus Rosae Laevigatae (*Jin Ying Zi*). If there is ascendant liver

yang hyperactivity with dizziness and tinnitus, add 12 grams each of Ramulus Uncariae Cum Uncis (*Gou Teng*), Radix Achyranthis Bidentatae (*Niu Xi*), Concha Margaritiferae (*Zhen Zhu Mu*), and Radix Albus Paeoniae Lactiflorae (*Bai Shao*) to level the liver and subdue yang. If there is blurred vision, add nine grams each of Semen Celosiae Argenteae (*Qing Xiang Zi*), Scapus Et Inflorescentia Eriocaulonis Seu Buergeriani (*Gu Jing Cao*), Thallus Algae (*Kun Bu*), and Semen Leonuri Heterophylli (*Chong Wei Zi*).

If there are night sweats due to yin vacuity with fire effulgence, one can use *Zhi Bai Di Huang Wan Jia Wei* (Anemarrhena & Phellodendron Rehmannia Pills with Added Flavors): Radix Polygoni Multiflori (*He Shou Wu*), 20g, Ramulus Loranthi Seu Visci (*Sang Ji Sheng*) and Radix Achyranthis Bidentatae (*Niu Xi*), 15g each, cooked Radix Rehmanniae (*Shu Di*) and Radix Dioscoreae Oppositae (*Shan Yao*), 12g each, and Cortex Eucommiae Ulmoidis (*Du Zhong*), Cortex Phellodendri (*Huang Bai*), Rhizoma Anemarrhenae Aspheloidis (*Zhi Mu*), Fructus Corni Officinalis (*Shan Zhu Yu*), Sclerotium Poriae Cocos (*Fu Ling*), Rhizoma Alismatis (*Ze Xie*), and Cortex Radicis Moutan (*Dan Pi*), 9g each.

ACUPUNCTURE & MOXIBUSTION: Same as pattern #1 above

ADDITIONS & SUBTRACTIONS: If there is concomitant yang vacuity, add moxibustion at *Qi Hai* (CV 6) and *Guan Yuan* (CV 4). If there is concomitant ascendant liver yang hyperactivity with dizziness and head distention and pain, add draining *Feng Chi* (GB 20), *Yi Feng* (TB 17), and *Bai Hui* (GV 20). For night sweats, add draining *Yin Xi* (Ht 6). If there is blurred vision, add even supplementing-even draining *Guang Ming* (GB 37) and *Jing Ming* (Bl 1). For numbness and tingling of the fingers, add even supplementing-even draining of *Ba Xie* (M-UE-22). For numbness and tingling of the lower extremities, add even supplementing-even draining of *Ba Feng* (M-LE-8).

3. PHLEGM & STASIS OBSTRUCTING & STAGNATING IN THE VESSELS & NETWORK VESSELS PATTERN

MAIN SYMPTOMS: Obesity, dizziness, heaviness, and distention of the head, a bitter taste in the mouth and/or a sticky feeling, heart palpitations, chest oppression, chest pain, heavy and/or numb limbs, stomach duct glomus, scanty appetite, dark-colored lips, a dark tongue or possible static macules or spots, a mostly fat tongue body, slimy, possibly yellow tongue fur, and a bowstring, slippery pulse

NOTE: Although the name of this pattern does not say so, the symptoms (a bitter taste in the mouth) and the formula given below suggest concomitant heat.

TREATMENT PRINCIPLES: Transform phlegm and dispel stasis, quicken the blood and free the flow of the network vessels

RX: *Jiang Zhi San Hao Fang* (Fat-lowering Formula No. 3)

INGREDIENTS: Herba Artemisiae Capillaris (*Yin Chen Hao*), Radix Salviae Miltiorrhizae (*Dan Shen*), and Fructus Crataegi (*Shan Zha*), 30g each, Fructus Trichosanthis Kirlowii (*Gua Lou*) and Rhizoma Alismatis (*Ze Xie*), 15g each, Radix Et Rhizoma Polygoni Cupidati (*Hu Zhang*), Rhizoma Atractylodis Macrocephalae (*Bai Zhu*), and Radix Ligustici Wallichii (*Chuan Xiong*), 12g each, Rhizoma Pinelliae Ternatae (*Ban Xia*), bile-treated Rhizoma Arisaematis (*Dan Nan Xing*), Tuber Curcumae (*Yu Jin*), Cortex Magnoliae Officinalis (*Hou Po*), and Pericarpium Citri Reticulatae (*Chen Pi*), 9g each, wine-fried Radix Et Rhizoma Rhei (*Da Huang*), 6-9g, and Rhizoma Coptidis Chinensis (*Huang Lian*), 6g

FORMULA ANALYSIS: *Huang Lian, Ban Xia, Dan Nan Xing,* and *Gua Lou* clear heat and transform phlegm. *Bai Zhu* and *Ze Xie* fortify the spleen and disinhibit dampness. *Yin Chen Hao* and *Hu Zhang* clear heat and disinhibit dampness. *Hou Po* and *Chen Pi* rectify the qi and transform phlegm. Wine-fried *Da Huang* frees the flow of the bowels and drains turbidity. *Dan Shen, Shan Zha, Chuan Xiong,* and *Yu Jin* quicken the blood, transform stasis, and free the flow of the network vessels.

ADDITIONS & SUBTRACTIONS: Without constipation, consider omitting *Da Huang*.

ACUPUNCTURE & MOXIBUSTION: *Zu San Li* (St 36), *Nei Guan* (Per 6), *Feng Long* (St 40), *Yin Ling Quan* (Sp 9), *San Yin Jiao* (Sp 6), *Xue Hai* (Sp 10)

FORMULA ANALYSIS: Draining *Yin Ling Quan* rectifies the triple burner, *i.e.*, the water pathways of the entire body, and disinhibits dampness. Draining *Feng Long* harmonizes the stomach and transforms phlegm. Together, these two points are a main combination for treating phlegm dampness. Supplementing *Zu San Li* fortifies the spleen and boosts the qi, transforms dampness and prevents phlegm accumulation. The first two points treat the branch repletion, *i.e.*, the phlegm; the latter point treats

the root vacuity, *i.e.*, the spleen. Draining *Nei Guan* moves the qi to disperse the phlegm. Draining *Xue Hai* and even supplementing-even draining *San Yin Jiao* quickens the blood and transforms stasis.

ADDITIONS & SUBTRACTIONS: If there is concomitant liver depression, add *Tai Chong* (Liv 3) and *Zhang Men* (Liv 13). If there is severe qi vacuity, add *Tai Bai* (Sp 3) and *Pi Shu* (Bl 20). If there is blood vacuity, add *Xin Shu* (Bl 15), *Ge Shu* (Bl 17), and *Gan Shu* (Bl 18). If there is dizziness and headache, add *Feng Chi* (GB 20). If there is nausea, poor appetite, or stomach duct glomus, add *Gong Sun* (Sp 4) and, if necessary, *Zhong Wan* (CV 12). If there is phlegm heat, add draining *Yang Ling Quan* (GB 34) and *Xing Jian* (Liv 2).

4. LIVER-GALLBLADDER QI STAGNATION & BLOOD STASIS PATTERN

MAIN SYMPTOMS: Emotional tension, chest and rib-side distention, fullness, aching, and pain, a bitter taste in the mouth, a sticky, slimy feeling in the mouth, heaviness of the head and/or body, stomach duct glomus, torpid intake, possible nausea and vomiting, a tendency towards obesity, cholecystitis or cholelithiasis, dark lips, a dark tongue with thick, slimy or yellow, slimy fur, and a deep, bowstring pulse

NOTE: As with the pattern above, an element of heat is implied by the signs and symptoms as well as the Chinese medicinal formula below even though neither the name of the pattern nor the treatment principles include references to this heat. In real-life, some sort of heat evils complicate virtually all cases of diabetes.

TREATMENT PRINCIPLES: Course the liver and disinhibit the gallbladder, rectify the qi and quicken the blood

RX: *Jiang Zhi Si Hao Fang* (Fat-lowering Formula No. 4)

INGREDIENTS: Herba Artemisiae Capillaris (*Yin Chen Hao*) and Radix Salviae Miltiorrhizae (*Dan Shen*), 30g each, Radix Et Rhizoma Polygoni Cuspidati (*Hu Zhang*), Radix Albus Paeoniae Lactiflorae (*Bai Shao*), Radix Rubrus Paeoniae Lactiflorae (*Chi Shao*), and Rhizoma Alismatis (*Ze Xie*), 15g each, Radix Bupleuri (*Chai Hu*), Fructus Citri Aurantii (*Zhi Ke*), Fructus Immaturus Citri Aurantii (*Zhi Shi*), Radix Polygoni Multiflori (*He Shou Wu*), Cortex Magnoliae Officinalis (*Hou Po*), and Radix Scutellariae Baicalensis (*Huang*

Qin), 9g each, wine-fried Radix Et Rhizoma Rhei (*Da Huang*), 6-9g

FORMULA ANALYSIS: *Chai Hu, Yin Chen Hao, Huang Qin,* and *Hu Zhang* course the liver and disinhibit the gallbladder, clear heat and eliminate dampness. *Hou Po, Zhi Ke, Zhi Shi, Dan Shen, Chi Shao,* and *Bai Shao* rectify the qi and quicken the blood. *Da Huang* and *Ze Xie* free the flow of the bowels and drain turbidity.

ADDITIONS & SUBTRACTIONS: If there is stomach duct glomus, torpid intake, and loose stools, omit *Da Huang* and add nine grams each of Rhizoma Atractylodes Macrocephalae (*Bai Zhu*) and Pericarpium Citri Reticulatae (*Chen Pi*) and 21 grams of Semen Coicis Lachryma-jobi (*Yi Yi Ren*) in order to fortify the spleen, rectify the qi, and transform dampness. If there is liver-gallbladder qi counterflow with stomach loss of harmony and downbearing resulting in nausea and vomiting, add nine grams each of Flos Inulae Racemosae (*Xuan Fu Hua*) and Rhizoma Pinelliae Ternatae (*Ban Xia*) and 2-3 slices of uncooked Rhizoma Zingiberis (*Sheng Jiang*) to harmonize the stomach, downbear counterflow, and stop vomiting. If there is marked bilateral rib-side aching and pain, add 12 grams each of Rhizoma Corydalis Yanhusuo (*Yan Hu Suo*) and Fructus Meliae Toosendan (*Chuan Lian Zi*) and 15 grams of Cortex Albizziae Julibrissinis (*He Huan Pi*) to soothe the liver and regulate the qi. If there is simultaneous cholelithiasis, add nine grams each of Endothelium Corneum Gigeriae Galli (*Ji Nei Jin*) and Tuber Curcumae (*Yu Jin*) and 15 grams of Herba Desmodii Seu Lysimachiae (*Jin Qian Cao*) to disinhibit the gallbladder and expel stones.

ACUPUNCTURE & MOXIBUSTION: *Tai Chong* (Liv 3), *Yang Ling Quan* (GB 34), *He Gu* (LI 4), *San Yin Jiao* (Sp 6), *Xue Hai* (Sp 10)

FORMULA ANALYSIS: Draining *Tai Chong* and *He Gu* courses the liver and rectifies the qi. Draining *Yang Ling Quan* clears heat and disinhibits the gallbladder. Draining *San Yin Jiao* and *Xue Hai* quickens the blood and transforms stasis.

ADDITIONS & SUBTRACTIONS: For stomach duct glomus, nausea, and vomiting, add draining *Nei Guan* (Per 6) and *Zhong Wan* (CV 12). For diarrhea, add supplementing *Pi Shu* (Bl 20), *Wei Shu* (Bl 21), *Tian Shu* (St 25), and *Da Chang Shu* (Bl 25). For rib-side distention and pain, add draining *Zhang Men* (Liv 13) and *Qi Men* (Liv 14). For more marked heat, needle *Tai Chong* through to *Xing Jian* (Liv 2) with draining method.

ABSTRACTS OF REPRESENTATIVE CHINESE RESEARCH:

Xu Zhu-ting, "The Treatment of 76 Cases of Diabetes Accompanied by Hyperlipidemia with Self-composed *Jiu Wei Jiang Zhi Tang* (Nine Flavors Lower Fat Decoction)," *Shang Hai Zhong Yi Yao Za Zhi* (*Shanghai Journal of Chinese Medicine & Medicinals*), #12, 1999, p. 30-31: One hundred fourteen patients were included in this study, all of whom had type 2 diabetes complicated by hyperlipidemia. Fasting blood glucose and total cholesterol was equal to or more than 6.0mmol/L and triglycerides were equal to or more than 1.69mmol/L in all cases. These 114 patients were divided into two groups, the treatment group and the comparison group. Of the 76 patients in the treatment group, 42 were male and 34 were female aged 39-75, with an average age of 58.25 years. Fifteen patients also had high blood pressure, 10 also had coronary heart disease, and nine had concomitant retinopathy. In the comparison group, there were 21 males and 17 females aged 42-75, with an average age of 60.12 years. Three cases had concomitant hypertension, seven had coronary heart disease, and four had accompanying retinopathy. Two weeks before the commencement of treatment, all 114 patients stopped taking cholesterol-lowering medication. However, they continued taking 1-2 types of Western hypoglycemic medicines.

The treatment group was given the following Chinese medicinals: processed Radix Polygoni Multiflori (*He Shou Wu*), Rhizoma Alismatis (*Ze Xie*), and Radix Puerariae (*Ge Gen*), 30g each, Fructus Ligustri Lucidi (*Nu Zhen Zi*), Fructus Lycii Chinensis (*Gou Qi Zi*), and Herba Sargassii (*Hai Zao*), 15g each, Herba Artemisiae Capillaris (*Yin Chen Hao*) and Semen Pruni Persicae (*Tao Ren*), 12g each, and Hirudo Seu Whitmania (*Shui Zhi*), 3g. If there was headache or dizziness, 15 grams each of Rhizoma Gastrodiae Elatae (*Tian Ma*) and Ramulus Uncariae Cum Uncis (*Gou Teng*) were added. If there was chest oppression and heart palpitations, 30 grams of Radix Salviae Miltiorrhizae (*Dan Shen*) and 15 grams of Tuber Curcumae (*Yu Jin*) were added. If there was blurred vision, 12 grams of Scapus Et Inflorescentia Eriocaulonis Buergeriani (*Gu Jing Cao*) and 10 grams of Flos Immaturus Buddleiae Officinalis (*Mi Meng Hua*) were added. One *ji* was decocted in water and administered orally per day in two divided doses. The comparison group received 2.7g of niacin in pill form two times per day. Three months equaled one course of treatment for both groups.

A marked effect was defined as a reduction of total cholesterol equal to or more than 20%, a reduction in triglycerides equal to or more than 40%, or an increase in high density lipids by more than 0.26mmol/L. Some effect meant that total cholesterol was reduced 10-20%, trigylcerides were reduced 20-40%, or high density lipids increased 0.11-0.26mmol/L. No effect meant that these criteria were not met. Based on these criteria, 10 cases (13.16%) in the treatment group were judged to have gotten a marked effect, 52 cases (68.42%) got some effect, and 14 cases (18.42%) got no effect, for a total amelioration rate of 81.58%. In the comparison group, three cases (7.89%) got a marked effect, 20 cases (52.63%) got some effect, and 15 cases (39.47%) got no effect, for a total amelioration rate of 60.53%. Further, in the treatment group, mean total cholesterol was 6.98 ± 0.21mmol/L before treatment and 5.14 ± 0.37mmol/L after treatment compared to 6.88 ± 0.34mmol/L before treatment and 5.75 + 0.39mmol/L in the comparison group. Mean triglycerides went from 2.85 ± 0.35mmol/L before treatment to 1.78 ± 0.27mmol/L after treatment in the treatment group and from 2.91 ± 0.31mmol/L to 2.47 ± 0.38mmol/L in the comparison group. And mean high density lipids went from 1.02 ± 0.28mmol/L to 1.49 ± 0.21mmol/L in the treatment group and from 1.05 ± 0.31mmol/L to 1.21 ± 0.37mmol/L after treatment in the comparison group. Thus there were significant differences in total cholesterol, triglycerides, and high density lipids pre- and post-treatment in the treatment group, but only a significant difference in total cholesterol pre- and post-treatment in the comparison group. This study suggests that this formula is more effective at lowering total cholesterol and triglycerides and raising high density lipids than niacin. In addition, it also has definite effects in lowering glucose and lowering blood pressure.

REPRESENTATIVE CASE HISTORIES:

CASE 1[6]

The patient was a 46 year old male who, for the last month, was having extreme thirst with dry tongue and mouth. He was not able to satisfy his thirst, and sticky white froth formed at the corners of his mouth. In addition, there was profuse urination, even during the night, constipation, dry stools, aching muscle pain in the arms and legs, a clamorous stomach, and great appetite. His blood sugar was 17.3 mmol/L (310 mg/dL), and his serum cholesterol was 5.52mmol/L. The tongue was dark red with thick, white, slimy fur and a grayish black area at the center of the root. His pulse was bowstring and slippery.

Based on these signs and symptoms, the man's Chinese medical pattern was categorized as stomach fire effulgence

drying the intestines and damaging fluids. The treatment principles were to clear heat and drain fire, supplement yin and engender fluids. The formula prescribed included: uncooked Gypsum Fibrosum (Shi Gao), 30g, Rhizoma Anemarrhenae Aspheloidis (Zhi Mu), 10g, uncooked Radix Glycyrrhizae (Gan Cao), 3g, uncooked Radix Rehmanniae (Sheng Di), 15g, Tuber Ophiopogonis Japonici (Mai Dong), 15g, Radix Trichosanthis Kirlowii (Tian Hua Fen), 10g, Herba Dendrobii (Shi Hu), 15g, Radix Salviae Miltiorrhizae (Dan Shen), 10g, Cortex Radicis Moutan (Mu Dan Pi), 10g, Semen Cannabis Sativae (Huo Ma Ren), 15g, and Semen Pruni (Yu Li Ren) 15g.

After the patient had taken seven ji of the above medicinals, the tongue fur became thin, yellow, and slimy. He was drinking less, his eating habits normalized, and his urination and bowels resumed their normal functions. However, the patient's the mouth was still dry, and his aching limbs caused the patient distress. His blood sugar was 15.7mmol/L (282 mg/dL). Therefore, uncooked Fructus Crataegi (Shan Zha), 15g, and Herba Eupatorii Fortunei (Pei Lan), 10g, were added to the basic formula, and another seven ji were administered. After that, the man's tongue fur became thin and white and overall yellowish but without the thick sliminess, while the tongue body was light red. The dry mouth had lessened, as had the frequency of the nocturia, and the patient's diet was stabilized. After taking altogether 21 ji, the patient's blood sugar lowered to 8 mmol/L (144 mg/dL), and his serum cholesterol lowered to 3.8 mmol/L.

CASE 2[7]

The patient was a 62 year old female who presented with frequent, profuse urination. Her urine was turbid, she experienced low back and knee soreness and limpness, tinnitus with a heavy sensation in her head, tidal reddening of the face, constant thirst and hunger, and dry stools. The patient's blood sugar level was 9.8 mmol/L (176 mg/dL), and her serum cholesterol was 6.3 mmol/L. The tongue was peeled with scanty fur and a central fissure. The pulse was fine and rapid.

Based on the above, the Chinese medical pattern was categorized as liver blood-kidney yin vacuity with kidney essence depletion below and liver yang hyperactivity above. The treatment plan was to enrich water to moisten wood, boost the essence and supplement the blood, moisten dryness and stop thirst. The prescription included: uncooked Radix Rehmanniae (Sheng Di), 15g, cooked Radix Rehmanniae (Shu Di), 15g, Fructus Corni Officinalis

(*Shan Zhu Yu*), 10g, Radix Dioscoreae Oppositae (*Shan Yao*), 30g, Sclerotium Poriae Cocos (*Fu Ling*), 10g, Radix Salviae Miltiorrhizae (*Dan Shen*), 10g, Cortex Radicis Moutan (*Mu Dan Pi*), 10g, Tuber Ophiopogonis Japonici (*Mai Dong*), 20g, Tuber Asparagi Cochinensis (*Tian Men Dong*), 20g, Herba Dendrobii (*Shi Hu*), 30g, Radix Astragali Membranacei (*Huang Qi*), 20g, Concha Haliotidis (*Shi Jue Ming*), 30g, Fructus Lycii Chinensis (*Gou Qi Zi*), 12g, Semen Cassiae Torae (*Jue Ming Zi*), 20g, and Semen Cannabis Sativae (*Huo Ma Ren*), 10g.

After seven *ji* of the above medicinals, the tongue was still red in color, but the fur at the tip was thin and white. The thirst had lessened, the heaviness in the head and the tinnitus were relieved, and the woman's bowels and urination were normal. *Shi Jue Ming* was removed from the original formula, and uncooked Fructus Crataegi (*Shan Zha*), 15g and Radix Et Rhizoma Polygoni Cuspidati (*Hu Zhang*), 30g, were added. After six months of continuous administration of these medicinals, the patient's blood sugar and cholesterol levels were normal.

REMARKS:

1. In real life, there will almost always be a liver-spleen disharmony in patients with diabetic dyslipidemia. In that case, medicinals which harmonize the liver and spleen, such as Fructus Citri Sacrodactylis (*Fo Shou*), Radix Auklandiae Lappae (*Mu Xiang*), Folium Perillae Frutescentis (*Zi Su Ye*), and Fructus Pruni Mume (*Wu Mei*) may be added to appropriate formulas as well as spleen supplements, such as Radix Codonopsitis Pilosulae (*Dang Shen*), Radix Pseudostellariae Heterophyllae (*Tai Zi Shen*), Rhizoma Polygonati (*Huang Jing*), Radix Dioscoreae Oppositae (*Shan Yao*), and Sclerotium Poriae Cocos (*Fu Ling*). Because most cases of diabetes involve some element of yin fluid insufficiency or dryness, care should be taken when using acrid, windy qi-rectifying medicinals. For instance, while Radix Bupleuri (*Chai Hu*) may be used in some cases of diabetes, it should be used with care due to its reputation for plundering yin.

2. The following are those Chinese medicinals which have all demonstrated pronounced empirical abilities to lower fat and treat hyperlipoproteinemia. Most formulas for this condition will include several of these medicinals depending on the patient's pattern discrimination.

MEDICINALS WHICH QUICKEN THE BLOOD: Fructus Crataegi (*Shan Zha*), Pollen Typhae (*Pu Huang*), Radix Pseudoginseng (*San Qi*), Rhizoma Curcumae Longae (*Jiang Huang*), Semen Leonuri Heterophylli (*Chong Wei Zi*)

MEDICINALS WHICH MOVE THE QI: Pericarpium Citri Reticulatae (*Chen Pi*), Tuber Curcumae (*Yu Jin*)

MEDICINALS WHICH CLEAR HEAT: Bombyx Batryticatus (*Jiang Can*), Cornu Bubali (*Shui Niu Jiao*), Flos Chrysanthemi Morifolii (*Ju Hua*), Radix Et Rhizoma Polygoni Cuspidati (*Hu Zhang*), Radix Et Rhizoma Rhei (*Da Huang*), Radix Ilicis Pubescentis (*Mao Dong Qing*), Semen Cassiae Torae (*Jue Ming Zi*), Flos Lonicerae Japonicae (*Jin Yin Hua*)

MEDICINALS WHICH DISINHIBIT DAMPNESS: Herba Artemisiae Capillaris (*Yin Chen Hao*), Herba Cephalanoploris Segeti (*Xiao Ji*), Herba Plantaginis (*Che Qian Cao*), Rhizoma Alismatis (*Ze Xie*), Semen Abutilonis Seu Malvae (*Dong Kui Zi*), Folium Nelumbinis Nuciferae (*He Ye*)

MEDICINALS WHICH SUPPLEMENT: Cordyceps Sinensis (*Dong Chong Xia Cao*), Cortex Eucommiae Ulmoidis (*Du Zhong*), Fructus Lycii Chinensis (*Gou Qi*), Ganoderma Lucidum (*Ling Zhi*), Radix Angelicae Sinensis (*Dang Gui*), Radix Astragali Membranacei (*Huang Qi*), Ramulus Loranthi Seu Visci (*Sang Ji Sheng*), Rhizoma Polygonati (*Huang Jing*), Rhizoma Polygonati Odorati (*Yu Zhu*)

OTHERS MEDICINALS: Bulbus Allii Sativi (*Da Suan*), Fructus Rosae Laevigatae (*Jin Ying Zi*), Rhizoma Acori Graminei (*Shi Chang Pu*), Semen Euryalis Ferocis (*Qian Shi*), Succinum (*Hu Po*), Thallus Algae (*Kun Bu*), Radix Puerariae (*Ge Gen*)

3. Three acupuncture points have especially demonstrated incontestable effectiveness for hyperlipoproteinemia: *Zu San Li* (St 36), *Feng Long* (St 40), and *Nei Guan* (Per 6).

4. In Chinese medicine, certain foods are reputed to help regulate serum cholesterol. These include garlic, shiitake mushroom, soybeans, various types of seaweed, black Chinese tree fungus, and water chestnuts.

ENDNOTES:

[1] www.postgradmed.com/issues/1999/02_99/bohannon.htm
[2] www.nmsr.labmed.umn.edu/~relson/atpch4_1.html#diabeticdyslipidemia
[3] www.postgradmed.com, op. cit.*op. cit.*
[4] *Ibid.*
[5] *Ibid.*
[6] Kang Lu-wa, "The Treatment of Diabetes by Pattern Identification of the Tongue", *Zhong Yi Za Zhi* (*Journal of Traditional Chinese Medicine*), #9, 1999, p. 530-1.
[7] *Ibid.*

17

DIABETIC RETINOPATHY

Diabetic retinopathy is a potentially blinding microvascular complication of both type 1 and type 2 diabetes that damages the retina of the eye. It occurs when diabetes damages the tiny blood vessels in the retina. In terms of its pathophysiology, it is a complex disease and probably does not stem from a single retinal change. Instead, it is probably triggered by a combination of biochemical, metabolic, and hematologic abnormalities. For instance, a chronic increase in normal blood glucose levels may gradually alter cell metabolism in the retinal blood vessels, while diabetes-related biochemical changes may make circulating blood platelets abnormally sticky. Further, hematologic changes may cause the retinal blood vessels to constrict. These abnormalities may cause certain cells within the retinal blood vessels to die, thus leading to altered blood flow, increased blood vessel permeability, and the growth of certain blood vessel components. As a result, tiny out-croppings called microaneurysms may bulge from the weakened blood vessel walls. If these microaneurysms leak blood onto the central retina or macula, they may cause macular edema[1] and probable loss of vision. This condition is generally suspected when loss of visual acuity is not corrected by glasses.

In fact, there are three stages to this disease. The earliest phase is known as background diabetic retinopathy (BDR). In this phase, due to the death of the pericytes which line the vascular endothelium, the arteries in the retina become weakened and leak, forming small, dot-like hemorrhages as described above. In addition, hard exudates due to the leakage of proteins and lipids may form as ring-like structures around the leaking capillaries. Background diabetic retinopathy may be asymptomatic. Eighty percent of people who have had diabetes for over 20 years have some BDR, but only about one out of every 4-5 of those with BDR will eventually suffer measurable

vision impairment. The next stage is known as preproliferative diabetic retinopathy. Preproliferative diabetic retinopathy is a more advanced stage of damage to the eye than the early signs found in BDR. In this stage, intraretinal microvascular abnormalities (IRMA) are present. These are irregularly shaped blood vessels that appear in a localized area of the retina as squiggly lines. They signify irregular dilation of the retinal blood vessels in response to poor blood circulation. In addition, there may be cotton wool spots or exudates which are microinfarcts. These are seen as pale white areas in the retina where the blood vessels have become blocked and the nerves in the localized areas have been damaged. Once this stage is present, vision may worsen rapidly. The third stage of this disease is proliferative diabetic retinopathy (PDR). In this stage, circulation problems cause areas of the retina to become oxygen-deprived or ischemic. New, fragile vessels develop as the circulatory system attempts to maintain adequate oxygen levels within the retina. This is called neovascularization. Unfortunately, these delicate vessels hemorrhage easily, and blood may leak into the retina and vitreous, causing spots or floaters along with decreased vision. In the later phase of this disease, continued abnormal vessel growth and scar tissue may cause serious problems, such as retinal detachment and glaucoma. As a result, severe visual loss or blindness will occur.[2, 3]

For many people with diabetic retinopathy, there are no early symptoms. There is no pain, no blurred vision, and no ocular inflammation. In fact, many people do not develop any visual impairment until the disease has advanced well into its proliferative stage. At this point the vision has been lost and cannot be restored. However, some people in the early and advanced stages of diabetic retinopathy may notice a change in their central and/or color vision. The loss of central vision results from macular edema which can often be effectively treated. Many diabetics notice blurred vision when their blood sugar is particularly high or low. This blurred vision is due to changes in the shape of the lens of the eye and usually reverses when the blood sugar returns to normal. It is not a symptom of diabetic retinopathy.

The incidence of diabetic retinopathy is strongly correlated to the duration of disease and age of onset. After 20 years of diabetes, nearly all patients with type 1 diabetes and more than 60% of patients with type 2 diabetes have some degree of retinopathy. Vision-threatening retinopathy virtually never appears in type 1 patients in the first 3-5 years of diabetes or before puberty. However, in the subsequent two decades, nearly all type 1 patients develop retinopathy. For instance, after having diabetes for 15 years, about 80% of type 1 diabetics have some degree of diabetic retinopathy, and 50% have PDR. Up to 21% of patients with type 2 diabetes have been found to have retinopathy at the time of first diagnosis of diabetes, and most develop some retinopathy over subsequent decades. Overall, diabetic retinopathy is estimated to be the most frequent cause of blindness among adults aged 20-74 years.[4, 5]

The Western medical diagnosis of diabetic retinopathy primarily consists of ophthalmoscopy with magnification and illumination of the retina subsequent to pupil dilation looking for leaking blood vessels, macular edema, cotton wool patches, or any other changes in the blood vessels of the retina. If there is macular edema, flourescein angiography is usually performed. Flourescein angiography is a technique which involves injecting a dye (fluorescein) into the veins and taking a series of photographs of the retina while the dye circulates through the retinal vessels. Ultrasound imaging of the eyes may also sometimes be used.

The Western medical prevention of this condition consists of careful control of blood sugar levels through attention to diet, exercise, and medications, monitoring for and control of hypertension, avoidance of smoking, and early detection and treatment of diabetic retinopathy. The Diabetes Control and Complications Trial (DCCT) has shown that better control of blood sugar levels slow the onset and progression of retinopathy and lessen the need for laser surgery for severe retinopathy. The United Kingdom Prospective Diabetes Study (UKPDS) conclusively demonstrated that improved blood glucose control in type 2 diabetics reduces the rate of development of retinopathy. The National Eye Institute's Early Treatment Diabetic Retinopathy Study (ETDRS) showed that a daily dose of aspirin has no significant effect on preventing retinopathy.

Remedial treatment in any particular case depends upon multiple factors, including the type and degree of retinopathy, associated ocular factors such as cataract or vitreous hemorrhage, and the medical history of the patient. Treatment options include laser photocoagulation, kyrotherapy, and pars plana vitrectomy surgery (i.e., the removal of the vitreous gel along with blood, scar tissue, etc. and its replacement with a clear saline solution). As mentioned above, patients with diabetes are at greater risk for developing retinal tears and detachment. Such tears are often sealed with laser surgery. Retinal detachment requires surgical treatment to reattach the retina to the back of the eye. Current treatment guidelines are so successful that even people with proliferative retinopathy have a 90% chance of maintaining their vision.[6, 7] In terms of experimental treatments, an oral inhibitor of protein kinase C, a substance involved in the stimulation of certain growth hormones, is already in Phase II/Phase III clinical trials, and other growth hormone antagonists are also being looked at by researchers. The development of such an oral medication would avoid the inherently destructive properties of current laser treatments. The heparin analogue, beta-cyclodextrin tetradecasulfate, may prevent proliferative retinopathy.

CHINESE MEDICAL DISEASE CATEGORIZATION: If symptomatic, this condition corresponds to *hua yan*, blurred (literally, flowery) vision, or *qing mang*, clear-eyed blindness.

CHINESE DISEASE MECHANISMS:

In Chinese medicine, there are two main disease mechanisms of diabetic retinopathy. These are yin vacuity with dryness and heat leading to essence and blood depletion and detriment not nourishing the eyes and static blood obstructing the network vessels of the eyes. In diabetes, there are three main disease causes leading to yin vacuity with dryness and heat. First, overeating fats and sweets and drinking alcohol may result in accumulation of heat brewing internally which transforms dryness and damages fluids. Secondly, due to emotional stress and frustration, liver depression may transform fire which disperses and burns yin fluids. And third, habitual bodily yin vacuity compounded by aging, overtaxation, and unregulated bedroom affairs (i.e., too much sex) may also damage yin fluids. If any of these three factors result in enduring yin fluid depletion and consumption, essence and blood may suffer detriment. According to the *Nei Jing (Inner Classic)*, the eyes can see only if they obtain blood, and the *Ling Shu (Spiritual Axis)* says, "The essence of the five viscera and six bowels flows upward to the eyes and makes their essence." Thus the eyes' function of sight is dependent on receiving sufficient blood and essence to moisten, enrich, and nourish them, and, therefore, conversely, a liver blood-kidney yin vacuity is a major mechanism of vision problems. In addition, if yin vacuity gives rise to fire effulgence, vacuity fire may flame upward, burning and damaging the network vessels in the eyes and forcing the blood in the eyes to move outside its vessels.

It is also possible for any of a number of other disease mechanisms associated with diabetes to result in blood stasis. If there is a spleen qi vacuity failing to upbear, the blood may lack the power to move to and through the network vessels in the eyes, instead becoming static there. Since the qi moves the blood, it is also possible for enduring liver depression qi stagnation to result in blood stasis. If overeating thick-flavored, fatty foods leads to gumming up of the qi mechanism, clear and turbid will not be separated, and phlegm, dampness, and turbidity may impede and block the free and easy flow of qi and blood to the eyes. Likewise, if yin blood is scanty and insufficient to nourish the vessels, this may lead to blood stasis since the vessels will not be able to perform their proper function in terms of the circulation of blood. And finally, if yin and/or qi vacuity reaches yang, yang vacuity may lead to cold congealing the blood and, hence, blood stasis. In other words, any or all these disease mechanisms may ultimately result in the formation of static blood within the network vessels, thus depriving the eyes of proper nourishment. Since diabetic retinopathy is a chronic, enduring condition, based on the saying, "Enduring diseases enter the network vessels," most cases of diabetic retinopathy are complicated by at least an element of blood stasis. For instance, in one group of 46 Chinese patients with diabetic retinopathy, 91.3% met the criteria for the diagnosis of blood stasis.[8]

TREATMENT BASED ON PATTERN DISCRIMINATION:

1. YIN VACUITY WITH DRYNESS & HEAT PATTERN

MAIN SYMPTOMS: This pattern is mostly seen in patients with first stage diabetic retinopathy or BDR before there are any symptoms of visual disturbance. The clinical signs and symptoms of this pattern include dry mouth, polydipsia, polyphagia and easy hungering, an emaciated body, frequent, profuse urination, dry, bound stools, a red tongue with thin, yellow fur, and a bowstring, fine or surging, slightly rapid pulse.

TREATMENT PRINCIPLES: Enrich yin and engender fluids, clear heat and moisten dryness

RX: *Zeng Ye Tang* (Increase Fluids Decoction) plus *Bai Hu Tang* (White Tiger Decoction) with additions and subtractions

INGREDIENTS: Uncooked Radix Rehmanniae (*Sheng Di*), Radix Scrophulariae Ningpoensis (*Xuan Shen*), and uncooked Gypsum Fibrosum (*Shi Gao*), 30g each, Radix Trichosanthis Kirlowii (*Tian Hua Fen*), 20g, Tuber Ophiopogonis Japonici (*Mai Men Dong*) and Rhizoma Anemarrhenae Aspheloidis (*Zhi Mu*), 9g each, and Radix Glycyrrhizae (*Gan Cao*), 6g

FORMULA ANALYSIS: *Sheng Di, Xuan Shen,* and *Mai Men Dong* enrich yin and engender fluids. Uncooked *Shi Gao, Zhi Mu,* and *Tian Hua Fen* clear and discharge lung-stomach dryness and heat, engender fluids and stop thirst.

ADDITIONS & SUBTRACTIONS: If there is retinal bleeding, add nine grams each of Cortex Radicis Moutan (*Dan Pi*), carbonized Flos Immaturus Sophorae Japonicae (*Huai Hua Mi*), and uncooked Pollen Typhae (*Pu Huang*) to cool the blood and stop bleeding. For bowel repletion constipation, add nine grams each of uncooked Radix Et Rhizoma Rhei (*Da Huang*), Fructus Immaturus Citri Aurantii (*Zhi Shi*), and Fructus Trichosanthis Kirlowii (*Gua Lou*) to free the flow of the bowels and discharge heat. If there is lung-stomach dryness and heat with polydipsia and polyphagia, increase the dose of *Tian Hua Fen* and add nine grams each of Calcitum (*Han Shui Shi*) and Herba Dendrobii (*Shi Hu*) to further clear heat and engender fluids. If there is concomitant qi stagnation, add 18 grams of Radix Albus Paeoniae Lactiflorae (*Bai Shao*) and nine grams each of Radix Bupleuri (*Chai Hu*), Fructus Citri Aurantii (*Zhi Ke*), and Fructus Trichosanthis Kirlowii (*Gua Lou*). If there is simultaneous blood stasis, one can add 30 grams of Radix Salviae Miltiorrhizae (*Dan Shen*), 15 grams of Radix Ligustici Wallichii (*Chuan Xiong*), and nine grams each of Flos Carthami Tinctorii (*Hong Hua*), Radix Rubrus Paeoniae Lactiflorae (*Chi Shao*), Cortex Radicis Moutan (*Dan Pi*), and uncooked Pollen Typhae (*Pu Huang*).

ACUPUNCTURE & MOXIBUSTION: *Jing Ming* (Bl 1), *Qiu Hou* (M-HN-8), *Feng Chi* (GB 20), *Tai Xi* (Ki 3), *San Yin Jiao* (Sp 6), *Guang Ming* (GB 37), *Ge Shu* (Bl 17), *Gan Shu* (Bl 18)

FORMULA ANALYSIS: Supplementing *Tai Xi, San Yin Jiao, Guang Ming, Ge Shu,* and *Gan Shu* nourishes the blood, enriches the kidneys, and brightens the eyes. *Guang Ming* is the connecting point between the gallbladder channel and a channel divergence of the liver, therefore, this pathway is how liver qi and blood ascend to the eyes. Even supplementing-even draining *Jing Ming* and *Qiu Hou* moves the qi and quickens the blood in the network vessels of the eyes. Draining *Feng Chi* clears heat from the head and eyes.

ADDITIONS & SUBTRACTIONS: If there is oral dryness and polydipsia, add supplementing *Zhao Hai* (Ki 6) and even supplementing-even draining *Lie Que* (Lu 7). If there is polyphagia and easy hungering, add draining *Nei Tong* (St 44) and *He Gu* (LI 4). If there is liver depression, add even supplementing-even draining *Tai Zhong* (Liv 3) and draining *He Gu*. For liver depression transforming heat, add even supplementing-even draining *Xing Jian* (Liv 2) through to *Tai Zhong*.

2. LUNG-STOMACH QI & YIN DUAL VACUITY PATTERN

MAIN SYMPTOMS: This pattern is mostly seen in preproliferative and the early stage of proliferative diabetic retinopathy. The clinical signs and symptoms of this pattern include dry mouth and polydipsia, polyphagia and easy hungering, fatigue, lack of strength, low back and knee soreness and limpness, dizziness, tinnitus, a dark red or dark, fat tongue with white, possibly scanty fur, and a surging and slippery or deep, fine, possibly rapid pulse.

TREATMENT PRINCIPLES: Supplement the lungs and boost the qi, enrich and supplement kidney yin

RX: *Sheng Mai San* (Engender the Pulse Powder) plus *Qi Ju Di Huang Tang* (Lycium & Chrysanthemum Rehmannia Decoction) with additions and subtractions

INGREDIENTS: Radix Scrophulariae Ningpoensis (*Xuan Shen*), 20g, Radix Codonopsitis Pilosulae (*Dang Shen*), Radix Dioscoreae Oppositae (*Shan Yao*), uncooked Radix Rehmanniae (*Sheng Di*), and cooked Radix Rehmanniae (*Shu Di*), 15g each, Sclerotium Poriae Cocos (*Fu Ling*), 12g, Tuber Ophiopogonis Japonici (*Mai Men Dong*), Rhizoma Alismatis (*Ze Xie*), Fructus Corni Officinalis (*Shan Zhu Yu*), Cortex Radicis Moutan (*Dan Pi*), Flos Chryanthemi Morifolii (*Ju Hua*), and Fructus Lycii Chinensis (*Gou Qi Zi*), 9g each

FORMULA ANALYSIS: *Dang Shen, Mai Men Dong, Sheng Di* and *Xuan Shen* boost the qi and nourish yin. *Gou Qi Zi* and *Ju Hua* nourish the liver and brighten the eyes, while *Shu Di* enriches the kidneys and fosters essences. *Shan Zhu Yu* supplements the liver and kidneys at the same time as it astringes the essence. *Shan Yao* supplements and boosts the kidney qi, fortifies the spleen and disinhibits damp-

ness. *Ze Xie* drains kidney fire and protects against *Shu Di's* enriching sliminess. *Dan Pi* clears and discharges liver fire and controls *Shan Zhu Yu's* warmth.

ADDITIONS & SUBTRACTIONS: If retinal bleeding has endured and cannot be stopped, one can add nine grams each of Radix Salviae Miltiorrhizae (*Dan Shen*) and uncooked Pollen Typhae (*Pu Huang*) and three grams of powdered Radix Pseudoginseng (*San Qi*) swallowed with the decoction to cool the blood and stop bleeding. If there is macular edema, add more *Fu Ling* and *Ze Xie* as well as nine grams each of Semen Plantaginis (*Che Qian Zi*) and Radix Salviae Miltiorrhizae (*Dan Shen*) to quicken the blood and disinhibit water. For more pronounced macular sclerosis and leakage, add nine grams each of Thallus Algae (*Kun Bu*), Herba Sargassii (*Hai Zao*), Concha Ostreae (*Mu Li*), and Fructus Crataegi (*Shan Zha*) to soften and scatter binding, quicken the blood and transform stasis. If there is concomitant qi stagnation, add 18 grams of Radix Albus Paeoniae Lactiflorae (*Bai Shao*) and nine grams each of Radix Bupleuri (*Chai Hu*), Fructus Citri Aurantii (*Zhi Ke*), and Fructus Trichosanthis Kirlowii (*Gua Lou*).

ACUPUNCTURE & MOXIBUSTION: *Jing Ming* (Bl 1), *Qiu Hou* (M-HN-8), *Zu San Li* (St 36), *San Yin Jiao* (Sp 6), *Fei Shu* (Bl 13), *Ge Shu* (Bl 17), *Gan Shu* (Bl 18), *Shen Shu* (Bl 23), *Tai Xi* (Ki 3), *Guang Ming* (GB 37), *Feng Chi* (GB 20)

FORMULA ANALYSIS: Supplementing *Zu San Li, San Yin Jiao, Fei Shu, Ge Shu, Gan Shu, Shen Shu, Tai Xi,* and *Guang Ming* supplements the lungs, spleen, liver, and kidneys, nourishes the blood, enriches yin, and brightens the eyes. Even supplementing-even draining *Jing Ming* and *Qiu Hou* moves the qi and quickens the blood in the network vessels of the eyes. Draining *Feng Chi* clears heat from the head and eyes.

ADDITIONS & SUBTRACTIONS: If there is marked liver depression, add even supplementing-even draining *Tai Chong* (Liv 3) and draining *He Gu* (LI 4). If there is marked blood stasis, add even supplementing-even draining *Xue Hai* (Sp 10) and draining *He Gu* (LI 4). For heat in the stomach with dry mouth and oral thirst, add draining *Nei Ting* (St 44) and change supplementing *Zu San Li* to even supplementing-even draining *Zu San Li*.

3. YIN & YANG DUAL VACUITY PATTERN

MAIN SYMPTOMS: This pattern is mostly seen in proliferative diabetic retinopathy. The clinical signs and symptoms of this pattern include fear of cold, chilled limbs, shortness of breath, lack of strength, superficial edema, a bright white facial complexion, a dark fat tongue, and a deep, fine, weak pulse.

NOTE: Although the name of this pattern does not say so, there is also a pronounced qi vacuity.

TREATMENT PRINCIPLES: Foster yin and warm yang, quicken the blood and scatter binding or nodulation

RX: Jin Gui Shen Qi Wan Jia Jian (Golden Cabinet Kidney Qi Pills with Additions & Subtractions)

INGREDIENTS: Radix Astragali Membranacei (Huang Qi) and Radix Salviae Miltiorrhizae (Dan Shen), 30g each, cooked Radix Rehmanniae (Shu Di) and Radix Disocoreae Oppositae (Shan Yao), 15g each, Sclerotium Poriae Cocos (Fu Ling), 12g, Fructus Corni Officinalis (Shan Zhu Yu), Rhizoma Alismatis (Ze Xie), Cortex Radicis Moutan (Dan Pi), Thallus Algae (Kun Bu), and Semen Plantaginis (Che Qian Zi), 9g each, and Ramulus Cinnamomi Cassiae (Gui Zhi), 6g

FORMULA ANALYSIS: Shu Di and Shan Zhu Yu supplement the liver and kidneys, while Huang Qi and Shan Yao supplement the spleen and kidneys. Fu Ling, Ze Xie, and Che Qian Zi seep dampness and lead ministerial fire downward along the yin tract. Gui Zhi warms and supplements kidney yang. Dan Shen, Dan Pi, and Kun Bu quicken the blood and scatter nodulation.

ADDITIONS & SUBTRACTIONS: If there is marked sclerosis and cotton wool patches, add nine grams each of Herba Saragassii (Hai Zao), Bulbus Fritillariae Thunbergii (Zhe Bei Mu), uncooked Fructus Crataegi (Shan Zha), and uncooked Pollen Typhae (Pu Huang) to increase the effect of quickening the blood, transforming stasis, and scattering nodulation. If there is marked phlegm dampness, add nine grams each of Fructus Trichosanthis Kirlowii (Gua Lou) and Rhizoma Pinelliae Ternatae (Ban Xia). If there is concomitant qi stagnation, add 18 grams of Radix Albus Paeoniae Lactiflorae (Bai Shao) and nine grams each of Radix Bupleuri (Chai Hu), Fructus Citri Aurantii (Zhi Ke), and Fructus Trichosanthis Kirlowii (Gua Lou).

If there is marked kidney yin depletion and vacuity with vacuity fire flaming upward, one can use Er Zhi Wan (Two Ultimates Pills) plus Zhi Bai Di Huang Wan (Anemarrhena & Phellodendron Rehmannia Pills) with added flavors: Herba Ecliptae Prostratae (Han Lian Cao) and Fructus Ligustri Lucidi (Nu Zhen Zi), 15g each, cooked Radix Rehmanniae (Shu Di) and Sclerotium Poriae Cocos (Fu Ling), 12g each, Fructus Corni Officinalis (Shan Zhu Yu), Radix Dioscoreae Oppositae (Shan Yao), Cortex Radicis Moutan (Dan Pi), Rhizoma Alismatis (Ze Xie), Rhizoma Anemarrhenae Aspheloidis (Zhi Mu), and Cortex Phellodendri (Huang Bai), 9g each, and Cortex Cinnamomi Cassiae (Rou Gui), 3-6g.

ACUPUNCTURE & MOXIBUSTION: Jing Ming (Bl 1), Qiu Hou (M-HN-8), Feng Chi (GB 20), Zu San Li (St 36), San Yin Jiao (Sp 6), Tai Xi (Ki 3), Pi Shu (Bl 20), Shen Shu (Bl 23), Ming Men (GV 4), Qi Hai (CV 6), Guan Yuan (CV 4)

FORMULA ANALYSIS: Supplementing Zu San Li, San Yin Jiao, and Pi Shu supplements the spleen and upbears the clear, while supplementing Tai Xi and San Yin Jiao supplements the kidneys and enriches yin. Moxaing Shen Shu, Ming Men, Qi Hai, and Guan Yuan warms and invigorates yang. Even supplementing-even draining Jing Ming and Qiu Hou moves the qi and quickens the blood in the network vessels of the eyes, while draining Feng Chi clears heat in the head and eyes.

ADDITIONS & SUBTRACTIONS: For simultaneous liver depression, add even supplementing-even draining Tai Chong (Liv 3) and draining He Gu (LI 4). For simultaneous blood stasis, add draining Xue Hai (Sp 10) and He Gu (LI 4).

ABSTRACTS OF REPRESENTATIVE CHINESE RESEARCH:

Zhang Hong-ming, "The Treatment of 50 Cases of Diabetic Retinopathy with Jiang Tang Yin (Lower Sugar Drink)," Si Chuan Zhong Yi (Sichuan Chinese Medicine), #3, 1999, p. 45: Of the 50 patients described in this study, 38 were male and 12 were female. They ranged in age from 42-71 years, with a median age of 52.5 years of age. The course of their disease had lasted from 5-21 years. All were diagnosed with type 2 (i.e., NIDDM) diabetic retinopathy according to the criteria promulgated at the 1985 National Eye Disease Symposium. Symptoms included decreased visual acuity, abnormal changes in the visual field, and abnormal changes in the eye ground. Twenty-eight cases had non-proliferative retinopathy, while 22 cases had the proliferative type.

Jiang Tang Yin consisted of: uncooked Radix Rehmanniae (Sheng Di), Radix Trichosanthis Kirlowii (Tian Hua Fen), and Semen Leonuri Heterophylli (*Chong Wei Zi*), 30g each, Rhizoma Anemarrhenae Aspheloidis (*Zhi Mu*), Tuber Ophiopogonis Japonici (*Mai Dong*), Fructus Pruni Mume (*Wu Mei*), Cortex Radicis Lycii Chinensis (*Di Gu Pi*), Cortex Radicis Moutan (*Dan Pi*), and Radix Rubrus Paeoniae Lactiflorae (*Chi Shao*), 15g each, uncooked Radix Dioscoreae Oppositae (*Shan Yao*), 60g, uncooked Gypsum Fibrosum (*Shi Gao*), 90g, Radix Scrophulariae Ningpoensis (*Xuan Shen*), 20-30g, Radix Salviae Miltiorrhizae (*Dan Shen*), 15-20g, Semen Cassiae Torae (*Cao Jue Ming*), 25g, and Flos Chrysanthemi Morifolii (*Ju Hua*), 10g. If there was qi vacuity, Radix Astragali Membranacei (*Huang Qi*) and Radix Pseudostellariae (*Tai Zi Shen*) were added. If there was skin itching, Cortex Radicis Dictamnia Dasycarpi (*Bai Xian Pi*) and Periostracum Cicadae (*Chan Tui*) were added. If there were skin infections, Flos Lonicerae Japonicae (*Yin Hua*), Fructus Forsythiae Suspensae (*Lian Qiao*), and Herba Taraxaci Mongolici Cum Radice (*Gong Ying*) were added. If there was relatively pronounced seepage, Rhizoma Atractylodis (*Cang Zhu*), Rhizoma Atractylodis Macrocephalae (*Bai Zhu*), and Semen Coicis Lachryma-jobi (*Yi Yi Ren*) were added. The above were decocted in water and administered internally two times per day. Thirty days equaled one course of treatment.

Cure was defined as a return to normal visual acuity and visual field. Any microanuerysms, bleeding, or seepage in the eye ground basically disappeared. Marked effect meant that visual acuity improved by three competencies or more and the visual field enlarged by 10-15E. Bleeding and seepage were either completely eliminated or greatly improved. Fair effect meant that visual acuity increased by two competencies, the visual filed enlarged by 5-10E, and any areas of bleeding and seepage shrunk. No effect meant that there was no marked change from before to after treatment. Based on the above criteria, six cases were deemed cured, 18 got a marked effect, 21 got a fair effect, and five got no effect. Thus the total amelioration rate was 90%.

Liu Li, "A Survey of the Treatment Efficacy of *Qing Ying Tang* (Clear the Constructive Decoction) as the Main Treatment for Bleeding of the Fundus of the Eye," *Zhong Yi Za Zhi* (*Journal of Chinese Medicine*), #2, 2001, p. 101-102: This study describes the treatment of 68 out patients with bleeding in the fundus of their eyes. Among these, there were 36 men and 32 women, 16 of whom had diabetic eye fundus bleeding. *Qing Ying Tang* was administered to all 68 patients based on the principles of clearing the constructive and out-thrusting heat, cooling the blood and dispelling stasis, and blandly seeping and eliminating dampness. The formula consisted of: Sclerotium Poriae Cocos (*Fu Ling*), 20g, uncooked Radix Rehmanniae (*Sheng Di*), Radix Salviae Miltiorrhizae (*Dan Shen*), Herba Lycopi Lucidi (*Ze Lan*), Lumbricus (*Di Long*), and Radix Scrophulariae Ningpoensis (*Xuan Shen*), 15g each, Fructus Forsythiae Suspensae (*Lian Qiao*), Herba Lophatheri Gracilis (*Dan Zhu Ye*), and Flos Lonicerae Japonicae (*Jin Yin Hua*), 12g each, and Rhizoma Coptidis Chinensis (*Huang Lian*), 3g. During the early stage of this condition, only this formula was administered. During the middle stage, based on the treatment principles of clearing the constructive and out-thrusting heat, quickening the blood and transforming stasis, and blandly seeping and eliminating dampness, *Sheng Di* was removed, 20 grams of Radix Astragali Membranacei (*Huang Qi*), 15 grams each of Flos Carthami Tinctorii (*Hong Hua*) and Radix Ligustici Wallichii (*Chuan Xiong*), and 1.5 grams of Radix Psuedoginseng (*San Qi*) were added. The *San Qi* was administered in 0.5 gram capsules, one capsule three times per day. During the latter stage, based on the principles of clearing the constructive and out-thrusting heat, enriching yin and dispelling stasis, softening the hard and scattering nodulation, *Huang Lian* and *Sheng Di* were removed and 30 grams each of Herba Sargassii (*Hai Zao*) and Thallus Algae (*Kun Bu*), 20 grams of Concha Ostreae (*Mu Li*), 15 grams each of Tuber Ophiopogonis Japonici (*Mai Men Dong*) and Radix Glehniae Littoralis (*Sha Shen*), and 10 grams of mix-fried Radix Glycyrrhizae (*Gan Cao*) were added. In addition modifications were also made on the basis of each patient's pattern discrimination in terms of liver-kidney insufficiency, ascendant liver yang hyperactivity, yin vacuity fire effulgence, qi vacuity, and internal exuberance of phlegm turbidity.

Cure was defined as marked improvement in the symptoms, complete resolution of retinal bleeding, disappearance of edema, and increase in visual acuity by three ormore degrees. Marked effect was defined as improvement of subjective symptoms, resolution of the greater part of retinal hemorrhage, disappearance of edema, and increase in visual acuity. Good effect meant that the subjective symptoms markedly improved and retinal bleeding was somewhat resolved. No effect meant that there was no improvement in subjective symptoms or possible worsening, decreased visual acuity, and worsening of ophthalmoscopic findings. Based on these criteria, 56 patients were judged cured, eight got a marked effect, and four got a good or fair effect. In terms of the outcomes amongst the 16 diabetic patients, 15 of these were judged cured and the other got a marked effect.

Cao Su-lan *et al.*, "The Treatment of Diabetic Retinopathy with *Zeng Shi Jiao Nang* (Improve the Vision Gelatin

Capsules)," *Shan Dong Zhong Yi Za Zhi (Shandong Journal of Chinese Medicine)*, #5, 2000, p. 281-282: From 1993-1999, the authors treated 52 cases of diabetic retinopathy using self-composed *Zeng Shi Jiao Nang*. The oldest patient was 78 years old and the youngest 35 years old. Thirty patients were male and 22 were female. The longest duration of diabetes was 30 years, the shortest duration was five years, and the average duration was 12.5 years. Of these 52 cases, 43 cases were affected in both eyes, while nine cases were affected in only one eye. In all of these cases, the pattern was primarily qi and yin dual vacuity with phlegm and stasis mutually binding. Six to eight capsules of *Zeng Shi Jiao Nang* were administered each time, three times per day. One month was considered one course of treatment, and, generally, three courses were administered. The treatment principles were to boost the qi and nourish yin, engender fluids and stop thirst, quicken the blood and transform stasis, and disinhibit water and transform phlegm. The formula consisted of: uncooked Radix Astragali Membranacei (*Huang Qi*), Fructus Lycii Chinensis (*Gou Qi Zi*), Radix Dioscoreae Oppositae (*Shan Yao*), Radix Puerariae (*Ge Gen*), and Radix Salviae Miltiorrhizae (*Dan Shen*), 30g each, uncooked Radix Rehmanniae (*Sheng Di*), Fructus Leonuri (*Chong Wei Zi*), Thallus Algae (*Kun Bu*), and Herba Sargassii (*Hai Zao*), 20g each, Rhizoma Alismatis (*Ze Xie*), 15g, Fructus Citri Aurantii (*Zhi Ke*), 12g, and powdered Radix Pseudoginseng (*San Qi*), 5g.

Of these 52 cases, 82.6% experienced a marked effect. When those patients with moderate improvement were also included, the total amelioration rate rose to 100%. In addition, before treatment, the fasting blood sugar level was lower than 8.33mmol/L for only 31.73% of the 52 cases, but, after treatment, 68.27% of the 52 cases had a blood sugar level lower than 8.33mmol/L.

Liu Ling & Guo Xia, "The Treatment of Diabetic Retinopathy with *Tang Mu Qing* (Diabetic Eye-clearing Decoction)," *Shan Dong Zhong Yi Za Zhi (Shandong Journal of Chinese Medicine)*, #3, 2000, p. 145-146: In this study, there were a total of 58 patients with diabetic retinopathy divided into two groups: a treatment group of 30 cases receiving *Tang Mu Qing* and a control group of 28 cases receiving *Qi Ju Di Huang Wan* (Lycium & Chrysanthemum Rehmannia Pills). In the treatment group, the ages ranged from 50-70 years old, with an average age of 58.6 years. There were nine men and 21 women in this group, and the duration of their diabetes was from 0.5-23 years, with an average duration of 10.38 years. The duration of the retinopathy was from 0.5-24 months, with an average duration of 5.7 months. In the control group, the ages

ranged from 42-70 years old, with an average age of 59.6 years. There were eight men and 20 women in this group. The duration of the diabetes was from 1-18 years, with an average duration of 9.39 years. The duration of the retinopathy was from 2-23 months, with an average duration of 7.5 months.

Tang Mu Qing consisted of: Radix Astragali Membranacei (*Huang Qi*), uncooked Radix Rehmanniae (*Sheng Di*), Herba Epimedii (*Xian Ling Pi*), Radix Angelicae Sinensis (*Dang Gui*), Tuber Ophiopogonis Japonici (*Mai Men Dong*), Fructus Lycii Chinensis (*Gou Qi Zi*), Herba Gynostemmae (*Jiao Gu Lan*), Cortex Radicis Lycii Chinensis (*Di Gu Pi*), Rhizoma Alismatis (*Ze Xie*), Radix Puerariae (*Ge Gen*), and Radix Et Rhizoma Polygoni Cuspidati (*Hu Zhang*). These medicinals were boiled in water, and one *ji* was administered in two divided doses, morning and evening, every day. Thirty days was considered one course of treatment. After the symptoms were alleviated, the same presciption was administered in capsule form, 15 grams each time, two times per day for another 30 days. If the bleeding in the fundus was heavy and the blood fresh, then *Ge Gen* and *Xian Ling Pi* were omitted from the basic formula, and Herba Cephalanoploris Segeti (*Xiao Ji*), Radix Rubiae Cordifoliae (*Qian Cao Gen*), and powdered Radix Pseudoginseng (*San Qi*) were added. If the fundus showed a large amount of seepage, then Herba Lycopi Lucidi (*Ze Lan*), Thallus Algae (*Kun Bu*), Herba Sargassii (*Hai Zao*), and Radix Salviae Miltiorrhizae (*Dan Shen*) were added. If there were yellow spots or severe edema, then Sclerotium Poriae Cocos (*Fu Ling*), Rhizoma Atractylodis (*Cang Zhu*), and Semen Coicis Lachryma-jobi (*Yi Yi Ren*) were added. If the bleeding was not severe, the blood vessels were thin, and the retina was pale in color, then Radix Morindae Officinalis (*Ba Ji Tian*), cooked Radix Rehmanniae (*Shu Di*), Radix Pseudostellariae Heterophyllae (*Tai Zi Shen*), and Radix Albus Paeoniae Lactiflorae (*Bai Shao*) were added. The control group received *Qi Ju Di Huang Wan*, nine grams each time, three times per day. One month was considered one course of treatment, and both groups were treated for six months. The treatment group had an amelioration rate of 93.1%, while the rate for the comparison group was only 82%.

Wang Da-qian, "The Treatment of 161 Cases of Diabetic Retinal Bleeding with *Dan Qi Di Huang Tang* (Salvia, Pseudoginseng & Rehmannia Decoction)," *Bei Jing Zhong Yi (Beijing Chinese Medicine)*, #5, 1999, p. 25-26: The author of this study treated 161 patients in two groups of 106 and 55. In the treatment group of 106 cases, 65 were men and 41 were women. Their ages ranged from 48-70 years old, with an average age of 56.76. The duration of disease was 5-24 years, with an average duration of 14.67 years. The treatment group received *Dan Qi Di Huang Tang* which consisted of: Radix Salviae Miltiorrhizae (*Dan Shen*), 30g, uncooked Radix Rehmanniae (*Sheng Di*), 20g, stir-fried Pollen Typhae (*Pu Huang*) and Herba Dendrobii (*Shi Hu*), 15g each, Radix Rubrus Paeoniae Lactiflorae (*Chi Shao*), 12g, Cortex Radicis Moutan (*Dan Pi*), 10g, Rhizoma Cimicifugae (*Sheng Ma*), 6g, and powdered Radix Pseudoginseng (*San Qi*), 3g, taken with the decocted medicinals. These medicinals were administered orally, one *ji* per day, 200ml each time in the morning and evening. The control group received *Yun Nan Bai Yao Jiao Nang* (Yunnan White Medicine Gelatin Capsules) together with *Tong Sai Mai Pian* (Free the Flow of Blocked Vessels Tablets) at a dosage of two tablets each time, two times per day for one month. For both groups, one month was considered one course of treatment.

In the treatment group, 39.62% had marked improvement, 42.45% had moderate improvement, and 17.86% had no improvement. Thus the total amelioration rate in that group was 82.14%. In the control group, 32.26% had marked improvement, and 41.91% had moderate improvement. Therefore, the total amelioration rate in that group was only 74.19%.

Ling Bi-da, "The Treatment of Diabetic Retinal Bleeding with Integrated Chinese-Western Medicine," *Bei Jing Zhong Yi (Beijing Chinese Medicine)*, #3, 1999, p. 17-18: The author of this study treated 27 type 2 patients with diabetes retinopathy in a total of 36 individual eyes. Twenty-two of these had extensive areas of bleeding in the retina, 10 had bleeding due to proliferated vessels, and four had bleeding in the vitreous body. There were nine men in the study and 18 women. Their ages ranged from 55-76 years old, with an average age of 62.5 years. The duration of disease ranged from 3-16 years, with an average duration of 9.7 years. The patients were divided into two patterns: 1) liver-kidney yin vacuity with frenetic movement of hot blood (20 patients with 25 individual eyes) and 2) qi and yin dual vacuity with blood spilling outside the vessels (seven patients with 11 individual eyes). The Chinese medicinal formulas were administered orally, one *ji* per day, with 30 days as one course of treatment. Both patient groups continued with the Chinese medicinals for three months.

The patients in the liver-kidney yin vacuity with frenetic movement of blood pattern presented with dizziness, tinnitus, tidal reddening of the face, a dry mouth with a sour taste, heart vexation, insomnia, low back and knee soreness and limpness, and diminished vision or sudden flashes of red in front of the eye. Their tongues were dark red with thin, white or thin, yellow fur, and their pulses were bowstring and fine. The treatment principles for this group were to enrich and nourish the liver and kidneys, quicken the blood and transform stasis. The medicinals used were: uncooked Radix Rehmanniae (*Sheng Di*), 20g, Fructus Lycii Chinensis (*Gou Qi Zi*), Radix Scrophulariae Ningpoensis (*Yuan Shen*), Ramulus Loranthi Seu Visci (*Sang Ji Sheng*), Radix Achyranthis Bidentatae (*Niu Xi*), Radix Salviae Miltiorrhizae (*Dan Shen*), and Semen Cassiae Torae (*Cao Jue Ming*), 15g each, Flos Chrysanthemi Morifolii (*Ju Hua*) and Radix Puerariae (*Ge Gen*), 12g each, Radix Angelicae Sinensis (*Dang Gui*), Radix Rubrus Paeoniae Lactiflorae (*Chi Shao*), and Herba Dendrobii (*Shi Hu*), 10g each, and powdered Radix Pseudoginseng (*San Qi*), 3g, taken with the decocted medicinals.

The patients in the qi and yin dual vacuity with blood spilling outside the vessels presented with lack of strength, lassitude of spirit, dizziness, spontaneous perspiration, a sallow yellow facial complexion, a weak voice and/or disinclination to speak, and declining vision with sudden flashes of redness in front of the eyes or complete loss of vision. Their tongues were pale red and enlarged with thin, white fur, and their pulses were deep and fine. The treatment principles in this group were to boost the qi and nourish yin, quicken the blood and transform stasis. The medicinals prescribed were: Radix Pseudostellariae Heterophyllae (*Tai Zi Shen*), 30g, uncooked Radix Astralagi Membranacei (*Huang Qi*), 20g, uncooked Radix Rehmanniae (*Sheng Di*), Radix Scrophulariae Ningpoensis (*Yuan Shen*), Fructus Lycii Chinensis (*Gou Qi Zi*), Semen Cassiae Torae (*Cao Jue Ming*), and Radix Salviae Miltiorrhizae (*Dan Shen*), 15g each, Flos Chrysanthemi Morifolii (*Ju Hua*), 12g, Radix Anemarrhenae Aspheloidis (*Zhi Mu*), Herba Dendrobii (*Shi Hu*), and Radix Angelicae Sinensis (*Dang Gui*), 10g each, and powdered Radix Pseudoginseng (*San Qi*), 3g, taken with the decocted medicinals. The patients in both groups also took oral doses of blood sugar controlling drugs to maintain their blood sugar levels in the range of 6-8mmol/L, together with vitamins C and E. The total amelioration rate for the 27 patients in this study after three months of treatment was 75%.

Yang Hai-yan & Yang Jian-hua, "Clinical & TCD Observations on Frequency Spectrum of Ophthalmic Arterial Blood Flow in 61 Eyes with Diabetic Retinopathy Treated with *Yi Shen Huo Xue Fang* (Boost the Kidneys & Quicken the Blood Formula)," *Zhe Jiang Zhong Yi Za Zhi*

(*Zhejiang Journal of Chinese Medicine*), #1, 2001, p. 30-31: There were 60 patients in this study who were divided into two groups, a treatment group and a comparison group. Among these 60 patients, 29 were male and 31 were female. They ranged in age from 51-75 years, with an average age of 61.2 years. Their course of disease had lasted from 4-20 years, with an average duration of 8.5 years. After division, there was no significant differences in terms of sex, age, or disease course between the two groups. All these patients had type 2 diabetes and retinopathy. Patients with type 1 diabetes, other endocrine disorders, or serious organic heart, liver, lung, or kidney diseases were excluded. The comparison group was treated with typical oral hypoglycemic drugs, such as glyburide. The treatment group also received these typical Western hypoglycemic medications as well as the following Chinese medicinal formula: Concha Haliotidis (*Shi Jue Ming*), 24g, Radix Scrophulariae Ningpoensis (*Xuan Shen*), 20g, uncooked Radix Rehmanniae (*Sheng Di*), cooked Radix Rehmanniae (*Shu Di*), Rhizoma Polygonati (*Huang Jing*), and Fructus Lycii Chinensis (*Gou Qi Zi*), 15g each, and Herba Dendrobii (*Shi Hu*), Radix Angelicae Sinensis (*Dang Gui*), Flos Carthami Tinctorii (*Hong Hua*), Radix Puerariae (*Ge Gen*), Caulis Milletiae Seu Spatholobi (*Ji Xue Teng*), Radix Achyranthis Bidentatae (*Niu Xi*), Cortex Eucommiae Ulmoidis (*Du Zhong*), and Fructus Citri Aurantii (*Zhi Ke*), 10g each. One *ji* of these medicinals was decocted in water and administered per day for one month.

In terms of outcomes, marked effect was defined as visual acuity increasing by more than three steps, complete disappearance of eye ground blood vessel tumors, bleeding, and seepage or disappearance of at least the major portion of these, and improvement of peripheral vision by 10-15E or more. Improvement means that visual acuity increased 1-3 steps or grades, eye ground blood vessel tumors, bleeding, and seepage partially disappeared, and peripheral vision increased 5-10E. No effect meant that the preceding criteria were not met or that the condition worsened. Based on these criteria, out of a total of 61 eyes in the treatment group, 27 eyes (44.26%) got a marked effect, 25 eyes (40.98%) improved, and nine eyes (14.75%) got no effect. In the comparison group, 13 eyes (25.00%) got a marked effect, 19 eyes (36.54%) improved, and 20 eyes (38.46%) got no effect. Hence there was a marked statistical difference in treatment outcomes between these two groups suggesting that Chinese medicinals combined with Western oral hypoglycemic agents is more effective for diabetic retinopathy than Western oral hypoglycemics alone.

Wu De-yin, "The Treatment of 32 Cases of Diabetic Retinopathy Mainly by Quickening the Blood & Transforming Stasis," *Zhe Jiang Zhong Yi Za Zhi* (*Zhejiang Journal of Chinese Medicine*), #4, 2000, p. 158: There were 32 patients in this study, 21 men and 11 women aged 38-62, with an average age of 52.6 years and a disease course of 3-18 years, with an average disease duration of 9.3 years. There were 19 cases of background DR, five cases of yellow macule pathological changes, six cases of preproliferative DR, and two cases of proliferative DR. Twenty-one cases presented the Chinese medical pattern of blood stasis and yin vacuity, and 11 presented blood stasis and qi vacuity. In addition to typical Western oral hypoglycemic agents, patients received the following Chinese medicinals: Radix Salviae Miltiorrhizae (*Dan Shen*), 30g, Pollen Typhae (*Pu Huang*), Herba Ecliptae Prostratae (*Han Lian Cao*), and Radix Rubiae Cordifoliae (*Qian Cao Gen*), 15g each, Radix Ligustici Wallichii (*Chuan Xiong*), Radix Rubrus Paeoniae Lactiflorae (*Chi Shao*), Semen Pruni Persicae (*Tao Ren*), Radix Bletillae Striatae (*Bai Ji*), and uncooked Radix Rehmanniae (*Sheng Di*), 12g each, and Flos Carthami Tinctorii (*Hong Hua*), 10g. If there was accompanying yin vacuity, 15 grams of Radix Trichosanthis Kirlowii (*Tian Hua Fen*) and 12 grams each of Tuber Ophiopogonis Japonici (*Mai Men Dong*), Radix Scrophulariae Ningpoensis (*Xuan Shen*), Cortex Phellodendri (*Huang Bai*), and Radix Achyranthis Bidentatae (*Niu Xi*) were added. If there was simultaneous qi vacuity, 18 grams of Radix Astragali Membranacei (*Huang Qi*), 15 grams of Radix Codonopsitis Pilosulae (*Dang Shen*), and 12 grams each of Radix Pseudostellariae Heterophyllae (*Tai Zi Shen*), Rhizoma Atractylodis Macrocephalae (*Bai Zhu*), and Radix Dioscoreae Oppositae (*Shan Yao*) were added. If there was seepage into the eye ground, 30 grams of Fructus Crataegi (*Shan Zha*), 12 grams each of Endothelium Corneum Gigeriae Galli (*Ji Nei Jin*) and Massa Medica Fermentata (*Shen Qu*), and 10 grams of Fructus Amomi (*Sha Ren*) were added. If there was eye ground edema, 30 grams of Semen Coicis Lachyrma-jobi (*Yi Yi Ren*), 15 grams of Sclerotium Poriae Cocos (*Fu Ling*), and 12 grams of Semen Plantaginis (*Che Qian Zi*) were added. Patients were treated with this protocol from two weeks to three months, with an average length of treatment of 36 days.

Cure was defined as increase in visual acuity equal or more than 0.6 degrees and complete control of eye ground bleeding and/or edema. Improvement was defined as recovery of visual acuity two steps or stages or more, basic control of eye ground bleeding and/or edema, and a reduction in seepage. No effect meant that recovery of visual acuity was less than two steps or that there was no improvement in eye ground bleeding, edema, and/or seepage. Based on these criteria, 23 cases with background DR were cured and five improved. Three cases with yellow macule pathological changes were cured, four improved, and one got no effect. Five cases with preproliferative DR were cured and four improved. One case with proliferative DR improved and one got no effect. Hence, a total of 31 cases were cured and 14 improved using this protocol.

Zhao Hong, "The Treatment of Diabetic Retinopathy Based on Pattern Discrimination," *He Nan Zhong Yi (Henan Chinese Medicine)*, #3, 2001, p. 54: There were 70 patients in this study with diabetic retinopathy, 44 men and 26 women aged 45-66 years old. All had suffered from diabetes for 8-20 years, and all had disease changes in both eyes. In addition to hypoglycemic and antidiabetic medications, these patients were administered *Zhi Bai Di Huang Tang Jia Jian* (Anemarrhena & Phellodendron Rehmannia Decoction with Additions & Subtractions): Radix Salviae Miltiorrhizae (*Dan Shen*), Radix Puerariae (*Ge Gen*), Rhizoma Alismatis (*Ze Xie*), Sclerotium Poriae Cocos (*Fu Ling*), and Radix Scrophulariae Ningpoensis (*Xuan Shen*), 30g each, Rhizoma Anemarrhenae Aspheloidis (*Zhi Mu*), Cortex Radicis Moutan (*Dan Pi*), uncooked Radix Rehmanniae (*Sheng Di*), Radix Dioscoreae Oppositae (*Shan Yao*), Fructus Corni Officinalis (*Shan Zhu Yu*), Radix Trichosanthis Kirlowii (*Tian Hua Fen*), and Semen Leonuri Heterophylli (*Chong Wei Zi*), 20g each, and Cortex Phellodendri (*Huang Bai*) and Lumbricus (*Di Long*), 15g each.

Prior to treatment, 17 cases had visual acuity less than 0.1 degree, 16 had 0.1-0.3 degrees, 13 had 0.4-0.6 degrees, and 24 had 0.6 to less than 1.0 degrees. After treatment, nine had visual acuity less than 0.1 degree, seven had 0.1-0.3 degrees, 11 had 0.4-0.6 degrees, and 43 had visual acuity of more than 0.6 degrees. Altogether, 88% of the patients in this study experienced an increase in their visual acuity. Among these, 10 cases of vision increased 1-3 steps, 16 improved 4-5 steps, and 15 improved more than five steps or grades. Only nine cases failed to experience a marked improvement in visual acuity from before to after this treatment.

REPRESENTATIVE CASE HISTORIES:

CASE 1[9]

The patient was a 50 year old female who had had diabetes for eight years and had experienced blurred vision for three years. Previously, the patient had been taking three tablets of glibenclamide[10] orally per day. That and controlling her diet had managed to keep her blood sugar

11.2-16.5mmol/L, her urine glucose (++-+), and her urine ketone (-). The patient's symptoms at the time of her initial examination were polydipsia, polyphagia, and polyuria, dizziness, blurred vision, dry stools, a red tongue with scanty fur, and a fine, rapid pulse. In the last few days, the woman's vision was more blurry than usual. Ophthalmic examination confirmed diabetic retinopathy in both eyes complicated by cataracts.

Based on the above signs and symptoms, the woman's Chinese pattern discrimination was categorized as yin fluid depletion and vacuity with dryness and heat. Therefore she was prescribed *Qi Ju Di Huang Wan Jia Jian* (Lycium & Chrysanthemum Rehmannia Pills with Additions & Subtractions): Herba Ecliptae Prostratae (*Han Lian Cao*) and Rhizoma Imperatae Cyclindricae (*Bai Mao Gen*), 30g each, Rhizoma Atractylodis (*Cang Zhu*), 20g, uncooked Radix Rehmanniae (*Sheng Di*), Radix Dioscoreae Oppositae (*Shan Yao*), and Rhizoma Alismatis (*Ze Xie*), 15g each, Fructus Lycii Chinensis (*Gou Qi Zi*), Radix Scrophulariae Ningpoensis (*Xuan Shen*), and Fructus Corni Officinalis (*Shan Zhu Yu*), 12g each, Flos Chrysanthemi Morifolii (*Ju Hua*), Scapus Et Inflorescentia Eriocaulonis Buergeriani (*Gu Jing Cao*), Cortex Radicis Moutan (*Dan Pi*), and carbonized Herba Seu Flos Schizonepetae Tenuifoliae (*Jing Jie Sui*), 9g each. One *ji* was decocted in water and administered orally per day. In addition, the woman was also prescribed 80mg of glibenclamide three times per day.

After one half month of this regime, the woman's symptoms of diabetes were decreased with less frequent and less profuse urination and clearer vision. Her blood glucose was 11.2mmol/L and her urine glucose was (++). Ophthalmic examination showed that fresh retinal bleeding had stopped and the exudate was reduced. Twelve grams of Fructus Ligustri Lucidi (*Nu Zhen Zi*) were added to the original formula and this was administered continuously for another four months. At the end of that time, the woman's blood glucose was 8.4mmol/L and her urine glucose was (+). Eye examination showed no fresh bleeding and reabsorption of part of the extravasated blood.

CASE 2[11]

The patient was a 41 year old male who had been diabetic for eight years. Vision in both his eyes had declined over the last two years even though he had taken oral medications regularly for diabetes. During the previous week, he would suddenly lose his sight in both eyes and could only see his hands in front of his eyes. Examination revealed that the corpus vitreum contained accumulated blood and that the patient had little or no vision. He was also emaciated. This patient was given *Dan Qi Di Huang Tang* (Salvia, Pseudoginseng & Rehmannia Decoction) which consisted of: Radix Salviae Miltiorrhizae (*Dan Shen*), 30g, uncooked Radix Rehmanniae (*Sheng Di*), 20g, stir-fried Pollen Typhae (*Pu Huang*) and Herba Dendrobii (*Shi Hu*), 15g each, Radix Rubrus Paeoniae Lactiflorae (*Chi Shao*), 12g, Cortex Radicis Moutan (*Dan Pi*), 10g, Rhizoma Cimicifugae (*Sheng Ma*), 6g, and powdered Radix Pseudoginseng (*San Qi*), 3g, taken with the decocted liquid. The prescription was administered orally, one *ji* per day in two divided doses, 200ml each time in the morning and evening.

After seven days of these medicinals, the man's vision in his right eye was 0.1 and in his left eye, 0.2. Both eyes showed that the accumulated blood had been absorbed and blood vessels could be seen in the area of the fundus. After an additional week of this prescription, the vision in the patient's right eye tested at 0.4 and in the left, at 0.5. One year later, both eyes tested at 0.3, but the retinal bleeding had not recurred.

CASE 3[12]

The patient was a 63 year old woman who had had diabetes for 12 years. During the previous two months, dark shadowy shapes would appear from the side of this woman's left eye. Examination revealed that the vision in the right eye was 1.0, but in the left eye was 0.04. Both eyes contained crystals and turbidity. She was given *Dan Qi Di Huang Tang* (Salvia, Pseudoginseng & Rehmannia Decoction) which consisted of: Radix Salviae Miltiorrhizae (*Dan Shen*), 30g, uncooked Radix Rehmanniae (*Sheng Di*), 20g, stir-fried Pollen Typhae (*Pu Huang*) and Herba Dendrobii (*Shi Hu*), 15g each, Radix Rubrus Paeoniae Lactiflorae (*Chi Shao*), 12g, Cortex Radicis Moutan (*Dan Pi*), 10g, Rhizoma Cimicifugae (*Sheng Ma*), 6g, and powdered Radix Pseudoginseng (*San Qi*), 3g, taken with the decocted liquid. The prescription was administered orally, one *ji* per day in two divided doses, 200ml each time in the morning and evening. After 14 days on this prescription, the bleeding in the entire region of the fundus was absorbed, the woman's vision improved to 0.6, and her vision did not decline even six months after stopping taking these medicinals.

CASE 4[13]

The patient was a 60 year old woman who had had diabetes for three years. While she was taking oral medications, her blood sugar levels remained close to 7mmol/L.

Thinking that she no longer needed to observe good eating habits, the woman went off her diabetic diet, thinking that taking the orally administered blood sugar lowering medications was enough. However, after two months, her blood sugar levels rose to 18.1mmol/L. Again, the oral dosages were adjusted to lower the blood sugar to 10mmol/L. Six months later, she experienced sudden flashes of redness in front of her eyes, her vision declined, and she was diagnosed with retinal bleeding. The Chinese medical pattern discrimination was liver-kidney yin vacuity with frenetic movement of blood, and the treatment principles were to enrich and nourish the liver and kidneys, quicken the blood and transform stasis.

The medicinals used were: uncooked Radix Rehmanniae (*Sheng Di*) 20g, Fructus Lycii Chinensis (*Gou Qi Zi*), 15g, Radix Scrophulariae Ningpoensis (*Yuan Shen*), Ramulus Loranthi Seu Visci (*Sang Ji Sheng*), Radix Achyranthis Bidentatae (*Niu Xi*), Radix Salviae Miltiorrhizae (*Dan Shen*), and Semen Cassiae Torae (*Cao Jue Ming*), 15g each, Flos Chrysanthemi Morifolii (*Ju Hua*) and Radix Puerariae (*Ge Gen*), 12g each, Radix Angelicae Sinensis (*Dang Gui*), Radix Rubrus Paeoniae Lactiflorae (*Chi Shao*), and Herba Dendrobii (*Shi Hu*), 10g each, and powdered Radix Pseudoginseng (*San Qi*), 3g, taken with the decocted medicinals.

After taking this prescription for one month, much of the retinal bleeding had stopped, and, after an additional month on these medicinals, the bleeding had stopped completely and the vision was returned to its initial condition. In addition, the woman's blood sugar levels remained normal. Then, for the next six months, this patient used this prescription without powdered *San Qi* with no recurrence of the problem.

CASE 5[14]

The patient was a 72 year old woman who had had diabetes for 12 years. Her dosage of oral hypoglycemic medication was 2.5mg each time, two times per day. Her blood sugar levels averaged between 6-7mmol/L, but, even so, she suddenly experienced a decline in her vision and red flashes in front of her eyes. Opthalmologic examination revealed bleeding anterior to the retina. The woman's Chinese medical pattern discrimination was qi and yin dual vacuity with blood spilling outside the vessels, and the treatment principles were to boost the qi and nourish yin, quicken the blood and transform stasis. The medicinals prescribed were: Radix Pseudostellariae (*Tai Zi Shen*) 30g, uncooked Radix Astralagi Membranacei (*Huang Qi*) 20g, uncooked Radix Rehmanniae (*Sheng Di*) and Radix

Scrophulariae Ningpoensis (*Yuan Shen*), Fructus Lycii Chinensis (*Gou Qi Zi*), Semen Cassiae Torae (*Cao Jue Ming*), and Radix Salviae Miltiorrhizae (*Dan Shen*), 15g each, Flos Chrysanthemi Morifolii (*Ju Hua*), 12g, Radix Anemarrhenae Aspheloidis (*Zhi Mu*), Herba Dendrobii (*Shi Hu*), and Radix Angelicae Sinensis (*Dang Gui*), 10g each, and powdered Radix Pseudoginseng (*San Qi*), 3g, taken with the decocted medicinals. After two months on this prescription, the bleeding finally stopped and the woman's vision was restored to 0.1.

CASE 6[15]

The patient was a 56 year old woman who had had diabetes for 26 years. After pulmonary surgery five years previously, the woman's blood sugar had become uncontrolled even after years of taking biguanide phenformin and Chinese medicinals. She had had three laser treatments for retinopathy, but the effects of each of the procedures had only lasted a few months. The patient presented with an emaciated body, a red facial complexion, a thin, red tongue with slimy, yellow fur, and a slippery, fine, rapid pulse. Medicinals to boost the qi and enrich yin were prescribed but were ineffective. Then, *Wen Dan Tang Jia Wei* (Warm the Gallbladder Decoction with Added Flavors) was prescribed as follows: Flos Chrysanthemi Morifolii (*Ju Hua*) and Sclerotium Poriae Cocos (*Fu Ling*), 15g each, Caulis Bambusae In Taeniis (*Zhu Ru*), Cortex Radicis Moutan (*Mu Dan Pi*), and bile-processed Rhizoma Arisaematis (*Dan Nan Xing*), 10g each, and Rhizoma Pinelliae Ternatae (*Ban Xia*), Pericarpium Citri Reticulatae (*Chen Pi*), and Fructus Citri Aurantii (*Zhi Ke*), 6g each. After 17 *ji*, the patient's facial complexion returned to normal, but her tongue was slightly red with thin, white fur.

Therefore, the prescribing physician thought that it was appropriate to nourish yin and supplement the kidneys. Hence, *Zhi Bai Di Huang Tang Jia Jian* (Anemarrhena & Phellodendron Rehmannia Decoction with Additions & Subtractions) was prescribed: Herba Ecliptae Prostratae (*Han Lian Cao*), 30g, Radix Pseudostellariae Heterophyllae (*Tai Zi Shen*) and Flos Chrysanthemi Morifolii (*Ju Hua*), 20g each, Sclerotium Poriae Cocos (*Fu Ling*), 15g, uncooked Radix Rehmanniae (*Sheng Di*), Radix Dioscoreae Oppositae (*Shan Yao*), Cortex Radicis Moutan (*Dan Pi*), and Radix Anemarrhenae Aspheloidis (*Zhi Mu*), 10g each, Cortex Phellodendri (*Huang Bai*) and Pericarpium Citri Reticulatae (*Chen Pi*), 6g each, and mix-fried Radix Glycyrrhizae (*Gan Cao*), 3g. The patient took this prescription continuously for three more months, at which time her blood sugar levels remained normal and her eyesight was stable.

REMARKS:

1. Effective treatment of diabetic retinopathy with Chinese medicine depends on simultaneous effective control of glucose levels.

2. Like many contemporary Chinese authors, Li Zhenzhong et al.[16] identify the disease mechanisms of diabetic retinopathy as qi and yin dual vacuity with insufficiency of the liver and kidneys and enduring blood stasis obstructing the network vessels of the eyes. However, they give an interesting series of modifications for various ophthalmoscopic indications. For instance, 30 grams of calcined Concha Ostreae (*Mu Li*) and 15 grams of Thallus Algae (*Kun Bu*) can be added to various formulas to treat retinal bleeding. When the corpus vitreum is unclear or contains accumulated blood, one can add 30 grams of calcined Concha Ostreae (*Mu Li*), 15 grams each of Thallus Algae (*Kun Bu*) and Spica Prunellae Vulgaris (*Xia Ku Cao*), and nine grams each of Squama Manitis Pentadactylis (*Chuan Shan Jia*), Radix Achyranthis Bidentatae (*Niu Xi*), Bombyx Batryticatus (*Jiang Can*), Herba Sargasii (*Hai Zao*), and Bulbus Fritillariae (*Bei Mu*). If there is fresh bleeding in the corpus vitreum or anterior to the retina, add 15 grams each of Herba Cirsii Japonici (*Da Ji*) and Herba Cephalanoploris Segeti (*Xiao Ji*) and nine grams each of Radix Rubiae Cordifoliae (*Qian Cao Gen*), Flos Immaturus Sophorae Japonicae (*Huai Hua Mi*), and Radix Rubrus Paeoniae Lactiflorae (*Chi Shao*). If the bleeding is in a deep layer of the retina and is accompanied by seepage of blood, add nine grams each of Herba Lycopi Lucidi (*Ze Lan*) and Tuber Curcumae (*Yu Jin*), six grams of Flos Carthami Tinctorii (*Hong Hua*), and three grams of powdered Radix Pseudoginseng (*San Qi*) taken with the decocted liquid. If the seepage of blood is considerable or the exudate is white or yellow in color, add nine grams each of Fructus Crataegi (*Shan Zha*) and Endothelium Coreum Gigeriae Galli (*Ji Nei Jin*). If there is accompanying retinal edema, add 12 grams of Sclerotium Poriae Cocos (*Fu Ling*) and 20 grams of Semen Coicis Lachryma-jobi (*Yi Yi Ren*). If retinal proliferation is extensive, add nine grams each of Radix Rubiae Cordifoliae (*Qian Cao Gen*), Flos Immaturus Sophorae Japonicae (*Huai Hua Mi*), Radix Rubrus Paeoniae Lactiflorae (*Chi Shao*), and Tuber Curcumae (*Yu Jin*). When this condition is accompanied by peripheral neuropathy, add nine grams each of Cortex Erythriniae (*Hai Tong Pi*), Herba Siegesbeckiae (*Xi Xian Cao*), Caulis Millettiae Seu Spatholobi (*Ji Xue Teng*), and Radix Clematidis Chinensis (*Wei Ling Xian*). For albuminuria, add 30 grams of Radix Astragali Membranacei (*Huang*

Qi), 18 grams of Herba Oldenlandiae Diffusae Cum Radice (*Bai Hua She She Cao*), and nine grams each of Rhizoma Imperatae Cylindricae (*Bai Mao Gen*) and Radix Dioscoreae Oppositae (*Shan Yao*). For swelling in the lower limbs, add nine grams each of Radix Achyranthis Bidentatae (*Niu Xi*) and Semen Plantaginis (*Che Qian Zi*). For concomitant constipation, add 3-9 grams of uncooked Radix Et Rhizoma Rhei (*Da Huang*) and nine grams of Semen Pruni (*Yu Li Ren*).

3. Vision degeneration problems are often difficult to treat satisfactorily with either fine needle acupuncture or internally administered Chinese medicinals. One explanation for this is that there is blood stasis in the grandchild network vessels which nourish the eyes, and fine needles are not so good for freeing the flow of the network vessels, especially in this region. Therefore, daily local self-massage, including tapotement around the orbits of the eyes, is recommended as local adjunctive therapy. Likewise, cupping, *gua sha*, and bleeding therapy may also be helpful adjunctively as these are more successful for freeing the flow of the network vessels and dispelling stasis.

4. If there is diabetic retinopathy and generalized signs and symptoms are not marked, this is mainly due to blood stasis. In that case, one should quicken the blood and transform stasis using formulas such as *Tao Hong Si Wu Tang* (Persica & Carthamus Four Materials Decoction) or *Tong Qiao Huo Xue Tang* (Free the Flow of the Orifices & Quicken the Blood Decoction) with additions and subtractions. According to Liu Li, whose study on fundal bleeding is presented above, this condition is intimately associated with blood stasis no matter what the other presenting patterns. The blood-quickening medicinals that Liu favors for the treatment of this condition are Radix Salviae Miltiorrhizae (*Dan Shen*), Herba Lycopi Lucidi (*Ze*

Lan), Lumbricus (*Di Long*), Radix Pseudoginseng (*San Qi*), Flos Carthami Tinctorii (*Hong Hua*), and Radix Ligustici Wallichii (*Chuan Xiong*).

5. Daily supplementation of 1,000IU of vitamin E has been shown to help prevent retinal hemorrhage in patients with diabetic retinopathy. However, ingestion of 3,000IU of vitamin E per day may actually cause or promote retinal hemorrhage.

ENDNOTES:

[1] www.nei.nih.gov/nehep/dedfacts.htm
[2] www.diabetesnet.com/eyes.htm
[3] www.nei.nih.gov, *op. cit.*
[4] http://journal.diabetes.org/FullText/Supplements/DiabetesCare/Supplement100/s73.htm
[5] www.konnections.com/eyedoc/drstart.htm
[6] www.nei.nih.gov, op. cit.
[7] http://204.5.4.24/ISSUE/0998F8.htm
[8] Gao Yan-bin, *Zhong Guo Tang Niao Bing Fang Zhi Tie Se (The Characteristics of the Chinese National Prevention & Treatment of Diabetes)*, Heilongjiang Science & Technology Publishing Co., Harbin, 1995, p. 518
[9] Chen Jin-ding, *The Treatment of Diabetes with Traditional Chinese Medicine*, trans. by Sun Ying-kui & Zhou Shu-hui and revised by Lu Yu-bin, Shandong Science & Technology Publishing Co., Jinan, 1994, p. 170-171
[10] A.k.a. glyburide
[11] Wang Da-qian, "A Clinical Audit of the Treatment of 161 Cases of Diabetic Retinal Bleeding with *Dan Qi Di Huang Tang* (Salvia & Pseudoginseng Rehmannia Decoction)," *Bei Jing Zhong Yi (Beijing Chinese Medicine)*, #5, 1999, p. 25-26
[12] *Ibid.*, p. 26
[13] Ling Bi-da, "The Treatment of Diabetic Eye Ground Bleeding with Integrated Chinese Western Medicine," *Bei Jing Zhong Yi (Beijing Chinese Medicine)*, #3, 1999, p. 17-18
[14] *Ibid.*, p. 18
[15] Gao Lu-wen, "*Wen Dan Tang* (Warm the Gallbladder Decoction) & Diabetic Retinopathy," *Zhong Yi Za Zhi (Journal of Chinese Medicine)*, #2, 2000, p. 20-22
[16] Li Zhen-zhong *et al.*, "The Disease Causes and Mechanisms of Diabetic Proliferative Retinopathy," *Jiang Su Zhong Yi (Jiangsu Chinese Medicine)*, #3, 2000, p. 12-13

18

DIABETIC NEUROPATHY

Diabetic neuropathy is a heterogenous group of clinical disorders manifested by a variety of somatic and autonomic nerve cell defects caused by diabetes. All types of nerve fibers can be involved in diabetic neuropathy. With progression of the neuropathy comes progressive axonal degeneration and loss of myelinated fibers. Diabetic peripheral polyneuropathy, the most common of these disorders, is characterized by loss or reduction of sensation and vibration in the feet and, in some cases, the hands as well as pain and weakness in the feet. Nerve damage caused by diabetes can also lead to problems with autonomic neuropathy involving the digestive tract, heart, and sexual organs, leading to delayed gastric emptying, diarrhea, constipation, dizziness, bladder paralysis, and impotence. Clinical presentation varies based on the distribution and types of nerves involved, and some patients have signs and symptoms that cannot be ascribed to any one neuropathic category. In general, nerve fiber degeneration and neuropathy associated with diabetes affects 60-70% of both type 1 and type 2 diabetes patients. Neuropathy is one of the earliest detectable signs of long-term glucotoxicity during the "silent" prediabetes stage.[1, 2]

Three mechanisms have been postulated to explain the neurodestructive effects of prolonged hyperglycemia: 1) the production of destructive metabolic products, such as sorbitol, 2) protein glycation, and 3) damage resulting from vascular dysfunction, such as increased vascular resistance, abnormal thickening of endoneural blood vessel walls and atherosclerosis, resulting in ischemia. It is also thought by some that immunologic factors may play a part in some diabetic neuropathies, especially autonomic neuropathies. Researchers have suggested that, in diabetic neuropathy, the immune system may target an antigen specific for the peripheral nerve and, possibly, the pancreas. In addition, lymphocytic infiltration in the nerves of some diabetics with neuropathy suggests an immunogenic pathogenesis.[3]

The Western medical classification of diabetic neuropathies is based on the anatomic distribution of the affected nerves, keeping in mind that many diabetes patients have overlapping clinical features and may not be easily exclusively categorized.

A. MONONEUROPATHIES

1. Peripheral mononeuropathy refers to isolated peripheral nerve lesions most commonly seen in older individuals with type 2 diabetes. However, this is not a commonly seen condition. Patients with this type of diabetic neuropathy present with acute onset of pain, paresthesia, and motor weakness along the distribution of the affected nerve. This type of peripheral neuropathy often occurs at sites of external pressure. The peroneal, median, ulnar, sciatic, and femoral nerves are often affected. This type of neuropathy has a high degree of spontaneous reversibility.

2. Cranial mononeuropathy refers to an isolated lesion of cranial nerves III, IV, or VI which control pupillary response and eye movements. The patient presents with unilateral forehead pain, eye pain, and diplopia that develops over a few hours. These neuropathies often gradually improve during the course of 6-12 weeks without treatment other than good glycemic control. However, this type of neuropathy must be differentiated from other potentially life-threatening conditions, such as cerebral aneurysm or tumor, which produce similar symptoms but on a different time scale.

3. Mononeuropathy multiplex refers to impairment of two or more single motor neurons involved at different times.

Patients develop lesions in the femoral, sciatic, and upper limb nerves which are accompanied by asymmetrical weakness, muscle wasting, and progressive sensory loss. This syndrome often occurs simultaneously with distal polyneuropathy. Mononeuropathy multiplex may improve with time but recovery is not always complete.

4. Entrapment neuropathy refers to carpal tunnel, cubital tunnel, and ulnar entrapment syndromes which occur more frequently in diabetes patients and in those with hypothyroidism.

B. POLYNEUROPATHIES

1. Distal sensory neuropathy is the most common of all diabetic neuropathies and is often referred to as "stocking-glove" neuropathy. Its presentations may range from no symptoms at all to excruciating pain and may include painless foot ulceration. Many patients report that the pain, if present, is worse at night. Symptoms usually begin in the feet and spread proximally. Distal sensory neuropathy usually occurs bilaterally and is fairly symmetric. Although symptoms are primarily sensory, there may also be motor weakness, reduced ankle reflexes, reduced vibratory sensation, and impaired peripheral autonomic function.

2. Diabetic amyotrophy is also called diabetic proximal motor neuropathy and diabetic polyradiculoneuropathy. Patients with this syndrome usually present with pain and weakness in the proximal large muscles of the legs and pelvic area. Hence, this condition resembles primary muscle disease. Muscle wasting may be either unilateral or bilateral but is usually asymmetric with bilateral involvement. Patients complain of severe pain in the lumbosacral region, and many patients report loss of appetite, weight loss, and depression. Improvement may take from six months to two years.

3. Thoracoabdominal radiculopathy refers to a rare condition which may, nevertheless, present at the initial diagnosis of diabetes. Nerve roots T8-12 are commonly affected, and patients complain of a tight, band-like or constricting pain in the chest and/or abdomen. Abdominal muscle weakness many lead to herniation and an asymmetric bulge in the abdominal wall. Prognosis is usually good, and most patients recover within several months.

C. AUTONOMIC NEUROPATHIES

Symptomatic diabetic autonomic neuropathy (DAN) occurs in up to 30% of patients with either type 1 or type 2 diabetes. However, many patients with autonomic dysfunction have only mild or subclinical symptoms. Often,

DAN occurs in conjunction with diabetic polyneuropathies. Diabetic autonomic neuropathy may affect any organ or system relying on autonomic innervation.

1. Cardiovascular dysautonomia is a subtype of DAN. The first sign of this species of diabetic autonomic neuropathy is resting tachycardia or chronotropic incompetence (tested with valsalva-related EKG tracing). As cardiac dysautonomia progresses, orthostatic hypotension develops. Symptoms suggestive of orthostatic hypotension include light-headedness, cognitive impairment, blurred vision, and generalized weakness. Orthostatic hypotension may become so severe that the patient becomes bedridden. Cardiac involvement increases the risk for a malignant arrhythmia, such as complete block.

2. Gastrointestinal dysautonomia is often characterized by constipation. Diabetic gastroparesis is common as well, with patients often complaining of intermittent nausea, vomiting, early satiety, epigastric pain, and postprandial abdominal distention. A complication of this type of gastrointestinal dysautonomia is intermittent diabetic autonomic diarrhea (characteristically nocturnal) with episodes of profuse, watery diarrhea and even possible fecal incontinence which lasts for several days.

3. Genitourinary dysautonomia is usually first evidenced in diabetic men as erectile dysfunction. Erectile failure is only partial at first but often becomes complete by two years. Other genitourinary complications include residual urine in the bladder leading to retention, overflow incontinence, and frequent secondary urinary tract infections due to large post-voiding urine residue.

4. Sudomotor dysautonomia refers to various forms of abnormal perspiration, such as hyperhidrosis or anhidrosis of the extremities or gustatory sweating accompanied by venous congestion, pain, and redness of the feet.

DIABETIC NEUROPATHIC FOOT ULCERATION

The risk of lower limb amputation in patients affected with diabetes is 15-40 times higher than in non-diabetic patients, and ulceration of the foot is often the initiating lesion leading to such amputation.[4] At least 15% of all people with diabetes eventually have a foot ulcer, and six out of every 1,000 people with diabetes have an amputation.[5] Patients with diabetes are particularly vulnerable to foot ulceration due to the coexistence of peripheral neuropathy (PN) and peripheral vascular disease (PVD). Sensory neuropathy leads to unperceived, excessive, and repetitive pressure on plantar bony prominences resulting in skin ulceration. Autonomic dysfunction results in dry, cracked, and scaly skin that is prone to fissure and subsequent ulcer formation. Corns and calluses develop due to persistent friction and often ulcerate with little perception by patients with neuropathy. Additionally, ingrown nails and unperceived foreign bodies in the foot lead to ulceration and possible infection. For the Chinese medical pattern discrimination and treatment of diabetic foot ulceration, see the chapter on Diabetic Arteriosclerosis Obliterans and Acromelic Gangrene below.

The Western medical diagnosis of diabetic neuropathy is based on the patient's symptoms and a physical exam which includes checking muscle strength, reflexes, and sensitivity to position, vibration, temperature, and light touch. In addition, nerve conduction studies check the flow of electrical current through a nerve, and electromyography may be used to see how well muscles respond to electrical impulses transmitted by nearby nerves. Ultrasound can be used to determine how well the bladder and other parts of the urinary tract are functioning. Nerve biopsies are usually only conducted in research settings. Patients suspected of autonomic neuropathy may be referred to a gastroenterologist for additional tests.[6] Diabetic neuropathy has a wide array of presentation that must be differentiated from other disorders that may have similar features, and as many as 10% of patients with diabetes have an alternative cause for the neuropathy.[7]

The Western medical treatment of diabetic neuropathy consists of tight and stable glycemic control. Some studies suggest that the stability of glycemic control may be more important for relieving neuropathic pain than the actual level of blood glucose.[8] However, intensive insulin therapy increases the risk of symptomatic hypoglycemia and weight gain two to three-fold.[9] For burning, tingling, or numbness, doctors may suggest such analgesics as aspirin, acetaminophen, or anti-inflammatory drugs, such as ibuprofen. Tricyclic antidepressants, such as amitriptyline alone or in combination with fluphenazine, or anticonvulsant medications, such as carbamazepine, may be helpful. Codeine is sometimes prescribed for short-term use to relieve severe pain. Other treatments for pain relief include topical creams containing capsicum, transcutaneous electronic nerve stimulation (TENS), hypnosis, biofeedback, and relaxation training. For mild symptoms of delayed gastric emptying, Western medical doctors usually suggest eating small, frequent meals and avoiding fat. For severe gastroparesis, they may prescribe metoclopramide which speeds digestion and helps relieve nausea. To relieve diarrhea, immodium may be used. For other bowel problems, antibiotics or clonidine HCl are sometimes effective. For orthostatic hypotension, salt-retaining hormones, such as fludrocortisone, may be prescribed as well as full length elastic stockings. Muscle weakness and loss of coordination caused by diabetic neuropathy can often be helped by physical therapy. For erectile dysfunction in diabetic men, Western medical treatments include the prescription of sildenafil citrate (Viagra), use of mechanical vacuum devices or injection of vasodilators into the penis before sex, or surgical implantation of inflatable or semirigid devices in the penis. For diabetic foot and lower limb ulceration, topical antibiotics, such as silver sulfadiazine and mupirocin, may be tried, and recently, becaplermin gel, a genetically engineered recombinant human platelet-derived growth factor, has shown promise in the promotion of ulcer healing in patients with diabetes. Experimental drugs under research for the treatment of diabetic neuropathy at the time of this writing include myoinositaol and aminoguanidine.

In terms of prognosis, it depends largely on the optimal management of the underlying condition of diabetes. Tight glycemic control may halt the progression of the neuropathy and even improve its symptoms. However, recovery, when that is possible, tends to be slow.[10]

CHINESE DISEASE MECHANISMS:

As with diabetes in general, the root disease mechanisms of diabetic neuropathy are a qi and yin vacuity (complicated by liver depression), while the branch disease mechanisms are lung-stomach dryness and heat. Over time, this core qi and yin vacuity may give rise to either or both a blood vacuity or yang vacuity. Qi and blood are mutually related. Qi is able to engender the blood. Therefore, if there is a qi vacuity, the engenderment of blood may be insufficient. On the one hand, if the spleen qi is vacuous and weak, the latter heaven source of transformation of the blood may be insufficient. On the other, if the kidney qi is vacuous and weak, a former heaven kidney essence insufficiency will not be able to transform the blood. Thus either of these two qi vacuity scenarios may result in blood vacuity. Furthermore, since fluids and blood share a common source, if yin fluids become depleted and are consumed, this may also result in a constructive and blood insufficiency leading to a blood vacuity.

If yin and yang both become vacuous and qi and blood are depleted and consumed, the physiological activities of the viscera and bowels will be lowered or diminished. For instance, a yang qi vacuity externally may lead to the defensive yang not securing, the blood vessels losing their smooth and easy flow, and inability to warm and shine the skin and flesh. Internally, such a yang qi vacuity may lead to the functions of respiration of the great qi and the digestion of water and grains being lowered. Hence one may see fear of cold, chilled limbs, lassitude of the spirit, lack of strength, a bright white facial complexion, shortness of breath, spontaneous perspiration, and easy contraction of external evils. On the other hand, if yin blood become sdepleted and consumed, then the viscera and bowels, the formal body, the channels and network vessels, the five officials (i.e., the five senses), and the nine orifices may all lose their moistening and nourishment, thus gradually leading to desiccation and wilting (or atrophy). Due to these pathological changes, the vision may become blurred, the hands and feet may become numb, movement may lack force, the flesh and muscles may become atrophied, and there may be easy fatigue and taxation. In addition, one's thinking may become slowed and confused, thus leading to feeblemindedness, impaired memory, insomnia, anxiety, and susceptibility to fright.

In terms of simultaneous branch repletions, these include dampness, heat, phlegm, and turbidity as well as qi stagnation and blood stasis. If there is a lung-spleen qi vacuity, the movement of water dampness will lose its free flow and regulation. If there is a kidney qi vacuity, the kidney-bladder qi will not transform water. In either case, if dampness accumulates and endures, it may become phlegm. If phlegm turbidity brews and accumulates, over time it may transform heat. Thus damp heat, phlegm, and turbidity may congest in the center of the chest, leading to heart chest glomus, oppression, distention, and fullness, heart palpitations, and shortness of breath. If these disease evils stagnate in the middle burner, this may lead to devitalized eating and drinking, epigastric glomus and fullness, nausea, and upward counterflow. If these disease evils ascend and mist the clear orifices, they may result in head and eye dimness and misting, essence spirit depression, heaviness of the head, and somnolence. If damp heat pours downward, one may see inhibited urination and non-crisp defecation.

If emotional depression is not soothed, if there is phlegm and stasis obstructing and stagnating, and/or there is viscera and bowel qi vacuity, movement and transportation will lose their force, the qi will stagnate, and the movement of blood will not be free-flowing. In addition, yin vacuity with burning heat may boil and stew the blood and fluids causing the blood to become thickened, making its flow all the more difficult. Any or all of these disease mechanisms may result in blood stasis, and, if there is qi stagnation and blood stasis, one may see chest oppression and pain or abdominal fullness, distention, and pain. If phlegm and stasis impede

and obstruct the channels and vessels in the four extremities, this may also lead to numbness and pain of the extremities as well as inhibited walking.

In terms of the viscera and bowel location of the disease mechanisms of diabetic neuropathy, these are mainly located in the four viscera of the heart, spleen, liver, and kidneys. In terms of the heart, this may include the mechanisms of heart, qi, blood, yin, and/or yang vacuities, heart blood stasis, and phlegm turbidity obstructing and stagnating in the heart orifices. The clinical symptoms of these heart-based disease mechanisms are chest oppression and pain, heart palpitations, fearful throbbing, shortness of breath, and head and eye dimming and misting. The disease mechanisms located in the spleen include central qi vacuity weakness, spleen yang devitalization, qi and blood dual vacuity, and phlegm turbidity obstructing the center, thus giving rise to devitalized eating and drinking, fatigue, lack of strength, emaciation of the flesh and muscles, nausea, abdominal distention, stomach venter glomus and fullness, diarrhea, and/or constipation. The disease mechanisms centered in the liver include liver qi depression and binding, qi stagnation not smoothly flowing, liver blood depletion and vacuity, liver qi attacking the spleen, and liver channel damp heat. Clinically, these disease mechanisms are responsible for chest and rib-side distention and fullness, emotional depression, dizziness and vertigo, blurred vision, spasm and contraction of the sinew vessels, numbness and pain of the extremities, a bitter taste in the mouth, and torpid intake. As for the disease mechanisms located in the kidneys, these include kidney qi vacuity, kidney yin vacuity and depletion, kidney yang vacuity, kidney essence depletion and detriment, and lower burner damp heat. The clinical signs and symptoms produced by these mechanisms are low back and knee soreness and limpness, impotence, inhibited urination, dizziness and vertigo, psychological disturbances, dementia, and muscular atrophy. In real life, it is common to find disease mechanisms involving two or more viscera as well as vacuities compounded by repletion. Thus the clinical manifestations of diabetic neuropathy are many and varied depending on the age, sex, and constitution of the patient and their personal mix of disease mechanisms.

TREATMENT BASED ON PATTERN DISCRIMINATION:

PERIPHERAL NEUROPATHY

1. QI & BLOOD DEPLETION & VACUITY PATTERN

MAIN SYMPTOMS: Numbness and pain of the four limbs, cramping and spasms, lack of strength, possible flesh and muscle emaciation, a sallow yellow, lusterless facial complexion, pale white lips and nails, profuse or scanty sweating, fatigue, lassitude of the spirit, shortness of breath, disinclination to speak and/or faint, weak voice, heart palpitations, dizziness, a pale tongue with thin, white fur, and a fine, forceless pulse

TREATMENT PRINCIPLES: Regulate and supplement the qi and blood

RX: *Huang Qi Gui Zhi Wu Wu Tang Jia Jian* (Astragalus & Cinnamon Twigs Five Materials Decoction with Additions & Subtractions)

INGREDIENTS: Radix Astragali Membranacei (*Huang Qi*), 30g, Radix Albus Paeoniae Lactiflorae (*Bai Shao*) and Radix Achyranthis Bidentatae (*Niu Xi*), 15g each, Radix Angelicae Sinensis (*Dang Gui*), 12g, Ramulus Cinnamomi Cassiae (*Gui Zhi*), Radix Gentianae Macrocphyllae (*Qin Jiao*), and Ramulus Mori Albi (*Sang Zhi*), 9g each

FORMULA ANALYSIS: A heavy dose of *Huang Qi* supplements qi vacuity, while the combination of it plus *Dang Gui* and *Bai Shao* supplements blood vacuity. *Gui Zhi, Qin Jiao,* and *Sang Zhi* warm, free the flow, and extend or spread the qi and blood to the four corners (*i.e.,* the four extremities).

ADDITIONS & SUBTRACTIONS: If there is mostly qi vacuity, use *Bu Zhong Yi Qi Tang Jia Wei* (Supplement the Center & Boost the Qi Decoction with Added Flavors): Astragali Membranacei (*Huang Qi*), 30g, Radix Angelicae Sinensis (*Dang Gui*), 12g, Radix Codonopsitis Pilosulae (*Dang Shen*), Rhizoma Atractylodis Macrocephalae (*Bai Zhu*), Radix Clematidis Chinensis (*Wei Ling Xian*), Rhizoma Curcumae Longae (*Jiang Huang*), and Cortex Radicis Acanthopanacis Gracilistylis (*Wu Jia Pi*), 9g each, Pericarpium Citri Reticulatae (*Chen Pi*) and mix-fried Radix Glycyrrhizae (*Gan Cao*), 6g each, Rhizoma Cimicifugae (*Sheng Ma*), 4.5g, and Radix Bupleuri (*Chai Hu*) and Radix Lateralis Praeparatus Aconiti Carmichaeli (*Fu Zi*), 3g each.

For predominantly blood vacuity, use *Si Wu Tang Jia Wei* (Four Materials Decoction with Added Flavors): Radix Astragali Membranacei (*Huang Qi*), 30g, Radix Albus Paeoniae Lactiflorae (*Bai Shao*), 18g, cooked Radix Rehmanniae (*Shu Di*) and Radix Angelicae Sinensis (*Dang Gui*), 12g each, Radix Ligustici Wallichii (*Chuan Xiong*), Radix Codonopsitis Pilosulae (*Dang Shen*), and Ramulus Cinnamomi Cassiae (*Gui Zhi*), 9g each.

If there is concomitant blood stasis, one can add nine grams each of Flos Carthami Tinctorii (*Hong Hua*) and Semen Pruni Persicae (*Tao Ren*) to any of the above formulas.

ACUPUNCTURE & MOXIBUSTION: *Ge Shu* (Bl 17), *Gan Shu* (Bl 18), *Pi Shu* (Bl 20), *Zu San Li* (St 36), *San Yin Jiao* (Sp 6), local points depending on the site of pain or numbness

FORMULA ANALYSIS: Supplementing *Ge Shu* and *Gan Shu* supplements the liver and nourishes the blood. Supplementing *Pi Shu, Zu San Li,* and *San Yin Jiao* supplements the spleen, the latter heaven root of the engenderment and transformation of qi and blood. In addition, *Zu San Li* is the main point for all diseases of the lower extremities. Even supplementing-even draining the local points moves the qi and quickens the blood in the network vessels.

ADDITIONS & SUBTRACTIONS: If there is pain in the heel, needle *Kun Lun* (Bl 60). If there is tingling or burning on the sole of the foot, add *Yong Quan* (Ki 1). If there is pain, tingling, or numbness of the toes, needle the *Ba Feng* (M-LE-8).

2. QI STAGNATION & BLOOD STASIS PATTERN

MAIN SYMPTOMS: Numbness of the four extremities accompanied by distention and pain or pain like being pricked by a needle which is soothed when it is pressed, dry, scaly skin, a dark, dusky facial complexion, purplish lips, a dark or purple tongue or possible static macules or spots on the tongue with thin, somewhat dryish fur, and a bowstring, choppy pulse

NOTE: In real life, this pattern mostly complicates other patterns of diabetic peripheral neuropathy. It is rarely, if ever, met in this simple, discrete form.

TREATMENT PRINCIPLES: Move the qi, quicken the blood, and free the flow of the network vessels

RX: *Si Ni San* (Four Counterflows Powder) plus *Tao Hong Si Wu Tang* (Persica & Carthamus Four Materials Decoction) with additions and subtractions

INGREDIENTS: Radix Salviae Miltiorrhizae (*Dan Shen*), 30g, cooked Radix Rehmanniae (*Shu Di*), Radix Ligustici Wallichii (*Chuan Xiong*), and Radix Albus Paeoniae Lactiflorae (*Bai Shao*), 15g each, Radix Angelicae Sinensis (*Dang Gui*), 12g, Radix Bupleuri (*Chai Hu*), Fructus Immaturus Citri Aurantii (*Zhi Shi*), Semen Pruni

Persicae (*Tao Ren*), and Flos Carthami Tinctorii (*Hong Hua*), 9g each, and Radix Glycyrrhizae (*Gan Cao*), 6g

FORMULA ANALYSIS: *Chai Hu* upbears yang and soothes depression. *Zhi Shi* descends the qi and breaks binding. Together, these two medicinals move the qi and free the flow of extension or spreading. *Bai Shao* is an essential medicinal for harmonizing the blood, while *Tao Ren*, *Hong Hua*, and *Dan Shen* quicken the blood and free the flow of the network vessels. *Dang Gui*, *Bai Shao*, *Chuan Xiong*, and *Shu Di* both move and nourish the blood.

ADDITIONS & SUBTRACTIONS: If qi stagnation is predominant with numbness that comes and goes, slight aching and pain, a dark tongue but no static spots or macules, and a bowstring pulse, use *Qiang Huo Xing Bi Tang* (Notopterygium Move Impediment Decoction): Radix Gentianae Macrophyllae (*Qin Jiao*) and Radix Dipsaci (*Xu Duan*), 15g each, Radix Angelicae Sinensis (*Dang Gui*), 12g, Radix Clematidis Chinensis (*Wei Ling Xian*), Radix Et Rhizoma Notopterygii (*Qiang Huo*), and Radix Ledebouriellae Divaricatae (*Fang Feng*), 9g each, and Flos Carthami Tinctorii (*Hong Hua*), Resina Olibani (*Ru Xiang*), and Resina Myrrhae (*Mo Yao*), 6g each.

If there is more serious blood stasis with numbness and aching and pain which never gets less, cyanotic lips, definite static macules or spots on the tongue, and a deep, choppy pulse, use *Shen Tong Zhu Yu Tang* (Body Pain Dispel Stasis Decoction): Radix Gentianae Macrophyllae (*Qin Jiao*), 15g, Radix Achyranthis Bidentatae (*Niu Xi*), Radix Angelicae Sinensis (*Dang Gui*), and Radix Et Rhizoma Notpterygii (*Qiang Huo*), 12g each, Semen Pruni Persicae (*Tao Ren*), Flos Carthami Tinctorii (*Hong Hua*), Feces Trogopterori Seu Pteromi (*Wu Ling Zhi*), Rhizoma Cyperi Rotundi (*Xiang Fu*), and Lumbricus (*Di Long*), 9g each, Lignum Aquilariae Agallochae (*Chen Xiang*), 6g, and Radix Glycyrrhizae (*Gan Cao*), 3g.

ACUPUNCTURE & MOXIBUSTION: *Xue Hai* (Sp 10), *San Yin Jiao* (Sp 6), *Tai Chong* (Liv 3), *He Gu* (LI 4), *Zu San Li* (St 36), local points depending on the location of the pain and/or numbness

FORMULA ANALYSIS: Draining *Xue Hai*, *San Yin Jiao*, and *He Gu* quickens the blood and dispels stasis, while draining *Tai Chong* and *He Gu* courses the liver and rectifies the qi. *Zu San Li* is the main point for treating all diseases of the lower extremities. Draining the local points frees the flow of the qi and blood in the network vessels.

ADDITIONS & SUBTRACTIONS: If there is pain in the

heel, needle *Kun Lun* (Bl 60). If there is tingling or burning on the sole of the foot, add *Yong Quan* (Ki 1). If there is pain, tingling, or numbness of the toes, needle the *Ba Feng* (M-LE-8).

3. LIVER BLOOD-KIDNEY YIN VACUITY PATTERN

MAIN SYMPTOMS: A long, slow disease course with gradual but progressive atrophy, weakness, and loss of use of the upper or lower limbs, low back and knee soreness and limpness, emaciation, numbness and tingling of the hands and feet, dizziness, tinnitus, blurred vision, tidal heat, night sweats, a dry mouth and a parched throat, hoarse voice, a red crimson tongue with scanty fluids and teethmarks on its edges with possible cracks and fissures, and a fine, rapid or fine, bowstring, and rapid pulse

TREATMENT PRINCIPLES: Supplement the liver and boost the kidneys, diffuse impediment and harmonize the network vessels

RX: *Hu Qian Wan Jia Jian* (Hidden Tiger Pills with Additions & Subtractions)

INGREDIENTS: Plastrum Testudinis (*Gui Ban*), cooked Radix Rehmanniae (*Shu Di*), and Ramulus Mori Albi (*Sang Zhi*), 30g each, Radix Cyathulae (*Chuan Niu Xi*), 15g, Radix Angelicae Sinensis (*Dang Gui*), processed Radix Polygoni Multiflori (*He Shou Wu*), Radix Rubrus Paeoniae Lactiflorae (*Chi Shao*), and Radix Et Rhizoma Notopterygii (*Qiang Huo*), 12g each, and Cortex Phellodendri (*Huang Bai*), Rhizoma Anemarrhenae Asphelodis (*Zhi Mu*), and Gelatinum Corii Asini (*E Jiao*), 9g each

ANALYSIS OF FORMULA: *Gui Ban*, *Shu Di*, *He Shou Wu*, *Dang Gui*, and *E Jiao* nourish liver blood and enrich kidney yin. In addition, *Gui Ban* strengthens the sinews and reinforces the bones. *Huang Bai* and *Zhi Mu* clear and descend vacuity heat. *Sang Zhi* and *Qiang Huo* dispel wind, eliminate dampness, and free the flow of impediment. *Chuan Niu Xi*, *Dang Gui*, and *Chi Shao* quicken the blood and free the flow of the network vessels.

ADDITIONS & SUBTRACTIONS: If yin vacuity has reached yang with chilled limbs, a pale tongue, and a deep, fine pulse, add nine grams each of Gelatinum Cornu Cervi (*Lu Jiao Jiao*), Fructus Psoraleae Corylifoliae (*Bu Gu Zhi*), Cortex Cinnamomi Cassiae (*Rou Gui*), and Radix Lateralis Praeparatus Aconiti Carmichaeli (*Fu Zi*). If there is concomitant qi vacuity with fatigue and lack of strength, add 30 grams of Radix Astragali Membranacei

(*Huang Qi*) and nine grams of Radix Psuedostellariae Heterophyllae (*Tai Zi Shen*). If there is numbness in the lower extremities, add nine grams each of Radix Achyranthis Bidentatae (*Niu Xi*) and Fructus Chaenomelis Lagenariae (*Mu Gua*). If there is heavy dampness and diarrhea, delete *Shu Di* and add 21 grams of Semen Coicis Lachyrma-jobi (*Yi Yi Ren*) and nine grams each of Rhizoma Atractylodis Macrocephalae (*Bai Zhu*) and Rhizoma Atractylodis (*Cang Zhu*). If there is simultaneous blood stasis, add 30 grams of Radix Salviae Miltiorrhizae (*Dan Shen*) and nine grams each of Flos Carthami Tinctorii (*Hong Hua*), Semen Pruni Persicae (*Tao Ren*), and Radix Rubrus Paeoniae Lactiflorae (*Chi Shao*). If there is enduring disease and recalcitrant phlegm, add nine grams each of Buthus Martensis (*Quan Xie*), Scolopendra Subspinipes (*Wu Gong*), and Zaocys Dhumnades (*Wu Shao She*).

If there is vexatious heat in the five hearts, insomnia, restlessness, and heat in the feet with desiccation and wilting, use *Zhi Bai Di Huang Tang Jia Wei* (Anemarrhena & Phellodendron Rehmannia Decoction with Added Flavors): Radix Gentianae Macrophyllae (*Qin Jiao*), 18g, Radix Achyranthis Bidentatae (*Niu Xi*), Gelatinum Cornu Cervi (*Lu Jiao Jiao*), and Plastrum Testudinis (*Gui Ban*), 15g each, cooked Radix Rehmanniae (*Shu Di*) and Fructus Lycii Chinensis (*Gou Qi Zi*), 12g each, and Radix Dioscoreae Oppositae (*Shan Yao*), Fructus Corni Officinalis (*Shan Zhu Yu*), Sclerotium Poriae Cocos (*Fu Ling*), Rhizoma Alismatis (*Ze Xie*), Rhizoma Anemarrhenae Aspheloidis (*Zhi Mu*), and Cortex Phellodendri (*Huang Bai*), 9g each.

If there is simultaneous qi and blood vacuity, use *Du Huo Ji Sheng Tang Jia Jian* (Angelica Pubescens & Loranthus Decoction with Additions & Subtractions): Gentianae Macrophyllae (*Qin Jiao*), 15g, cooked Radix Rehmanniae (*Shu Di*), Ramulus Loranthi Seu Visci (*Sang Ji Sheng*), Radix Codonopsitis Pilosulae (*Dang Shen*), and Sclerotium Poriae Cocos (*Fu Ling*), 12g each, Radix Angelicae Pubescentis (*Du Huo*), Radix Ledebouriellae Divaricatae (*Fang Feng*), Cortex Eucommiae Ulmoidis (*Du Zhong*), Radix Achyranthis Bidentatae (*Niu Xi*), Radix Angelicae Sinensis (*Dang Gui*), Radix Ligustici Wallichii (*Chuan Xiong*), Radix Albus Paeoniae Lactiflorae (*Bai Shao*), Ramulus Cinnamomi Cassiae (*Gui Zhi*), and Fructus Chaenomelis Lagenariae (*Mu Gua*), 9g each, and Radix Glycyrrhizae (*Gan Cao*), 6g. If there is concomitant blood stasis, add nine grams each of Flos Carthami Tinctorii (*Hong Hua*) and Semen Pruni Persicae (*Tao Ren*).

ACUPUNCTURE & MOXIBUSTION: *San Yin Jiao* (Sp 6),

Tai Xi (Ki 3), *Fu Liu* (Ki 7), *Zu San Li* (St 36), *Xue Hai* (Sp 10), local points depending on the site of pain or numbness

ANALYSIS OF FORMULA: Supplementing *San Yin Jiao*, *Tai Xi*, and *Fu Liu* supplements the kidneys and enriches yin. Supplementing *San Yin Jiao* and *Zu San Li* supplements the spleen and boosts the qi. In addition, needling *Zu San Li* frees the flow of qi and blood in the lower extremities. Draining *Xue Hai* quickens the blood and dispels stasis. Even supplementing-even draining the local points frees the flow of the qi and blood in the network vessels.

ADDITIONS & SUBTRACTIONS: For more marked spleen qi vacuity, add *Pi Shu* (Bl 20) and *Wei Shu* (Bl 21). For marked kidney vacuity, add *Shen Shu* (Bl 23). If there is concomitant yang vacuity, moxa *Shen Shu* (Bl 23) and *Ming Men* (GV 4). If there is tingling or burning on the sole of the foot, add *Yong Quan* (Ki 1). If there is pain, tingling, or numbness of the toes, needle the *Ba Feng* (M-LE-8).

4. DAMP HEAT OBSTRUCTING THE NETWORK VESSELS PATTERN

MAIN SYMPTOMS: Lower limb numbness and tingling accompanied by a burning hot, painful sensation, possible redness and swelling of the affected areas, a dark red tongue with yellow-white, slimy fur, and a bowstring, slippery, rapid or soggy, rapid pulse

TREATMENT PRINCIPLES: Clear heat, disinhibit dampness, and quicken the blood

RX: *Jia Wei Er Miao San Jia Jian* (Added Flavors Two Wonders Powder with Additions & Subtractions)

INGREDIENTS: Semen Coicis Lachryma-jobi (*Yi Yi Ren*), 30g, Sclerotium Poriae Cocos (*Fu Ling*) and Radix Achyranthis Bidentatae (*Niu Xi*), 15g each, Fructus Chaenomelis Lagenariae (*Mu Gua*), 12g, and Extremtias Radicis Angelicae Sinensis (*Dang Gui Wei*), Rhizoma Atractylodis (*Cang Zhu*), Cortex Phellodendri (*Huang Bai*), Radix Stephaniae Tetrandrae (*Han Fang Ji*), Plastrum Testudinis (*Gui Ban*), Radix Scutellariae Baicalensis (*Huang Qin*), Rhizoma Alismatis (*Ze Xie*), and Radix Gentianae Macrophyllae (*Qin Jiao*), 9g each

FORMULA ANALYSIS: *Huang Bai* and *Huang Qin* clear heat and eliminate dampness. *Cang Zhu* dries dampness. *Fu Ling* and *Ze Xie* disinhibit dampness. *Qin Jiao*, *Niu Xi*, *Yi Yi Ren*, and *Han Fang Ji* abduct dampness and heat and move it downward. *Dang Gui Wei* quickens the blood.

ADDITIONS & SUBTRACTIONS: If there is flesh and muscle emaciation, burning heat in both feet, heart vexation, a red tongue tip, or peeled fur, and a fine, rapid pulse signifying that damp heat has damaged yin, add 12 grams each of Tuber Ophiopogonis Japonici (*Mai Men Dong*), Radix Glehniae Littoralis (*Sha Shen*), Radix Trichosanthis Kirlowii (*Tian Hua Fen*), and Radix Dioscoreae Oppositae (*Shan Yao*) to clear heat and engender fluids.

ACUPUNCTURE & MOXIBUSTION: *Xue Hai* (Sp 10), *Yin Ling Quan* (Sp 9), *San Yin Jiao* (Sp 6), *Zu San Li* (St 36), local points depending on the area of pain or numbness

ANALYSIS OF FORMULA: Draining *Xue Hai* quickens the blood and dispels stasis. Draining *Yin Ling Quan* clears heat and eliminates dampness, especially from the lower half of the body. When *San Yin Jiao* is combined with *Yin Ling Quan*, it strengthens the function of clearing and eliminating dampness and heat from the lower limbs. *Zu San Li* is a main point for treating all diseases of the lower limbs. Draining the local points moves and quickens the qi and blood in the network vessels.

ADDITIONS & SUBTRACTIONS: If there is pain in the heel, needle *Kun Lun* (Bl 60). If there is tingling or burning on the sole of the foot, add *Yong Quan* (Ki 1). If there is pain, tingling, or numbness of the toes, needle the *Ba Feng* (M-LE-8). If there is concomitant spleen vacuity, supplement *Pi Shu* (Bl 20) and *Wei Shu* (Bl 21). If damp heat has damaged yin, supplement *Shen Shu* (Bl 23) and *Tai Xi* (Ki 3). If there is concomitant liver depression, add draining *Tai Chong* (Liv 3) and *He Gu* (LI 4). If there is concomitant phlegm turbidity, add draining *Feng Long* (St 40).

POLYRADICULONEUROPATHY

1. DAMP HEAT ATTACKING & EXCESSIVENESS PATTERN

MAIN SYMPTOMS: Cramping and numbness of the limbs, abnormal sensations, possible fatigue and lack of strength, bodily heat, encumbered limbs, heavy-headedness as if the head were wrapped, chest and duct glomus and oppression, sticky, turbid, non-crisp stools, reddish, choppy urination with heat and pain, a red, enlarged tongue with slimy, yellow fur, and a slippery, rapid pulse

TREATMENT PRINCIPLES: Clear heat and dry dampness

RX: *Jia Wei Er Miao San Jia Jian* (Added Flavors Two Wonders Powder with Additions & Subtractions)

INGREDIENTS: Radix Achyranthis Bidentatae (*Niu Xi*) and Rhizoma Dioscoreae Hypoglaucae (*Bie Xie*), 15g each, Rhizoma Atractylodis (*Cang Zhu*), Cortex Phellodendri (*Huang Bai*), Radix Angelicae Sinensis (*Dang Gui*), Plastrum Testudinis (*Gui Ban*), and Radix Stephaniae Tetrandrae (*Han Fang Ji*), 9g each

FORMULA ANALYSIS: *Huang Bai* and *Cang Zhu* transform dampness and clear heat. *Han Fang Ji* and *Bie Xie* disinhibit dampness. *Dang Gui* and *Niu Xi* quicken the blood, and *Gui Ban* enriches yin.

ADDITIONS & SUBTRACTIONS: If there is simultaneous external contraction of evils, add nine grams each of Radix Ledebouriellae Divaricatae (*Fang Feng*), Radix Bupleuri (*Chai Hu*), and Radix Angelicae Pubescentis (*Du Huo*). If the urination is red, choppy, hot, and painful and dribbles and drips without stopping, add 12 grams each of Sclerotium Poriae Cocos (*Fu Ling*) and Sclerotium Polypori Umbellati (*Zhu Ling*) and nine grams each of Rhizoma Alismatis (*Ze Xie*), Fructus Gardeniae Jasminoidis (*Zhi Zi*), and Semen Plantaginis (*Che Qian Zi*) to clear and disinhibit lower burner dampness and heat.

If damp heat endures for a long time and is accompanied by liver-kidney depletion and vacuity, use *Qi Wei Cang Bai San* (Seven Flavors Atractylodes & Phellodendron Powder) to clear heat and disinhibit dampness at the same time as supplementing the kidneys and strengthening the bones: Rhizoma Atractylodis (*Cang Zhu*), Cortex Phellodendri (*Huang Bai*), Radix Angelicae Sinensis (*Dang Gui*), Cortex Eucommiae Ulmoidis (*Du Zhong*), Radix Ligustici Wallichii (*Chuan Xiong*), Fructus Psoraleae Corylifoliae (*Bu Gu Zhi*), and Rhizoma Atractylodis Macrocephalae (*Bai Zhu*), 9g each.

ACUPUNCTURE & MOXIBUSTION: *Yin Ling Quan* (Sp 9), *Yang Ling Quan* (GB 34), *Huan Tiao* (GB 30), *Ba Liao* (Bl 31-34), *Zu San Li* (St 36), local points depending on the site of numbness, pain, or weakness

FORMULA ANALYSIS: Draining *Yin Ling Quan* needled through to *Yang Ling Quan* clears heat and disinhibits dampness. Draining *Huan Tiao* and the *Ba Liao* moves the qi and quickens the blood in the lumbosacral area. *Zu San Li* is the main point for all diseases of the lower extremities.

ADDITIONS & SUBTRACTIONS: If there is concomitant blood stasis, add draining *Xue Hai* (Sp 10) and *San Yin Jiao* (Sp 6). If there is concomitant liver depression qi stagnation, add draining *Tai Chong* (Liv 3) and *He Gu* (LI

4). For lumbar pain, add *Shen Shu* (Bl 23) and *Da Chang Shu* (Bl 25).

2. STATIC BLOOD OBSTRUCTING & STAGNATING PATTERN

MAIN SYMPTOMS: Limpness, weakness, and lack of strength of the four limbs, possible numbness and insensitivity, possible spasm and cramping, inhibited bending and stretching, dry, scaly skin, cyanotic lips, a purplish tongue, possible static macules or spots on the tongue, and a slow, choppy, stagnant pulse

TREATMENT PRINCIPLES: Quicken the blood and transform stasis

RX: *Tao Hong Si Wu Tang Jia Jian* (Persica & Carthamus Four Materials Decoction with Additions & Subtractions)

INGREDIENTS: Radix Achyranthis Bidentatae (*Niu Xi*), Radix Astragali Membranacei (*Huang Qi*), Radix Albus Paeoniae Lactiflorae (*Bai Shao*), Radix Ligustici Wallichii (*Chuan Xiong*), and cooked Radix Rehmanniae (*Shu Di*), 15g each, Radix Angelicae Sinensis (*Dang Gui*), 12g, Semen Pruni Persicae (*Tao Ren*) and Flos Carthami Tinctorii (*Hong Hua*), 9g each

FORMULA ANALYSIS: *Shu Di, Dang Gui, Chuan Xiong,* and *Bai Shao* supplement the blood. *Tao Ren* and *Hong Hua* quicken the blood and transform stasis. *Huang Qi* boosts the qi in order to strengthen the quickening of the blood, and *Niu Xi* quickens the blood and strengthens the bones.

ADDITIONS & SUBTRACTIONS: If there is simultaneous damp heat, add nine grams each of Rhizoma Atractylodis (*Cang Zhu*) and Cortex Phellodendri (*Huang Bai*) to dry dampness and clear heat. If phlegm is mixed with blood stasis, add 12 grams each of Rhizoma Pinelliae Ternatae (*Ban Xia*) and Sclerotium Poriae Cocos (*Fu Ling*), nine grams of Pericarpium Citri Reticulatae (*Chen Pi*), and three slices of uncooked Rhizoma Zingiberis (*Sheng Jiang*). If enduring disease has entered the network vessels, add nine grams each of Buthus Martensis (*Quan Xie*), Euployphaga Seu Opistoplatiae (*Tu Bei Chong*), and Zaocys Dhumnades (*Wu Shao She*) to free the flow of the network vessels.

ACUPUNCTURE & MOXIBUSTION: *Xue Hai* (Sp 10), *He Gu* (LI 4), *Tai Chong* (Liv 3), local points depending on the affected areas

FORMULA ANALYSIS: Draining *Xue Hai* quickens the blood and transforms stasis. Draining *Tai Chong* and *He Gu* courses the liver and rectifies the qi, remembering that the qi moves the blood. Draining the local points frees the flow of the network vessels.

ADDITIONS & SUBTRACTIONS: One may guasha the affected areas and/or bleed any visibly engorged venules in order to free the flow of the network vessels.

NOTE: Fine needle treatment by itself is not very effective for treating blood stasis.

3. LIVER-KIDNEY DEPLETION & VACUITY PATTERN

MAIN SYMPTOMS: Single-sided or bilateral lower extremity disturbances in sensation, pain which comes and goes, inhibition of bending and stretching the lower extremities, possible atrophy and loss of function, numbness of the skin, lower and upper back wilting and limpness, dizziness, tinnitus, impotence, menstrual irregularities, a pale red tongue with scanty fur, and a deep, fine or fine and rapid pulse

TREATMENT PRINCIPLES: Enrich and supplement the liver and kidneys

RX: *Hu Qian Wan Jia Jian* (Crouching Tiger Pills with Additions & Subtractions)

INGREDIENTS: Cooked Radix Rehmanniae (*Shu Di*), Radix Albus Paeoniae Lactiflorae (*Bai Shao*), and Radix Achyranthis Bidentatae (*Niu Xi*), 15g each, Radix Angelicae Sinensis (*Dang Gui*) and Gelatinum Cornu Cervi (*Lu Jiao Jiao*), 12g each, Plastrum Testudinis (*Gui Ban*), Cortex Phellodendri (*Huang Bai*), Rhizoma Anemarrhenae Aspheloidis (*Zhi Mu*), and Herba Cynomorii Songarici (*Suo Yang*), 9g each

FORMULA ANALYSIS: *Suo Yang* supplements the kidneys and strengthens the bones. *Shu Di, Gui Ban, Huang Bai,* and *Zhi Mu* enrich yin and clear heat. *Niu Xi* strengthens the sinews and bones. *Lu Jiao Jiao* nourishes the blood at the same time as it invigorates yang, while *Dang Gui* and *Bai Shao* also supplement the liver and nourish the blood.

ADDITIONS & SUBTRACTIONS: If yin vacuity is marked, add 12 grams each of Radix Scrophulariae Ningpoensis (*Xuan Shen*) and Radix Dioscoreae

Oppositae (*Shan Yao*) and nine grams of Fructus Lycii Chinensis (*Gou Qi Zi*). If enduring disease and detriment of yin has reached yang, and yin and yang are both vacuous, add nine grams of Herba Epimedii (*Xian Ling Pi*), Fructus Psoraleae Corylifoliae (*Bu Gu Zhi*), and Radix Morindae Officinalis (*Ba Ji Tian*).

If there is kidney yang vacuity, one can use *Jin Gui Shen Qi Wan* (*Golden Cabinet* Kidney Qi Pills): cooked Radix Rehmanniae (*Shu Di*), 15g, Radix Dioscoreae Oppositae (*Shan Yao*), 12g, Fructus Corni Officinalis (*Shan Zhu Yu*), Sclerotium Poriae Cocos (*Fu Ling*), Rhizoma Alismatis (*Ze Xie*), and Cortex Radicis Moutan (*Dan Pi*), 9g each, Ramulus Cinnamomi Cassiae (*Gui Zhi*), 6-9g, and Radix Lateralis Praeparatus Aconiti Carmichaeli (*Fu Zi*), 3-6g.

If there is kidney yang depletion and detriment with relatively mild simultaneous lower limb water swelling, one can use *Ji Sheng Shen Qi Wan* (*Aid the Living* Kidney Qi Pills): cooked Radix Rehmanniae (*Shu Di*), 15g, Radix Dioscoreae Oppositae (*Shan Yao*), 12g, Fructus Corni Officinalis (*Shan Zhu Yu*), Sclerotium Poriae Cocos (*Fu Ling*), Rhizoma Alismatis (*Ze Xie*), Radix Cyathulae (*Chuan Niu Xi*), Cortex Radicis Moutan (*Dan Pi*), and Semen Plantaginis (*Che Qian Zi*), 9g each, Cortex Cinnamomi Cassiae (*Rou Gui*) and Radix Lateralis Praeparatus Aconiti Carmichaeli (*Fu Zi*), 3-6g each. If lower limb edema is relatively heavy, one can add 15 grams each of Rhizoma Atractylodis Macrocephalae (*Bai Zhu*) and Sclerotium Poriae Cocos (*Fu Ling*), nine grams of Radix Albus Paeoniae Lactiflorae (*Bai Shao*), and three slices of uncooked Rhizoma Zingiberis (*Sheng Jiang*).

ACUPUNCTURE & MOXIBUSTION: *San Yin Jiao* (Sp 6), *Qu Quan* (Liv 8), *Tai Xi* (Ki 3), *Ge Shu* (Bl 17), *Gan Shu* (Bl 18), *Shen Shu* (Bl 23), local points depending on the affected area

FORMULA ANALYSIS: Supplementing *Qu Quan*, *Ge Shu*, and *Gan Shu* supplements the liver and nourishes the blood. Supplementing *Tai Xi* and *Shen Shu* supplements the liver and enriches yin. Supplementing *San Yi Jiao* supplements both the liver and kidneys and enriches yin. Even supplementing-even draining the local points moves the qi and blood to and through the affected area.

ADDITIONS & SUBTRACTIONS: If there is concomitant liver depression, add even supplementing-even draining *Tai Chong* (Liv 3) and draining *He Gu* (LI 4). If there is concomitant blood stasis, add draining *Xue Hai* (Sp 10) and bleed any visibly engorged venules. If there is simultaneous damp heat damaging yin, add draining *Yin Ling*

Quan (Sp 9). If yin vacuity has reached yang, add moxibustion at *Shen Shu*, *Qi Hai* (CV 6) and *Guan Yuan* (CV 4). For dizziness and tinnitus, add even supplementing-even draining *Feng Chi* (GB 20) and *Yi Feng* (TB 17). For menstrual irregularities, add even supplementing-even draining *Qi Hai* (CV 6), *Shui Dao* (St 28), and *Gui Lai* (St 29).

AUTONOMIC NEUROPATHIES

CARDIOVASCULAR AUTONOMIC NEUROPATHY

1. HEART QI VACUITY & DETRIMENT PATTERN

MAIN SYMPTOMS: Heart palpitations, restlessness, a bright white facial complexion, chest fullness, shortness of breath, lassitude of the spirit, lack of strength, pale white lips, lack of warmth in the hands and feet, a susceptibility to laugh or to greatly sigh, spontaneous perspiration, disinclination to speak and/or a faint, weak voice, a pale red tongue with thin, white fur, and a fine, weak pulse

NOTE: Although the name of this pattern says nothing about spleen vacuity, the heart qi comes from the spleen qi. Likewise, although the name of the pattern says nothing about yin vacuity, the Chinese medicinal treatment plan given below assumes an element of yin vacuity.

TREATMENT PRINCIPLES: Nourish the heart and boost the qi, quiet the spirit and stabilize the mind

RX: *Wu Wei Zi Tang Jia Jian* (Schisandra Decoction with Additions & Subtractions)

INGREDIENTS: Cortex Albizziae Julibrissinis (*He Huan Pi*) and Radix Astragali Membranacei (*Huang Qi*), 15g each, Tuber Ophiopogonis Japonici (*Mai Men Dong*) and Semen Zizyphi Spinosae (*Suan Zao Ren*), 12g each, Fructus Schisandrae Chinensis (*Wu Wei Zi*), Radix Panacis Ginseng (*Ren Shen*), and Semen Biotae Orientalis (*Bai Zi Ren*), 9g each, and mix-fried Radix Glycyrrhizae (*Gan Cao*), 6g

FORMULA ANALYSIS: *Ren Shen*, *Huang Qi*, and mix-fried *Gan Cao* supplement and boost the heart qi. *Wu Wei Zi* and *Mai Men Dong* boost the qi and nourish yin. *Suan Zao Ren*, *Bai Zi Ren*, and *He Huan Pi* nourish the heart and boost the qi. *Ren Shen*, *Gan Cao*, *Suan Zao Ren*, *Bai Zi Ren*, and *He Huan Pi* all quiet the spirit and calm the mind.

ADDITIONS & SUBTRACTIONS: If there is simultaneous heart yang vacuity with fear of cold and chilled limbs, one can use *Bao Yuan Tang* (Protect the Source Decoction): Radix Astragali Membranacei (*Huang Qi*), 15g, Radix Panacis Ginseng (*Ren Shen*), 9g, mix-fried Radix Glycyrrhizae (*Gan Cao*), 3-9g, and Cortex Cinnamomi Cassiae (*Rou Gui*), 3-6g. If there is yang vacuity with inhibition of qi transformation and rheum collecting below the heart, thirst but no desire to drink, and scanty urination, add 9-12 grams each of Rhizoma Atractylodis Macrocephalae (*Bai Zhu*) and Sclerotium Poriae Cocos (*Fu Ling*).

ACUPUNCTURE & MOXIBUSTION: *Jue Yin Shu* (Bl 14), *Xin Shu* (Bl 15), *Dan Zhong* (CV 17), *Shen Men* (Ht 7), *Nei Guan* (Per 6), *Zu San Li* (St 36)

FORMULA ANALYSIS: Supplementing *Jue Yin Shu, Xin Shu, Dan Zhong,* and *Shen Men* supplements the heart qi. In addition, supplementing *Shen Men* and even supplementing-even draining *Nei Guan* quiets the spirit. Supplementing *Zu San Li* supplements and boosts the qi.

ADDITIONS & SUBTRACTIONS: For water rheum collecting below the heart, add draining *Shang Wan* (CV 13), *Guan Yuan* (CV 4) and/or *Zhong Ji* (CV 3), and *Yin Ling Quan* (Sp 9). For concomitant yang vacuity, add moxibustion at *Jue Yin Shu* and *Xin Shu* and add moxaing *Shen Shu* (Bl 23) and *Ming Men* (GV 4).

2. HEART YIN INSUFFICIENCY PATTERN

MAIN SYMPTOMS: Heart palpitations, vexation and agitation, dizziness and vertigo, red cheeks, tinnitus, a dry mouth and itchy throat, insomnia, profuse dreams, low-grade fever, night sweats, a red tongue with scanty fur or a bright, peeled tongue, and a fine, rapid pulse

TREATMENT PRINCIPLES: Enrich yin and downbear fire, calm the heart and quiet the spirit

RX: *Tian Wang Bu Xin Dan Jia Jian* (Heavenly Emperor Supplement the Heart Elixir with Additions & Subtractions)

INGREDIENTS: Radix Salviae Miltiorrhizae (*Dan Shen*), 30g, uncooked Radix Rehmanniae (*Sheng Di*) and Radix Scrophulariae Ningpoensis (*Xuan Shen*), 15g each, Sclerotium Poriae Cocos (*Fu Ling*), Radix Angelicae Sinensis (*Dang Gui*), Tuber Asparagi Cochinensis (*Tian Men Dong*), Tuber Ophiopogonis Japonici (*Mai Men Dong*), and Semen Zizyphi Spinosae (*Suan Zao Ren*), 12g each, Fructus Schisandrae Chinensis (*Wu Wei Zi*), Radix

Polygalae Tenuifoliae (*Yuan Zhi*), Radix Platycodi Grandiflori (*Jie Geng*), and Semen Biotae Orientalis (*Bai Zi Ren*), 9g each, Radix Panacis Ginseng (*Ren Shen*), 6g, and Succinum (*Hu Po*), 3g

FORMULA ANALYSIS: *Tian Men Dong, Mai Men Dong, Xuan Shen,* and *Sheng Di* enrich and nourish heart yin. The latter three ingredients also clear vacuity heat from the heart if necessary. *Dang Gui* and *Dan Shen* supplement and nourish heart blood as well as quicken the blood if necessary. *Ren Shen* and *Fu Ling* supplement the heart qi and quiet the spirit. *Suan Zao Ren, Bai Zi Ren, Wu Wei Zi,* and *Yuan Zhi* nourish the heart and quiet the spirit. *Hu Po* also quiets the spirit, quickens the blood, and disinhibits water if necessary.

ADDITIONS & SUBTRACTIONS: If there is simultaneous constipation, add nine grams of Semen Trichosanthis Kirlowii (*Gua Lou Ren*) and double the amount of *Sheng Di*. If there is yin vacuity tidal heat, add nine grams each of Cortex Radicis Lycii Chinensis (*Di Gu Pi*) and Radix Cynanchi Baiwei (*Bai Wei*). If there is yin vacuity with fire blazing internally resulting in heart-liver fire effulgence with heart vexation, tension and agitation, and easy anger, add nine grams of Fructus Gardeniae Jasminoidis (*Zhi Zi*) and 3-6 grams of Rhizoma Coptidis Chinensis (*Huang Lian*).

If there is simultaneous liver-kidney yin vacuity, one can use *Yi Guan Jian* (One Link Decoction) plus *Suan Zao Ren Tang* (Zizyphus Decoction): uncooked Radix Rehmanniae (*Sheng Di*) and Semen Zizyphi Spinosae (*Suan Zao Ren*), 15g each, Radix Glehniae Littoralis (*Sha Shen*), Tuber Ophiopogonis Japonici (*Mai Men Dong*), and Sclerotium Poriae Cocos (*Fu Ling*), 12g each, Rhizoma Anemarrhenae Aspheloidis (*Zhi Mu*), Radix Angelicae Sinensis (*Dang Gui*), Radix Ligustici Wallichii (*Chuan Xiong*), and Fructus Lycii Chinensis (*Gou Qi Zi*), 9g each, Fructus Meliae Toosendan (*Chuan Lian Zi*), 6g, and Radix Glycyrrhizae (*Gan Cao*), 3-6g.

ACUPUNCTURE & MOXIBUSTION: *Jue Yin Shu* (Bl 14), *Xin Shu* (Bl 15), *Dan Zhong* (CV 17), *Shen Men* (Ht 7), *Nei Guan* (Per 6), *San Yin Jiao* (Sp 6)

FORMULA ANALYSIS: Supplementing *Jue Yin Shu, Xin Shu, Dan Zhong,* and *Shen Men* supplements the heart. In addition, supplementing *Shen Men* and even supplementing-even draining *Nei Guan* quiets the spirit, while supplementing *San Yin Jiao* enriches yin.

ADDITIONS & SUBTRACTIONS: If there is simultaneous liver-kidney yin vacuity, add supplementing *Gan Shu* (Bl 18) and *Shen Shu* (Bl 23). If there is heart fire effulgence, drain *Shen Men*, delete *Nei Guan*, and add draining *Lao Gong* (Per 8). If there is liver fire effulgence, add draining *Xing Jian* (Liv 2).

3. HEART BLOOD-SPLEEN QI VACUITY PATTERN

MAIN SYMPTOMS: Heart palpitations, fearful throbbing, a lusterless facial complexion, insomnia, lassitude of the spirit, fatigue, lack of strength in the hands and feet, devitalized essence spirit, pale lips and white nails, a pale tongue with thin, white fur, and a fine, weak pulse

TREATMENT PRINCIPLES: Nourish the heart and supplement the blood, quiet the spirit and stabilize the mind

RX: *Gui Pi Tang* (Restore the Spleen Decoction)

INGREDIENTS: Radix Astragali Membranacei (*Huang Qi*), 15g, Arillus Euphoriae Longanae (*Long Yan Rou*) and Semen Zizyphi Spinosae (*Suan Zao Ren*), 12g each, Sclerotium Pararadicis Poriae Cocos (*Fu Shen*), Rhizoma Atractylodis Macrocephalae (*Bai Zhu*), Radix Auklandiae Lappae (*Mu Xiang*), Radix Angelicae Sinensis (*Dang Gui*), and Radix Polygalae Tenuifoliae (*Yuan Zhi*), 9g each, and Radix Panacis Ginseng (*Ren Shen*) and mix-fried Radix Glycyrrhizae (*Gan Cao*), 6-9g each

FORMULA ANALYSIS: *Ren Shen, Huang Qi, Bai Zhu,* and mix-fried *Gan Cao* fortify the spleen and boost the qi. *Dang Gui* and *Long Yan Rou* supplement and nourish heart blood. *Suan Zao Ren, Fu Shen,* and *Yuan Zhi* nourish the heart and quiet the spirit, and *Mu Xiang* rectifies the qi and arouses the spleen, thus promoting supplementation without stagnation.

ADDITIONS & SUBTRACTIONS: If there is simultaneous low blood pressure, add 12 grams of Tuber Ophiopogonis Japonici (*Mai Men Dong*), nine grams of Fructus Schisandrae Chinensis (*Wu Wei Zi*), six grams of Pericarpium Citri Reticulatae (*Chen Pi*), 4.5 grams of Rhizoma Cimicifugae (*Sheng Ma*), and three grams of Radix Bupleuri (*Chai Hu*).

ACUPUNCTURE & MOXIBUSTION: *Xin Shu* (Bl 15), *Ge Shu* (Bl 17), *Pi Shu* (Bl 20), *Dan Zhong* (CV 17), *Shen Men* (Ht 7), *Nei Guan* (Per 6), *Zu San Li* (St 36)

FORMULA ANALYSIS: Supplementing *Xin Shu, Dan Zhong,* and *Shen Men* supplements the heart qi. In addition, supplementing *Shen Men* and even supplementing-

even draining *Nei Guan* quiets the spirit. Supplementing *Pi Shu* and *Zu San Li* fortifies the spleen and boosts the qi, and supplementing *Ge Shu* nourishes the blood.

ADDITIONS & SUBTRACTIONS: For low blood pressure, add moxa at *Bai Hui* (GV 20).

4. HEART, LUNGS, SPLEEN & KIDNEYS ALL VACUOUS PATTERN

MAIN SYMPTOMS: Heart palpitations, shortness of breath, inability to lie flat when resting, edematous swelling below the waist, counterflow chilling of the four limbs, chest and stomach duct distention and oppression, nausea, torpid intake, a tender, dark red tongue, and a deep, fine, rapid or possibly bound or regularly intermittent pulse

TREATMENT PRINCIPLES: Fortify the spleen and boost the qi, warm yang and disinhibit water

RX: *Shen Qi Zhen Wu Tang* (Ginseng & Astragalus True Warrior Decoction)

INGREDIENTS: Radix Astragali Membranacei (*Huang Qi*), 20g, Sclerotium Poriae Cocos (*Fu Ling*), 15g, Radix Albus Paeoniae Lactiflorae (*Bai Shao*), 12g, Radix Panacis Ginseng (*Ren Shen*), Rhizoma Atractylodis Macrocephalae (*Bai Zhu*), Radix Auklandiae Lappae (*Mu Xiang*), Semen Plantaginis (*Che Qian Zi*), Ramulus Cinnamomi Cassiae (*Gui Zhi*), and Radix Lateralis Praeparatus Aconiti Carmichaeli (*Fu Zi*), 9g each, and uncooked Rhizoma Zingiberis (*Sheng Jiang*), 3-5 slices

FORMULA ANALYSIS: *Ren Shen, Huang Qi,* and *Bai Zhu* fortify the spleen and boost the qi, thus supplementing the lung and heart qi. *Mu Xiang* harmonizes the liver and spleen and disperses distention, while *Sheng Jiang* harmonizes the stomach and stops nausea. *Bai Shao* and *Gui Zhi* harmonize the constructive and defensive, while *Gui Zhi* and *Fu Zi* warm spleen and kidney yang. *Fu Ling* and *Che Qian Zi* free the flow of urination, thus seeping water accumulated under the heart.

ADDITIONS & SUBTRACTIONS: This is a first aid treatment which is not typically modified.

ACUPUNCTURE & MOXIBUSTION: *Zu San Li* (St 36), *Guan Yuan* (CV 4)

FORMULA ANALYSIS: Strong moxibustion of *Zu San Li* and *Guan Yuan* supplements the qi of the entire body and stems desertion.

5. PHLEGM TURBIDITY OBSTRUCTION & STAGNATION PATTERN

MAIN SYMPTOMS: Heart palpitations, heart chest glomus, oppression, distention, and fullness, profuse phlegm, scanty eating, abdominal distention, possible nausea, slimy, white or glossy, slimy tongue fur, and a bowstring, slippery pulse

TREATMENT PRINCIPLES: Rectify the qi and transform phlegm, calm the heart and quiet the spirit

RX: *Dao Tan Tang Jia Jian* (Abduct Phlegm Decoction with Additions & Subtractions)

INGREDIENTS: Sclerotium Poriae Cocos (*Fu Ling*) and Semen Zizyphi Spinosae (*Suan Zao Ren*), 12g each, Rhizoma Pinelliae Ternatae (*Ban Xia*), Pericarpium Citri Reticulatae (*Chen Pi*), Fructus Immaturus Citri Aurantii (*Zhi Shi*), Radix Polygalae Tenuifoliae (*Yuan Zhi*), Semen Biotae Orientalis (*Bai Zi Ren*), Rhizoma Acori Graminei (*Shi Chang Pu*), and Tuber Curcumae (*Yu Jin*), 9g each, and bile-treated Rhizoma Arisaematis (*Dan Nan Xing*) and Radix Glycyrrhizae (*Gan Cao*), 6g each

FORMULA ANALYSIS: *Ban Xia* and *Chen Pi* rectify the qi and transform phlegm. *Fu Ling* fortifies the spleen and seeps dampness. *Zhi Shi* and *Dan Nan Xing* move the qi and eliminate phlegm. *Shi Chang Pu* and *Yu Jin* transform phlegm, free the flow of the network vessels, and open the orifices. *Sun Zao Ren*, *Bai Zi Ren*, and *Yuan Zhi* nourish the heart and quiet the spirit, and *Gan Cao* harmonizes the center and supplements earth.

ADDITIONS & SUBTRACTIONS: If there is phlegm heat harassing the heart, one can use *Huang Lian Wen Dan Tang* (Coptis Warm the Gallbladder Decoction): Rhizoma Pinelliae Ternatae (*Ban Xia*) and Sclerotium Poriae Cocos (*Fu Ling*), 12g each, Pericarpium Citri Reticulatae (*Chen Pi*), Fructus Immaturus Citri Aurantii (*Zhi Shi*), and Caulis Bambusae In Taeniis (*Zhu Ru*), 9g each, Radix Glycyrrhizae (*Gan Cao*), 3g, and Fructus Zizyphi Jujubae (*Da Zao*), 3-5 pieces.

If there is phlegm heat with simultaneous qi vacuity, one can use *Shi Wei Wen Dan Tang Jia Jian* (Eleven Flavors Warm the Gallbladder Decoction with Additions & Subtractions): Concha Ostreae (*Mu Li*) and Caulis Polygoni Multiflori (*Ye Jiao Teng*), 15g each, Sclerotium Poriae Cocos (*Fu Ling*) and Semen Zizyphi Spinosae (*Suan Zao Ren*), 12g each, Caulis Bambusae In Taeniis (*Zhu Ru*), Rhizoma Pinelliae Ternatae (*Ban Xia*), Rhizoma Acori Graminei (*Shi Chang Pu*), Radix Codonopsitis Pilosulae (*Dang Shen*), Fructus Schisandrae Chinensis (*Wu Wei Zi*), and Radix Angelicae Sinensis (*Dang Gui*), 9g each, Pericarpium Citri Reticulatae (*Chen Pi*), mix-fried Radix Glycyrrhizae (*Gan Cao*), Fructus Immaturus Citri Aurantii (*Zhi Shi*), and Radix Polygalae Tenuifoliae (*Yuan Zhi*), 6g each, Rhizoma Coptidis Chinensis (*Huang Lian*), 3-6g, Fructus Zizyphi Jujubae (*Da Zao*), 3-5 pieces, and uncooked Rhizoma Zingiberis (*Sheng Jiang*), 2-3 slices.

ACUPUNCTURE & MOXIBUSTION: *Feng Long* (St 40), *Dan Zhong* (CV 17), *Zhong Wan* (CV 12), *Nei Guan* (Per 6)

FORMULA ANALYSIS: Draining *Feng Long* transforms phlegm. Draining *Dan Zhong* loosens the chest. Draining *Zhong Wan* harmonizes the stomach and disperses distention, and draining *Nei Guan* loosens the chest, regulates the center, and quiets the spirit.

ADDITIONS & SUBTRACTIONS: If there is phlegm heat, add draining *Xing Jian* (Liv 2) and *Da Ling* (Per 7). If there is concomitant spleen vacuity, add even supplementing-even draining *Zu San Li* (St 36) and supplementing *Pi Shu* (Bl 20) and *Wei Shu* (Bl 21). If there is simultaneous blood stasis, add draining *Xue Hai* (Sp 10). If there is liver depression qi stagnation, add draining *Tai Chong* (Liv 3) and *He Gu* (LI 4).

6. HEART BLOOD STASIS & OBSTRUCTION PATTERN

MAIN SYMPTOMS: Heart palpitations, chest oppression, rib-side pain, if severe, pain radiating to the shoulder, dark, purplish face and lips, counterflow chilling of the four limbs, a dry mouth and parched throat, a bluish green tongue or possible static macules or spots and white or yellow fur, and a choppy, possibly bound or regularly intermittent pulse

TREATMENT PRINCIPLES: Move the qi and quicken the blood, transform stasis and free the flow of the network vessels

RX: *Xue Fu Zhu Yu Tang Jia Jian* (Blood Mansion Dispel Stasis Decoction with Additions & Subtractions)

INGREDIENTS: Radix Salviae Miltiorrhizae (*Dan Shen*), 30g, Radix Rubrus Paeoniae Lactiflorae (*Chi Shao*), 15g, Radix Angelicae Sinensis (*Dang Gui*), uncooked Radix Rehmanniae (*Sheng Di*), Radix Ligustici Wallichii (*Chuan Xiong*), and Radix Achyranthis Bidentatae (*Niu Xi*), 12g each, Flos Carthami Tinctorii (*Hong Hua*), Semen Pruni Persicae (*Tao Ren*), Fructus Immaturus Citri Aurantii (*Zhi*

Shi), and Radix Bupleuri (*Chai Hu*), 9g each, and Radix Platycodi Grandiflori (*Jie Geng*) and Radix Glycyrrhizae (*Gan Cao*), 6g each

FORMULA ANALYSIS: *Tao Ren, Hong Hua, Chuan Xiong, Chi Shao, Niu Xi,* and *Dan Shen* all quicken the blood and transform stasis. *Dang Gui* and *Sheng Di* nourish and quicken the blood. *Chai Hu, Zhi Shi,* and *Jie Geng* course the liver and rectify the qi, thus promoting the movement of the blood.

ADDITIONS & SUBTRACTIONS: If there is simultaneous qi vacuity, delete *Chai Hu, Jie Geng,* and *Zhi Shi* and add 15 grams of Radix Astragali Membranacei (*Huang Qi*) and 12 grams each of Radix Codonopsitis Pilosulae (*Dang Shen*) and Rhizoma Polygonati (*Huang Jing*) to supplement and boost the qi. If there is simultaneous blood vacuity, add 12 grams of cooked Radix Rehmanniae (*Shu Di*) and nine grams each of Fructus Lycii Chinensis (*Gou Qi Zi*) and Radix Polygoni Multiflori (*He Shou Wu*) to supplement and nourish the blood. If there is simultaneous yin vacuity, omit *Chai Hu, Jie Geng, Chuang Xiong,* and *Zhi Shi* and add 12 grams each of Tuber Ophiopogonis Japonici (*Mai Men Dong*), Fructus Ligustri Lucidi (*Nu Zhen Zi*), and Herba Ecl+iptae Prostratae (*Han Lian Cao*) and nine grams of Rhizoma Polygoni Odorati (*Yu Zhu*) to nourish yin and engender fluids. If there is simultaneous yang vacuity, delete *Chai Hu* and *Jie Geng* and add nine grams each of Herba Epimedii (*Xian Ling Pi*) and Radix Morindae Officinalis (*Ba Ji Tian*), six grams of Cortex Cinnamomi Cassiae (*Rou Gui*), and 3-6 grams of Radix Lateralis Praeparatus Aconiti Carmichaeli (*Fu Zi*) to warm the channels and invigorate yang.

ACUPUNCTURE & MOXIBUSTION: *Jue Yin Shu* (Bl 14), *Xin Shu* (Bl 15), *Dan Zhong* (CV 17), *Nei Guan* (Per 6), *Xue Hai* (Sp 10), *He Gu* (LI 4), *Tai Chong* (Liv 3)

FORMULA ANALYSIS: Draining *Jue Yin Shu, Xin Shu, Dan Zhong,* and *Nei Guan* drains the heart and loosens the chest. Draining *Xue Hai* quickens the blood and transforms stasis. Draining *He Gu* and *Tai Chong* courses the liver and rectifies the qi in order to move the blood.

ADDITIONS & SUBTRACTIONS: If there is simultaneous qi vacuity, change draining *Jue Yin Shu, Xin Shu,* and *Dan Zhong* to even supplementing-even draining and add supplementing *Shen Men* (Ht 7) and *Zu San Li* (St 36). If there is simultaneous blood vacuity, add supplementing *Ge Shu* (Bl 17) to the above modifications. If there is simultaneous yin vacuity, add supplementing *San Yin Jiao* (Sp 6) and *Tai Xi* (Ki 3) to the first set of modifications. If there is simultaneous yang vacuity, add moxibustion at *Shen Shu* (Bl 23) and *Guan Yuan* (GV 4) to the first set of

modifications. If there is concomitant phlegm, add draining *Feng Long* (St 40) and also *Zhong Wan* (CV 12) if there is abdominal fullness and nausea.

DIABETIC IMPOTENCE

1. KIDNEY YANG INSUFFICIENCY PATTERN

MAIN SYMPTOMS: Impotence, chilly genitalia, thin, clear, chilly semen, dizziness, tinnitus, a bright white facial complexion, essence spirit listlessness, low back and knee soreness and limpness, fear of cold, chilled limbs, shortness of breath, lack of strength, a fat, pale, moist tongue with possible teeth-marks on its edges, and a deep, fine, slow, weak pulse

TREATMENT PRINCIPLES: Warm and supplement kidney yang

RX: *You Gui Wan Jia Jian* (Restore the Right [Kidney] Pills with Additions & Subtractions)

INGREDIENTS: Radix Dioscoreae Oppositae (*Shan Yao*), 15g, cooked Radix Rehmanniae (*Shu Di*) and Radix Angelicae Sinensis (*Dang Gui*), 12g each, Gelatinum Cornu Cervi (*Lu Jiao Jiao*), Semen Cuscutae Chinensis (*Tu Si Zi*), Cortex Eucommiae Ulmoidis (*Du Zhong*), Fructus Corni Officinalis (*Shan Zhu Yu*), and Fructus Lycii Chinensis (*Gou Qi Zi*), 9g each, and Cortex Cinnamomi Cassiae (*Rou Gui*) and Radix Lateralis Praeparatus Aconiti Carmichaeli (*Fu Zi*), 6g each

FORMULA ANALYSIS: *Lu Jiao Jiao, Tu Si Zi, Du Zhong, Fu Zi,* and *Rou Gui* warm the kidneys and invigorate yang. *Shu Di, Dang Gui, Gou Qi Zi,* and *Shan Zhu Yu* nourish the blood and enrich yin, and yin and yang are mutually rooted. In addition, they help prevent warm supplementation from aggravating dryness and heat. *Shan Yao* supplements both spleen and kidney qi, remembering that the former and latter heavens mutually support and bolster each other.

ADDITIONS & SUBTRACTIONS: If there is concomitant liver depression, add nine grams each of Radix Bupleuri (*Chai Hu*), Radix Albus Paeoniae Lactiflorae (*Bai Shao*), and Fructus Citri Sacrodactylis (*Fo Shou*). If there is concomitant blood stasis, add 30 grams of Radix Salviae Miltiorrhizae (*Dan Shen*) and two strips of Scolopendra Subspinipes (*Wu Gong*).

ACUPUNCTURE & MOXIBUSTION: *Shen Shu* (Bl 23), *Zhi Shi* (Bl 47), *Ming Men* (GV 4), *Guan Yuan* (CV 4), *San Yin Jiao* (Sp 6)

FORMULA ANALYSIS: Moxaing *Shen Shu, Zhi Shi, Ming Men,* and *Guan Yuan* supplements the kidneys and invigorates yang. Supplementing *San Yin Jiao* supplements the spleen, liver, and kidneys and treats urogenital disorders.

ADDITIONS & SUBTRACTIONS: For concomitant liver depression, add draining *Tai Chong* (Liv 3) and *He Gu* (LI 4). For concomitant blood stasis, add draining *Xue Hai* (Sp 10) and use even supplementing-even draining technique at *San Yin Jiao.*

2. HEART-SPLEEN DUAL VACUITY PATTERN

MAIN SYMPTOMS: Impotence and inability to achieve and maintain an erection, devitalized essence spirit, heart palpitations, shortness of breath, fatigue, lassitude of the spirit, lack of strength, spontaneous perspiration, an emaciated body, insomnia, restlessness, poor appetite, a lusterless facial complexion, a pale tongue, and a deep, fine pulse

TREATMENT PRINCIPLES: Supplement the heart and fortify the spleen, boost the qi and nourish the blood

RX: *Gui Pi Tang Jia Jian* (Restore the Spleen Decoction with Additions & Subtractions)

INGREDIENTS: Radix Polygalae Tenuifoliae (*Yuan Zhi*), 21g, Radix Astragali Membranacei (*Huang Qi*), 15g, Sclerotium Pararadicis Poriae Cocos (*Fu Shen*), Semen Zizyphi Spinosae (*Suan Zao Ren*), Radix Angelicae Sinensis (*Dang Gui*), and Arillus Euphoriae Longanae (*Long Yan Rou*), 12g each, Rhizoma Atractylodis Macrocephalae (*Bai Zhu*), Radix Auklandiae Lappae (*Mu Xiang*), and Radix Panacis Ginseng (*Ren Shen*), 9g each, and mix-fried Radix Glycyrrhizae (*Gan Cao*), 6g

FORMULA ANALYSIS: *Huang Qi, Ren Shen, Bai Zhu, Fu Shen,* and mix-fried *Gan Cao* fortify the spleen and boost the qi. *Suan Zao Ren, Yuan Zhi,* and *Long Yan Rou* nourish the heart and quiet the spirit. *Dang Gui* supplements the blood, and *Mu Xiang* harmonizes the liver and spleen and rectifies the qi.

ADDITIONS & SUBTRACTIONS: For marked insomnia, add 12 grams each of Concha Ostreae (*Mu Li*), Dens Draconis (*Long Chi*), Caulis Polygoni Multiflori (*Ye Jiao Teng*), and Cortex Albizziae Julibrissinis (*He Huan Pi*). For simultaneous liver depression, add nine grams each of Radix Bupleuri (*Chai Hu*), Radix Albus Paeoniae Lactiflorae (*Bai Shao*), and Fructus Citri Sacrodactylis (*Fo Shou*). For concomitant blood stasis, add 30 grams of Radix Salviae Miltiorrhizae (*Dan Shen*) and nine grams

each of Flos Carthami Tinctorii (*Hong Hua*) and Semen Pruni Persicae (*Tao Ren*).

ACUPUNCTURE & MOXIBUSTION: *Xin Shu* (Ht 15), *Ge Shu* (Bl 17), *Pi Shu* (Bl 20), *Shen Men* (Ht 7), *Nei Guan* (Per 6), *Zu San Li* (St 36), *San Yin Jiao* (Sp 6)

FORMULA ANALYSIS: Supplementing *Xin Shu, Ge Shu,* and *Shen Men* supplements the heart and nourishes the blood, while supplementing *Zu San Li, Pi Shu,* and *San Yin Jiao* fortifies the spleen and boosts the qi. Even supplementing-even draining *Nei Guan* harmonizes the liver and spleen and quiets the spirit. In addition, *San Yin Jiao* has a known empirical effect for treating urogenital diseases.

ADDITIONS & SUBTRACTIONS: For marked liver depression, add draining *Tai Chong* (Liv 3) and *He Gu* (LI 4). For concomitant blood stasis, add draining *Xue Hai* (Sp 10) and use even supplementing-even draining technique at *San Yin Jiao.* For concomitant liver-stomach heat, add draining *Xing Jian* (Liv 2) and/or *Nei Ting* (St 44).

3. DAMP HEAT POURING DOWNWARD PATTERN

MAIN SYMPTOMS: Complete impotence or partial flaccidity, scrotal dampness, foul-smelling urine or itching and pain on urination, lower limb soreness and encumbrance, short, reddish urination, slimy, yellow tongue fur, and a soggy, rapid or slippery, rapid pulse

NOTE: This pattern rarely presents in diabetic patients as the main pattern of impotence. In most cases of diabetic impotence, damp heat complicates other disease mechanisms.

TREATMENT PRINCIPLES: Clear heat and disinhibit dampness

RX: *Long Dan Xie Gan Tang Jia Jian* (Gentiana Drain the Liver Decoction with Additions & Subtractions)

INGREDIENTS: Semen Coicis Lachyrma-jobi (*Yi Yi Ren*), 30g, uncooked Radix Rehmanniae (*Sheng Di*), 15g, Radix Scutellariae Baicalensis (*Huang Qin*), Fructus Gardeniae Jasminoidis (*Zhi Zi*), Rhizoma Alismatis (*Ze Xie*), Semen Plantaginis (*Che Qian Zi*), Radix Angelicae Sinensis (*Dang Gui*), and Radix Bupleuri (*Chai Hu*), 9g each, and Radix Gentianae Scabrae (*Long Dan Cao*) and Radix Glycyrrhizae (*Gan Cao*), 6g each

FORMULA ANALYSIS: *Long Dan Cao, Huang Qin,* and

Zhi Zi clear the liver and drain fire. *Chai Hu* courses the liver and out-thrusts depression. *Yi Yi Ren, Che Qian Zi,* and *Ze Xie* clear and disinhibit dampness and heat. *Dang Gui* and *Sheng Di* nourish yin, quicken and cool the blood.

ADDITIONS & SUBTRACTIONS: If there is concomitant spleen vacuity, add nine grams each of Radix Codonopsitis Pilosulae (*Dang Shen*) and Rhizoma Atractylodis Macrocephalae (*Bai Zhu*). If heat has damaged lung-stomach yin, add 12 grams each of Tuber Ophiopogonis Japonici (*Mai Men Dong*) and Radix Glehniae Littoralis (*Sha Shen*). If there is concomitant blood stasis, add 15 grams each of Herba Patriniae Heterophyllae Cum Radice (*Bai Jiang Cao*) and Caulis Sargentodoxae (*Hong Teng*).

ACUPUNCTURE & MOXIBUSTION: *Zhong Ji* (CV 3), *Yin Ling Quan* (Sp 9), *San Yin Jiao* (Sp 6), *Ba Liao* (Bl 31-34)

FORMULA ANALYSIS: Draining *Zhong Ji, Yin Ling Quan, San Yin Jiao,* and the *Ba Liao* clears heat from and disinhibits dampness in the lower burner.

ADDITIONS & SUBTRACTIONS: If there is concomitant liver depression transforming heat, needle *Tai Chong* (Liv 3) through to *Xing Jian* (Liv 2) and use draining technique. If enduring heat has damaged lung-stomach yin, add even supplementing-even draining of *Zhao Hai* (Ki 6), *Lie Que* (Lu 7), and/or *Nei Ting* (St 44). If there is concomitant spleen vacuity, add supplementing *Pi Shu* (Bl 20) and *Wei Shu* (Bl 21) and use even supplementing-even draining at *San Yin Jiao.* If there is concomitant kidney yin vacuity, add supplementing *Tai Xi* (Ki 3) and *Shen Shu* (Bl 23). If there is simultaneous blood stasis, add draining *Xue Hai* (Sp 10) and use even supplementing-even draining at *San Yin Jiao.*

4. LIVER DEPRESSION QI STAGNATION PATTERN

MAIN SYMPTOMS: Impotence and inability to consummate union, emotional depression or easy stimulation, irritability, a dark tongue with white fur, and a bowstring pulse

NOTE: This pattern mostly complicates other patterns of diabetic impotence. However, it may be the main pattern in patients whose disease has led them to become depressed and anxious about their sexual performance. As the treatment principles evidence below, this pattern of diabetic impotence is usually complicated by an element of blood stasis.

TREATMENT PRINCIPLES: Course the liver and rectify the qi assisted by quickening the blood

RX: *Si Ni San Jia Jian* (Four Counterflows Powder with Additions & Subtractions)

INGREDIENTS: Fructus Citri Sacrodactylis (*Fo Shou*) and Radix Albus Paeoniae Lactiflorae (*Bai Shao*), 12g each, Radix Bupleuri (*Chai Hu*), Fructus Immaturus Citri Aurantii (*Zhi Shi*), Radix Angelicae Sinensis (*Dang Gui*), and Corium Erinacei (*Ci Wei Pi*), 9g each, Radix Glycyrrhizae (*Gan Cao*), 6g, and Scolopendra Subspinipes (*Wu Gong*), 2 strips

FORMULA ANALYSIS: *Chai Hu* and *Zhi Shi* course the liver and rectify the qi. *Dang Gui* and *Bai Shao* nourish and quicken the blood. *Fo Shou* and *Ci Wei Pi* rectify the qi and quicken the blood. In addition, *Ci Wei Pi* secures the essence to help prevent premature ejaculation. *Wu Gong* enters the liver channel where it helps to spread and out-thrust the liver qi, thus insuring that the channels and network vessels are freely and smoothly flowing. It both strengthens *Chai Hu* and *Zhi Shi*'s function of coursing the liver and rectifying the qi and *Dang Gui* and *Bai Shao*'s function of quickening the blood.

ADDITIONS & SUBTRACTIONS: If there is even more marked blood stasis, add 30 grams of Salviae Miltiorrhizae (*Dan Shen*) and nine grams each of Flos Carthami Tinctorii (*Hong Hua*) and Semen Pruni Persicae (*Tao Ren*). If there is concomitant spleen vacuity, add nine grams each of Radix Codonopsitis Pilosulae (*Dang Shen*), Rhizoma Atractylodis Macrocephalae (*Bai Zhu*), and Sclerotium Poriae Cocos (*Fu Ling*). If there is concomitant lung-stomach fluid dryness, add 12 grams each of Tuber Ophiopogonis Japonici (*Mai Men Dong*), Radix Trichosanthis Kirlowii (*Tian Hua Fen*), and Radix Puerariae (*Ge Gen*). If there is simultaneous liver-kidney yin vacuity, add 12 grams each of cooked Radix Rehmanniae (*Shu Di*) and Fructus Lycii Chinensis (*Gou Qi Zi*). If there is simultaneous kidney yang vacuity, add nine grams each of Semen Cuscutae Chinensis (*Tu Si Zi*), Gelatinum Cornu Cervi (*Lu Jiao Jiao*), and Cortex Eucommiae Ulmoidis (*Du Zhong*). If there is liver-stomach depressive heat, add nine grams each of Radix Scutellariae Baicalensis (*Huang Qin*) and Fructus Gardeniae Jasminoidis (*Zhi Zi*).

ACUPUNCTURE & MOXIBUSTION: *Tai Chong* (Liv 3), *Nei Guan* (Per 6), *He Gu* (LI 4), *San Yin Jiao* (Sp 6), *Qi Hai* (CV 6)

FORMULA ANALYSIS: Draining *Tai Chong* and *He Gu*

courses the liver and rectifies the qi. Draining *Nei Guan* harmonizes the liver and spleen, quiets the spirit and tranquilizes the mind. Draining *Qi Hai* rectifies the qi of the lower burner, while even supplementing-even draining *San Yin Jiao* treats urogenital diseases.

ADDITIONS & SUBTRACTIONS: If there is concomitant yin vacuity, add supplementing *Shen Shu* (Bl 23) and *Tai Xi* (Ki 3). If there is concomitant spleen vacuity, add supplementing *Pi Shu* (Bl 20) and *Wei Shu* (Bl 21). If there is simultaneous blood stasis, add draining *Xue Hai* (Sp 10). If there is simultaneous blood vacuity, add supplementing *Ge Shu* (Bl 17) and even supplementing-even draining *Gan Shu* (Bl 18). If there is concomitant lung-stomach fluid dryness, add even supplementing-even draining of *Zhao Hai* (Ki 6), *Lie Que* (Lu 7), and/or *Nei Ting* (St 44). If there is concomitant kidney yang vacuity, add moxa at *Shen Shu*, *Ming Men* (GV 4), and *Guan Yuan* (CV 4). If there is concomitant liver depression transforming heat, add draining *Xing Jian* (Liv 2) and *Yang Ling Quan* (GB 34).

DIABETIC NEUROGENIC BLADDER

1. CENTRAL QI INSUFFICIENCY PATTERN

MAIN SYMPTOMS: Lower abdominal sagging and distention, occasional desire to urinate and inability to, lassitude of the spirit, shortness of breath, devitalized eating and drinking, reduced appetite, faint, weak voice, a pale tongue with thin, white fur, and a deep, weak pulse

TREATMENT PRINCIPLES: Supplement the center and boost the qi, transform the qi and move water

Rx: *Bu Zhong Yi Qi Tang* (Supplement the Center & Boost the Qi Decoction) plus *Chun Ze Tang* (Spring Pond Decoction)

INGREDIENTS: Sclerotium Polypori Umbellati (*Zhu Ling*), 30g, Radix Astragali Membranacei (*Huang Qi*), 15g, Sclerotium Poriae Cocos (*Fu Ling*), 12g, Radix Panacis Ginseng (*Ren Shen*), Radix Angelicae Sinensis (*Dang Gui*), Pericarpium Citri Reticulatae (*Chen Pi*), Rhizoma Atractylodis Macrocephalae (*Bai Zhu*), Radix Bupleuri (*Chai Hu*), Ramulus Cinnamomi Cassiae (*Gui Zhi*), and Rhizoma Alismatis (*Ze Xie*), 9g each, and Rhizoma Cimicifugae (*Sheng Ma*) and Radix Glycyrrhizae (*Gan Cao*), 6g each

FORMULA ANALYSIS: *Huang Qi*, *Ren Shen*, and *Bai Zhu* fortify the spleen and boost the qi. *Dang Gui* nourishes the blood in order to better supplement the qi at the same

time as it emolliates and harmonizes the liver and thus, indirectly, promotes coursing and discharge. *Zhu Ling*, *Fu Ling*, and *Ze Xie* seep dampness and disinhibit water. *Chen Pi* disinhibits the qi mechanism and transforms dampness. *Chai Hu* and *Sheng Ma* upbear yang and lift the fallen. *Gui Zhi* promotes qi transformation, and *Gan Cao* harmonizes all the other medicinals in the formula.

ADDITIONS & SUBTRACTIONS: If there is urinary dribbling and dripping, redness, and choppiness, add nine grams each of Herba Pyrrosiae (*Shi Wei*) and Semen Plantaginis (*Che Qian Zi*).

ACUPUNCTURE & MOXIBUSTION: *Zu San Li* (St 36), *Bai Hui* (GV 20), *Yin Ling Quan* (Sp 9), *San Yin Jiao* (Sp 6), *Zhong Ji* (CV 3)

FORMULA ANALYSIS: Supplementing *Zu San Li* and *San Yin Jiao* fortifies the spleen and boosts the qi. Moxaing *Bai Hui* upbears yang and lifts the fallen. Even supplementing-even draining *Yin Ling Quan* and *Zhong Ji* rectifies and regulates the qi of the bladder and seeps dampness.

ADDITIONS & SUBTRACTIONS: If there is marked fatigue and loose stools, add supplementing *Pi Shu* (Bl 20) and *Wei Shu* (Bl 21). If there is liver depression, add draining *Tai Chong* (Liv 3) and *He Gu* (LI 4). If there is concomitant kidney yang vacuity, add moxa at *Shen Shu* (Bl 23) and *Ming Men* (GV 4). If there is concomitant yin vacuity, add supplementing *Tai Xi* (Ki 3) and *Shen Shu* (Bl 23).

2. KIDNEY QI INSUFFICIENCY PATTERN

MAIN SYMPTOMS: Lower abdominal distention and fullness, urine expelled without force, possible dribbling and dripping and uneasy flow, even possible urinary incontinence, low back and knee soreness and aching, lack of warmth in the four limbs, a pale tongue with thin, white fur, and a deep, fine, slow, weak pulse

NOTE: The above signs and symptoms describe a simple, discrete kidney qi shading into a kidney yang vacuity pattern. In real-life Western patients with diabetes, such a pure kidney vacuity pattern is not commonly seen. Therefore, the above signs and symptoms will be modified by other disease mechanisms, especially any sort of heat evils or yang hyperactivity.

TREATMENT PRINCIPLES: Supplement the kidneys, transform the qi, and disinhibit urination

Rx: *Ji Sheng Shen Qi Wan Jia Jian* (*Aid the Living* Kidney Qi Pills with Additions & Subtractions)

INGREDIENTS: Radix Dioscoreae Oppositae (*Shan Yao*) and Sclerotium Poriae Cocos (*Fu Ling*), 15g each, cooked Radix Rehmanniae (*Shu Di*) and Radix Cyathulae (*Chuan Niu Xi*), 12g each, Cortex Cinnamomi Cassiae (*Rou Gui*), Cortex Radicis Moutan (*Dan Pi*), Semen Plantaginis (*Che Qian Zi*), Rhizoma Alismatis (*Ze Xie*), and Fructus Corni Officinalis (*Shan Zhu Yu*), 9g each, and Radix Lateralis Praeparatus Aconiti Carmichaeli (*Fu Zi*), 6g

FORMULA ANALYSIS: *Rou Gui* and *Fu Zi* supplement lower burner yang in order to promote the transformation of the kidney qi. *Shu Di, Shan Yao,* and *Shan Zhu Yu* supplement the kidneys and enrich yin. *Fu Ling, Ze Xie,* and *Che Qian Zi* seep dampness and disinhibit urination. *Chuan Niu Xi* and *Dan Pi* quicken the blood and guide it and, therefore, fluids to move downward.

ADDITIONS & SUBTRACTIONS: If there is urinary incontinence, add nine grams of Fructus Rosae Laevigatae (*Jin Ying Zi*) and Semen Euryalis Ferocis (*Qian Shi*).

If there is a tendency to yin depletion and vacuity, use *Liu Wei Di Huang Wan* (Six Flavors Rehmannia Pills) with *Zhu Ling Tang* (Polyporus Decoction): Sclerotium Polypori Umbellati (*Zhu Ling*), Sclerotium Poriae Cocos (*Fu Ling*), and Radix Dioscoreae Oppositae (*Shan Yao*), 15g each, cooked Radix Rehmanniae (*Shu Di*) and Gelatinum Corii Asini (*E Jiao*), 12g each, and Fructus Corni Officinalis (*Shan Zhu Yu*), Cortex Radicis Moutan (*Dan Pi*), Rhizoma Alismatis (*Ze Xie*), and Talcum (*Hua Shi*), 9g each. If there is damp heat in the lower burner, add nine grams each of Rhizoma Anemarrhenae Aspheloidis (*Zhi Mu*) and Cortex Phellodendri (*Huang Bai*) to clear heat and harden yin.

If there is yin vacuity and yang is not transforming the qi, one can use *Zi Shen Tong Guan Wan* (Enrich the Kidneys & Free the Flow of the Bar Pills): Rhizoma Anemarrhenae Aspheloidis (*Zhi Mu*) and Cortex Phellodendri (*Huang Bai*), 9g each, and Cortex Cinnamomi Cassiae (*Rou Gui*), 6g.

ACUPUNCTURE & MOXIBUSTION: *Shen Shu* (Bl 23), *Tai Xi* (Ki 3), *San Yin Jiao* (Sp 6), *Qi Hai* (CV 6), *Guan Yuan* (CV 4)

FORMULA ANALYSIS: Supplementing *Shen Shu* and *Tai Xi* supplements the kidneys. Supplementing *Qi Hai* and *Guan Yuan* supplements and secures the qi of the lower burner. Supplementing *San Yin Jiao* supplements the kidneys and treats urinary disorders.

ADDITIONS & SUBTRACTIONS: For urinary incontinence, add supplementing *Zhi Shi* (Bl 47). If there is kidney yang vacuity, moxa *Shen Shu, Qi Hai,* and *Guan Yuan* and add moxibustion at *Ming Men* (GV 4). If there is spleen-kidney yang vacuity, also add moxa at *Pi Shu* (Bl 20) and *Wei Shu* (Bl 21). If there is concomitant liver depression, add draining *Tai Chong* (Liv 3) and *He Gu* (LI 4). If there is concomitant blood stasis, add draining *Xue Hai* (Sp 10) and use even supplementing-even draining at *San Yin Jiao.*

3. LOWER BURNER DAMP HEAT PATTERN

MAIN SYMPTOMS: Difficult, spotting and dripping urination which is scanty in amount, dark yellow or reddish in color, and burning hot and painful, urinary frequency and urgency, lower abdominal distention and cramping, a bitter taste and a sticky feeling in the mouth, possible thirst but no desire to drink, possible uneasy defecation, a red tongue with slimy, yellow fur at its root, and a deep, rapid or soggy, rapid pulse

TREATMENT PRINCIPLES: Clear heat and disinhibit dampness, free the flow and disinhibit urination

Rx: *Ba Zheng San Jia Jian* (Eight [Ingredients] Correcting Powder with Additions & Subtractions)

INGREDIENTS: Herba Pyrrosiae (*Shi Wei*), 30g, Talcum (*Hua Shi*), 15g, Semen Plantaginis (*Che Qian Zi*), 12g, Cortex Phellodendri (*Huang Bai*), Herba Dianthi (*Qu Mai*), Herba Polygoni Avicularis (*Bian Xu*), and Fructus Gardeniae Jasminoidis (*Zhi Zi*), 9g each, and Extremitas Radicis Glycyrrhizae (*Gan Cao Xiao*), Medulla Tetrapanacis Papyriferi (*Tong Cao*), and Radix Et Rhizoma Rhei (*Da Huang*), 6g each

FORMULA ANALYSIS: *Shi Wei, Che Qian Zi, Bian Xu,* and *Qu Mai* free the flow of blockage and disinhibit urination. *Huang Bai* and *Zhi Zi* clear and transform damp heat from the three burners. *Hua Shi* and *Gan Cao Xiao* clear and disinhibit heat and transform dampness in the lower burner, and *Da Huang* frees the flow of the stools and drains fire.

ADDITIONS & SUBTRACTIONS: If the tongue fur is thick and slimy, add nine grams of Rhizoma Atractylodis (*Cang Zhu*) to strengthen the clearing of heat and transformation of dampness. If there is simultaneous heart vexation and sores and ulcers in the mouth and on the tongue due to heart fire, one can also add the ingredients of *Dao Chi San* (Abduct the Red Powder), *i.e.*, uncooked Radix Rehmanniae (*Sheng Di*), 12-15g, and Caulis Akebiae (*Mu Tong*) and Herba Lophatheri Gracilis (*Dan Zhu Ye*), 9g each.

If damp heat lingering in the lower burner has damaged yin, one can use *Zi Shen Tong Guan Wan Jia Wei* (Enrich the Kidneys & Free the Flow of the Bar Pills with Added Flavors) to enrich kidney yin, clear and eliminate dampness and heat, and promote qi transformation: uncooked Radix Rehmanniae (*Sheng Di*), 12-15g, Rhizoma Anemarrhenae Aspheloidis (*Zhi Mu*), Cortex Phellodendri (*Huang Bai*), Radix Achyranthis Bidentatae (*Niu Xi*), and Semen Plantaginis (*Che Qian Zi*), 9g each, and Cortex Cinnamomi Cassiae (*Rou Gui*), 6g.

If there is a spleen-kidney vacuity with concomitant damp heat, one can use *Zhi Bai Wu Bi Shan Yao Wan Jia Jian* (Anemarrhena & Phellodendron No Comparison Dioscorea Pills with Additions & Subtractions): uncooked Radix Sanguisorbae (*Di Yu*), 30g, Radix Codonopsitis Pilosulae (*Dang Shen*), 15g, cooked Radix Rehmanniae (*Shu Di*), Radix Dioscoreae Oppositae (*Shan Yao*), Sclerotium Poriae Cocos (*Fu Ling*), Rhizoma Alismatis (*Ze Xie*), Cortex Eucommiae Ulmoidis (*Du Zhong*), Cortex Phellodendri (*Huang Bai*), and Rhizoma Anemarrhenae Aspheloidis (*Zhi Mu*), 9g each, and Semen Ginkgonis Bilobae (*Bai Guo*), 10 pieces.

If damp heat is brewing and binding in the three burners and the qi transformation is inhibited, with extremely scanty urination, a dark, stagnant facial complexion, chest oppression, vexation and agitation, nausea and vomiting, and, if severe, spirit dimming, one can use *Huang Lian Wen Dan Tang Jia Wei* (Coptis Warm the Gallbladder Decoction with Added Flavors) to downbear turbidity and harmonize the stomach, clear heat and transform dampness: Rhizoma Imperatae Cyclindricae (*Bai Mao Gen*), 15g, Semen Plantaginis (*Che Qian Zi*), Rhizoma Pinelliae Ternatae (*Ban Xia*), and Sclerotium Poriae Cocos (*Fu Ling*), 12g each, Pericarpium Citri Reticulatae (*Chen Pi*), Caulis Bambusae In Taeniis (*Zhu Ru*), and Caulis Akebiae (*Mu Tong*), 9g each, Radix Glycyrrhizae (*Gan Cao*) and Rhizoma Coptidis Chinensis (*Huang Lian*), 3-6g each, and Fructus Zizyphi Jujubae (*Da Zao*), 3-5 pieces.

ACUPUNCTURE & MOXIBUSTION: *Yin Ling Quan* (Sp 9), *San Yin Jiao* (Sp 6), *Zhong Ji* (CV 3), *Ba Liao* (Bl 31-34)

FORMULA ANALYSIS: Draining *Yin Ling Quan*, *Zhong Ji*,

and the *Ba Liao* seeps dampness and frees the flow of urination. Even supplementing-even draining *San Yin Jiao* treats urogenital disorders.

ADDITIONS & SUBTRACTIONS: If there is concomitant liver depression, add draining *Tai Chong* (Liv 3) and *He Gu* (LI 4). If there is concomitant spleen vacuity, add supplementing *Pi Shu* (Bl 20) and *Wei Shu* (Bl 21). If enduring heat has damaged liver-kidney yin, add supplementing *Tai Xi* (Ki 3), *Qu Quan* (Liv 8), and *Shen Shu* (Bl 23) and use supplementing technique at *San Yin Jiao*. If there is nausea and vomiting, add draining *Zhong Wan* (CV 12), *Nei Guan* (Per 6), and *Zu San Li* (St 36). If there is lung-stomach fluid dryness, add even supplementing-even draining *Zhao Hai* (Ki 6), *Lie Que* (Lu 7), and/or *Nei Ting* (St 44). For heart-liver fire effulgence, add draining *Shao Fu* (Ht 8) and *Xing Jian* (Liv 2).

4. LIVER-STOMACH DEPRESSIVE HEAT PATTERN

MAIN SYMPTOMS: Non-freely flowing urination or freely flowing urination which is, nonetheless, not crisp, incomplete emptying of the bladder, urinary frequency and urgency, emotional depression, profuse vexation, easy anger, insomnia, restlessness, rib-side and abdominal distention and fullness, a bitter taste in the mouth, possible acid eructations, polyphagia, rapid hungering, a red tongue with thin, yellow fur, and a bowstring, rapid pulse

TREATMENT PRINCIPLES: Course the liver, resolve depression, and clear heat from the liver and stomach, free the flow and disinhibit urination

RX: *Chen Xiang San Jia Jian* (Eagleswood Powder with Additions & Subtractions)

INGREDIENTS: Herba Pyrrosiae (*Shi Wei*), 30g, Talcum (*Hua Shi*) and Radix Albus Paeoniae Lactiflorae (*Bai Shao*), 15g each, Radix Angelicae Sinensis (*Dang Gui*) and Semen Vaccariae Segetalis (*Wang Bu Liu Xing*), 12g each, Radix Bupleuri (*Chai Hu*), Pericarpium Citri Reticulatae (*Chen Pi*), Fructus Gardeniae Jasminoidis (*Zhi Zi*), and Semen Abutilonis Seu Malvae (*Dong Gui Zi*), 9g each, Radix Gentianae Scabrae (*Long Dan Cao*) and Extremitas Radicis Glycyrrhizae (*Gan Cao Xiao*), 6g each, and powdered Lignum Aquilariae Agallochae (*Chen Xiang*), 3g, swallowed with the decoction

FORMULA ANALYSIS: *Chen Xiang*, *Chai Hu*, and *Chen Pi* course and out-thrust the liver qi. When combined with *Dang Gui* and *Wang Bu Liu Xing*, they are able to move the qi and blood of the lower burner. *Shi Wei*, *Dong Gui Zi*, and *Hua Shi* free the flow and disinhibit the water passageways, while *Zhi Zi* and *Long Dan Cao* clear heat from the liver and three burners. *Gan Cao Xiao* both helps clear and disinhibit dampness and heat and harmonizes all the other medicinals in the formula.

ADDITIONS & SUBTRACTIONS: If there is concomitant spleen vacuity, add 15 grams of Radix Astragali Membranacei (*Huang Qi*) and 12 grams of Sclerotium Poriae Cocos (*Fu Ling*). If there is lung-stomach fluid dryness, add 12 grams each of Tuber Ophiopogonis Japonici (*Mai Men Dong*) and Radix Glehniae Littoralis (*Sha Shen*). If there is concomitant blood stasis, add 30 grams of Radix Salviae Miltiorrhizae (*Dan Shen*) and 12 grams of Herba Leonuri Heterophylli (*Yi Mu Cao*).

ACUPUNCTURE & MOXIBUSTION: *Tai Chong* (Liv 3) through to *Xing Jian* (Liv 2), *Yang Ling Quan* (GB 34) through to *Yin Ling Quan* (Sp 9), *San Yin Jiao* (Sp 6), *Qi Hai* (CV 6), *Zhong Ji* (CV 3)

FORMULA ANALYSIS: Draining *Tai Chong-Xing Jian* and *Yang Ling Quan-Yin Ling Quan* courses the liver, resolves depression, and clears heat. Draining *Qi Hai* and *Zhong Ji* rectifies the qi of the lower burner and disinhibits urination. Even supplementing-even draining *San Yin Jiao* treats urogenital disorders.

ADDITIONS & SUBTRACTIONS: For concomitant heat in the stomach, add draining *Nei Ting* (St 44). For concomitant thirst, add even supplementing-even draining *Zhao Hai* (Ki 6) and *Lie Que* (Lu 7). For concomitant blood stasis, add draining *Xue Hai* (Sp 10) and use even supplementing-even draining at *San Yin Jiao*. If there is simultaneous spleen vacuity, add even supplementing-even draining *Zu San Li* (St 36) and supplementing *Pi Shu* (Bl 20) and *Wei Shu* (Bl 21). If there is simultaneous kidney yin vacuity, add supplementing *Tai Xi* (Ki 3) and *Shen Shu* (Bl 23). If there is simultaneous kidney yang vacuity, add moxa at *Shen Shu* and *Ming Men* (GV 4). If there is heart fire effulgence, add draining *Shao Fu* (Ht 8).

DIABETIC ESOPHAGEAL & STOMACH HYPOTONIA

1. LIVER-STOMACH DEPRESSIVE HEAT PATTERN

MAIN SYMPTOMS: Difficulty swallowing, retrosternal discomfort, thirst with a desire for chilled drinks, vexation and agitation, easy anger, a burning heat sensation within the chest, a red tongue with sticky, yellow fur, and a bowstring, slippery or bowstring, rapid pulse

TREATMENT PRINCIPLES: Clear and drain the liver and stomach

RX: *Yu Nu Jian Jia Jian* (Jade Maiden Decoction with Additions & Subtractions)

INGREDIENTS: Uncooked Gypsum Fibrosum (*Shi Gao*), 30g, uncooked Radix Rehmanniae (*Sheng Di*), 15g, Radix Achyranthis Bidentatae (*Niu Xi*) and Tuber Ophiopogonis Japonici (*Mai Men Dong*), 12g each, Rhizoma Anemarrhenae Aspheloidis (*Zhi Mu*), Radix Bupleuri (*Chai Hu*), and Radix Scutellariae Baicalensis (*Huang Qin*), 9g each

FORMULA ANALYSIS: *Shi Gao* and *Zhi Mu* clear stomach heat. *Sheng Di* enriches yin. *Mai Men Dong* clears heat and nourishes yin. *Niu Xi* abducts heat and moves it downward. *Chai Hu* and *Huang Qin* course the liver and clear liver heat.

ADDITIONS & SUBTRACTIONS: If there is simultaneous qi vacuity, add 9-15 grams of Radix Codonopsitis Pilosulae (*Dang Shen*). If there is simultaneous qi stagnation, add nine grams each of Rhizoma Cyperi Rotundi (*Xiang Fu*), Fructus Meliae Toosendan (*Chuan Lian Zi*), and Flos Inulae Racemosae (*Xuan Fu Hua*).

If there is simultaneous yin vacuity, one can use *Yi Guan Jian Jia Wei* (One Link Decoction with Added Flavors): uncooked Gypsum Fibrosum (*Shi Gao*), 30g, uncooked Radix Rehmanniae (*Sheng Di*), 15g, Tuber Ophiopogonis Japonici (*Mai Men Dong*), 12g, Rhizoma Anemarrhenae Aspheloidis (*Zhi Mu*), Radix Glehniae Littoralis (*Sha Shen*), Radix Angelicae Sinensis (*Dang Gui*), Fructus Lycii Chinensis (*Gou Qi Zi*), and Fructus Meliae Toosendan (*Chuan Lian Zi*), 9g each. If there is constipation, add nine grams of Semen Trichosanthis Kirlowii (*Gua Lou Ren*). If there is abdominal pain, add 18 grams of Radix Albus Paeoniae Lactiflorae (*Bai Shao*) and six grams of Radix Glyucyrrhizae (*Gan Cao*). If there is concomitant blood stasis, add 30 grams of Radix Salviae Miltiorrhizae (*Dan Shen*) and 12 grams of Carapax Amydae Sinensis (*Bei Jia*).

ACUPUNCTURE & MOXIBUSTION: *Xing Jian* (Liv 2), *He Gu* (LI 4), *Nei Ting* (St 44), *Nei Guan* (Per 6), *Dan Zhong* (CV 17), *Zhong Wan* (CV 12)

FORMULA ANALYSIS: Draining *Xing Jian* drains liver heat, while draining *Nei Ting* drains stomach heat. Draining *He Gu* and *Zhong Wan* disinhibits the qi mechanism and harmonizes the stomach, while draining *Nei Guan* and *Zhong Wan* regulates and rectifies the qi and loosens the chest.

ADDITIONS & SUBTRACTIONS: If there is simultaneous yin vacuity, add supplementing *Tai Xi* (Ki 3), *Shen Shu* (Bl 23), and *San Yin Jiao* (Sp 6). If there is constipation, add draining *Tian Shu* (St 25), *Da Chang Shu* (Bl 25), *Zhi Gou* (TB 6), and *Yang Ling Quan* (GB 34) and supplementing *Zhao Hai* (Ki 6). If there is concomitant blood stasis, add draining *Xue Hai* (Sp 10) and even supplementing-even draining *San Yin Jiao* (Sp 6).

2. SPLEEN VACUITY & PHLEGM CONGELATION PATTERN

MAIN SYMPTOMS: Difficulty swallowing, stomach duct glomus and oppression, scanty intake, bodily fatigue, nausea, profuse phlegm, sticky, slimy tongue fur, and a soggy, moderate (*i.e.*, relaxed or slightly slow) pulse

TREATMENT PRINCIPLES: Fortify the spleen and transform phlegm, disinhibit the qi mechanism and harmonize the stomach

RX: *Si Jun Zi Tang* (Four Gentlemen Decoction) plus *Er Chen Tang* (Two Aged [Ingredients] Decoction) with additions and subtractions

INGREDIENTS: Radix Codonopsitis Pilosulae (*Dang Shen*) and Sclerotium Poriae Cocos (*Fu Ling*), 12g each, Rhizoma Atractylodis Macrocephalae (*Bai Zhu*), Pericarpium Citri Reticulatae (*Chen Pi*), and Rhizoma Pinelliae Ternatae (*Ban Xia*), 9g each, and Cortex Magnoliae Officinalis (*Hou Po*) and Radix Glycyrrhizae (*Gan Cao*), 6g each

FORMULA ANALYSIS: *Dang Shen, Bai Zhu, Fu Ling*, and *Gan Cao* all fortify the spleen and supplement the qi. *Ban Xia* and *Chen Pi* rectify the qi and transform phlegm, harmonize the stomach and stop vomiting. *Hou Po* also rectifies the qi and transforms turbidity, while *Gan Cao* harmonizes all the other medicinals in the formula.

ADDITIONS & SUBTRACTIONS: If there are loose stools and poor appetite, add nine grams each of Radix Dioscoreae Oppositae (*Shan Yao*), Semen Nelumbinis Nuciferae (*Lian Zi Rou*), and Endothelium Corneum Gigeriae Galli (*Ji Nei Jin*). If there is simultaneous qi stagnation, add nine grams each of Radix Bupleuri (*Chai Hu*), Fructus Immaturus Citri Aurantii (*Zhi Shi*), Radix Auklandiae Lappae (*Mu Xiang*), and Fructus Citri Sacrodactylis (*Fo Shou*) to rectify the qi and open depression.

ACUPUNCTURE & MOXIBUSTION: *Pi Shu* (Bl 20), *Wei Shu* (Bl 21), *Zu San Li* (St 36), *Feng Long* (St 40), *Zhong Wan* (CV 12)

FORMULA ANALYSIS: Supplementing *Pi Shu, Wei Shu*, and *Zu San Li* fortifies the spleen and supplements the qi, while even supplementing-even draining *Feng Long* and *Zhong Wan* transforms phlegm.

ADDITIONS & SUBTRACTIONS: If there are loose stools, add supplementing *Tian Shu* (St 25) and *Da Chang Shu* (Bl 25). If there is simultaneous liver depression qi stagnation, add draining *Tai Chong* (Liv 3) and *He Gu* (LI 4).

3. SPLEEN-STOMACH VACUITY WEAKNESS PATTERN

MAIN SYMPTOMS: Chest and epigastric discomfort, glomus, congestion, distention, and fullness, drum distention after meals, decreased appetite, a liking for heat and a liking for pressure, obtaint of warmth leading to soothing, lack of warmth in the four extremities, shortness of breath, lack of strength, bodily fatigue, disinclination to speak and/or a faint, weak voice, loose stools, a pale tongue with white fur, and a deep, fine, or vacuous, large, forceless pulse

TREATMENT PRINCIPLES: Fortify the spleen and supplement the qi, upbear the clear and downbear the turbid

RX: *Bu Zhong Yi Qi Tang* (Supplement the Center & Boost the Qi Decoction)

INGREDIENTS: Radix Astragali Membranacei (*Huang Qi*) and Radix Codonopsitis Pilosulae (*Dang Shen*), 15g each, Rhizoma Atractylodis Macrocephalae (*Bai Zhu*), 12g, Radix Angelicae Sinensis (*Dang Gui*), Pericarpium Citri Reticulatae (*Chen Pi*), and Radix Bupleuri (*Chai Hu*), 9g each, and mix-fried Radix Glycyrrhizae (*Gan Cao*) and Rhizoma Cimicifugae (*Sheng Ma*), 6g each

FORMULA ANALYSIS: *Huang Qi, Dang Shen, Bai Zhu*, and mix-fried *Gan Cao* supplement the spleen and boost the qi. *Chen Pi* rectifies the qi and transforms stagnation, while *Chai Hu* and *Sheng Ma* upbear and lift clear yang.

ADDITIONS & SUBTRACTIONS: If there is simultaneous yang vacuity, one can add 3-9 grams of Radix Lateralis Praeparatus Aconiti Carmichaeli (*Fu Zi*). If dampness is exuberant, add 12 grams of Sclerotium Poriae Cocos (*Fu Ling*) and nine grams of Rhizoma Alismatis (*Ze Xie*). If center cold is severe, add 9-12 grams of Fructus Evodiae Rutecarpae (*Wu Zhu Yu*) and 18-21 grams of uncooked Rhizoma Zingiberis (*Sheng Jiang*). If there is simultaneous liver depression qi stagnation, add 9-18 grams of Radix

Albus Paeoniae Lactiflorae (*Bai Shao*). If stomach intake is torpid, add 6-9 grams of Massa Medica Fermentata (*Shen Qu*) and 3-4.5 grams of Fructus Amomi (*Sha Ren*).

If there is spleen-kidney dual vacuity, use *Li Zhong Wan Jia Wei* (Rectify the Center Pills with Added Flavors): Radix Panacis Ginseng (*Ren Shen*), 9-15g, Rhizoma Atractylodis Macrocephalae (*Bai Zhu*), 9g, dry Rhizoma Zingiberis (*Gan Jiang*), 6-9g, and mix-fried Radix Glycyrrhizae (*Gan Cao*), Radix Lateralis Praeparatus Aconiti Carmichaeli (*Fu Zi*), and Cortex Cinnamomi Cassiae (*Rou Gui*), 3-6g each.

If there is spleen vacuity and cold at the same time as there is dampness and heat in the stomach and intestines, use *Ban Xia Xie Xin Tang* (Pinelliae Drain the Heart Decoction): Radix Codonopsitis Pilosulae (*Dang Shen*) and Rhizoma Pinelliae Ternatae (*Ban Xia*), 12g each, Radix Scutellariae Baicalensis (*Huang Qin*) and dry Rhizoma Zingiberis (*Gan Jiang*), 9g each, mix-fried Radix Glycyrrhizae (*Gan Cao*), 6g, Rhizoma Coptidis Chinensis (*Huang Lian*), 3-6g, and Fructus Zizyphi Jujubae (*Da Zao*), 3-5 pieces. If there is a spleen-heart dual vacuity, increase the mix-fried *Gan Cao* up to 15 grams. If there is water and heat both binding in the center, substitute 3-5 slices of uncooked Rhizoma Zingiberis (*Sheng Jiang*) for *Gan Jiang*.

ACUPUNCTURE & MOXIBUSTION: *Pi Shu* (Bl 20), *Wei Shu* (Bl 21), *Zu San Li* (St 36), *Zhong Wan* (CV 12), *Tian Shu* (St 25)

FORMULA ANALYSIS: Supplementing *Pi Shu, Wei Shu, Zu San Li, Zhong Wan,* and *Tian Shu* supplements the spleen and harmonizes the stomach and intestines.

ADDITIONS & SUBTRACTIONS: If there is simultaneous center cold or spleen yang vacuity, add moxibustion at *Zhong Wan, Pi Shu,* and *Wei Shu*. If there is spleen-kidney dual vacuity, also add moxibustion at *Shen Shu* (Bl 23), *Ming Men* (GV 4), and *Guan Yuan* (CV 4). If there is simultaneous liver depression, add draining at *Tai Chong* (Liv 3) and *He Gu* (LI 4). If there is heat in the stomach and intestines, add draining *Nei Ting* (St 44) and even supplementing-even draining *Da Chang Shu* (Bl 25) and use even supplementing-even draining at *Zhong Wan, Tian Shu,* and *Zu San Li*.

4. PHLEGM DAMPNESS OBSTRUCTING INTERNALLY PATTERN

MAIN SYMPTOMS: Chest and epigastric glomus, congestion, fullness, oppression, and discomfort, dizziness and vertigo, devitalized eating and drinking, nausea and vomiting, a heavy body, fatigue, possible cough with profuse phlegm, loose stools, turbid, slimy tongue fur, and a slippery pulse

TREATMENT PRINCIPLES: Eliminate dampness and transform phlegm, normalize the flow of qi and loosen the center

RX: *Er Chen Tang Jia Jian* (Two Aged [Ingredients] Decoction with Additions & Subtractions)

INGREDIENTS: Sclerotium Poriae Cocos (*Fu Ling*), 12g, Rhizoma Pinelliae Ternatae (*Ban Xia*), Pericarpium Citri Reticulatae (*Chen Pi*), Rhizoma Atractylodis (*Cang Zhu*), Cortex Magnoliae Officinalis (*Hou Po*), Fructus Immaturus Citri Aurantii (*Zhi Shi*), and Fructus Amomi (*Sha Ren*), 9g each, and Radix Glycyrrhizae (*Gan Cao*), 6g

FORMULA ANALYSIS: *Cang Zhu* dries dampness and fortifies the spleen, while *Hou Po* eliminates fullness and loosens the chest. *Chen Pi* and *Zhi Shi* rectify the qi and transform phlegm. *Ban Xia* dries dampness and transforms phlegm. *Fu Ling* and *Sha Ren* boost the spleen and open the stomach, while *Gan Cao* harmonizes the center and supplements vacuity.

ADDITIONS & SUBTRACTIONS: If there is cough with profuse phlegm, add nine grams each of Folium Perillae Frutescentis (*Zi Su Ye*) and Radix Platycodi Grandiflori (*Jie Geng*). If there is nausea, add nine grams each of Flos Inulae Racemosae (*Xuan Fu Hua*) and Haemititum (*Dai Zhi Shi*). If there is chest oppression, add nine grams each of Bulbus Allii Fistulosi(*Cong Bai*) and Radix Bupleuri (*Chai Hu*).

ACUPUNCTURE & MOXIBUSTION: *Feng Long* (St 40), *Shang Qiu* (Sp 5), *Nei Guan* (Per 6), *Shang Wan* (CV 13), *Zhong Wan* (CV 12), *Xia Wan* (CV 10)

FORMULA ANALYSIS: Draining *Feng Long* transforms phlegm. Draining *Shang Qiu* eliminates damp encumbrance from the spleen. Draining *Nei Guan* harmonizes the stomach and downbears counterflow, while draining *Shang Wan, Zhong Wan,* and *Xia Wan* strongly disinhibits the qi mechanism and divides clear from turbid.

ADDITIONS & SUBTRACTIONS: If there is chest oppression, add draining *Dan Zhong* (CV 17). If there is liver depression qi stagnation, add draining *Tai Chong* (Liv 3) and *He Gu* (LI 4). If there is cough, add draining *Kong Zui* (Lu 6) and *Fei Shu* (Bl 13).

5. LIVER DEPRESSION QI STAGNATION PATTERN

MAIN SYMPTOMS: Chest and epigastric discomfort, glomus, congestion, fullness, and oppression, devitalized eating and drinking, easy anger, rib-side distention and pain, occasional sighing, thin, white tongue fur, and a bowstring pulse

---

NOTE: This pattern rarely presents in such a simple, discrete form. However, it complicates most patterns of most chronic diseases.

TREATMENT PRINCIPLES: Course the liver and resolve depression, rectify the qi and disperse stagnation

RX: *Chai Hu Shu Gan Yin Jia Jian* (Bupleurum Course the Liver Drink with Additions & Subtractions)

INGREDIENTS: Radix Albus Paeoniae Lactiflorae (*Bai Shao*), 12g, Radix Bupleuri (*Chai Hu*), Pericarpium Citri Reticulatae (*Chen Pi*), Fructus Citri Aurantii (*Zhi Ke*), Radix Ligustici Wallichii (*Chuan Xiong*), Rhizoma Cyperi Rotundi (*Xiang Fu*), and Tuber Curcumae (*Yu Jin*), 9g each, and Radix Glycyrrhizae (*Gan Cao*), 6g

FORMULA ANALYSIS: *Chai Hu, Xiang Fu, Zhi Ke,* and *Chen Pi* course the liver and rectify the qi. *Chuan Xiong* and *Yu Jin* are qi within the blood medicinals which are also able to rectify the qi and resolve depression. *Bai Shao* and *Gan Cao* relax tension and soothe the spleen.

ADDITIONS & SUBTRACTIONS: If there is damp exuberance, add 12 grams of Sclerotium Poriae Cocos (*Fu Ling*) and nine grams of Rhizoma Alismatis (*Ze Xie*). If there is profuse phlegm, add nine grams each of Rhizoma Pinelliae Ternatae (*Ban Xia*) and Rhizoma Atractylodis (*Cang Zhu*). If there is simultaneous food stagnation, add nine grams each of Massa Medica Fermentatae (*Shen Qu*) and Fructus Crataegi (*Shan Zha*). If there is qi depression transforming fire, add three grams of Fructus Evodiae Rutecarpae (*Wu Zhu Yu*), 3-9 grams of Rhizoma Coptidis Chinensis (*Huang Lian*), and nine grams of Fructus Meliae Toosendan (*Chuan Lian Zi*).

If there is qi stagnation and blood stasis with piercing stomach duct pain which is fixed in location, chest and rib-side distention and fullness, a dark red tongue, and choppy pulse, one can use *Shi Xiao San* (Loose a Smile Powder) plus *Dan Shen Yin* (Salvia Drink) with additions and subtractions: Radix Salviae Miltiorrhizae (*Dan Shen*), 15g, Feces Trogopterori Seu Pteromi (*Wu Ling Zhi*) and uncooked Pollen Typhae (*Pu Huang*), 9g each, Lignum Santali Albi (*Bai Tan Xiang*), 6g, and Fructus Amomi (*Sha Ren*), 3g.

ACUPUNCTURE & MOXIBUSTION: *Tai Chong* (Liv 3),

He Gu (LI 4), *Nei Guan* (Per 6), *Dan Zhong* (CV 17), *Zhong Wan* (CV 12)

FORMULA ANALYSIS: Draining *Tai Chong* and *He Gu* courses the liver and rectifies the qi. Draining *Nei Guan, Dan Zhong,* and *Zhong Wan* resolves depression and eliminates distention.

ADDITIONS & SUBTRACTIONS: If there is simultaneous rib-side distention and pain, add draining *Wai Guan* (TB 5), *Zu Lin Qi* (GB 41), and *Zhang Men* (Liv 13). If there is damp exuberance, add draining *Shang Qiu* (Sp 5). If there is profuse phlegm, add draining *Feng Long* (St 40). If there is concomitant food stagnation, add draining *Liang Men* (St 21). If there is qi depression transforming fire, add draining *Yang Ling Quan* (GB 34) and *Xing Jian* (Liv 2) by needling through from *Tai Chong*. If there is concomitant stomach fire, add draining *Nei Ting* (St 44). If there is hard, fixed, piercing epigastric pain, add draining *Xue Hai* (Sp 10).

DIABETIC CONSTIPATION

1. STOMACH & INTESTINES REPLETE HEAT PATTERN

MAIN SYMPTOMS: Dry bound stools, short, reddish urination, a red facial complexion, heart vexation, possible bodily heat, a dry mouth, bad breath, abdominal distention and possible pain, a red tongue with dry, yellow fur, and a slippery, rapid pulse

TREATMENT PRINCIPLES: Clear heat, moisten the intestines, and free the flow of the stools

RX: *Ma Zi Ren Wan Jia Jian* (Cannabis Seed Pills with Additions & Subtractions)

INGREDIENTS: Semen Cannabis Sativae (*Huo Ma Ren*) and Radix Albus Paeoniae Lactiflorae (*Bai Shao*), 12g each, Semen Pruni Armeniacae (*Xing Ren*), Fructus Immaturus Citri Aurantii (*Zhi Shi*), Cortex Magnoliae Officinalis (*Hou Po*), and Mel (*Feng Mi*), 9g each, Radix Et Rhizoma Rhei (*Da Huang*), 6-9g, and Radix Glycyrrhizae (*Gan Cao*), 6g

FORMULA ANALYSIS: *Da Huang* and *Huo Ma Ren* discharge heat, moisten the intestines, and free the flow of the stools. *Xing Ren* downbears the qi and moistens the intestines, while *Bai Shao* nourishes yin. *Zhi Shi* and *Hou Po* descend and break the qi, move the qi and eliminate fullness. *Gan Cao* harmonizes the center, and *Feng Mi* strengthens the effect of moistening the intestines.

ADDITIONS & SUBTRACTIONS: If the stools are hard, add 3-6 grams of Mirabilitum (*Mang Xiao*) to soften the hard and scatter binding, drain heat and free the flow of the stools. If there is a dry mouth and tongue due to damaged and consumed fluids and humors, add 12 grams of uncooked Radix Rehmanniae (*Sheng Di*) and nine grams each of Radix Scrophulariae Ningpoensis (*Xuan Shen*) and Herba Dendrobii (*Shi Hu*) to nourish yin and engender fluids. If there are simultaneous hemorrhoids and hemafecia, add 15 grams of Flos Immaturus Sophorae Japonicae (*Huai Hua Mi*) and nine grams of Radix Sanguisorbae (*Di Yu*) to clear the intestines and stop bleeding. If there is simultaneous depression and anger damaging the liver with red eyes, irritability, and a bowstring, rapid pulse, add 12 grams of Herba Aloes (*Lu Hui*) to clear the liver and free the flow of the stools. If there is phlegm heat congesting in the lungs resulting in large intestine heat binding, one can add nine grams each of Radix Scutellariae Baicalensis (*Huang Qin*) and Semen Trichosanthis Kirlowii (*Gua Lou Ren*) to clear the lungs, moisten the intestines, and discharge heat.

ACUPUNCTURE & MOXIBUSTION: *He Gu* (LI 4), *Nei Ting* (St 44), *Tian Shu* (St 25), *Da Chang Shu* (Bl 25)

FORMULA ANALYSIS: Draining *He Gu* and *Nei Ting* drains the hand and foot yang ming. Draining *Tian Shu* and *Da Chang Shu* drains the large intestine and frees the flow of the stools.

ADDITIONS & SUBTRACTIONS: If there is simultaneous liver depression qi stagnation, add draining *Yang Ling Quan* (GB 34) and *Zhi Gou* (TB 6). If there is a dry mouth and tongue due to damaged fluids, add supplementing *Zhao Hai* (Ki 6).

2. SPLEEN VACUITY & QI WEAKNESS PATTERN

MAIN SYMPTOMS: Dry bound or soft stools which only move once every so many days, lack of force and difficulty in expelling the feces even though one feels like having a bowel movement, possible sweating during defecation, fatigue which worsens after a bowel movement, disinclination to speak and/or a faint, weak voice, no lower abdominal distention or pain, but possible rectal prolapse or hemorrhoids, a cold body and a white facial complexion, lusterless lips and nails, a pale, tender tongue with thin, white fur, and a vacuous, weak pulse

NOTE: This pattern of constipation rarely presents by itself. However, spleen qi vacuity may and, in the case of diabetic constipation, usually does complicate either of the other two patterns presented here.

TREATMENT PRINCIPLES: Fortify the spleen and supplement the qi, moisten the intestines and free the flow of the stools

RX: *Huang Qi Tang Jia Jian* (Astragalus Decoction with Additions & Subtractions)

INGREDIENTS: Radix Astragali Membranacei (*Huang Qi*), 30g, Pericarpium Citri Reticulatae (*Chen Pi*), Semen Cannabis Sativae (*Huo Ma Ren*), and Mel (*Feng Mi*), 9g each

FORMULA ANALYSIS: *Huang Qi* supplements the qi of the lungs and spleen, while *Huo Ma Ren* and *Feng Mi* moisten the intestines and free the flow of the stools. *Chen Pi* rectifies the qi and downbears turbidity.

ADDITIONS & SUBTRACTIONS: If there is anal prolapse, hemorrhoids, and/or orthostatic hypotension due to downward falling of the central qi, add nine grams of Radix Platycodi Grandiflori (*Jie Geng*), six grams of Radix Panacis Ginseng (*Ren Shen*) or 9-12 grams of Radix Codonopsitis Pilosulae (*Dang Shen*), 4.5 grams of Rhizoma Cimicifugae (*Sheng Ma*), and 3-9 grams of Radix Bupleuri (*Chai Hu*). If there is concomitant lung qi vacuity with enduring cough and shortness of breath, add 12 grams of Tuber Ophiopogonis Japonici (*Mai Men Dong*), nine grams each of Fructus Schisandrae Chinensis (*Wu Wei Zi*) and Radix Asteris Tatarici (*Zi Wan*), and 6-9 grams of Radix Panacis Ginseng (*Ren Shen*). If there is concomitant kidney yang vacuity, add nine grams each of Herba Cistanchis Deserticolae (*Rou Cong Rong*) and Herba Cynomorii Songarici (*Suo Yang*). If there is spleen vacuity and qi stagnation, one can add nine grams each of Semen Arecae Catechu (*Bin Lan*), Radix Auklandiae Lappae (*Mu Xiang*), Rhizoma Cyperi Rotundi (*Xiang Fu*), and Tuber Curcumae (*Yu Jin*).

ACUPUNCTURE & MOXIBUSTION: *He Gu* (LI 4), *Zu San Li* (St 36), *Da Heng* (Sp 15), *Tian Shu* (St 25), *Pi Shu* (Bl 20), *Wei Shu* (Bl 21), *Da Chang Shu* (Bl 25)

FORMULA ANALYSIS: Supplementing *Zu San Li*, *Pi Shu*, and *Wei Shu* fortifies the spleen and boosts the qi. Supplementing *Da Heng*, *Tian Shu*, and *Da Chang Shu* supplements the large intestine qi and frees the flow of the stools. Even supplementing-even draining *He Gu* supplements the large intestine and downbears the turbid.

ADDITIONS & SUBTRACTIONS: If there is concomitant liver depression, add draining *Qi Hai* (CV 6), *Zhi Gou* (TB 6), and *Yang Ling Quan* (GB 34). If there is concomitant kidney yang vacuity, add moxibustion at *Shen Shu* (Bl 23), *Ming Men* (GV 4), and *Pi Shu* and *Wei Shu*. If there is anal prolapse, hemorrhoids, or orthostatic hypotension, moxa *Bai Hui* (GV 20).

3. BLOOD VACUITY & YIN DEPLETION CONSTIPATION PATTERN

MAIN SYMPTOMS: Dry stools which are difficult to expel, an emaciated body, a dry throat with scanty fluids, a sallow yellow or pale, white lusterless facial complexion, heart palpitations, dizziness, pale white lips and nails, a pale or possibly red tongue with scanty fluids depending on whether blood or yin vacuity predominate, and a fine or fine, rapid, forceless pulse

TREATMENT PRINCIPLES: Nourish the blood and enrich yin, moisten dryness and free the flow of the stools

RX: *Run Chang Tang Jia Jian* (Moisten the Intestines Decoction with Additions & Subtractions)

INGREDIENTS: Uncooked Radix Rehmanniae (*Sheng Di*), 20g, Semen Trichosanthis Kirlowii (*Gua Lou Ren*), 15g, Radix Angelicae Sinensis (*Dang Gui*) and Semen Cannabis Sativae (*Huo Ma Ren*), 12g each, and Semen Pruni Persicae (*Tao Ren*) and Fructus Citri Aurantii (*Zhi Ke*), 9g each

FORMULA ANALYSIS: *Dang Gui* and *Sheng Di* supplement the blood and enrich yin. *Huo Ma Ren, Tao Ren,* and *Gua Lou Ren* moisten the intestines and free the flow of the stools. *Zhi Ke* breaks the qi and moves it downward.

ADDITIONS & SUBTRACTIONS: If there is simultaneous heat, add nine grams each of Radix Polygoni Multiflori (*He Shou Wu*), Rhizoma Polygonati Odorati (*Yu Zhu*), Radix Scrophulariae Ningpoensis (*Xuan Shen*), and Rhizoma Anemarrhenae Aspheloidis (*Zhi Mu*) to engender fluids and clear heat.

ACUPUCNTURE & MOXIBUSTION: *San Yin Jiao* (Sp 6), *Zhao Hai* (Ki 6), *Ge Shu* (Bl 17), *Gan Shu* (Bl 18), *Shen Shu* (Bl 23), *Da Chang Shu* (Bl 25)

FORMULA ANALYSIS: Supplementing *San Yin Jiao* nourishes and enriches the liver and kidneys. Supplementing *Zhao Hai* moistens dryness and clears vacuity heat. Supplementing *Ge Shu, Gan Shu, Shen Shu,* and *Da Chang*

Shu nourishes the blood and enriches yin, moistens the intestines and frees the flow of the stools.

ADDITIONS & SUBTRACTIONS: If there is concomitant liver depression qi stagnation, add draining *He Gu* (LI 4), *Zhi Gou* (TB 6), *Qi Hai* (CV 6), and *Yang Ling Quan* (GB 34). If there is concomitant spleen qi vacuity, add supplementing *Zu San Li* (St 36). If there is concomitant kidney yang vacuity, add moxibustion at *Shen Shu, Ming Men* (GV 4), and *Guan Yuan* (CV 4).

DIABETIC DIARRHEA

1. DAMP HEAT OBSTRUCTING THE CENTER PATTERN

MAIN SYMPTOMS: Abdominal pain and diarrhea, urgent, forceful diarrhea, foul-smelling stools, bright yellow or dark colored stools, possible burning heat around the anus, oral thirst, slimy, yellow tongue fur, and a slippery, rapid pulse

TREATMENT PRINCIPLES: Clear heat, transform dampness, and stop diarrhea

RX: *Ge Gen Qin Lian Tang Jia Jian* (Pueraria, Scutellaria & Coptis Decoction with Additions & Subtractions)

INGREDIENTS: Radix Puerariae (*Ge Gen*) and stir-fried Semen Plantaginis (*Che Qian Zi*), 15g each, Radix Scutellariae Baicalensis (*Huang Qin*), Radix Auklandiae Lappae (*Mu Xiang*), and Herba Agastachis Seu Pogostemi (*Huo Xiang*), 9g each, Rhizoma Coptidis Chinensis (*Huang Lian*) and Radix Glycyrrhizae (*Gan Cao*), 6g each

FORMULA ANALYSIS: *Ge Gen* engenders fluids and stops thirst, upbears the clear and stops diarrhea. *Huang Qi* and *Huang Lian* clear heat and eliminate dampness from the stomach and intestines. *Mu Xiang* and *Huo Xiang* aromatically transform turbidity and arouse the spleen, while *Gan Cao* harmonizes all the other medicinals in the formula.

ADDITIONS & SUBTRACTIONS: If there is concomitant food stagnation, add nine grams each of Massa Medica Fermentata (*Shen Qu*), Fructus Crataegi (*Shan Zha*), and Fructus Germinatus Horedi Vulgaris (*Mai Ya*). If there is concomitant spleen qi vacuity, add nine grams each of Radix Codonopsitis Pilosulae (*Dang Shen*), Rhizoma Atractylodis Macrocephalae (*Bai Zhu*), and Sclerotium Poriae Cocos (*Fu Ling*) and use mix-fried *Gan Cao*. If smoldering damp heat has damaged yin fluids, add

12 grams each of Tuber Ophiopogonis Japonici (*Mai Men Dong*) and Radix Glehniae Littoralis (*Sha Shen*).

ACUPUNCTURE & MOXIBUSTION: *He Gu* (LI 4), *Shang Ju Xu* (St 37), *Nei Ting* (St 44), *Tian Shu* (St 25), *Da Chang Shu* (Bl 25)

FORMULA ANALYSIS: Draining *He Gu, Shang Ju Xu, Nei Ting, Tian Shu*, and *Da Chang Shu* clear heat and eliminates dampness from the stomach and intestines.

ADDITIONS & SUBTRACTIONS: If there is concomitant food stagnation, add draining *Liang Men* (St 21) and *Zhong Wan* (CV 12). If there is concomitant qi stagnation, add draining *Qi Hai* (CV 6) and *Yang Ling Quan* (GB 34). For simultaneous spleen vacuity, add supplementing *Pi Shu* (Bl 20) and *Wei Shu* (Bl 21) and even supplementing-even draining *Zu San Li* (St 36) and delete *Shang Ju Xu*. If dampness is marked, add draining *Yin Ling Quan* (Sp 9) to seep dampness.

2. LIVER-SPLEEN DISHARMONY PATTERN

MAIN SYMPTOMS: Diarrhea precipitated or worsened by emotional stress possibly accompanied by cramping and pain, chest, epigastric, and/or rib-side distention, fullness, oppression, and/or pain, devitalized eating and drinking, acid eructation, hiccup, flatulence, a fat, enlarged, possibly pale but yet dark tongue with teeth-marks on its edges and thin, white fur, and a bowstring pulse

TREATMENT PRINCIPLES: Course the liver and rectify the qi, fortify the spleen and supplement the qi, stop diarrhea

RX: *Tong Xie Yao Fang Jia Wei* (Essential Formula for Painful Diarrhea with Added Flavors)

INGREDIENTS: Rhizoma Atractylodis Macrocephalae (*Bai Zhu*), 15g, Radix Albus Paeoniae Lactiflorae (*Bai Shao*), 12g, Pericarpium Citri Reticulatae (*Chen Pi*), Caulis Perillae Frutescentis (*Su Gen*), Rhizoma Cyperi Rotundi (*Xiang Fu*), and Radix Auklandiae Lappae (*Mu Xiang*), 9g each, and Radix Ledebouriellae Divaricatae (*Fang Feng*), 6g

FORMULA ANALYSIS: *Bai Zhu* fortifies the spleen and dries dampness. *Bai Shao* nourishes the blood and emolliates the liver. *Chen Pi* rectifies the qi and arouses the spleen. *Su Gen* and *Xiang Fu* also rectify the qi and disperse fullness and distention. *Mu Xiang* harmonizes the liver and spleen, and *Fang Feng* scatters the liver and soothes the spleen.

ADDITIONS & SUBTRACTIONS: If spleen vacuity is more severe, double the amount of *Bai Zhu* and add nine grams each of Radix Dioscoreae Oppositae (*Shan Yao*), Semen Dolichoris Lablab (*Bai Bian Dou*), and Semen Nelumbinis Nuciferae (*Lian Zi Rou*) and 4.5 grams of Fructus Amomi (*Sha Ren*).

ACUPUNCTURE & MOXIBUSTION: *Tai Chong* (Liv 3), *He Gu* (LI 4), *Zu San Li* (St 36), *San Yin Jiao* (Sp 6), *Tian Shu* (St 25), *Qi Hai* (CV 6), *Pi Shu* (Bl 20), *Wei Shu* (Bl 21), *Da Chang Shu* (Bl 25)

FORMULA ANALYSIS: Draining *Tai Chong, He Gu*, and *Qi Hai* courses the liver and regulates the qi. Supplementing *Zu San Li, San Yin Jiao, Pi Shu*, and *Wei Shu* fortifies the spleen and supplements the qi. Even supplementing-even draining *Tian Shu* and *Da Chang Shu* regulates the intestines and stops diarrhea.

ADDITIONS & SUBTRACTIONS: If depression has transformed heat, needle *Tai Chong* through to *Xing Jian* (Liv 2). If there is concomitant stomach heat, add draining *Nei Ting* (St 44).

3. SPLEEN VACUITY & DAMP EXUBERANCE PATTERN

MAIN SYMPTOMS: Sometimes loose stools, sometimes frank diarrhea, a long disease course with frequent relapses, untransformed grains in the stools, decreased appetite, abdominal fullness, distention, and discomfort after meals, marked aggravation of loose stools and diarrhea after eating greasy, oily foods, lassitude of the spirit, fatigue, lack of strength, a sallow yellow facial complexion, a pale, fat tongue with teeth-marks on its edges and white, possibly slimy fur, and a fine, forceless, possibly soggy, soft pulse

TREATMENT PRINCIPLES: Fortify the spleen and boost the qi, disinhibit dampness and stop diarrhea

RX: *Shen Ling Bai Zhu San* (Ginseng, Poria & Atractylodes Powder)

INGREDIENTS: Semen Coicis Lachryma-jobi (*Yi Yi Ren*) and Radix Dioscoreae Oppositae (*Shan Yao*), 30g each, Sclerotium Poriae Cocos (*Fu Ling*), Semen Dolichoris Lablab (*Bai Bian Dou*), Rhizoma Atractylodis Macrocephalae (*Bai Zhu*), and Semen Nelumbinis Nuciferae (*Lian Zi Rou*), 15g each, Radix Panacis Ginseng (*Ren Shen*), Pericarpium Citri Reticulatae (*Chen Pi*), and Fructus Amomi (*Sha Ren*), 9g each, and Radix Platycodi Grandiflori (*Jie Geng*) and mix-fried Radix Glycyrrhizae (*Gan Cao*), 6g each

FORMULA ANALYSIS: *Ren Shen, Bai Zhu, Fu Ling,* and *Gan Cao* fortify the spleen and boost the qi. *Sha Ren, Chen Pi, Jie Geng, Bai Bian Dou, Shan Yao, Lian Zi Rou,* and *Yi Yi Ren* fortify the spleen, rectify the qi, and transform dampness. When dampness is eliminated, the diarrhea automatically stops.

ADDITIONS & SUBTRACTIONS: If dampness is exuberant, add 12 grams of Sclerotium Polypori Umbellati (*Zhu Ling*) and nine grams of Rhizoma Alismatis (*Ze Xie*).

If there is spleen yang vacuity and decline, one can use *Fu Zi Li Zhong Tang* (Aconite Rectify the Center Decoction) to warm the center and scatter cold: Rhizoma Atractylodis Macrocephalae (*Bai Zhu*), 15g, Radix Panacis Ginseng (*Ren Shen*) and dry Rhizoma Zingiberis (*Gan Jiang*), 9g each, mix-fried Radix Glycyrrhizae (*Gan Cao*) and Radix Lateralis Praeparatus Aconiti Carmichaeli (*Fu Zi*), 6g each.

If diarrhea has endured for a long time and not healed and there is downward falling of the central qi, one can use *Bu Zhong Yi Qi Tang* (Supplement the Center & Boost the Qi Decoction) to fortify the spleen and stop diarrhea: Radix Astragali Membranacei (*Huang Qi*), 18-30g, Radix Codonopsitis Pilosulae (*Dang Shen*) and Rhizoma Atractylodis Macrocephalae (*Bai Zhu*), 12g each, Pericarpium Citri Reticulatae (*Chen Pi*), 9g, Radix Angelicae Sinensis (*Dang Gui*) and mix-fried Radix Glycyrrhizae (*Gan Cao*), 6g each, Rhizoma Cimicifugae (*Sheng Ma*), 4.5g, and Radix Bupleuri (*Chai Hu*), 3g.

ACUPUNCTURE & MOXIBUSTION: *Zu San Li* (St 36), *Shang Qiu* (Sp 5), *Zhong Wan* (CV 12), *Tian Shu* (St 25), *Pi Shu* (Bl 20), *Wei Shu* (Bl 21), *Da Chang Shu* (Bl 25)

FORMULA ANALYSIS: Supplementing *Zu San Li, Pi Shu,* and *Wei Shu* fortifies the spleen and supplements the qi. Supplementing *Zhong Wan, Tian Shu,*and *Da Chang Shu* supplements the stomach and intestines and stops diarrhea. Even supplementing-even draining *Shang Qiu* disinhibits dampness. If there is downward falling of the central qi, add moxibustion at *Bai Hui* (GV 20).

ADDITIONS & SUBTRACTIONS: If there is concomitant liver depression, add draining *Tai Chong* (Liv 3) and *He Gu* (LI 4).

4. SPLEEN-KIDNEY YANG VACUITY PATTERN

MAIN SYMPTOMS: Periumbilical pain, borborygmus preceding diarrhea, possible cockcrow diarrhea, fatigue, lassitude of the spirit, a cold body and chilled limbs and especially cold feet, polyuria, nocturia, long, clear urination, low back and knee soreness and limpness, decreased sexual desire, a pale tongue with white fur, and a deep, fine pulse

NOTE: The above signs and symptoms are that of a pure yang vacuity pattern. When spleen-kidney yang vacuity combines with any sort of heat, be it depressive heat, damp heat, or vacuity heat, heat signs will take precedence over cold signs in the tongue and pulse.

TREATMENT PRINCIPLES: Warm and supplement the spleen and kidneys, secure, astringe, and stop diarrhea

RX: *Li Zhong Tang* (Rectify the Center Decoction) plus *Si Shen Wan* (Four Spirits Pills) with additions and subtractions

INGREDIENTS: Radix Codonopsitis Pilosulae (*Dang Shen*), Rhizoma Atractylodis Macrocephalae (*Bai Zhu*), and Semen Myristicae Fragrantis (*Rou Dou Kou*), 15g each, Fructus Psoraleae Corylifoliae (*Bu Gu Zhi*), Fructus Evodiae Rutecarpae (*Wu Zhu Yu*), and Fructus Schisandrae Chinensis (*Wu Wei Zi*), 9g each, and dry Rhizoma Zingiberis (*Gan Jiang*) and mix-fried Radix Glycyrrhizae (*Gan Cao*), 6g each

FORMULA ANALYSIS: *Bu Gu Zhi* warms and supplements kidney yang. *Rou Dou Kou, Gan Jiang,* and *Wu Zhu Yu* warm the center and scatter cold. *Wu Wei Zi* restrains, contains, and stops diarrhea. *Dang Shen* fortifies the spleen and supplements the qi, while *Bai Zhu* and mix-fried *Gan Cao* fortify the spleen and boost the qi.

ADDITIONS & SUBTRACTIONS: If, due to enduring diarrhea, the central qi is falling downward, add 15-30 grams of Radix Astragali Membranacei (*Huang Qi*) and nine grams each of Fructus Terminaliae Chebulae (*He Zi*) and Hallyositum Rubrum (*Chi Shi Zhi*).

ACUPUNCTURE & MOXIBUSTION: *Zu San Li* (St 36), *Zhong Wan* (CV 12), *Tian Shu* (St 25), *Guan Yuan* (CV 4), *Pi Shu* (Bl 20), *Wei Shu* (Bl 21), *Shen Shu* (Bl 23), *Ming Men* (GV 4), *Da Chang Shu* (Bl 25)

FORMULA ANALYSIS: Supplementing and moxaing *Zu San Li, Zhong Wan, Pi Shi,* and *Wei Shu* fortifies the spleen and warms yang. Supplementing and moxaing *Guan Yuan, Shen Shu,* and *Ming Men* supplements the kidneys and invigorates yang. Supplementing and moxaing *Tian Shu* and *Da Chang Shu* secures the intestines and stops diarrhea.

ADDITIONS & SUBTRACTIONS: If there is concomitant liver-kidney yin vacuity, add supplementing *Tai Xi* (Ki 3) and *San Yin Jiao* (Sp 6). If there is concomitant liver depression, add draining *Tai Chong* (Liv 3).

DIABETIC ABNORMAL PERSPIRATION

1. YIN & YANG LOSS OF HARMONY PATTERN

MAIN SYMPTOMS: Profuse sweating from the upper half of the body and no or scanty perspiration from the lower half, dread of chill as well as aversion to heat, insomnia, profuse dreams, perspiration easily caused by emotional stress, if severe, sweat dribbling and dripping, a dark but pale tongue, and a deep, fine pulse

NOTE: It is specifically heart yin and yang which have lost their harmony in this case due to liver depression causing a failure to nourish the heart and construct the spirit.

TREATMENT PRINCIPLES: Regulate and harmonize yin and yang

RX: *Gui Zhi Jia Long Gu Mu Li Tang Jia Wei* (Cinnamon Twig Plus Dragon Bone & Oyster Shell Decoction with Added Flavors)

INGREDIENTS: Concha Ostreae (*Mu Li*), Os Draconis (*Long Gu*), and Fructus Levis Tricitic Aestivi (*Fu Xiao Mai*), 30g each, Radix Albus Paeoniae Lactiflorae (*Bai Shao*), 15g, Fructus Schisandrae Chinensis (*Wu Wei Zi*), 9g, and Ramulus Cinnamomi Cassiae (*Gui Zhi*) and mix-fried Radix Glycyrrhizae (*Gan Cao*), 6g each

FORMULA ANALYSIS: *Gui Zhi* and *Bai Shao* regulate and harmonize the constructive and defensive. *Long Gu, Mu Li,* and *Fu Xiao Mai* restrain yin and stop sweating. Mix-fried *Gan Cao* boosts the qi, nourishes the heart, and stops sweating.

ADDITIONS & SUBTRACTIONS: For concomitant fire effulgence, add nine grams each of Rhizoma Anemarrhenae Aspheloidis (*Zhi Mu*) and Cortex Phellodendri (*Huang Bai*). For concomitant qi vacuity, add 15-18 grams of Radix Astragali Membranacei (*Huang Qi*) and 9-12 grams of Radix Codonopsitis Pilosulae (*Dang Shen*). For insomnia, add 15 grams each of Cortex Albizziae Julibrissinis (*He Huan Pi*) and Caulis Polygoni Multiflori (*Ye Jiao Teng*).

ACUPUNCTURE & MOXIBUSTION: *Shen Men* (Ht 7), *Yin Xi* (Ht 6), *He Gu* (LI 4), *Zu San Li* (St 36)

FORMULA ANALYSIS: Even supplementing-even draining *Shen Men* and *Yin Xi* supplements the heart, quiets the spirit, and stops sweating. Supplementing *He Gu* and *Zu San Li* supplements the defensive qi in the upper part of the body to control the opening and closing of the pores.

ADDITIONS & SUBTRACTIONS: If there is yin vacuity with fire effulgence, add supplementing *Tai Xi* (Ki 3) and *Shen Shu* (Bl 23) and draining *Yin Ling Quan* (Sp 9) to enrich yin and downbear fire by leading yang into the yin tract via urination.

2. LUNG-SPLEEN QI VACUITY PATTERN

MAIN SYMPTOMS: Sweating from the head and chest in the region of the heart which is made worse by eating, a bright white facial complexion, fatigue, lassitude of the spirit, shortness of breath, lack of strength, heart palpitations, impaired memory, torpid intake, loose stools, a pale, tender tongue, and a vacuous, weak pulse

NOTE: This pattern actually does contain heart qi vacuity signs and symptoms. However, no mention is made of the heart in order to differentiate this pattern from the preceding one.

TREATMENT PRINCIPLES: Supplement and boost the spleen and lungs, secure the exterior and stop sweating

RX: *Yu Ping Feng San Jia Wei* (Jade Windscreen Powder with Added Flavors)

INGREDIENTS: Radix Astragali Membranacei (*Huang Qi*), Rhizoma Polygonati (*Huang Jing*), Concha Ostreae (*Mu Li*), and Os Draconis (*Long Gu*), 30g each, Rhizoma Atractylodis Macrocephalae (*Bai Zhu*) and Radix Codonopsitis Pilosulae (*Dang Shen*), 12g each, Radix Ledebouriellae Divaricatae (*Fang Feng*), 9g, and mix-fried Radix Glycyrrhizae (*Gan Cao*), 6g

FORMULA ANALYSIS: *Dang Shen, Huang Jing,* and mix-fried *Gan Cao* boost the qi, secure the exterior, and stop sweating. *Bai Zhu* fortifies the spleen and transforms dampness. *Fang Feng* gently out-thrusts any lingering evils lodged in the exterior. *Long Gu* and *Mu Li* constrain yin and stop sweating.

ADDITIONS & SUBTRACTIONS: If sweating is profuse, one can add 30 grams of Fructus Levis Tritici Aestivi (*Fu Xiao Mai*) and 9-15 grams of Radix Ephedrae (*Ma Huang Gen*).

ACUPUNCTURE & MOXIBUSTION: *Gao Huang Shu* (Bl 43), *Da Zhui* (GV 14), *Zu San Li* (St 36)

FORMULA ANALYSIS: Supplementing *Gao Huang Shu* and *Da Zhui* supplements the yang qi in the upper body in general and the upper sea of qi in particular. Supplementing *Zu San Li* fortifies the spleen and boosts the qi.

ADDITIONS & SUBTRACTIONS: If intake is decreased, add even supplementing-even draining *Zhong Wan* (CV 12). If there is abdominal distention, add even supplementing-even draining *Zhong Wan* and *Gong Sun* (Sp 4). If there are loose stools, add supplementing *Tian Shu* (St 25), *Pi Shu* (Bl 20), *Wei Shu* (Bl 21), and *Da Chang Shu* (Bl 25). If there is concomitant kidney yang vacuity, add supplementing *Fu Liu* (Ki 7).

3. HEART-KIDNEY YIN VACUITY PATTERN

MAIN SYMPTOMS: Sweating from the heart region of the chest, night sweats, vacuity vexation, insomnia, profuse dreams, heart palpitations, impaired memory, dizziness, tinnitus, dry mouth and parched throat, low back and knee soreness and limpness, steaming bones, tidal heat, short, reddish urination, a red tongue with scanty fur, and a fine, rapid pulse

TREATMENT PRINCIPLES: Supplement and boost the heart and kidneys, constrain yin and stop sweating

RX: *Liu Wei Di Huang Wan Jia Wei* (Six Flavors Rehmannia Pills with Added Flavors)

INGREDIENTS: Fructus Corni Officinalis (*Shan Zhu Yu*) and Radix Dioscoreae Oppositae (*Shan Yao*), 15g each, cooked Radix Rehmanniae (*Shu Di*) and Sclerotium Poriae Cocos (*Fu Ling*), 12g each, and Cortex Radicis Moutan (*Dan Pi*), Rhizoma Alismatis (*Ze Xie*), Fructus Schisandrae Chinensis (*Wu Wei Zi*), Radix Stellariae Dichotomae (*Yin Chai Hu*), and Cortex Radicis Lycii Chinensis (*Di Gu Pi*), 9g each

FORMULA ANALYSIS: *Shan Zhu Yu*, *Shu Di*, and *Shan Yao* supplement the heart and kidneys and enrich true yin. *Fu Ling* and *Ze Xie* fortify the spleen and disinhibit urination based on the former and latter heavens supporting and bolstering each other and the prevention of damp evils when enriching yin. *Dan Pi* quickens and cools the blood, based on enduring diseases commonly being complicated by blood stasis and the prevention of upward flaring of ministerial fire. *Yin Chai Hu* and *Di Gu Pi* recede or abate vacuity heat and stop sweating.

ADDITIONS & SUBTRACTIONS: If there is simultaneous qi vacuity, add 15-30 grams of Radix Astragali Membranacei (*Huang Qi*) to boost the qi and secure the exterior.

If enduring disease has caused lung-kidney yin depletion, one can use *Mai Wei Di Huang Wan Jia Wei* (Ophiopogon & Schisandra Rehmannia Pills with Added Flavors): Concha Ostreae (*Mu Li*) and Os Draconis (*Long Gu*), 30g each, cooked Radix Rehmanniae (*Shu Di*), 15g, Tuber Ophiopogonis Japonici (*Mai Men Dong*), Radix Dioscoreae Oppositae (*Shan Yao*), and Fructus Corni Officinalis (*Shan Zhu Yu*), 12g each, Sclerotium Poriae Cocos (*Fu Ling*), Fructus Schisandrae Chinensis (*Wu Wei Zi*), Rhizoma Alismatis (*Ze Xie*), and Cortex Radicis Moutan (*Dan Pi*), 9g each.

ACUPUNCTURE & MOXIBUSTION: *Fei Shu* (Bl 13), *Fu Liu* (Ki 7), *San Yin Jiao* (Sp 6)

FORMULA ANALYSIS: Supplementing *Fei Shu* supplements the lung-defensive qi to secure the exterior. Even supplementing-even draining *Fu Liu* enriches yin and downbears fire. Supplementing *San Yin Jiao* supplements the yin of the liver and kidneys.

ADDITIONS & SUBTRACTIONS: If vacuity heat is effulgent above, add draining *Da Zhui* (GV 14). If there is concomitant spleen-kidney yang vacuity, add supplementing *Zu San Li* (St 36) and *Shen Shu* (Bl 23).

DIABETIC BLOOD VESSEL CIRCULATORY DISORDERS

1. LIVER-KIDNEY DEPLETION & DETRIMENT PATTERN

MAIN SYMPTOMS: Bilateral heel pain or pain in the center of the foot, lack of redness or swelling in the affected area, remission of pain during the day when active with worsening of the pain at night, low back and knee soreness and limpness, lassitude of the spirit, lack of strength in the limbs, a pale tongue, and a fine pulse (as long as liver blood vacuity is predominant and yin vacuity has not given rise to vacuity heat)

TREATMENT PRINCIPLES: Enrich and supplement the liver and kidneys

RX: *Zuo Gui Wan Jia Jian* (Restore the Left [Kidney] Pills with Additions & Subtractions)

INGREDIENTS: Radix Dioscoreae Oppositae (*Shan Yao*), 15g, cooked Radix Rehmanniae (*Shu Di*), Fructus Corni

Officinalis (*Shan Zhu Yu*), and Radix Achyranthis Bidentatae (*Niu Xi*), 12g each, and Gelatinum Cornu Cervi (*Lu Jiao Jiao*), Gelatinum Plastri Testudinis (*Gui Ban Jiao*), Semen Cuscutae Chinensis (*Tu Si Zi*), and Fructus Lycii Chinensis (*Gou Qi Zi*), 9g each

FORMULA ANALYSIS: *Shu Di*, *Shan Yao*, *Gou Qi Zi*, and *Shan Zhu Yu* supplement and nourish kidney yin, while *Lu Jiao Jiao* and *Tu Si Zi* warmly supplement kidney yang, thus leading to yin via yang. *Gui Ban Jiao* enriches yin and downbears fire, while *Niu Xi* strengthens the low back and knees.

ADDITIONS & SUBTRACTIONS: If yin vacuity with fire effulgence is marked, use *Zhi Bai Di Huang Wan Jia Wei* (Anemarrhena & Phellodendron Rehmannia Pills with Added Flavors): Radix Dioscoreae Oppositae (*Shan Yao*), 15g, cooked Radix Rehmanniae (*Shu Di*), Fructus Corni Officinalis (*Shan Zhu Yu*), and Radix Achyranthis Bidentatae (*Niu Xi*), 12g each, and Gelatinum Plastri Testudinis (*Gui Ban Jiao*), Rhizoma Anemarrhenae Aspheloidis (*Zhi Mu*), Cortex Phellodendri (*Huang Bai*), Sclerotium Poriae Cocos (*Fu Ling*), Rhizoma Alismatis (*Ze Xie*), and Cortex Radicis Moutan (*Dan Pi*), 9g each.

If kidney yang vacuity is predominant, use *You Gui Wan Jia Jian* (Restore the Right [Kidney] Pills with Additions & Subtractions): cooked Radix Rehmanniae (*Shu Di*), 30g, Radix Dioscoreae Oppositae (*Shan Yao*) and Fructus Corni Officinalis (*Shan Zhu Yu*), 15g each, Fructus Lycii Chinensis (*Gou Qi Zi*) and Radix Achyranthis Bidentatae (*Niu Xi*), 12g each, Semen Cuscutae Chinensis (*Tu Si Zi*), Gelatinum Cornu Cervi (*Lu Jiao Jiao*), Radix Angelicae Sinensis (*Dang Gui*), and Cortex Eucommiae Ulmoidis (*Du Zhong*), 9g each, and Radix Lateralis Praeparatus Aconiti Carmichaeli (*Fu Zi*) and Cortex Cinnamomi Cassiae (*Rou Gui*), 3-9g each.

ACUPUNCTURE & MOXIBUSTION: *Qu Quan* (Liv 8), *Tai Xi* (Ki 3), *San Yin Jiao* (Sp 6), *Shen Shu* (Bl 23)

FORMULA ANALYSIS: Supplementing *Qu Quan* nourishes liver blood, while supplementing *Tai Xi* and *Shen Shu* enriches kidney yin. Supplementing *San Yin Jiao* supplements and nourishes the liver and kidneys.

ADDITIONS & SUBTRACTIONS: If there is concomitant kidney yang vacuity, add moxibustion at *Shen Shu*, *Ming Men* (GV 4), and *Guan Yuan* (CV 4). If there is concomitant spleen qi vacuity, add supplementing at *Zu San Li* (St 36) and *Pi Shu* (Bl 20). If there is concomitant liver depression, add draining *Tai Chong* (Liv 3) and *He Gu* (LI 4). If there is concomitant blood stasis, add draining *Xue*

Hai (Sp 10) and use even supplementing-even draining at *San Yin Jiao*.

2. COLD DAMP CONGELATION & STAGNATION PATTERN

MAIN SYMPTOMS: Heel pain which is worsened by cold and pain which feels like being pierced by a needle, lower limb heaviness, encumbrance, and lack of strength, lower leg swelling and distention, chilly skin which is somber white gradually turning purple and dark, a pale tongue with white fur, and a fine pulse

TREATMENT PRINCIPLES: Warm the channels and scatter cold, eliminate dampness and stop pain

RX: *Dang Gui Si Ni Tang Jia Jian* (Dang Gui Four Counterflows Decoction with Additions & Subtractions)

INGREDIENTS: Radix Albus Paeoniae Lactiflorae (*Bai Shao*), 15g, Radix Angelicae Sinensis (*Dang Gui*) and Radix Achyranthis Bidentatae (*Niu Xi*), 12g each, Ramulus Cinnamomi Cassiae (*Gui Zhi*) and mix-fried Radix Glycyrrhizae (*Gan Cao*), 6g each, and Herba Asari Cum Radice (*Xi Xin*) and Medulla Tetrapanacis Papyriferi (*Tong Cao*), 3g each

FORMULA ANALYSIS: *Gui Zhi* and *Xi Xin* warm and scatter cold evils, free the flow of yang and stop pain. *Dang Gui* and *Bai Shao* nourish and harmonize the blood. *Shao Yao* and *Gan Cao* relax cramping and stop pain. *Tong Cao* frees the flow of the channels and vessels, while *Niu Xi* strengthens the bones especially in the lower limbs.

ADDITIONS & SUBTRACTIONS: Since this is a tip or branch treatment, this formula is not commonly modified for this condition. Rather, elements of this formula are usually added to other formulas treating the root of this condition.

ACUPUNCTURE & MOXIBUSTION: *Zu San Li* (St 36), *Yin Ling Quan* (Sp 9), *Kun Lun* (Bl 60), *Huan Tiao* (GB 30)

FORMULA ANALYSIS: *Zu San Li* is the main point for treating diseases of the lower limbs. When combined with *Yin Ling Quan* and treated with warm needle technique, these two points fortify the spleen and transform dampness to disperse swelling and stop pain. Warm needling *Kun Lun* frees the flow of the channels and network vessels and stops pain, while warm needling *Huan Tiao* dispels wind, scatters cold, and stops pain.

ADDITIONS & SUBTRACTIONS: Warm needle local points as necessary in the affected area(s).

3. DAMP HEAT BREWING & BINDING PATTERN

MAIN SYMPTOMS: Lower limb aching and pain accompanied by burning heat sensations and, if severe, swelling and distention and red-colored skin, possible emission of heat, oral thirst, vexation, oppression, and restlessness, a red tongue with slimy, yellow fur and scanty fluids, and a slippery, rapid pulse

TREATMENT PRINCIPLES: Clear heat and eliminate dampness

RX: *Xuan Bi Tang Jia Jian* (Assuage Impediment Decoction with Additions & Subtractions)

INGREDIENTS: Caulis Lonicerae Japonicae (*Ren Dong Teng*), Semen Phaseoli Calcarati (*Chi Xiao Dou*), and Semen Coicis Lachyrma-jobi (*Yi Yi Ren*), 30g each, Caulis Milletiae Seu Spatholobi (*Ji Xue Teng*) and Talcum (*Hua Shi*), 15g each, and Fructus Gardeniae Jasminoidis (*Zhi Zi*), Radix Stephaniae Tetrandrae (*Han Fang Ji*), Semen Pruni Armeniacae (*Xing Ren*), Bombyx Batryticatus (*Jiang Can*), Rhizoma Pinelliae Ternatae (*Ban Xia*), Rhizoma Curcumae Longae (*Jiang Huang*), and Cortex Erythiniae (*Hai Tong Pi*), 9g each

FORMULA ANALYSIS: *Ren Dong Teng, Zhi Zi, Yi Yi Ren,* and *Han Fang Ji* clear heat and disinhibit dampness. *Xing Ren* diffuses the lungs and disinhibits the qi. *Jiang Can, Ban Xia,* and *Chi Xiao Dou* disinhibit dampness and transform turbidity. *Jiang Huang, Ji Xue Teng,* and *Hai Tong Pi* quicken the blood, free the flow of the network vessels, and stop pain.

ADDITIONS & SUBTRACTIONS: One can add nine grams of any of the following to increase the effect of clearing heat and eliminating dampness, dispelling wind and freeing the flow of the network vessels: Rhizoma Dioscoreae Hypoglaucae (*Bie Xie*), Cortex Phellodendri (*Huang Bai*), Rhizoma Atractylodis (*Cang Zhu*), Fructus Chaenomelis Lagenariae (*Mu Gua*), and Lumbricus (*Di Long*).

ACUPUNCTURE & MOXIBUSTION: *Zhong Du* (Liv 6), *Qi Men* (Sp 11), *Yin Ling Quan* (Sp 9), *Yang Ling Quan* (GB 34), *Yang Fu* (GB 38), *Yong Quan* (Ki 1)

FORMULA ANALYSIS: Draining *Zhong Du* and *Qi Men* frees the flow of the network vessels and stops pain.

Draining *Yin Ling Quan, Yang Ling Quan,* and *Yang Fu* clears heat and disinhibits dampness. Even supplementing-even draining *Yong Quan* leads heat to move downwards.

ADDITIONS & SUBTRACTIONS: For fever and thirst, add draining *Qu Chi* (LI 11) and even supplementing-even draining *San Yin Jiao* (Sp 6). For tidal heat due to enduring heat damaging yin, add supplementing *Tai Xi* (Ki 3). For concomitant blood stasis, add draining *Xue Hai* (Sp 10) and even supplementing-even draining *San Yin Jiao.*

CRANIAL NERVE LESIONS

1. QI VACUITY & BLOOD STASIS PATTERN

MAIN SYMPTOMS: Bodily fatigue, lack of strength, a bright white facial complexion, blurred vision, possible double vision, drooping eyelids, a dark, fat tongue with white fur, and a deep, fine pulse

TREATMENT PRINCIPLES: Boost the qi and quicken the blood

RX: *Bu Yang Huan Wu Tang Jia Jian* (Supplement Yang & Restore Five [Tenths] Decoction with Additions & Subtractions)

INGREDIENTS: Radix Astragali Membranacei (*Huang Qi*), 30g, Radix Rubrus Paeoniae Lactiflorae (*Chi Shao*) and Radix Ligustici Wallichii (*Chuan Xiong*), 15g each, Extremitas Radicis Angelicae Sinensis (*Dang Gui Wei*) and Lumbricus (*Di Long*), 12g each, and Bombyx Batryticatus (*Jiang Can*), Flos Chrysanthemi Morifolii (*Ju Hua*), and Scapus Et Inflorescentia Eriocaulonis Buergeriani (*Gu Jing Cao*), 9g each

FORMULA ANALYSIS: *Huang Qi* supplements the qi, while *Dang Gui Wei, Chuan Xiong, Di Long,* and *Chi Shao* quicken the blood and transform stasis. *Jiang Can* dispels wind, and *Ju Hua* and *Gu Jing Cao* clear the liver and brighten the eyes.

ADDITIONS & SUBTRACTIONS: If damage to yin is marked, add 12 grams each of uncooked Radix Rehmanniae (*Sheng Di*), Radix Scrophulariae Ningpoensis (*Xuan Shen*), and Tuber Ophiopogonis Japonici (*Mai Men Dong*) and nine grams of Herba Dendrobii (*Shi Hu*). If liver depression qi stagnation is marked, add nine grams each of Radix Bupleuri (*Chai Hu*), Radix Scutellariae Baicalensis (*Huang Qin*), and Fructus Immaturus Citri Aurantii (*Zhi Shi*).

ACUPUNCTURE & MOXIBUSTION: *Zu San Li* (St 36), *San Yin Jiao* (Sp 6), *He Gu* (LI 4), *Xue Hai* (Sp 10)

FORMULA ANALYSIS: Supplementing *Zu San Li* boosts the qi, while draining *Xue Hai* quickens the blood and transforms stasis. Even supplementing-even draining *San Yin Jiao* supplements liver-kidney yin at the same time as it helps quicken the blood and transform stasis. *He Gu* is the main point for treating diseases of the head. Even supplementing-even draining *He Gu* clears heat from the head at the same time as it upbears the clear.

ADDITIONS & SUBTRACTIONS: For blurred or double vision, add even supplementing-even draining *Jing Ming* (Bl 1) and supplementing *Ge Shu* (Bl 17), *Gan Shu* (Bl 18), and *Guang Ming* (GB 37). For marked yin and fluid vacuity dryness, add supplementing *Tai Xi* (Ki 3) and *Shen Shu* (Bl 23). For concomitant stomach heat, add draining *Nei Ting* (St 44). For concomitant liver depression, add draining *Tai Chong* (Liv 3). For liver depression transforming heat, needle *Tai Chong* through to *Xing Jian* (Liv 2).

2. LIVER BLOOD-KIDNEY YIN VACUITY WITH BLOOD STASIS PATTERN

MAIN SYMPTOMS: Decreased visual acuity, possible eye-screen, possible bilateral dryness and scratchiness of the eyes, possible double vision, low back and knee soreness and limpness, dizziness, tinnitus, a pale but dark tongue with white fur, and a deep, fine pulse (as long as yin vacuity has not given rise to vacuity heat)

TREATMENT PRINCIPLES: Enrich and supplement the liver and kidneys while simultaneously quickening the blood

RX: *Qi Ju Di Huang Wan Jia Wei* (Lycium & Chrysanthemum Rehmannia Pills with Added Flavors)

INGREDIENTS: Radix Salviae Miltiorrhizae (*Dan Shen*), 30g, Radix Dioscoreae Oppositae (*Shan Yao*) and Fructus Corni Officinalis (*Shan Zhu Yu*), 15g each, cooked Radix Rehmanniae (*Shu Di*), Radix Angelicae Sinensis (*Dang Gui*), and Radix Ligustici Wallichii (*Chuan Xiong*), 12g each, and Flos Chrysanthemi Morifolii (*Ju Hua*), Fructus Lycii Chinensis (*Gou Qi Zi*), Rhizoma Alismatis (*Ze Xie*), Cortex Radicis Moutan (*Dan Pi*), and Sclerotium Poriae Cocos (*Fu Ling*), 9g each

FORMULA ANALYSIS: Within this formula, the ingredients of *Liu Wei Di Huang Wan* (Six Flavors Rehmannia Pills) enrich and supplement the liver and kidneys. *Ju Hua* and *Gou Qi Zi* supplement the liver and kidneys and

brighten the eyes. *Dan Shen*, *Dang Gui*, and *Chuan Xiong* quicken the blood, transform stasis, and free the flow of the network vessels.

ADDITIONS & SUBTRACTIONS: If, due to yin vacuity, fire is effulgent, add 12 grams of Plastrum Testudinis (*Gui Ban*) and nine grams each of Rhizoma Anamarrhenae Aspheloidis (*Zhi Mu*) and Cortex Phellodendri (*Huang Bai*) to enrich yin and downbear fire. If yin vacuity has reached yang resulting in kidney yang vacuity and decline, one can add 15 grams of Gelatinum Cornu Cervi (*Lu Jiao Jiao*), nine grams each of Cortex Eucommiae Ulmoidis (*Du Zhong*) and Semen Cuscutae Chinensis (*Tu Si Zi*), and 3-9 grams each of Cortex Cinnamomi Cassiae (*Rou Gui*) and Radix Lateralis Praeparatus Aconiti Carmichaeli (*Fu Zi*).

ACUPUNCTURE & MOXIBUSTION: *Jing Ming* (Bl 1), *Tai Yang* (M-HN-9), *Guang Ming* (GB 37), *Tai Xi* (Ki 3), *San Yin Jiao* (Sp 6), *Gan Shu* (Bl 18), *Shen Shu* (Bl 23)

FORMULA ANALYSIS: Supplementing *Tai Xi*, *San Yin Jiao*, *Gan Shu*, and *Shen Shu* nourishes and supplements the liver and kidneys. Even supplementing-even draining *Jing Ming* and *Tai Yang* frees the flow of the channels and network vessels of the eyes, while supplementing *Guang Ming* nourishes the liver and brightens the eyes.

ADDITIONS & SUBTRACTIONS: If there is concomitant kidney yang vacuity, add moxibustion at *Shen Shu*, *Ming Men* (GV 4), and *Guan Yuan* (CV 4). If there is blood stasis, add draining *Xue Hai* (Sp 10) and use even supplementing-even draining at *San Yin Jiao*. For stomach heat damaging yin, add draining *Nei Ting* (St 44). If there are dry, rough-feeling eyes, add draining *Si Bai* (St 1). If there is lung heat damaging yin, add draining *Chi Ze* (Lu 5).

BRAIN LESIONS

1. LIVER DEPRESSION QI STAGNATION PATTERN

MAIN SYMPTOMS: Emotional tension and depression, agitation, easy anger, possible stomach duct distention and oppression, a normal or dark-colored tongue with thin, white fur, and a deep, bowstring pulse

NOTE: In diabetic neuropathic brain lesions, this pattern never presents in such a simple discrete form. However, it complicates any other pattern where there is irritability, tension, and easy anger.

TREATMENT PRINCIPLES: Course the liver and resolve depression

RX: *Chai Hu Shu Gan Yin Jia Jian* (Bupleurum Course the Liver Drink with Additions & Subtractions)

INGREDIENTS: Radix Albus Paeoniae Lactiflorae (*Bai Shao*), 15g, Radix Bupleuri (*Chai Hu*), Pericarpium Citri Reticulatae (*Chen Pi*), Rhizoma Cyperi Rotundi (*Xiang Fu*), Fructus Immaturus Citri Aurantii (*Zhi Shi*), Radix Ligustici Wallichii (*Chuan Xiong*), Fructus Citri Sacrodactylis (*Fo Shou*), and Radix Auklandiae Lappae (*Mu Xiang*), 9g each, and mix-fried Radix Glycyrrhizae (*Gan Cao*), 6g

FORMULA ANALYSIS: *Chai Hu, Chen Pi, Xiang Fu, Mu Xiang, Fo Shou,* and *Zhi Shi* course the liver and rectify the qi. *Bai Shao* emolliates and harmonizes the liver, while *Chuan Xiong* moves the qi within the blood. In addition, *Chuan Xiong* as a messenger medicinal guides the effects of the other medicinals to the region of the head and brain. The combination of *Bai Shao* and mix-fried *Gan Cao* is well known for relaxing tension at the same time as *Gan Cao* harmonizes all the other medicinals in this formula.

ADDITIONS & SUBTRACTIONS: If there is no thought for eating or drinking, one can add 3-4.5 grams of Fructus Amomi (*Sha Ren*) to open the stomach. If there is concomitant phlegm and heat, one can add nine grams each of Rhizoma Pinelliae Ternatae (*Ban Xia*), Radix Scutellariae Baicalensis (*Huang Qin*), and Radix Trichosanthis Kirlowii (*Tian Hua Fen*).

ACUPUNCTURE & MOXIBUSTION: *Tai Chong* (Liv 3), *He Gu* (LI 4), *Nei Guan* (Per 6)

FORMULA ANALYSIS: Draining *Tai Chong* and *He Gu* courses the liver and rectifies the qi. Draining *Nei Guan* harmonizes the liver and spleen, loosens the chest, and quiets the spirit.

ADDITIONS & SUBTRACTIONS: If liver depression has transformed heat, needle *Tai Chong* through to *Xing Jian* (Liv 2) and add draining *Yang Ling Quan* (GB 34). If there is concomitant stomach heat, add draining *Nei Ting* (St 44). If there is abdominal distention and lack of appetite, add draining *Zu San Li* (St 36) and *Zhong Wan* (CV 12). If there is concomitant spleen vacuity, add even supplementing-even draining *Zu San Li* and supplementing *Pi Shu* (Bl 20) and *Wei Shu* (Bl 21). If there is concomitant phlegm, add draining *Feng Long* (St 40) and *Zhong Wan* (CV 12).

2. PHLEGM & DAMPNESS OBSTRUCTING THE ORIFICES PATTERN

MAIN SYMPTOMS: Essence spirit depression, a dull, stagnant, torpid affect, chest and rib-side distention and fullness, somnolence, impaired memory, phlegm drool flowing from the mouth, white, slimy tongue fur, and a deep, slippery pulse

TREATMENT PRINCIPLES: Sweep away phlegm and open the orifices

RX: *Dao Tan Tang Jia Jian* (Abduct Phlegm Decoction with Additions & Subtractions)

INGREDIENTS: Rhizoma Pinelliae Ternatae (*Ban Xia*) and Sclerotium Poriae Cocos (*Fu Ling*), 12g each, Pericarpium Citri Reticulatae (*Chen Pi*), Fructus Immaturus Citri Aurantii (*Zhi Shi*), Rhizoma Acori Graminei (*Shi Chang Pu*), and Radix Polygalae Tenuifoliae (*Yuan Zhi*), 9g each, and bile-treated Rhizoma Arisaematis (*Dan Nan Xing*) and Radix Glycyrrhizae (*Gan Cao*), 6g each

FORMULA ANALYSIS: *Ban Xia* and *Chen Pi* rectify the qi and transform phlegm. *Fu Ling* fortifies the spleen and seeps dampness. *Gan Cao* harmonizes the center and strengthens earth. *Zhi Shi, Dan Nan Xing,* and *Shi Chang Pu* move the qi and dispel phlegm. *Yuan Zhi* arouses the spirit and opens the orifices.

ADDITIONS & SUBTRACTIONS: If phlegm turbidity has brewed and accumulated, transforming heat, one can use *Huang Lian Wen Dan Tang Jia Wei* (Coptis Warm the Gallbladder Decoction with Added Flavors): Rhizoma Pinelliae Ternatae (*Ban Xia*) and Sclerotium Poriae Cocos (*Fu Ling*), 12g each, Pericarpium Citri Reticulatae (*Chen Pi*), Caulis Bambusae In Taeniis (*Zhu Ru*), Fructus Immaturus Citri Aurantii (*Zhi Shi*), Rhizoma Acori Graminei (*Shi Chang Pu*), and Radix Polygalae Tenuifoliae (*Yuan Zhi*), 9g each, bile-treated Rhizoma Arisaematis (*Dan Nan Xing*) and Radix Glycyrrhizae (*Gan Cao*), 6g each, and Rhizoma Coptidis Chinensis (*Huang Lian*), 3g. If there is marked insomnia, agitation, and restlessness, add 12 grams each of Concha Margaritiferae (*Zhen Zhu Mu*) and Caulis Polygoni Multiflori (*Ye Jiao Teng*).

If there is concomitant heart-spleen vacuity, one can use *Shi Wei Wen Dan Tang Jia Wei* (Ten Flavors Warm the Gallbladder Decoction with Added Flavors): Rhizoma Pinelliae Ternatae (*Ban Xia*), cooked Radix Rehmanniae (*Shu Di*), Semen Zizyphi Spinosae (*Suan Zao Ren*), and

Sclerotium Poriae Cocos (*Fu Ling*), 12g each, Pericarpium Citri Reticulatae (*Chen Pi*), Fructus Immaturus Citri Aurantii (*Zhi Shi*), Rhizoma Acori Graminei (*Shi Chang Pu*), Fructus Schisandrae Chinensis (*Wu Wei Zi*), and Radix Polygalae Tenuifoliae (*Yuan Zhi*), 9g each, Radix Panacis Ginseng (*Ren Shen*) and mix-fried Radix Glycyrrhizae (*Gan Cao*), 6g each, Fructus Zizyphi Jujubae (*Da Zao*), 5 pieces, and uncooked Rhizoma Zingiberis (*Sheng Jiang*), 2-3 slices.

ACUPUNCTURE & MOXIBUSTION: *Feng Long* (St 40), *Zhong Wan* (CV 12), *Nei Guan* (Per 6), *Tai Chong* (Liv 3), *He Gu* (LI 4), *Feng Chi* (GB 20)

FORMULA ANALYSIS: Even supplementing-even draining *Feng Long* and *Zhong Wan* transforms phlegm. Draining *Tai Chong* and *He Gu* courses the liver and rectifies the qi. Draining *Nei Guan* loosens the chest and quiets the spirit, and draining *Feng Chi* opens the orifices.

ADDITIONS & SUBTRACTIONS: If liver depression has transformed heat, needle *Tai Chong* through to *Xing Jian* (Liv 2). If there is stomach heat, add draining *Nei Ting* (St 44). If there is lung heat, add draining *Chi Ze* (Lu 5). If there is heart heat, add draining *Da Ling* (Per 7). If there is concomitant spleen qi vacuity, add even supplementing-even draining *Zu San Li* (St 36) and supplementing *Pi Shu* (Bl 20) and *Wei Shu* (Bl 21).

3. QI DEPRESSION & BLOOD VACUITY PATTERN

MAIN SYMPTOMS: Essence spirit abstraction, susceptibility to fright, worry and anxiety, chest oppression, tension and agitation, possible visual hallucinations, talking in one's sleep, vacuity vexation, insomnia, a pale tongue, and a fine, bowstring pulse

TREATMENT PRINCIPLES: Rectify the qi and harmonize the blood

RX: *Xiao Yao San Jia Wei* (Rambling Powder with Added Flavors)

INGREDIENTS: Radix Albus Paeoniae Lactiflorae (*Bai Shao*), 15g, Sclerotium Poriae Cocos (*Fu Ling*), Caulis Polygoni Multiflori (*Ye Jiao Teng*), and Cortex Albizziae Julibrissinis (*He Huan Pi*), 12g each, Radix Angelicae Sinensis (*Dang Gui*), Radix Bupleuri (*Chai Hu*), and Rhizoma Atractylodis Macrocephalae (*Bai Zhu*), 9g each, and Herba Menthae Haplocalycis (*Bo He*) and mix-fried Radix Glycyrrhizae (*Gan Cao*), 6g each

FORMULA ANALYSIS: *Bai Shao* and *Dang Gui* supplement the blood and harmonize the liver. *Chai Hu* and *Bo He* course the liver and resolve depression. *Bai Zhu*, *Fu Ling*, and mix-fried *Gan Cao* fortify the spleen and supplement the qi in order to engender and transform the blood. *Ye Jiao Teng* and *He Huan Pi* resolve depression and quiet the spirit.

ADDITIONS & SUBTRACTIONS: If there is concomitant depressive heat, add nine grams each of Cortex Radicis Moutan (*Dan Pi*) and Fructus Gardeniae Jasminoidis (*Zhi Zi*). If there are more marked signs and symptoms of qi stagnation, add nine grams each of Rhizoma Cyperi Rotundi (*Xiang Fu*) and Tuber Curcumae (*Yu Jin*). If there is vacuity vexation, worry, and anxiety due to malnourishment and nonconstruction of the heart spirit, add 30 grams of Fructus Tritici Aestivi (*Xiao Mai*) and 10 pieces of Fructus Zizyphi Jujubae (*Da Zao*) and increase the mix-fried *Gan Cao* to 9-15 grams. If there is more marked blood vacuity, add 12 grams each of Radix Astragali Membranacei (*Huang Qi*), Arillus Euphoriae Longanae (*Long Yan Rou*), and Semen Zizyphi Spinosae (*Suan Zao Ren*) to boost the qi and supplement the blood.

ACUPUNCTURE & MOXIBUSTION: *Tai Chong* (Liv 3), *He Gu* (LI 4), *San Yin Jiao* (Sp 6), *Zu San Li* (St 36), *Ge Shu* (Bl 17), *Gan Shu* (Bl 18)

FORMULA ANALYSIS: Draining *Tai Chong* and *He Gu* courses the liver and rectifies the qi. Supplementing *San Yin Jiao* and *Zu San Li* supplements the spleen and liver, remembering that it is the spleen which engenders the blood and the liver which stores it. Supplementing *Ge Shu* and *Gan Shu* supplements the blood and harmonizes the liver.

ADDITIONS & SUBTRACTIONS: If there is marked spleen qi vacuity, add supplementing *Pi Shu* (Bl 20) and *Wei Shu* (Bl 21). If there is depressive heat, needle *Tai Chong* through to *Xing Jian* (Liv 2). If there is concomitant heart vacuity, add supplementing *Shen Men* (Ht 7) and *Xin Shu* (Bl 15). If there is stomach heat, add draining *Nei Ting* (St 44). If there is lung heat, add draining *Chi Ze* (Lu 5). If there is kidney yin vacuity, add supplementing *Tai Xi* (Ki 3) and *Shen Shu* (Bl 23).

4. KIDNEY QI INSUFFICIENCY PATTERN

MAIN SYMPTOMS: Dizziness and vertigo, tinnitus, deafness, impaired memory, difficulty collecting one's thoughts, occasional heart vexation and easy anger, low back and knee soreness and limpness, a pale red tongue with scanty fur, and a fine, possibly rapid pulse

TREATMENT PRINCIPLES: Supplement the kidneys and boost the qi

RX: *He Che Da Zao Wan* (Placenta Great Construction Pills)

INGREDIENTS: Uncooked Radix Rehmanniae (*Sheng Di*) and Placenta Hominis (*Zi He Che*), 15g each, Radix Achyranthis Bidentatae (*Niu Xi*), Tuber Ophiopogonis Japonici (*Mai Men Dong*), and Tuber Asparagi Cochinensis (*Tian Men Dong*), 12g each, Plastrum Testudinis (*Gui Ban*), Cortex Eucommiae Ulmoidis (*Du Zhong*), Radix Panacis Ginseng (*Ren Shen*), and Cortex Phellodendri (*Huang Bai*), 9g each

FORMULA ANALYSIS: *Zi He Che* strengthens the true origin and greatly supplements the essence and marrow. *Ren Shen, Sheng Di, Gui Ban, Du Zhong,* and *Niu Xi* enrich yin and boost the qi. *Tian Men Dong* and *Mai Men Dong* enrich lung yin in order to engender kidney water, and *Huang Bai* downbears fire due to yin vacuity.

ADDITIONS & SUBTRACTIONS: If the essence qi is greatly depleted, add 12 grams of Ramulus Loranthi Seu Visci (*Sang Ji Sheng*) and nine grams each of Radix Morindae Officinalis (*Ba Ji Tian*), Semen Cuscutae Chinensis (*Tu Si Zi*), and Fructus Psoraleae Corylifoliae (*Bu Gu Zhi*). If there is bone-steaming and tidal heat, add nine grams of Rhizoma Anemarrhenae Aspheloidis (*Zhi Mu*). If there is concomitant kidney yang vacuity, add 3-9 grams each of Cortex Cinnamomi Cassiae (*Rou Gui*) and Radix Lateralis Praeparatus Aconiti Carmichaeli (*Fu Zi*). If the use of such slimy, enriching medicinals results in stomach duct glomus and fullness and decreased appetite, add nine grams each of Pericarpium Citri Reticulatae (*Chen Pi*) and Cortex Magnoliae Officinalis (*Hou Po*) and 4.5-6 grams of Fructus Amomi (*Sha Ren*) to aid dispersion and transformation.

ACUPUNCTURE & MOXIBUSTION: *Zu San Li* (St 36), *Tai Xi* (Ki 3), *San Yin Jiao* (Sp 6), *Guan Yuan* (CV 4), *Pi Shu* (Bl 20), *Shen Shu* (Bl 23)

FORMULA ANALYSIS: Supplementing *Zu San Li* and *Pi Shu* banks earth and bolsters the latter heaven. Supplementing *Tai Xi* and *Shen Shu* supplements the kidneys and enriches yin. Supplementing *San Yin Jiao* supplements the spleen, liver, and kidneys, while supplementing *Guan Yuan* supplements the source and fosters essence.

ADDITIONS & SUBTRACTIONS: If there is concomitant spleen-kidney yang vacuity, moxa *Pi Shu, Shen Shu, Guan Yuan, Ming Men* (GV 4), and *Zhi Shi* (Bl 47).

DIABETIC MUSCULAR ATROPHY

1. QI & BLOOD DUAL VACUITY PATTERN

MAIN SYMPTOMS: Emaciation of the muscles and flesh, possible great cachexia, a somber white facial complexion, lassitude of the spirit, exhaustion and fatigue, dizziness, vertigo, heart palpitations, shortness of breath, spontaneous perspiration, night sweats, a pale tongue with scanty fur, and a fine, faint pulse

TREATMENT PRINCIPLES: Greatly supplement the original qi, enrich and nourish yin and blood

RX: *Ren Shen Yang Ying Tang Jia Jian* (Ginseng Nourish the Constructive Decoction with Additions & Subtractions)

INGREDIENTS: Radix Astragali Membranacei (*Huang Qi*), 30g, Radix Albus Paeoniae Lactiflorae (*Bai Shao*), 15g, cooked Radix Rehmanniae (*Shu Di*) and Sclerotium Poriae Cocos (*Fu Ling*), 12g each, Radix Panacis Ginseng (*Ren Shen*), Rhizoma Atractylodis Macrocephalae (*Bai Zhu*), Radix Angelicae Sinensis (*Dang Gui*), Pericarpium Citri Reticulatae (*Chen Pi*), Cortex Cinnamomi Cassiae (*Rou Gui*), Radix Polygalae Tenuifoliae (*Yuan Zhi*), and Fructus Schisandrae Chinensis (*Wu Wei Zi*), 9g each, and uncooked Rhizoma Zingiberis (*Sheng Jiang*) and mix-fried Radix Glycyrrhizae (*Gan Cao*), 6g each

FORMULA ANALYSIS: *Ren Shen, Huang Qi, Bai Zhu, Fu Ling, Yuan Zhi,* and *Gan Cao* supplement the qi. *Rou Gui* warms yang and boosts the qi. *Bai Shao, Dang Gui,* and *Shu Di* enrich yin and nourish the blood. *Wu Wei Zi* nourishes and constrains yin, while *Chen Pi* and *Sheng Jiang* move the qi to promote supplementation without stagnation.

ADDITIONS & SUBTRACTIONS: If there is predominant qi vacuity with lassitude of the spirit, lack of strength, and spontaneous perspiration, one can use *Bu Zhong Yi Qi Tang Jia Wei* (Supplement the Center & Boost the Qi Decoction with Added Flavors): Radix Astragali Membranacei (*Huang Qi*), 30-60g, Fructus Levis Tritici Aestivi (*Fu Xiao Mai*), 15-30g, Radix Codonopsitis Pilosulae (*Dang Shen*), 9-18g, Rhizoma Atractylodis Macrocephalae (*Bai Zhu*), 12g, Radix Angelicae Sinensis (*Dang Gui*) and Fructus Schisandrae Chinensis (*Wu Wei*

Zi), 9g each, Pericarpium Citri Reticulatae (Chen Pi) and mix-fried Radix Glycyrrhizae (Gan Cao), 6g each, Rhizoma Cimicifugae (Sheng Ma), 4.5g, and Radix Bupleuri (Chai Hu), 3g.

If there is predominant blood vacuity with a sallow yellow or pale white facial complexion and dizziness, one can use Gui Pi Tang Jia Wei (Restore the Spleen Decoction with Added Flavors): Radix Astragali Membranacei (Huang Qi), 15-30g, cooked Radix Rehmanniae (Shu Di), Semen Zizyphi Spinosae (Suan Zao Ren), and Arillus Euphroae Longanae (Long Yan Rou), 12g each, Sclerotium Poriae Cocos (Fu Ling), Radix Angelicae Sinensis (Dang Gui), and Radix Polygalae Tenuifoliae (Yuan Zhi), 9g each, Radix Auklandiae Lappae (Mu Xiang) and mix-fried Radix Glycyrrhizae (Gan Cao), 6g each, Fructus Zizyphi Jujubae (Da Zao), 3-5 pieces, and uncooked Rhizoma Zingiberis (Sheng Jiang), 2-3 slices.

ACUPUNCTURE & MOXIBUSTION: Zu San Li (St 36), San Yin Jiao (Sp 6), Ge Shu (Bl 17), Gan Shu (Bl 18), Pi Shu (Bl 20)

FORMULA ANALYSIS: Supplementing Zu San Li, San Yin Jiao, and Pi Shu fortifies the spleen, the latter heaven root of qi and blood engenderment and transformation, and boosts the qi. Supplementing Ge Shu and Gan Shu, the so-called Four Flowers, supplements the blood.

ADDITIONS & SUBTRACTIONS: If there is spontaneous perspiration, also supplement He Gu (LI 4). If there is dizziness, also supplement Da Zhui (GV 14) and moxa Bai Hui (GV 20). If there are heart palpitations, supplement Shen Men (Ht 7), Nei Guan (Per 6), and Xin Shu (Bl 15). If there is shortness of breath, add supplementing Tai Yuan (Lu 9) and Fei Shu (Bl 13).

2. KIDNEY ESSENCE INSUFFICIENCY PATTERN

MAIN SYMPTOMS: Wasting and emaciation of the muscles and flesh, lack of strength in the four limbs, possible forward dropping of the head, impaired memory, low back and knee soreness and limpness, dizziness and vertigo, a pale red tongue with scanty fur, and a deep, fine pulse

TREATMENT PRINCIPLES: Supplement the kidneys and foster the essence

RX: Liu Wei Di Huang Wan Jia Wei (Six Flavors Rehmannia Pills with Added Flavors)

INGREDIENTS: Rhizoma Polygonati (Huang Jing), 30g,

cooked Radix Rehmanniae (Shu Di) and Radix Dioscoreae Oppositae (Shan Yao), 15g each, Sclerotium Poriae Cocos (Fu Ling), 12g, and Fructus Corni Officinalis (Shan Zhu Yu), Cortex Radicis Moutan (Dan Pi), and Rhizoma Alismatis (Ze Xie), 9g each

FORMULA ANALYSIS: Shu Di, Shan Zhu Yu, and Shan Yao supplement and enrich kidney essence. Huang Jing supplements the qi at the same time as it enriches yin. Dan Pi quickens the blood and clears vacuity heat, while Fu Ling, and Ze Xie free the flow and disinhibit urination.

ADDITIONS & SUBTRACTIONS: To increase the effect of supplementing the essence, one can add nine grams each of Gelatinum Cornu Cervi (Lu Jiao Jiao) and Semen Cuscutae Chinensis (Tu Si Zi). If low back pain is pronounced, add nine grams each of Cortex Eucommiae Ulmoidis (Du Zhong), Radix Achyranthis Bidentatae (Niu Xi), and Fructus Psoraleae Corylifoliae (Bu Gu Zhi) and 15 grams of Ramulus Loranthi Seu Visci (Sang Ji Sheng).

If there is more kidney yin vacuity with fire effulgence, vexatious heat in the five hearts, night sweats, steaming bones, and tidal heat, use Zhi Bai Di Huang Wan Jia Wei (Anemarrhena & Phellodendron Rehmannia Pills with Added Flavors): Fructus Levis Tritici Aestivi (Fu Xiao Mai), 15-30g, cooked Radix Rehmanniae (Shu Di) and uncooked Concha Ostreae (Mu Li), 15g each, Rhizoma Anemarrhenae Aspheloidis (Zhi Mu), 12g, and Fructus Schisandrae Chinensis (Wu Wei Zi), Fructus Corni Officinalis (Shan Zhu Yu), Radix Dioscoreae Oppositae (Shan Yao), Sclerotium Poriae Cocos (Fu Ling), Rhizoma Alismatis (Ze Xie), and Cortex Radicis Moutan (Dan Pi), 9g each.

If yin vacuity has reached yang with chilled limbs and cold body, impotence, clear, long urination, and loose stools, use Jin Gui Shen Qi Wan Jia Wei (Golden Cabinet Kidney Qi Pills with Added Flavors): Radix Dioscoreae Oppositae (Shan Yao) and Fructus Corni Officinalis (Shan Zhu Yu), 15g each, cooked Radix Rehmanniae (Shu Di), 12g, Rhizoma Atractylodis Macrocephalae (Bai Zhu), Sclerotium Poriae Cocos (Fu Ling), Rhizoma Alismatis (Ze Xie), and Cortex Radicis Moutan (Dan Pi), 9g each, Radix Panacis Ginseng (Ren Shen) and Cortex Cinnamomi Cassiae (Rou Gui), 6g each, and Radix Lateralis Praeparatus Aconiti Carmichaeli (Fu Zi), 3g.

ACUPUNCTURE & MOXIBUSTION: Tai Xi (Ki 3), San Yin Jiao (Sp 6), Guan Yuan (CV 4), Shen Shu (Bl 23), Zhi Shi (Bl 52)

FORMULA ANALYSIS: Supplementing Tai Xi, Guan

Yuan, Shen Shu, and Zhi Shi supplements the kidneys and fills the essence. Supplementing San Yin Jiao nourishes the liver and supplements the kidneys, remembering that the blood and essence share a common source.

ADDITIONS & SUBTRACTIONS: If yin vacuity has reached yang, add moxibustion at Guan Yuan, Shen Shu, Zhi Shi, and Ming Men (GV 4).

ABSTRACTS OF REPRESENTATIVE CHINESE RESEARCH:

PERIPHERAL NEUROPATHY

Xu Sheng-sheng, "The Use of Yi Qi Zhu Yu Tong Mai Tang (Boost the Qi, Dispel Stasis & Free the Flow of the Vessels Decoction) in the Treatment of Diabetic Peripheral Neuropathy," Jiang Su Zhong Yi (Jiangsu Chinese Medicine), #3, 1999, p. 23: Altogether, there were 118 patients in this study, all of which met the World Health Organization (WHO) criteria for the diagnosis of diabetes mellitus. In addition, all displayed varying symptoms of diabetic peripheral neuropathy. These included lower extremity tingling and numbness, formication, vague pain, piercing pain, burning pain, and muscular loss of strength. In addition, patellar and Achilles reflexes were either weakened or absent.

These 118 patients were divided into two groups which were statistically similar in terms of age, sex, and basic symptoms. These two groups were the treatment group and the comparison group. The treatment group consisted of 86 patients, 45 of whom were male and 41 of whom were female. These patients ranged in age from 31-76, with a median age of 50.6 years. Eighty-four of these 86 patients were diagnosed with non-insulin dependent diabetes mellitus (NIDDM) and two with insulin dependent diabetes mellitus (IDDM). Of the 32 patients in the comparison group, 18 were male and 14 were female. These patients ranged in age from 29-74, with a median age of 52.8. Thirty-one of these patients had NIDDM, while one had IDDM.

In terms of treatment, in addition to dietary restrictions and blood sugar lowering medications, the patients in the treatment group were orally administered the basic formula of self-composed Yi Qi Zhu Yu Tong Mai Tang. This consisted of: uncooked Radix Astragali Membranacei (Huang Qi), 30g, Radix Dioscoreae Oppositae (Shan Yao), 10g, Radix Scrophuariae Ningpoensis (Xuan Shen), 10g, Rhizoma Atractylodis (Cang Zhu), 10g, Radix Angelicae Sinensis (Dang Gui), 12g, Radix Rubrus Paeoniae

Lactiflorae (Chi Shao), 12g, Flos Carthami Tinctorii (Hong Hua), 12g, Cortex Radicis Moutan (Dan Pi), 12g, Semen Pruni Persicae (Tao Ren), 12g, Caulis Milletiae Seu Spatholobi (Ji Xue Teng), 8g, dry Lumbricus (Di Long), 5g, Lignum Sappan (Su Mu), 6g, Radix Achyranthis Bidentatae (Huai Niu Xi), 9g, Radix Dipsaci (Chuan Duan), 10g, Fructus Chaenomelis Lagenariae (Mu Gua), 10g, Radix Gentianae Macricphyllae (Qin Jiao), 10g, Radix Pseudoginseng (San Qi), 6g, Hirudo (Shui Zhi), 3g. All except this last ingredient were decocted in water once per day and administered orally. Shui Zhi was powdered and taken orally in gelatin capsules. Twenty days of this regimen equaled one course of therapy.

Instead of the Chinese medicinals described above, the comparison group was administered 25mg of dipyridamole, 10mg of vitamin B_1, and 20mg of vitamin B_6 three times per day. Likewise, 20 days of this regimen equaled one course of treatment.

Marked effect was defined as a self-reported marked improvement in or disappearance of self-conscious symptoms and either normal or markedly improved patellar and Achilles reflexes. Some effect meant that there was some improvement in both self-conscious symptoms and patellar and Achilles reflexes. No effect meant that there was no improvement in self-conscious symptoms and no improvement in patellar and Achilles reflexes. Based on these criteria, 41 patients (47.7%) in the treatment group were judged to have gotten a marked effect. Another 38 patients (44.2%) got some effect, and only seven patients (8.1%) failed to register any effect. Therefore, the total amelioration rate in the treatment group was 91.9%. In the comparison group, only two patients (6.3%) were judged to have experienced a marked effect. Nine patients (28.1%) got some effect, and 21 patients (65.6%) got no effect. Thus the total amelioration rate in the comparison group was only 34.4%. Hence there was a very marked difference in statistical outcomes between these two groups (P<0.005).

Da Li, "The Treatment of 30 Cases of Diabetic Peripheral Neuropathy with Bu Yang Huan Wu Tang (Supplement Yang & Restore Five [Tenths, i.e., Half] Decoction," Si Chuan Zhong Yi (Sichuan Chinese Medicine), #3, 2000, p. 24: All 30 of the patients described in this study were diagnosed with diabetes mellitus according to WHO criteria. In addition, all were diagnosed with peripheral neuropathy. Their symptoms included numbness, piercing pain, burning sensations, formication, and lack of muscular strength in their extremities. Within this group, there were 19 men and 11 women whose ages ranged from 41-

75 years old. All had suffered from diabetes for 3-5 years and from PN for three months to three years.

Treatment consisted of oral administration of *Bu Yang Huan Wu Tang* which was comprised of: Radix Astragali Membranacei (*Huang Qi*), 60-120g, Extremitas Radicis Angelicae Sinensis (*Gui Wei*) and Radix Ligustici Wallichii (*Chuan Xiong*), 10-15g each, Radix Rubrus Paeoniae Lactiflorae (*Chi Shao*), Flos Carthami Tinctorii (*Hong Hua*), and Semen Pruni Persicae (*Tao Ren*), 10g each, and Lumbricus (*Di Long*), 15-30g. If lower extremity pain was severe, 15g of Radix Achyranthis Bidentatae (*Niu Xi*) were added. If blood stasis was severe, 10g of Squama Manitis Pentadactylis (*Chuan Shan Jia*) and 15g of Radix Salviae Miltiorrhizae (*Dan Shen*) were added. If qi and yin dual vacuity symptoms were marked, 10g of Radix Panacis Quinquefolii (*Xi Yang Shen*) were added. One *ji* of these medicinals were administered per day after having been decocted in water three times. The resulting 500ml of medicinal liquid was administered in three divided doses morning, noon, and night. One half month equaled one course of treatment, and 2-3 courses were administered continuously.

Marked effect was defined as disappearance of the pain with no recurrence within three months. Some effect was defined as marked decrease or disappearance of the pain, but recurrence within three months or less. No effect meant that there was no improvement in the pain. Based on the above criteria, 16 (53.3%) patients got a marked effect, 11 (36.6%) patients got some effect, and three patients (10%) experienced no effect. Thus the total amelioration rate was 90%.

Ding Li-feng, "The Treatment of 43 Cases of Diabetic Peripheral Neuropathy by the Methods of Boosting the Qi, Nourishing Yin, and Transforming Stasis," *Si Chuan Zhong Yi (Sichaun Chinese Medicine)*, #3, 2000, p. 26: Among these 43 cases, 19 were men and 24 were women. The youngest was 29 and the oldest was 73, with a median age of 53 ± 10 years. The course of disease had lasted from 2-19 years, with a median duration of 4.3 ± 3 years. Seven cases were diagnosed with insulin dependent diabetes mellitus (IDDM), and 36 cases were diagnosed with non-insulin dependent diabetes mellitus (NIDDM). All the patients in this study experienced varying degrees of pain, hot sensations, numbness and tingling, formication, muscular atrophy, and lack of strength, with lessening or disappearance of patellar and Achilles reflexes.

On top of a basis of controlling their diet and taking blood sugar lowering medications, the patients in this study were also orally administered the following Chinese medicinals: Radix Astragali Membranacei (*Huang Qi*), 40g, Rhizoma Atractylodis (*Cang Zhu*), Flos Carthami Tinctorii (*Hong Hua*), Tuber Curcumae (*Yu Jin*), and Ramulus Cinnamomi Cassiae (*Gui Zhi*), 10g each, Radix Dioscoreae Oppositae (*Shan Yao*), uncooked Fructus Crataegi (*Shan Zha*), and Radix Salviae Miltiorrhizae (*Dan Shen*), 30g each, Radix Scrophulariae Ningpoensis (*Xuan Shen*), Radix Ligustici Wallichii (*Chuan Xiong*), and Herba Leonuri Heterophylli (*Yi Mu Cao*), 15g each, and Radix Rubrus Paeoniae Lactiflorae (*Chi Shao*), 20g. One *ji* of these medicinals were boiled in water and given in divided doses morning and evening. In addition, they received 20ml of *Fu Fang Dan Shen Zhu She Ye* (Compound Salvia Injectible Liquid) in 250ml of 0.9% saline solution intravenously one time per day. Two weeks of this therapy equaled one course of treatment, three such courses were given, and a 4-7 days rest was allowed between each successive course.

Marked effect was defined as the disappearance of clinical symptoms and return to normal of ankle reflexes. Some effect was defined as marked decrease in clinical symptoms and varying degrees of recuperation of ankle reflexes. No effect was defined as no obvious improvement in clinical symptoms after four weeks of treatment and no improvement in Achilles reflexes. Based on the above criteria, 27 cases (62.8%) got a marked effect, 12 cases (27.9%) got some effect, and four cases (9.3%) experienced no effect. Thus the total amelioration rate was 90.7%.

Han Zhen-chong *et al.*, "The Treatment of Diabetic Peripheral Neuropathy by the Methods of Nourishing Yin, Boosting the Qi & Quickening the Blood," *Si Chuan Zhong Yi (Sichuan Chinese Medicine)*, #11, 1999, p. 20-21: There were 92 patients in all in this study divided into a treatment and a comparison group. Of the 55 patients in the treatment group, 29 were male and 26 were female. These patients ranged in age from 46-75 years, with an average age of 57.5 years. Their disease course had lasted from 2-18 years, with an average duration of 8.2 years. Twenty-four cases had concomitant cerebral infarction, coronary heart disease, retinopathy, and/or nephropathy. In the comparison group of 37 patients, there were 22 males and 15 females ranging in age from 37-75, with an average age of 55.6 years and an average disease duration of 7.5 years. Thirteen of these patients had the same complicating conditions as in the treatment group. All the patients in this study had NIDDM according to WHO diagnostic criteria, and all had been diagnosed by Western medicine as suffering from diabetic neuropathy. In terms of Chinese medicine, all had been discriminated as presenting qi and yin dual vacuities with simultaneous blood stasis. Symptoms included fatigue, lack of strength, dry mouth, dizziness, vertigo, spontaneous perspiration, hand and foot numbness and pain, burning or chilly pain, possible formication, wasting of the muscles, and/or paralysis.

Both groups were treated as inpatients and received 0.25mg of glyburide in the A.M. and 0.5mg of glyburide in the P.M. which had succeeded in reducing their blood sugar to 7.1mmol/L or less. In addition, the treatment group received *Yi Qi Yang Yin Huo Xue Tang* (Boost the Qi, Nourish Yin & Quicken the Blood Decoction): Radix Puerariae (*Ge Gen*), 30g, Radix Astragali Membranacei (*Huang Qi*), 24g, Radix Dioscoreae Oppositae (*Shan Yao*) and Radix Salviae Miltiorrhizae (*Dan Shen*), 15g each, Radix Albus Paeoniae Lactiflorae (*Bai Shao*), Radix Angelicae Sinensis (*Dang Gui*), and Radix Ligustici Wallichii (*Chuan Xiong*), 9g each, and Hirudo Seu Whitmania (*Shui Zhi*), 0.3g washed down with the decoction. One *ji* of these medicinals was administered orally per day in two divided doses. The comparison group also received intramuscular injections of 100mg of vitamin B$_1$ and 500mg of vitamin B$_{12}$ once per day. Thirty days equaled one course of treatment for both groups, after which they were examined again.

Cure was defined as disappearance of clinical symptoms with use of the limbs returning to normal, filling out of the muscles, and normal electromyogram. Improvement was defined as improvement in clinical symptoms, recovery of use of the limbs but still a slight degree of lack of strength, and an improved electromyogram. No effect meant that there was no change in symptoms, bodily shape and strength, or electromyogram. Based on these criteria, 24 cases in the treatment group were judged cured, 25 improved, and six got no result. Hence the total amelioration rate was 89.09%. In the comparison group, there were four cures, 10 improvements, and 23 no effects, for a total amelioration rate of 37.38%.

Gao Ai-ai, "The Treatment of 52 Cases of Diabetic Peripheral Neuropathy with *Xiao Ke Tong Luo Yin* (Wasting & Thirsting Free the Flow of the Network Vessels Drink)," *Bei Jing Zhong Yi (Beijing Chinese Medicine)*, #3, 2000, p. 19-20: There were 27 men and 25 women in this study who ranged in age from 53-81 years, with an average age of 66.4 years. These patients had suffered from diabetes for 7-25 years and from various neuropathies for two months to three years. Symptoms of neuropathy included lower limb numbness, formication, pins and needles pain, a sensation of burning heat, or limb limpness and lack of strength. Besides dietary modifica-

tions, oral hypoglycemics, and/or insulin injections, all the patients in this clinical audit received the following basic Chinese medicinal formula: Radix Astragali Membranacei (*Huang Qi*) and Radix Salviae Miltiorrhizae (*Dan Shen*), 30g each, uncooked Radix Rehmanniae (*Sheng Di*), Radix Angelicae Sinensis (*Dang Gui*), Radix Achyranthis Bidentatae (*Niu Xi*), and Fructus Chaenomelis Lagenariae (*Mu Gua*), 15g each, Radix Ligustici Wallichii (*Chuan Xiong*) and Lumbricus (*Di Long*), 10g each, Hirudo Seu Whitmania (*Shui Zhi*), 6g, and Buthus Martensis (*Quan Xie*), 3g. If the body was cold and the limbs were chilled, six grams of Radix Lateralis Praeparatus Aconiti Carmichaeli (*Fu Zi*) and three grams of Cortex Cinnamomi Cassiae (*Rou Gui*) were added. If there was oral thirst and polydipsia, 15 grams each of Radix Glehniae Littoralis (*Sha Shen*) and Tuber Ophiopogonis Japonici (*Mai Men Dong*) were added. If there was rapid hungering after meals, 15 grams of uncooked Gypsum Fibrosum (*Shi Gao*) and 10 grams of Rhizoma Anemarrhenae Aspheloidis (*Zhi Mu*) were added. If there was heaviness of the limbs, 15 grams each of Rhizoma Atractylodis (*Cang Zhu*) and Rhizoma Pinelliae Ternatae (*Ban Xia*) were added. After 2-3 months of this medicinal therapy, the patients were re-examined once every two weeks for 4-6 times.

In terms of outcomes, marked effect meant that the clinical symptoms disappeared and fasting blood sugar was less than 140mg/dL. Some effect meant that the clinical symptoms markedly improved and fasting blood sugar had decreased to almost normal. No effect meant that there was not obvious improvement in symptoms and fasting blood sugar had not significantly decreased. Based on these criteria, 23 patients were judged to have gotten a marked effect, 26 patients got some effect, and three patients got no effect, for a total amelioration rate of 94.23%.

Huang Zhen-peng, "The Treatment of 26 Cases of Diabetes & Accompanying Peripheral Neuropathy with *Xiao Ke Bi Tong Tang* (Wasting & Thirsting Painful Impediment Decoction)," *Xin Zhong Yi (New Chinese Medicine)*, #12, 1996, p. 21-22: Thirty-six patients were described in all in this study. There were 26 in the treatment group and 10 in the comparison group. In the treatment group, there were 14 men and 12 women. In the comparison group, there were six men and four women. All had been diagnosed as suffering from type 2 diabetes. In the treatment group, there were 11 patients aged 40-58 and 15 patients 59-76. In the comparison group, there were four patients 40-58, and six, 59-76. Average blood glucose in the treatment group was 13.2mmol/L, while, in the comparison group, it was 12.8mmol/L. The shortest course of disease in the treatment group was half a year and the longest was six years, with an average duration of 4.2 years. In the comparison group, it was five months and five years respectively, with an average duration of four years. In addition, all these patients had varying degrees of polyphagia, polydipsia, polyuria, and emaciation accompanied by varying degrees of numbness of the extremities, formication, and aching and pain which was worse at night. Further, their tongues were dark red with white fur, and their pulses were bowstring and fine or fine and choppy.

All the patients in this study were advised on dietary restrictions and administered an oral hypoglycemic agent in addition to being administered the following Chinese medicinals: Radix Astragali Membranacei (*Huang Qi*) and Caulis Milletiae Seu Spatholobi (*Ji Xue Teng*), 30g each, uncooked Radix Rehmanniae (*Sheng Di*), 20g, Radix Achyranthis Bidentatae (*Niu Xi*), Radix Ligustici Wallichii (*Chuan Xiong*), Radix Rubrus Paeoniae Lactiflorae (*Chi Shao*), Lumbricus (*Di Long*), and Fructus Corni Officinalis (*Shan Zhu Yu*), 15g each, Radix Angelicae Sinensis (*Dang Gui*), Semen Pruni Persicae (*Tao Ren*), and Radix Pseudoginseng (*San Qi*), 10g each, and Ramulus Cinnamomi Cassiae (*Gui Zhi*), 6g. If aching and pain were severe, three grams of Agkistrodon Seu Bungarus (*Bai Hua She*) were added. One *ji* was decocted in water and administered per day, with two months continuous administration equaling one course of treatment. Besides the oral hypoglycemics, the comparison group was given 20mg of vitamins B_1 and B_6 three times per day plus 40mg of uridine triphosphate, with two months also equaling one course of treatment.

Marked effects were defined as basic disappearance or marked decrease in numbness, formication, and aching and pain. Some effect was defined as lessening of the above symptoms, while no effect meant that there was no lessening and maybe even worsening of the above symptoms. Based on these criteria, 14 patients (53.8%) in the treatment group got a marked effect, 10 (38.5%) got some effect, and only two (7.7%) got no effect. Thus the total amelioration rate in the treatment group was 92.3%. In the comparison group, no patients got a marked effect, one (10%) got some effect, and nine (90%) got no effect. In addition, in the treatment group, the average reduction in blood sugar was 3.8mmol/L, while in the comparison group it was 2.1mmol/L.

Jiang Zhi-cheng *et al.*, "A Small Discussion of the Treatment of 42 Cases of Diabetic Peripheral Neuropathy with Integrated Chinese-Western Medicine," *Hu Nan Zhong Yi Za Zhi* (*Hunan Journal of Chinese Medicine*), #1, 2000, p. 8-9: Altogether, there were 84 patients in this study divided into two groups of 42 each. Among the 42 patients in the so-called treatment group, 21 were male and 21 were female. Their ages ranged from 38-82, with an average age of 59.8 years. The course of their disease ranged from 2-18 years, with an average duration of 5.54 years. In the comparison group, there were 20 males and 22 females ranging in age from 40-79, with an average age of 58.2 years. These patients' disease courses had lasted from six months to 12 years, with an average duration of 5.62 years. All the patients were diagnosed with type 2 diabetes according to WHO criteria, and all were diagnosed as suffering from peripheral neuropathy. Exclusion criteria consisted of serious heart, liver, or kidney function disorders, incidence of diabetic coma or serious infection within the previous month, other serious diabetic complications, such as retinopathy or malignant tumors, serious psychiatric disorders, or chronic alcoholism.

Members of both groups received 80mg of glyburide orally morning and evening plus 10mg of vitamin B_1 orally three times per day. Members of the treatment group additionally received self-composed *Huang Qi Gui Zhi Wu Wu Tang Jia Wei* (Astragalus & Cinnamon Twig Five Materials Decoction with Added Flavors): Radix Astragali Membranacei (*Huang Qi*), Radix Salviae Miltiorrhizae (*Dan Shen*), Radix Puerariae (*Ge Gen*), and Semen Coicis Lachyrma-jobi (*Yi Yi Ren*), 30g each, Radix Albus Paeoniae Lactiflorae (*Bai Shao*) and Radix Dioscoreae Oppositae (*Shan Yao*), 15g each, Ramulus Cinnamomi Cassiae (*Gui Zhi*), Rhizoma Atractylodis (*Cang Zhu*), Lumbicus (*Di Long*), and Fructus Chaenomlis Lagenariae (*Mu Gua*), 10g each, and Radix Lateralis Praeparatus Aconiti Carmichaeli (*Fu Zi*), 3g. One *ji* of these medicinals was decocted in water and administered orally per day. One month of administration of these medicines equaled one course of therapy, and all patients in this study received two courses.

Marked effect was defined as basic disappearance of the symptoms of neuropathy with an 80% or more decrease in other accompanying symptoms, and a fasting blood sugar level which was basically normal. Some effect meant that there was marked improvement in the symptoms of neuropathy, a 50% or more decrease in accompanying symptoms, and a decrease in fasting blood sugar of 3mmol/L or more. No effect meant that the patient's symptoms and fasting blood sugar did not meet the above criteria. Based on these criteria, 29 patients in the treatment group were judged to have experienced a marked effect, nine got some effect, and four got no effect, for a total amelioration rate of 90.48%. In the comparison group, nine got a marked effect, 13 got some effect, and 20 got no effect, for a total amelioration rate of 52.38%.

Bu Xian-chun & Zhou Shen, "A Study of the Efficacy of Treating 107 Cases of Diabetic Neuropathy by the Method of Foot Baths," *Hu Nan Zhong Yi Za Zhi* (*Hunan Journal of Chinese Medicine*), #9, 2000, p. 15-16: Likewise, this was a comparison study, with 107 patients in the treatment group and 53 patients in the comparison group. In the treatment group, there were 61 males and 46 females ranging from 40-70 years of age, with a median age of 54.1 ± 7.45 years and a median disease duration of 3.5 ± 2.14 years. In the comparison group, there were 33 males and 20 females, aged 43-69, with a median age of 56.3 ± 6.74 years and a median disease duration of 3.7 ± 2.64 years. There was no significant statistical difference in terms of age, sex, disease duration, or symptom severity between these two groups.

All the members of both groups were orally administered glyburide, 80mg BID, and all achieved a blood sugar level of 7.1mmol/L or less after one week. In addition, the treatment group took four foot baths per day for 30 minutes each time. These foot baths consisted of adding 30ml of *Xi Xian Cao Tong Luo Ye* (Siegesbeckia Free the Flow of the Network Vessels Liquid) to 3000ml of hot water (40-50EC). *Xi Xian Cao Tong Luo Ye* was prepared from: Herba Siegesbeckiae (*Xi Xian Cao*), 100g, Caulis Milletiae Seu Spatholobi (*Ji Xue Teng*), Caulis Lonicerae Japonicae (*Ren Dong Teng*), and Folium Artemisiae Argyii (*Ai Ye*), 60g each, Cortex Radicis Acanthopanacis Gracilistylis (*Wu Jia Pi*) and Herba Tougucao (*Tou Gu Cao*), 30g each, and Flos Carthami Tinctorii (*Hong Hua*), Radix Sophorae Flavescentis (*Ku Shen*), and Resina Myrrhae (*Mo Yao*), 20g each. These medicinals were decocted two times in order to get 1000ml of medicinal liquid which was decanted and reserved for use.

In terms of outcomes, clinical control meant that the clinical symptoms of neuropathy improved 91% or better and that the sensation function and conduction of the nerves returned to normal. Marked effect meant that clinical symptoms improved 70-90% and that the sensation function and conduction of the nerves returned to basically normal. Some effect meant that the clinical symptoms decreased 36-69% and that nerve sensation and conduction improved. No effect meant that improvement in clinical symptoms was 35% or less and there was no improvement in nerve sensation and conduction. Based on these criteria, 11 patients in the treatment group were judged clinically controlled, 64 got a marked effect, 23 got

some effect, and nine got no effect, for a total amelioration rate of 91.59%. In the comparison group, three patients were judged clinically controlled, 14 got a marked effect, 19 got some effect, and 17 got no effect, for a total amelioration rate of 67.92%.

RESTLESS LEG SYNDROME

He Gang, "The Treatment of 36 Cases of Diabetic Restless Leg with *San Ren Tang Jia Jian* (Three Seeds Decoction with Additions & Subtractions)," *Jiang Su Zhong Yi* (*Jiangsu Chinese Medicine*), #5, 1999, p. 17: In 1995, the author treated 36 cases of diabetic restless leg. Five of these patients were men, and 31 were women. Their ages ranged from 39-71 years, with an average age of 56.4 years. The course of the diabetes was from five months to 14 years, with an average duration of 6.7 years. The course of disease for restless leg syndrome ranged from 10 days to three years, with an average duration of 1.2 years. All the patients were diagnosed with type 2 diabetes. *San Ren Tan Jia Jian* consisted of: Semen Coicis Lachryma-jobi (*Yi Yi Ren*), Caulis Lonicerae Japonicae (*Ren Dong Teng*), and Ramulus Mori Albi (*Sang Zhi*), 30g each, Talcum (*Hua Shi*) and Radix Cyathulae (*Chuan Niu Xi*), 15g each, and Semen Pruni Armeniacae (*Xing Ren*), Fructus Amomi Cardamomi (*Bai Dou Kou*), Folium Lophatheri Gracilis (*Dan Zhu Ye*), Cortex Magnoliae Officinalis (*Hou Po*), Medulla Tetrapanacis Papyriferi (*Tong Cao*), Fructus Chaenomelis Lagenariae (*Mu Gua*), and Radix Gentianae Macrophyllae (*Qin Jiao*), 10g each.

If damp heat was prevalent, then 10 grams each of Rhizoma Atractylodis (*Cang Zhu*) and Cortex Phellodendri (*Huang Bai*) were added. If spasms and contractures of the lower limbs were prevalent, then 30 grams each of Herba Lycopodii Cum Radice (*Shen Jin Cao*) and Ramulus Uncariae Cum Uncis (*Gou Teng*) were added. If there were signs of static blood, 30 grams of Radix Salviae Miltiorrhizae (*Dan Shen*) and 15 grams of Radix Rubrus Paeoniae Lactiflorae (*Chi Shao*) were added. One *ji* of these medicinals was decocted in water and administered per day for 20 days. The patients continued with their Western medication to control blood sugar levels. Using this protocol, the restless leg syndrome was cured in 28 cases, five cases got some results, and three got no results. Thus the total amelioration rate was 91.67%. From 1993-1998, the author treated 1247 cases of diabetes, of which 69 demonstrated complications with restless leg syndrome. This constituted 5.53% of all patients with diabetes seen during this time.

IMPOTENCE

Liang Kai-fa, "The Treatment of 31 Cases of Diabetic

Impotence by the Combined Methods of Boosting the Kidneys, Quickening the Blood & Standing Up the Wilted," *Si Chuan Zhong Yi (Sichuan Chinese Medicine)*, #3, 2001, p. 35: In this study, there were 31 male out-patients 29-66 years of age. Eleven patients were 29-40, 14 were 41-50, and six were 51-66 years old. The shortest duration of impotence was three months and the longest was two years. All these patients had been diagnosed with diabetes of 1-10 years duration. Common accompanying symptoms included lassitude of the spirit, lack of strength, low back and knee soreness and limpness, fear of cold, chilled extremities, and uneasy urination which dribbled and dripped and would not stop. Any patients with incomplete sexual organ development or impotence due to medications were excluded.

The basic formula used in this study consisted of: Radix Salviae Miltiorrhizae (*Dan Shen*), 24g, Fructus Lycii Chinensis (*Gou Qi Zi*), Semen Cuscutae Chinensis (*Tu Si Zi*), Fructus Cnidii Monnieri (*She Chuang Zi*), Radix Polygoni Multiflori (*He Shou Wu*), and cooked Radix Rehmanniae (*Shu Di*), 15g each, and Fructus Schisandrae Chinensis (*Wu Wei Zi*), Herba Epimedii (*Xian Ling Pi*), and Radix Achyranthis Bidentatae (*Niu Xi*), 10g each. If yang vacuity was severe, Cortex Cinnamomi Cassiae (*Rou Gui*) and Rhizoma Curculiginis Orchioidis (*Xian Mao*) were added. If yin vacuity was severe, Plastrum Testudinis (*Gui Ban*) and Carapax Amydae Chinensis (*Bie Jia*) were added. If there was yin vacuity with fire effulgence or concomitant damp heat, Rhizoma Anemarrhenae Aspheloidis (*Zhi Mu*), Cortex Phellodendri (*Huang Bai*), and Fructus Gardeniae Jasminoidis (*Zhi Zi*) were added. If qi and blood were simultaneously vacuous, Radix Astragali Membranacei (*Huang Qi*), Radix Codonopsitis Pilosulae (*Dang Shen*), Radix Angelicae Sinensis (*Dang Gui*), and Arillus Euphoriae Longanae (*Long Yan Rou*) were added. If there was concomitant liver depression, Radix Bupleuri (*Chai Hu*) and Radix Albus Paeoniae Lactiflorae (*Bai Shao*) were added. One *ji* of these medicinals were decocted in water and adminstered per day in three divided doses, with one month equaling one course of treatment. At the same time, patients were instructed to massage their perineum daily and do Kegel exercises.

Cure was defined as disappearance of clinical symptoms and a return to normal of sexual function. Improvement meant that the penis was able to become erect and was able to function sometimes well and sometimes not so well. No effect meant that there was no improvement in any of the symptoms. Based on these criteria, 12 cases or 38.71% were judged to have been cured, 13 cases or 41.94% improved, and six cases or 19.35% got no effect. Thus the total ame-

lioration rate was 80.65%. The shortest course of treatment was two months and the longest was six.

NEUROGENIC BLADDER

Pang Shu-zhen, "The Treatment of 27 Cases of Diabetic Neurogenic Bladder with *Bu Zhong Yi Qi Tang* (Supplement the Center & Boost the Qi Decoction)," *Si Chuan Zhong Yi (Sichuan Chinese Medicine)*, #3, 2001, p. 42: There were 12 men and 15 women in this study, the oldest of whom was 78 and the youngest, 42 years. All had had NIDDM for the greater part of 10 years, and all had lower abdominal sagging and distention, lack of strength in expelling urine, and posturinary dribbling and dripping. If severe, there was urinary retention. In fact, all had 100ml or more of residual urine in their bladders. However, none had serious kidney function impairment.

Treatment consisted of lowering serum glucose to 9mmol/L or lower combined with *Bu Zhong Yi Qi Tang*: Radix Astragali Membranacei (*Huang Qi*), 30g, Rhizoma Atractylodis Macrocephalae (*Bai Zhu*), 12g, Radix Angelicae Sinensis (*Dang Gui*) and Pericarpium Citri Reticulatae (*Chen Pi*), 10g each, Radix Panacis Ginseng (*Ren Shen*), 9g, and mix-fried Radix Glycyrrhizae (*Gan Cao*), 6g. If there was simultaneous yang vacuity, nine grams of Ramulus Cinnamomi Cassiae (*Gui Zhi*) and six grams of Radix Lateralis Praeparatus Aconiti Carmichaeli (*Fu Zi*) were added. If there was simultaneous low back soreness, 12 grams of Fructus Lycii Chinensis (*Gou Qi Zi*) and 10 grams of cooked Radix Rehmanniae (*Shu Di*) were added. If there was simultaneous piercing pain or burning heat on urination, 10 grams of Fructus Gardeniae Jasminoidis (*Zhi Zi*) and nine grams of Talcum (*Hua Shi*) were added. One *ji* of these medicinals was administered per day in two divided doses, morning and evening, with 10 days equaling one course of treatment. Typically 2-3 such courses were necessary to achieve an effect.

Marked effect was defined as disappearance of clinical symptoms with retained urine in the bladder less than 20ml. Some effect meant that clinical symptoms markedly decreased and residual urine in the bladder was 20–50ml. No effect meant that after four weeks of treatment, there was no improvement in clinical symptoms and residual urine was as much as 100ml. Based on these criteria, 15 cases (55.6%) were judged to have gotten a marked effect, 10 cases (37%) got some effect, and two cases (7.4%) got no effect, for a total amelioration rate of 92.6%.

Li She-li & Cheng Yong, "The Treatment of 36 Cases of Diabetic Neurogenic Bladder with Integrated Chinese-

Western Medicine," *Zhong Yi Za Zhi* (*Journal of Chinese Medicine*), #2, 1999, p. 93-94: Of the 36 patients included in this study, 19 were male and 17 were female. They ranged in age from 38-65, with a median age of 52 years. Their course of disease had lasted from 4-22 years, with a median duration of 14 years. All the patients in this study were diagnosed as suffering from type 2 diabetes, and all were diagnosed with diabetic neurogenic bladder. This was characterized as difficulty and obstruction of expelling urine as well as possible concomitant urinary tract infection. All had a fasting blood glucose level of 8-9mmol/L which rose to 12-13mmol/L two hours after eating. The 36 patients in this study were divided into two groups: the treatment group and the comparison group. There was no statistically significant difference in age, sex, or disease nature or severity between these two groups.

All the participants in this study were put on a diabetic diet and were given dimethyldiguanide and/or other blood sugar regulating medications orally. The treatment group was also given a Chinese medicinal formula on the basis of the principles of supplementing the kidneys, boosting the qi, and quickening the blood. This formula consisted of: Radix Astragali Membranacei (*Huang Qi*), cooked Radix Rehmanniae (*Shu Di*), and Radix Trichosanthis Kirlowii (*Tian Hua Fen*), 30g each, uncooked Radix Rehmanniae (*Sheng Di*), processed Radix Polygoni Multiflori (*He Shou Wu*), and Radix Puerariae (*Ge Gen*), 15g each, Radix Achyranthis Bidentatae (*Niu Xi*) and Radix Ligustici Wallichii (*Chuan Xiong*), 10g each, and Herba Asari Cum Radice (*Xi Xin*), 5g. If the tongue was pale and fat with teeth-marks on its edges, six grams each of Ramulus Cinnamomi Cassiae (*Gui Zhi*) and Radix Lateralis Praeparatus Aconiti Carmichaeli (*Fu Zi*) were added. If the tongue fur was white and slimy, six grams of Fructus Amomi (*Sha Ren*) and 10 grams of Pericarpium Citri Reticulatae (*Chen Pi*) were added. One *ji* of these medicinals were decocted in water and administered orally per day. The members of the comparison group received 20mg of vitamin B_6 and 10mg of B_1 orally three times per day. In addition, they received 0.5mg of vitamin B_{12} via intramuscular injection two times per week.

After 12 weeks of the above treatment, members of both groups were re-examined in terms of urinary frequency per day, a comparison of the amount they drank per day versus the amount of urine voided each day, their two hour PPBG level, their glycosylated hemoglobin, and B-ultrasonagraphy of the amount of urine remaining in their bladders. There was a statistically significant difference between the treatment group and the comparison group from before to after treatment in terms of the number of times of urination

per day, the volume of urine excreted, and the amounts of residual urine in the bladder (P<0.05). Although the glycosylated hemoglobin and both FBG and two hour PPBG levels were lower in the treatment group than in the comparison group at the end of this study, these differences were not statistically significant (P>0.05).

GASTRIC PARESIS

Liu Chang-zheng, "The Treatment of 25 Cases of Diabetic Gastric Paresis with Acupuncture & Western Medicine," *Hu Nan Zhong Yi Za Zhi* (*Hunan Journal of Chinese Medicine*), #3, 2001, p. 33: Forty-four patients were divided into two groups: a treatment group of 25 and a comparison group of 19. In the treatment group, there were 16 men and nine women aged 52-74, with an average age of 56.8 years. These patients had a history of diabetes for 5-14 years. In the comparison group, there were 12 men and seven women aged 50-73, with an average age of 54.2 years and a history of diabetes for 4-12 years. All met WHO criteria for the diagnosis of diabetes. Clinical symptoms included varying degrees of upper abdominal distention, indigestion, postprandial heaviness, nausea, and vomiting. X-rays showed slowed peristalsis. All patients were examined to exclude stomach and duodenal obstruction or cancer.

The treatment method consisted of administering 10mg three times per day of domperidone (Motilium) combined with acupuncture at *Shou San Li* (LI 10), *Nei Guan* (Per 6), *Zhong Wan* (CV 12), and *Zu San Li* (St 36). Supplementing hand technique was used and the needles were retained for 30 minutes each time after obtaining the qi. At the same time, moxibustion was performed with a moxa roll at *Ming Men* (GV 4) and *Guan Yuan* (CV 4). Four weeks equaled one course of treatment. The comparison group only received the Motilium. In addition, all the patients received normal treatment for their diabetes which kept their fasting blood sugar between 5.0-7.0mmol/L and their two hour postprandial blood sugar between 6.0-8.0mmol/L.

In terms of outcomes, a good effect meant that the sensation of abdominal distention was eliminated. The amount of food eaten increased, and peristalsis sped up. A half hour after eating, the stomach was 3/5 empty or more. Some effect meant that abdominal distention markedly decreased, the amount of food increased, and peristalsis sped up somewhat less. A half hour after eating the stomach was less than 3/5 empty. No effect meant there was no marked change in the symptoms and a half hour after eating, the stomach was less than 3/5 empty.   Of the 25 patients in the treatment group, 14 were judged to have gotten a good effect, 10 got some effect, and only one got no effect. Thus the total amelioration rate in the treatment group was 96.0%. In the comparison group, eight got a good effect, seven got some effect, and four got no effect, for a total amelioration rate of 77.8%.

CONSTIPATION

Gan Li, "The Treatment of 58 Cases of Diabetic Constipation Using *Jia Wei Si Mo Tang* (Added Flavors Four Milled Ingredients Decoction)," *Zhe Jiang Zhong Yi Za Zhi (Zhejiang Journal of Chinese Medicine)*, #6, 1999, p. 384: During 1995, the author used *Jia Wei Si Mo Tang* to treat 58 cases of diabetic constipation by regulating the qi. This group was compared with a second group of 41 patients who were treated with Western drugs. All 99 cases were diagnosed with diabetes using WHO criteria, and the patients had come to clinic for treatment of constipation. For the most part, their diets were under control. When the oral hypoglycemic agents were not entirely effective in controlling blood glucose levels, then, in addition, insulin at 12-48u was prescribed by injection under the skin three times each day before meals. Blood glucose test results were closely monitored, and the dosage of insulin was adjusted when necessary. As a baseline, FBG ranges were 4.9-8.7mmol/L, and two hour PPBG ranges were 5.3-10.2mmol/L. In the treatment group of 58 patients, 35 were male and 23 were female. Their ages ranged from 42-81, with an average age of 60.2 years. The duration of diabetes was 3-9 years for 32 cases and over 10 years for 26 cases. The duration of the constipation was from six months to five years for 30 cases and over five years for 28 cases. In the comparison group of 41 patients, 24 were male and 17 were female. Their ages ranged from 40-79, with an average age of 59.4 years. The duration of diabetes was 3-9 years for 29 cases and over 10 years for 12 cases. The duration of the constipation was from six months to five years for 22 cases and over five years for 19 cases.

The treatment group was prescribed: Radix Codonopsitis Pilosulae (*Dang Shen*), 20g, Radix Trichosanthis Kirlowii (*Tian Hua Fen*) and uncooked Radix Rehmanniae (*Sheng Di*), 15g each, Herba Leonuri Heterophylli (*Yi Mu Cao*) and Radix Dioscoreae Oppositae (*Huai Shan Yao*), 12g each, Semen Arecae Catechu (*Bing Lang*) and Radix Linderae Strychnifoliae (*Wu Yao*), 10g each, and Lignum Aquilariae Agallochae (*Chen Xiang*), 8g. For exuberant stomach heat, Rhizoma Anemarrhenae Aspheloidis (*Zhi Mu*) and Fructus Gardeniae Jasminoidis (*Shan Zhi*) were added. For cases of lung-kidney qi and yin vacuity, Tuber

Asparagi Cochinensis (*Tian Dong*) and Tuber Ophiopogonis Japonici (*Mai Dong*) were added. For cases of spleen-stomach vacuity weakness, Radix Astragali Membranacei (*Huang Qi*) was added. One *ji* was decocted in water and administered each day, and one month equalled one course of treatment. In the control group of 41 patients, cisapride was prescribed at 5-10mg TID. Both groups were evaluated after one course of treatment.

The results were considered very good if the bowels were kept in control (diarrhea not occurring), one bowel movement every 1-2 days, free flowing and smooth, without discomfort. The results were considered moderately good if the bowels were kept in control, bowel movements twice a week, formed stools, or sometimes dry stools. No results meant that, even after receiving the formula, the bowels did not move at all and the condition remained the same as prior to treatment. Based on these criteria, 45 patients in the treatment group got very good results (77.6%), nine patients got moderately good results (15.5%), and four patients were without results (6.9%), for a total amelioration rate of 93.1%. After treatment, the number of bowel movements increased from once every 4-6 days to once every 1-2 days. In the comparison group taking cisapride, 29 got very good results (70.7%), eight patients got moderately good results (19.5%), and four patients got no results (9.8%), for a total amelioration rate of 90.2%. The number of bowel movements for this group before treatment was once every 4-5 days lowered to 1-2 days. Among these patients, five experienced an increase in the number of the bowel movements. Therefore, the dosage was lessened and the frequency became normal. Based on the above, both groups showed good results without much difference in outcomes.

He Gang, "The Treatment of 42 Cases of Diabetic Constipation Using *Yi Yu Tang* (Benefit & Foster Decoction)," *Ji Lin Zhong Yi Yao (Jilin Chinese Medicine & Medicinals)*, #3, 1999, p. 29: Of the 42 patients in this study, 19 were men and 23 were women. Their ages ranged from 34-75 years old, with an average age of 54.8 years. The duration of the diabetes was from 2-17 years, with an average duration of 8.2 years. The duration of the constipation was five months to two years, with an average duration of 11 months. All of the patients were diagnosed with type 2 diabetes. The basic formula included: Radix Astragali Membranacei (*Huang Qi*), uncooked Radix Rehmanniae (*Sheng Di*), and Radix Scrophulariae Ningpoensis (*Xuan Shen*), 30g each, Radix Pseudostellariae Heterophyllae (*Tai Zi Shen*), Radix Angelicae Sinensis (*Dang Gui*), and Radix Polygoni Multiflori (*He Shou Wu*), 15g each, and Radix Anemarrhenae Aspheloidis (*Zhi Mu*), Semen Cannabis

Sativae (*Huo Ma Ren*), and Rhizoma Polygonati Odorati (*Yu Zhu*), 10g each. For abdominal distention, 10 grams of Fructus Immaturus Citri Aurantii (*Zhi Shi*) and six grams of Semen Arecae Catechu (*Bing Lang*) were added. For blurred vision, 15 grams of Semen Cassiae Torae (*Jue Ming Zi*) and 12 grams of Flos Chrysanthemi Morifolii (*Ju Hua*) were added. When blood stasis was present, 15 grams of Radix Salviae Miltiorrhizae (*Dan Shen*) and 10 grams of Semen Pruni Persicae (*Tao Ren*) were added. For complications with phlegm dampness, 15 grams of Fructus Trichosanthis Kirlowii (*Gua Lou*) and 10 grams of Bombyx Batryticatus (*Jiang Can*) were added. When yang vacuity was present, then Radix Anemarrhenae Aspheloidis was omitted and 10 grams of Herba Cistanchis Deserticolae (*Rou Cong Rong*) and six grams of Cortex Cinnamomi Cassiae (*Rou Gui*) were added. One *ji* of these medicinals were decocted in water and administered per day divided into two doses. Twenty-seven (64.3%) of the patients had a bowel movement within two days of starting the formula, and the remaining 15 (35.7%) patients had bowel movements within three days.

Huang Yong-yan, "The Treatment of 32 Cases of Type II Diabetic Constipation with Heat Stasis Pattern," *Jiang Su Zhong Yi (Jiangsu Chinese Medicine)*, #11, 1999, p. 18: The author of this study used *Tao He Cheng Qi Tang Jia Wei* (Persica Order the Qi Decoction with Added Flavors) to treat diabetic constipation caused by stasis and heat mutually binding in the interior. Of the 32 patients in this study, 18 were men and 14 were women. Their ages ranged from 45-68 years old. All the patients were clinically diagnosed with type 2 diabetes, and the duration of the constipation was as short as five days and as long as six years. All of the patients experienced dry, bound stools, consumed much food and drink, and also had a dry mouth and throat. The patients' tongue bodies were dark purple, and their pulses were bowstring and choppy. Fasting blood glucose was higher than 10.0mmol/L.

All patients were given *Tao He Cheng Qi Tang Jia Wei* as the basic formula, consisting of: Semen Pruni Persicae (*Tao Ren*), 15g, Radix Et Rhizoma Rhei (*Da Huang*), 6-15g added at the end of decocting, Mirabilitum (*Mang Xiao*) mixed with water, and Radix Glycyrrhizae (*Gan Cao*), 10g each, and Ramulus Cinnamomi Cassiae (*Gui Zhi*), 6g. If qi vacuity was present, then Radix Astragali Membranacei (*Huang Qi*) and Radix Codonopsitis Pilosulae (*Dang Shen*) were added. For yin vacuity, uncooked Radix Rehmanniae (*Sheng Di*) and Radix Scrophulariae Ningpoensis (*Xuan Shen*) were added. For blood vacuity, Herba Cistanchis Deserticolae (*Rou Cong Rong*) and Extremitas Radicis Angelicae Sinensis (*Dang*

Gui Wei) were added. For qi fullness, Semen Arecae Catechu (*Bing Lang*) and Fructus Citri Aurantii (*Zhi Ke*) were added. One *ji* of this formula was decocted in water and administered per day in two divided doses. Twenty-two cases got very good results, with more than one bowel movement each day, and 10 cases got good results, with one bowel movement every 1-2 days.

Zhang Min, "A Survey of the Treatment Efficacy of Treating Diabetic Constipation by the Methods of Boosting the Qi & Nourishing Yin, Transforming Stasis & Freeing the Flow of the Network Vessels," *Xin Zhong Yi (New Chinese Medicine)*, 37, 2001, p. 11-12: Altogether, there were 65 patients in this study, all of whom had been diagnosed as suffering from diabetes based on 1985 WHO criteria and all had varying degrees of constipation. These 65 patients were divided into two groups: 35 patients in the so-called Chinese medicinal group and 30 patients in the Western medicinal group. In the Chinese medicinal group, there were 16 men and 19 women with a median age of 61.32 ± 3.41 years, a median disease duration of 9.81 ± 2.59 years, and median blood glucose of 8.42 ± 2.75mmol/L. In the Western medicinal group, there were 18 men and 12 women, with a median age of 60.63 ± 3.72 years, a median disease duration of 10.25 ± 2.41 years, and a median blood glucose of 8.91 ± 2.07mmol/L. Hence there was no marked statistical difference between these two groups in terms of sex, age, disease duration, or blood glucose.

The patients in the Chinese medicinal group received the following basic formula: Radix Astragali Membranacei (*Huang Qi*) and uncooked Radix Rehmanniae (*Sheng Di*), 30g each, Radix Pseudostellariae Heterophyllae (*Tai Zi Shen*), Rhizoma Polygonati (*Huang Jing*), and Fructus Lycii Chinensis (*Gou Qi Zi*), 20g each, Radix Salviae Miltiorrhizae (*Dan Shen*) and Semen Cannabis Sativae (*Huo Ma Ren*), 15g each, and Fructus Immaturus Citri Aurantii (*Zhi Shi*), Herba Cistanchis Deserticolae (*Rou Cong Rong*), and Semen Pruni Persicae (*Tao Ren*), 10g each. If the tongue fur was thick and slimy, Pericarpium Citri Reticulatae (*Chen Pi*), Rhizoma Atractylodis (*Cang Zhu*), Cortex Magnoliae Officinalis (*Hou Po*), and Fructus Cardamomi (*Bai Dou Kou*) were added. If yin vacuity was marked, Rhizoma Anemarrhenae Aspheloidis (*Zhi Mu*), Radix Scrophulariae Ningpoensis (*Xuan Shen*), Fructus Mori Albi (*Sang Shen Zi*), and Fructus Ligustri Lucidi (*Nu Zhen Zi*) were added. If there was yin and blood depletion and vacuity, Radix Polygoni Multiflori (*He Shou Wu*), Radix Angelicae Sinensis (*Dang Gui*), Fructus Corni Officinalis (*Shan Zhu Yu*), and Tuber Ophiopogonis Japonici (*Mai Men Dong*) were added. If there was severe abdominal distention and a bowel movement only once every four days and the patient's body was still strong, *Huo Ma Ren* was removed and 3-9 grams of Folium Sennae (*Fan Xie Ye*) was added. The patients in the Western medicinal group received 10mg of cisapride TID, 30 minutes before meals.

Ten patients in the Chinese medicinal group experienced a marked effect, 19 got some effect, and six got no effect. Thus the total amelioration rate in this group was 82.86%. In the Western medicinal group, three patients got a marked effect, 14 got some effect, and 13 got no effect, for a total amelioration rate of 56.67%. Thus these Chinese medicinals were superior to cisapride for increasing the number of bowel movements and softening the stools in these patients with diabetic constipation.

DIARRHEA

He Ya-lu, "The Treatment of 36 Cases of Diabetic Diarrhea with Chinese Medicinals Applied to the Navel," *Zhe Jiang Zhong Yi Za Zhi (Zhejiang Journal of Chinese Medicine)*, #8, 2000, p. 332: All 36 patients in this study had been diagnosed as suffering from type 2 diabetes. Among them, there were 21 males and 15 females aged 42-71, with an average age of 53.61 years and disease course of 2-13 years, with an average disease duration of 5.43 years. All the patients had had diarrhea from 1-11 months, with an average duration of that complaint of 4.65 months. Each day, they would have five or more watery stools. All had undergone various examinations to exclude any other etiologies, and all had been previously treated without effect.

Herba Ephedrae (*Ma Huang*), Fructus Alpiniae Oxyphyllae (*Yi Zhi Ren*), Cortex Cinnamomi Cassiae (*Rou Gui*), Galla Rhois (*Wu Bei Zi*), and dry Rhizoma Zingiberis (*Gan Jiang*), were powdered and mixed together in the following respective proportions: 2:1:1:2:1. This powder was then made into a paste by mixing with vinegar. After disinfecting the navel with 75% alcohol, this paste was applied to the navel and held in place with an adhesive plaster. Twenty-four hours later it was removed. This treatment was repeated every other day, with five times equaling one course of therapy. During this course of treatment, all other medicines for stopping diarrhea were suspended. However, doses of hypoglycemic agents were not changed. All the patients underwent 1-3 courses of treatment, with the average being 1.68 courses.

Seven patients were judged to be clinically controlled. This meant that they had no more than two bowel movements per day and the consistency of the stools was normal. Twenty-three patients got a marked effect. This meant that the number of bowel movements per day was reduced by 2/3 or more and the stools were basically formed. Four patients improved, meaning the number of bowel movements decreased 1/3-2/3 and the consistency of the stools improved. Two cases got no effect, meaning that reduction in number of bowel movements per day was less than 1/3 or none. Thus the total amelioration rate was 94.45%. Further, this treatment did not affect blood glucose, and there were no adverse reactions.

ORTHOSTATIC HYPOTENSION

Liang Ping-mao, "The Treatment of 31 Cases of Diabetic Orthostatic Hypotension with Integrated Chinese-Western Medicine," *Hu Nan Zhong Yi Za Zhi (Hunan Journal of Chinese Medicine)*, #3, 1998, p. 47-48: The author treated two groups of patients with type 2 diabetic orthostatic hypotension. One group was the treatment group of 31 cases, and the other group was a comparison group of 12 cases. Combined, there were 19 men and 24 women whose ages ranged from 46-59 years old, with the average age of 51.6 years. Their blood pressure when lying down was 18.4/10.6kPa, and their blood pressure while standing was 14/10.6kPa. Their FBG was 10.5mmol/L. The course of disease for diabetes was 7-15 years, with an average duration of 9.2 years. The course of disease for orthostatic hypotension was 1-6 years, with an average duration of 1.8 years. In addition, there were eight cases of diabetic nephropathy and nine cases of diabetic retinopathy.

The comparison group received 80mg of glyburide twice per day. The treatment group received *Sheng Ya Tang* (Upbear Pressure Decoction) which consisted of: Tuber Ophiopogonis Japonici (*Mai Dong*), 40g, Radix Salviae Miltiorrhizae (*Dan Shen*) and Radix Ligustici Wallichii (*Chuan Xiong*), 30g each, Gelatinum Cornu Cervi (*Lu Jiao Jiao*), dissolved, Plastrum Testudinis (*Gui Ban*), Fructus Lycii Chinensis (*Gou Qi Zi*), cooked Radix Rehmanniae (*Shu Di*), and Fructus Liquidambaris Taiwaniae (*Lu Lu Tong*), 20g each, Fructus Schisandrae Chinensis (*Wu Wei Zi*), 15g, Radix Panacis Ginseng (*Ren Shen*), decocted separately, and Rhizoma Cimicifugae (*Sheng Ma*), 10g each, and Fructus Zizyphi Jujubae (*Da Zao*), 10 pieces.

Before treatment with *Sheng Ya Tang*, the difference between the standing and reclining blood pressure was 4.4kPa for the treatment group. After treatment, it was 2.8kPa. The difference between the standing and reclining blood pressure for the comparison group before and after treatment with Western drugs was 4.5kPa and 4.3kPa respectively. In the treatment group, FBG before treatment was 9.8 ± 4.9mmol/L and after treatment was 5.5 ± 1.5mmol/L. In the comparison group, FBG before treatment was 10.8 ± 4.3mmol/L and after treatment was 5.8 ± 2.2mmol/L (P < 0.01).

REPRESENTATIVE CASE HISTORIES:

CASE 1[11]

The patient was a 41 year old female who was first seen for polydipsia, polyphagia, and bilateral extremity pain lasting for three months. The patient had a history of type 2 diabetes for three years and was being treated with hypoglycemic medicinals. Three months prior to her first visit, her symptoms had gotten worse, and she had begun to experience bilateral lower extremity numbness and pain and a burning sensation which was worse at night. The patient's tongue was pale red with static macules and thin, white fur. Her pulse was fine and bowstring. Therefore, her Chinese medical pattern discrimination was qi vacuity with blood stasis resulting in non-free flow of the vessels and network vessels. In this case, the requisite treatment principles were to boost the qi and quicken the blood, free the flow of the network vessels and stop the pain. Therefore, *Bu Yang Huan Wu Tang* was administered plus Radix Achyranthis Bidentatae (*Niu Xi*), 15g, and Squama Manitis Pentadactylis (*Chuan Shan Jia*), 10g. After one course of treatment, the woman's pain was decreased. After two courses, it had remitted. On follow-up after three months, there had been no recurrence.

CASE 2[12]

The patient was a 57 year old female agricultural worker who was first examined on Jul. 21, 1997. Six years earlier, she had begun to experience oral thirst, polydipsia, and increased urination and was diagnosed at her local hospital with type 2 diabetes. She was put on a restricted diet and orally administered hypoglycemic medication. Two years earlier, the patient had begun to experience bilateral lower extremity numbness and tingling, emission of coolness, and formication. Several doctors at different hospitals diagnosed this as diabetic PN and had prescribed orally administered ATP, vitamin B$_1$, glandular B$_{12}$, and a medication identified only as 654-2. However, none of these treatments achieved any effect. At the time of her examination, the patient was emaciated, had a sallow yellow facial complexion, lower limb wilting, weakness, and lack of strength, and numbness and insensitivity. Her tongue was pale red with scanty fur, and her pulse was

deep and fine.[13] Therefore, she was prescribed the above described basic formula plus Tuber Curcumae (*Yu Jin*), Herba Leonuri Heterophylli (*Yi Mu Cao*), and Radix Lateralis Praeparatus Aconiti Carmichaeli ((*Fu Zi*), 6g each. After two weeks of this formula, the woman's symptoms were decreased, her lower legs had strength, and her bodily coolness was less. However, she still experienced numbness and tingling and formication. Thus she was given 45 more ji of this basic formula with additions and subtractions along with intravenous drips (described above) for four weeks, at which time, all her symptoms disappeared. On follow-up after one year, there had been no recurrence.

CASE 3[14]

The patient was a 62 year old cadre who was first examined on Oct. 20, 1996. This man presented with bilateral numbness of the upper extremities with lack of strength in grasping for more than two months. The patient said he was fatigued and lacked strength. He also had oral thirst, polydipsia, dry stools, a red tongue with scanty fur, and a fine, rapid pulse. His fasting blood sugar was 8.8mmol/L. The man's Western medical diagnosis was type 2 diabetes with diabetic peripheral neuropathy. His Chinese medical pattern discrimination was categorized as qi and yin dual vacuity with phlegm and stasis obstructing the network vessels. Therefore, the treatment principles were to enrich yin and clear heat, quicken the blood and transform stasis, flush phlegm and free the flow of the network vessels. The formula Zhang Fa-rong administered this man consisted of: Radix Dioscoreae Oppositae (*Shan Yao*), Tuber Ophiopogonis Japonici (*Mai Men Dong*), and uncooked Radix Rehmanniae (*Sheng Di*), 30g each, Radix Pseudostellariae Heterophyllae (*Tai Zi Shen*), Rhizoma Anemarrhenae Aspheloidis (*Zhi Mu*), Radix Angelicae Sinensis (*Dang Gui*), Radix Albus Paeoniae Lactiflorae (*Bai Shao*), Radix Salviae Miltiorrhizae (*Dan Shen*), and Rhizoma Pinelliae Ternatae (*Ban Xia*), 15g each, Rhizoma Corydalis Yanhusuo (*Yan Hu Suo*), 12g, Semen Sinapis Albae (*Bai Jie Zi*), Ramulus Cinnamomi Cassiae (*Gui Zhi*), and Radix Glycyrrhizae (*Gan Cao*), 10g each, and Radix Pseudoginseng (*San Qi*), 3g swallowed with the decoction. One ji of these medicinals was decocted in water and administered orally per day. In addition, the man was instructed how to follow a diabetic diet, to get more exercise, and to control his weight.

On Nov. 10, the patient was re-examined after taking 20 ji of the above medicinals. His upper extremity pain and numbness was markedly decreased and he had more strength than before. His affect had improved and his oral thirst had remitted. The man's tongue was pale red with thin, yellow fur, and his pulse was harmonious and moderate or relaxed. His fasting blood sugar was 7.11mmol/L. At this point, Dr. Zhang prescribed a ready-made Chinese medicine designed by himself to free the flow of the network vessels plus another to treat the diabetes. On Mar. 5, 1998, the man was examined once again by Dr. Zhang. At this point in time, all the man's symptoms had disappeared, his fasting blood sugar was 6.59mmol/L, and his nerve conduction in both arms was normal.

CASE 4[15]

The patient was a 69 year old male retired cadre who was first examined on Nov. 24, 1997. This man had been diagnosed as suffering from diabetes for 16 years and regularly took orally glyburide and dimethyldiguanide. For the previous two years, the patient had experienced bilateral lower limb numbness. In the past two weeks, both feet had become swollen and distended with a burning hot, painful sensation which was worse at night. His Western medical diagnosis was diabetic peripheral neuropathy and he had taken vitamins for 10 days but without marked improvement. Accompanying symptoms included dry mouth, heart vexation, lack of strength, poor vision, and dry stools. The patient's FBG was 175mg/dL. His tongue was dark red with thin, yellow fur, and his pulse was deep, fine, and choppy.

Based on the above signs and symptoms, this patient's Chinese medical pattern was categorized as yin vacuity with fire effulgence and stasis and heat mutually binding. The treatment principles were to nourish yin and clear heat, quicken the blood and free the flow of the network vessels. Therefore, he was prescribed the following Chinese medicinals: Radix Astragali Membranacei (*Huang Qi*) and Radix Salviae Miltiorrhizae (*Dan Shen*), 30g each, Radix Glehniae Littoralis (*Sha Shen*), Tuber Ophiopogonis Japonici (*Mai Men Dong*), Radix Albus Paeoniae Lactiflorae (*Bai Shao*), Radix Rubrus Paeoniae Lactiflorae (*Chi Shao*), uncooked Radix Rehmanniae (*Sheng Di*), and Fructus Chaenomelis Lagenariae (*Mu Gua*), 15g each, Rhizoma Anemarrhenae Aspheloidis (*Zhi Mu*), Radix Ligustici Wallichii (*Chuan Xiong*), Lumbricus (*Di Long*), Radix Glycyrrhizae (*Gan Cao*), and Radix Achyranthis Bidentatae (*Niu Xi*), 10g each, and Hirudo Seu Whitmania (*Shui Zhi*), 6g. One *ji* of these medicinals was decocted in water and administered orally per day in two divided doses.

After taking a continuous 14 *ji* of these medicinals, the patient was re-examined. At that time, the burning pain had markedly decreased and his symptoms of oral thirst and heart vexation had also diminished. His fasting blood

sugar was 154mg/dL. After another 14 *ji*, the pain basically disappeared and the lower limb numbness also decreased. Now his fasting blood sugar was 136mg/dL. Again the man was prescribed 14 *ji* of the above medicinals. Now his fasting blood sugar was 129mg/dL, and, despite occasional lower limb numbness, there was no other discomfort. In order to consolidate the treatment effects, the patient was prescribed the same medicinals in the form of pills which he took continuously for one month. At that point, the numbness disappeared completely, nerve conduction in his lower extremities returned to normal, and his fasting blood sugar was 117mg/dL. On follow-up after one and a half years, there had been no recurrence of the peripheral neuropathy.

CASE 5[16]

The patient was a 39 year old agricultural worker who had been diagnosed with diabetes two years before. Four months after being diagnosed with diabetes, his blood sugar was under control. However, several times each month, the man experienced partial flaccidity of his penis during sex. This had continued for a year and gradually progressed to complete impotence. It was difficult for this man to have normal sex once every 1-2 months. When the man was first examined for this problem on Sept. 14, 1998, the accompanying signs and symptoms included lassitude of the spirit, low back and knee soreness and weakness, insomnia, profuse dreams, dizziness, tinnitus, a pale red tongue with scattered static spots on its edges, and a bowstring, fine, choppy pulse. Serum glucose and urine sugar were basically normal. For the previous half year, the man had been taking 5mg of glyburide per day with stable effect.

Based on the above signs and symptoms, the man's pattern was discriminated as kidney vacuity and blood stasis for which he was prescribed: Radix Salviae Miltiorrhizae (*Dan Shen*), 24g, Fructus Lycii Chinensis (*Gou Qi Zi*), Semen Cuscutae Chinensis (*Tu Si Zi*), Fructus Cnidii Monnieri (*She Chuang Zi*), Radix Polygoni Multiflori (*He Shou Wu*), and cooked Radix Rehmanniae (*Shu Di*), 15g each, and Fructus Schisandrae Chinensis (*Wu Wei Zi*), Herba Epimedii (*Xian Ling Pi*), Radix Albus Paeoniae Lactiflorae (*Bai Shao*), Arillus Euphoriae Longanae (*Long Yan Rou*), and Radix Achyranthis Bidentatae (*Niu Xi*), 10g each. He was also instructed to massage his perineum and do Kegel exercises every day. After one month of this therapy, the patient was able to achieve an erection and was able to consummate sexual intercourse one time. After another month of the same therapy, the man's sexual function returned to normal and he stopped taking the medicinal. However, he continued the perineal massage and Kegel exercises. On follow-up after one year, there were no reported abnormalities.

CASE 6[17]

The patient was a 60 year old male cadre who was first examined on Oct. 2, 1998. According to the patient, he had been diagnosed with type 2 diabetes 10 years before. Because he persisted in not abiding by his dietary restrictions and was not regular in taking his hypoglycemic medicines, the man's blood sugar was not stable, sometimes reaching 21.5mmol/L. In the previous two years, this man's urination had become difficult, its amount scanty, and its times numerous. After urination, there was dribbling and dripping which would not stop. Accompanying symptoms included lassitude of the spirit, lack of strength, fear of cold, chilled extremities, a white, lusterless facial complexion, a pale tongue with thin, white fur, and a fine, forceless pulse. Prostate examination was normal as was kidney function. However, there was 120ml of residual urine in his bladder.

The patient's Chinese medical pattern was categorized as central qi downward falling with simultaneous yang vacuity. Therefore, he was treated with *Bu Zhong Yi Qi Tang* (Supplement the Center & Boost the Qi Decoction): Radix Astragali Membranacei (*Huang Qi*), 30g, Rhizoma Atractylodis Macrocephalae (*Bai Zhu*), 12g, Radix Angelicae Sinensis (*Dang Gui*) and Pericarpium Citri Reticulatae (*Chen Pi*), 10g each, Ramulus Cinnamomi Cassiae (*Gui Zhi*) and Radix Panacis Ginseng (*Ren Shen*), 9g each, and mix-fried Radix Glycyrrhizae (*Gan Cao*) and Radix Lateralis Praeparatus Aconiti Carmichaeli (*Fu Zi*), 6g each. After 20 days of taking these medicinals, all his symptoms disappeared and the residual urine was down to 10ml. From that time forward, this man took 10 days of these medicinals once every three months. On follow-up after one year, there had been no recurrence.

CASE 7[18]

The patient was a 36 year old male shop assistant who was first examined on Jan. 13, 1987. The patient's main complaint was diarrhea for the previous two years which had become exacerbated in the last four days. The man had been suffering from polydipsia and polyuria since 1979. He was diagnosed as suffering from diabetes and blindness due to diabetic retinopathy in 1984. In 1985, he was diagnosed with diabetic nephropathy and gastrointestinal autonomic neuropathy. After being treated with insulin (50 units per day), his fasting serum glucose reduced by half and his urine glucose, which had been (+++) was negative or trace. However, the man complained of increasing frequency of bowel movements ranging from 3-10 per day and especially at night. The patient was prescribed 0.3-0.9g per day of berberine which reduced his bowel movements to 1-2 times per day. However, if he went off the berberine, his diarrhea recurred. Stool examination in 1986 was normal. At the time of examination, the man had been taking berberine constantly for two years. Nevertheless, in the past four days, the bowel movements had increased in spite of taking berberine. At this point in time, the man was having 10 watery stools per day to the point of fecal incontinence. Accompanying symptoms included aversion to cold, especially in the abdominal and lumbar areas, depression, and anxiety. There was thin, white tongue fur and a slippery pulse.

Based on the above signs and symptoms, this patient was diagnosed with wasting and thirsting and diarrhea with spleen-kidney dual vacuity. Therefore, treatment principles were to warm and invigorate the spleen and kidneys, nourish the liver and regulate the spleen qi. The formula consisted of: Radix Astragali Membranacei (*Huang Qi*) and calcined Concha Margaritiferae (*Zhen Zhu Mu*), 30g each, Radix Albus Paeoniae Lactiflorae (*Bai Shao*), 20g, Semen Cuscutae Chinensis (*Tu Si Zi*), 15g, Ramulus Cinnamomi Cassiae (*Gui Zhi*), Rhizoma Atractylodis Macrocephalae (*Bai Zhu*), Pericarpium Citri Reticulatae (*Chen Pi*), Fructus Psoraleae Corylifoliae (*Bu Gu Zhi*), and Fructus Schisandrae Chinensis (*Wu Wei Zi*), 10g each, dry Rhizoma Zingiberis (*Gan Jiang*) and Radix Ledebouriellae Divaricatae (*Fang Feng*), 8g each, and mix-fried Radix Glycyrrhizae (*Gan Cao*), 6g.

After taking 6 *ji* of the above formula, the patient's bowel movements were reduced to six per day. However, when he stopped taking the decoction, he had nocturnal diarrhea, up to eight times per night. Therefore, 30 grams each of Sclerotium Poriae Cocos (*Fu Ling*) and Semen Coicis Lachryma-jobi (*Yi Yi Ren*) and 15 grams of Cornu Cervi (*Lu Rong*) were added to the original formula and his insulin was decreased to 46 units per day. After taking this prescription for three months, the patient had only 1-2 bowel movements per day with formed stools. His insulin was reduced to 44 units and he continued to take decoctions for one year until his bowel movements were completely normal, at which point he stopped taking these medicinals and his symptoms of diarrhea as well as coldness in his low back, abdomen, and extremities did not return.

CASE 8[19]

The patient was a 63 year old female who had had type 2

diabetes for four years. The patient's bowels were habitually bound and not free-flowing. Although the patient
had the desire, she was unable to defecate. This was
accompanied by belching, stomach duct and abdominal
glomus and fullness, and torpid intake. She had been taking various purgative formulas, such as *Da Huang Su Da
Pian* (Rhubarb Preserve & Remove Pills), *Guo Dao Pian*
(Guiding Out Fruit Pills), and *Bian Sai Ting Pian* (Bowel
Stoppage Pills), but these fomulas had only made the illness worse. Upon examination, the patient's tongue fur
was thin and slimy, and her pulse was bowstring and mod-
erate (*i.e.*, relaxed or slightly slow). Her Chinese medical
pattern was categorized as liver depression and spleen
vacuity and the following medicinals were prescribed:
Radix Codonopsitis Pilosulae (*Dang Shen*), 20g, Radix
Trichosanthis Kirlowii (*Tian Hua Fen*) and uncooked
Radix Rehmanniae (*Sheng Di*), 15g each, Herba Leonuri
Heterophylli (*Yi Mu Cao*) and Radix Dioscoreae
Oppositae (*Huai Shan Yao*), 12g each, Semen Arecae
Catechu (*Bing Lang*) and Radix Linderae Strychnifoliae
(*Wu Yao*), 10g each, and Lignum Aquilariae Agallochae
(*Chen Xiang*), 8g. An additional 15 grams of Radix
Astragali Membranacei (*Huang Qi*) was included, and the
decoction was administered at one *ji* daily for two weeks.
The bowels moved after two *ji*, and, after two weeks, the
bowel movements were regular, moving once a day with
formed stools and without discomfort. At this point, the
constipation was considered cured.

CASE 9[20]

The patient was a 59 year old woman who had had diabetes
for six years. Her bowel movements were difficult, occuring
only once every five days, with dry, bound stools.
Accompanying symptoms included abdominal fullness and
distention with aching pain, vexation and agitation, dry
mouth, thirst, no desire for food, and inability to sleep. The
patient's tongue was purple with static macules, and her
pulse was bowstring and choppy. Her fasting blood glucose
was 12.8mmol/L. The patient's Chinese medical pattern
discrimination was heat stasis internally binding with fluid
damage intestinal dryness and non-freely flowing bowel qi.
The treatment principles were to clear heat and dispel stasis, free the flow of the bowels and preserve yin. The formula consisted of: uncooked Radix Rehmanniae (*Sheng
Di*), 24g, Radix Scrophulariae Ningpoensis (*Xuan Shen*),
Semen Pruni Persicae (*Tao Ren*), and Semen Arecae
Catechu (*Bing Lang*), 15g each, Radix Et Rhizoma Rhei
(*Da Huang*), added at the end of decocting, Mirabilitum
(*Mang Xiao*), mixed with water, and Radix Glycyrrhizae
(*Gan Cao*), 10g each, and Ramulus Cinnamomi Cassiae
(*Gui Zhi*), 6g. Three *ji* were prescribed, with one *ji* being

decocted in water and administered in two divided doses.
After the first *ji*, the patient had a bowel movement and her
abdominal distention and pain were alleviated. After three
ji, the bowels were free-flowing and the patient's dry mouth
and thirst were lessened. A week later, blood glucose was
reduced to 8.6mmol/L, and, on follow-up after three
months, the constipation had not recurred.

CASE 10[21]

The patient was a 56 year old female whose first examination was in August, 1996. She had had diabetes for
five years and took Western medications to lower her
blood sugar levels. For the last month, the patient had
experienced soreness, numbness, distention, and heaviness in her lower limbs. Exercising the legs or slapping or
massaging them gave only temporary relief. The pain
would awaken her from sleep at night, and the experience was severe. Restless leg syndrome was accompanied
by heart vexation, a bitter taste in the mouth, and
abdominal distention and fullness. The patient's tongue
was red, and the tongue fur was thin, yellow, and slimy,
while her pulse was bowstring, slippery, and rapid.
Neurological examination was normal. The woman's
fasting blood glucose was 6.9mmol/L and her urine glucose was negative. The disease diagnosis was diabetic
restless leg syndrome, and the Chinese medical pattern
was categorized as damp heat pouring downward.
Therefore, the treatment principles were to clear the
heat and disinhibit dampness, relax the sinews and
quicken the blood in the network vessels, for which *San
Ren Tang Jia Jian* (Three Seeds Decoction with
Additions & Subtractions) was prescribed: Semen
Coicis Lachryma-jobi (*Yi Yi Ren*), Caulis Lonicerae
Japonicae (*Ren Dong Teng*), and Ramulus Mori Albi
(*Sang Zhi*), 30g each, Talcum (*Hua Shi*) and Radix
Cyathulae (*Chuan Niu Xi*), 15g each, and Semen Pruni
Armeniacae (*Xing Ren*), Fructus Amomi Cardamomi
(*Bai Dou Kou*), Folium Lophatheri Gracilis (*Dan Zhu
Ye*), Cortex Magnoliae Officinalis (*Hou Po*), Medulla
Tetrapanacis Papyriferi (*Tong Cao*), Fructus
Chaenomelis Lagenariae (*Mu Gua*), Radix Gentianae
Macrophyllae (*Qin Jiao*), Cortex Phellodendri (*Huang
Bai*), and Pericarpium Citri Reticulatae (*Chen Pi*), 10g
each. One *ji* was decocted in water and administered per
day, and, after 14 days, the symptoms disappeared. On
follow-up after one year, there had been no recurrence of
restless leg syndrome.

REMARKS:

1. The overwhelming majority of Chinese medical

research on diabetic neuropathy is specifically on peripheral neuropathy. This preponderance is reflected in the above research abstracts and case histories.

2. Most peripheral neuropathy is associated with the patterns of qi and yin dual vacuity complicated by blood stasis. According to Dr. Zhang Fa-rong, diabetic peripheral neuropathy can be divided into three stages. In the initial stage, there is yin vacuity with dryness and heat and phlegm and stasis obstructing and stagnating. The primary disease mechanism is lung dryness and stomach heat with damage of yin by this dryness and heat. In the middle stage, yin vacuity, dryness, and heat have consumed the qi and damaged fluids. Therefore, symptoms of qi and yin vacuity are marked. In the late stage, there are symptoms of yin and yang dual vacuity. Generalized symptoms are worse and nerve detriment is heavier. Besides pain and numbness, there is marked lack of strength in the extremities. Chinese medical treatment is most effective in the first and middle stages and is not so good in the later stage.

3. Because the course of this disease is long, after initial results have been achieved by water-based decoctions of bulk-dispensed Chinese medicinals, it is advisable to switch patients to formulas made from desiccated extracts for long-term use.

4. As Bu Xian-chun and Zhou Shen's above study suggests, Chinese medicinal foot baths may be useful adjunctive therapies in the treatment of diabetic PN. When prescribing such medicinal baths, the practitioner should choose Chinese medicinals which mainly quicken the blood and free the flow of the network vessels, emphasizing treatment of the replete tips or branches as opposed to the underlying root vacuities. These underlying root vacuities should be treated with internally administered medicinals.

5. When needling the *Ba Feng* points (M-LE-8) for the treatment of diabetic PN, it is important to needle deeply enough into the interosseous space. To do this, one should use the fingers of the left hand to spread each successive set of toes, thus abducting the metatarsals. Squeamish needling of these extremely important points will not accomplish the desired results. For marked blood stasis and/or damp heat, it is also possible to bleed the *Ba Feng*.

6. One of the key nutrients for the prevention and treatment of diabetic neuropathy is gamma-linoleic acid (GLA). If essential fatty acid (EFA) metabolism is only broken in one place, then GLA supplementation can resolve the prostacyclin/prostaglandin deficiency problem

which some researchers believe is one of the key pathomechanisms of this disorder. However, it takes 8-10 weeks for GLA supplementation to start having an effect.[22] Good sources of GLAs are Evening Primrose oil and fish oil. Other useful supplements for the prevention and treatment of diabetic neuropathy are vitamins A, C, E, and B complex.

7. More than half of all patients with diabetes suffer from constipation. When Western drugs are used for the treatment of this condition, even though definite results are seen, there is often immediate diarrhea or intestinal spasm. Although the immediate cause of diabetic constipation is fluid insufficiency and large intestine dryness, this is typically secondary to a systemic yin vacuity. In addition, most cases of diabetic constipation are complicated by qi vacuity not expelling the stools. To make matters worse, this condition is typically a chronic, enduring one. Therefore, many, if not most cases of diabetic constipation are also complicated by blood stasis. Therefore, the treatment principles for treating diabetic constipation commonly include boosting the qi at the same time as nourishing yin, quickening the blood and dispelling stasis, and regulating the qi and freeing the flow of the bowels. Then the results are good without any negative reaction. Radix Codonopsitis Pilosulae (*Dang Shen*), uncooked Radix Rehmanniae (*Sheng Di*), and Fructus Trichosanthis Kirlowii (*Gua Lou*) all have blood sugar lowering properties and are also commonly useful for diabetes patients when constipation is present.

8. Liu De-hua has created a formula for diabetic peripheral neuropathy called *Si Teng Yi Xian Tang* (Four Vines & One Immortal Decoction). It consists of: Caulis Milletiae Seu Spatholobi (*Ji Xue Teng*), Caulis Trachelospermi Jasminoidis (*Luo Shi Teng*), Caulis Piperis Futokadsurae (*Hai Feng Teng*), Ramulus Uncariae Cum Uncis (*Gou Teng*), and Radix Clematidis Chinensis (*Wei Ling Xian*). This formula is primarily designed to free the flow of the network vessels in the lower extremities. Depending on how it is modified, it may be used to treat a number of the above patterns of PN as well as diabetic impotence. For instance, Liu adds Herba Cistanchis Deserticolae (*Rou Cong Rong*), Herba Epimedii (*Xian Ling Pi*), Herba Cynomorii Songarici (*Suo Yang*), Radix Lateralis Praeparatus Aconiti Carmichaeli (*Fu Zi*), and Cortex Cinnamomi Cassiae (*Rou Gui*) to treat diabetic impotence associated with kidney yang vacuity. He adds Radix Salviae Miltiorrhizae (*Dan Shen*), Radix Angelicae Sinensis (*Dang Gui*), Radix Ligustici Wallichii (*Chuan Xiong*), Semen Pruni Persicae (*Tao Ren*), Flos Carthami Tinctorii (*Hong Hua*), and Radix Cyathulae (*Chuan Niu*

Xi) to treat diabetic impotence associated with blood stasis, and he adds Radix Bupleuri (*Chai Hu*), Fructus Pruni Mume (*Wu Mei*), Flos Albizziae Julibrissinis (*He Huan Hua*), Caulis Polygoni Multiflori (*Ye Jiao Teng*), Tuber Asparagi Cochinensis (*Tian Men Dong*), Tuber Curcumae (*Yu Jin*), and Rhizoma Coptidis Chinensis (*Huang Lian*) to treat diabetic impotence associated with liver depression and fire harassing the heart spirit.

ENDNOTES:

[1] www.uspharmacist.com/NewLook/DisplayArticle.cfm?item_num=145
[2] www.pajournal.com/pajournal/cme/pa0007a.htm
[3] *Ibid.*
[4] www.uspharmacist.com, *op. cit.*
[5] www.niddk.nih.gov/health/diabetes/pubs/neuro/neuro.htm
[6] *Ibid.*
[7] www.pajournal.com, *op. cit.*
[8] Boulton, A.J.M & Malik, R.A., "Diabetic Neuropathy: Prevention and Treatment of Diabetes and Its Complications," *Med. Clin. North Am.*, Jul., 1998, p. 909-929
[9] Krendel, D.A. *et al.*, "Autoimmune Diabetic Neuropathy," *Neurologic Clinics*, Nov., 1997, p. 959-971
[10] www.ninds.nih.gov/health_and_medical/disorders/diabetic_doc.htm
[11] Da Li, "The Treatment of 30 Cases of Diabetic Peripheral Neuropathy with *Bu Yang Huan Wu Tang* (Supplement Yang & Restore Five [Tenths, *i.e.*, Half] Decoction)," *Si Chuan Zhong Yi (Sichuan Chinese Medicine)*, #3, 2000, p. 24
[12] Ding Li-feng, "The Treatment of 43 Cases of Diabetic Peripheral Neuropathy by the Methods of Boosting the Qi, Nourishing Yin, and Transforming Stasis," *Si Chuan Zhong Yi (Sichaun Chinese Medicine)*, #3, 2000, p. 26
[13] Jin Jie *et al.*, "Instructor Zhang Fa-rong's Experiences in the Treatment of Diabetic Peripheral Neuropathy," *Si Chuan Zhong Yi (Sichuan Chinese Medicine)*, #6, 2000, p. 2
[14] Gao Ai-ai, "The Treatment of 52 Cases of Diabetic Peripheral Neuropathy with *Xiao Ke Tong Luo Yin* (Wasting & Thirsting Free the Flow of the Network Vessels Drink)," *Bei Jing Zhong Yi (Beijing Chinese Medicine)*, #3, 2000, p. 19
[15] Liang Kai-fa, "The Treatment of 31 Cases of Diabetic Impotence by the Combined Methods of Boosting the Kidneys, Quickening the Blood & Standing Up the Wilted," *Si Chuan Zhong Yi (Sichuan Chinese Medicine)*, #3, 2001, p. 35
[16] Pang Shu-zhen, "The Treatment of 27 Cases of Diabetic Neurogenic Bladder with *Bu Zhong Yi Qi Tang* (Supplement the Center & Boost the Qi Decoction)," *Si Chuan Zhong Yi (Sichuan Chinese Medicine)*, #3, 2001, p. 42
[17] Chen Ke-ji, *Traditional Chinese Medicine: Clinical Case Studies*, Foreign Languages Press, Beijing, 1994, p. 171-174
[18] Gan Li, "The Treatment of 58 Cases of Diabetic Constipation Using *Jia Wei Si Mo Tang* (Added Flavors Four Milled Ingredients Decoction)," *Zhejiang Zhong Yi Za Zhi (Zhejiang Journal of Traditional Chinese Medicine)*, #6, 1999, p. 384
[19] Huang Yong-yan, "The Treatment of 32 Cases of Type II Diabetic Constipation Based Stasis Heat," *Jiang Su Zhong Yi (Jiangsu Chinese Medicine)*, #11, 1999, p. 18
[20] He Gang, "The Treatment of 36 Cases of Diabetic Restless Leg with *San Ren Tan Jia Jian* (Modified Three Kernels Decoction)," *Jiang Su Zhong Yi (Jiangsu Journal of Chinese Medicine)*, #5, 1999, p. 17
[21] www.geocities.com/bsy53/dn/neuropat.htm

19

DIABETIC ARTERIOSCLEROSIS OBLITERANS & ACROMELIC GANGRENE

Arteriosclerosis refers to a number of pathological conditions in which there is thickening, hardening, and loss of elasticity of the walls of the arteries. Arteriosclerosis obliterans (ASO), also known as peripheral vascular disease (PVD), refers specifically to occlusive arterial disease of the lower limbs. In terms of Western medicine, the cause of arteriosclerosis obliterans is unknown. However, aging, altered lipid metabolism, and other factors, including gender, the environment, psychological, physiological, as well as genetic influences are thought to be contributory to the likelihood of developing this condition. Risk factors include hypertension, increased blood lipids (particularly cholesterol and triglycerides), obesity, cigarette smoking, diabetes, inability to cope with stress, a family history of early-onset atherosclerosis, physical inactivity, and the male sex. (Women may be protected from this disease by estrogen.) Recent research has also shown that diabetic patients with ASO tend to have higher insulin resistance than those without.[1] Arteriosclerosis is a common disorder, usually affecting men over 50 years of age, and those with diabetes are at higher risk.[2]

The manifestations of this condition include effort-related leg pain which is relieved by rest (called intermittent claudication), numbness of the legs or feet when at rest, muscle pains in the legs or feet, loss of hair on the lower extremities, change of color (especially paleness or cyanosis) and coldness of the legs and feet, the presence of open sores or ulcers on the feet and toes (in advanced stages, gangrene), and walking or gait abnormalities.[3] Depending on which arteries are diseased, there may be pain in the hips and thighs.[4] Physical examination may reveal arterial bruits (whooshing sounds heard with the stethoscope held over the artery), decreased or absent pulse, and decreased blood pressure in the affected extremity. A lipid profile may show hyperlipidemia. In addition, angiography of the arteries of the legs, Doppler ultrasound examination of the extremity, rheological studies, and magnetic resonance imaging (MRI) may all be of diagnostic importance.

The Western medical treatment of arteriosclerosis obliterans includes medical management, surgery, balloon angioplasty, and/or laser ablation. Pentoxifylline may be used to help relieve the pain of claudication by facilitating the passage of eythrocytes through sites of obstruction. If there is diabetes, hypertension, and/or high cholesterol, pharmaceuticals for reducing blood sugar, blood pressure, and serum cholesterol are useful. Surgery is usually only performed in severe cases when the ability to work or perform essential activities is affected or there is resting pain.[5] This may consist of surgical removal of the lining of the artery (endarterectomy), repair or replacement of the vessel (grafting), or, most commonly, by pass surgery using a vein or synthetic graft. Balloon angioplasty or laser ablation may be used as alternatives to surgery. However, the effects of balloon angioplasty are not fully satisfactory, and it is best reserved for patients with small segments of blockage since the area quickly becomes restenosed in approximately 30% of all cases, requiring a second intervention within one to two years.[6]

Acromelic gangrene refers to dystrophy of tissue of an extremity due to impaired blood supply secondary to injury and/or disease. Acromelic gangrene is a not uncommon complication of PVD in diabetics due to simultaneous neuropathy and abnormal leukocyte function.[7] Due to neuropathy, the patient may be unaware of painless injuries to the lower extremities, while immunosuppression may lead to easy infection. This, combined with arterial obstruction and reduced blood flow to the extremities results in chronic nonhealing sores which may progress to acromelic gangrene. This syndrome is commonly called diabetic foot. The Western medical treatment of gangrene consists of surgical removal of the necrotic tissue, including possible amputation of the extremity, by pass surgery to improve circulation, hyperbaric oxygen therapy, and/or intravenous antibiotics.[8] Approximately 15% of all patients with diabetes develop a foot or leg ulceration at some time during the course of their disease. Lower extremity amputation (LEA) is a major complication of diabetes and is preceded by foot ulceration in approximately 80% of cases. In 1994, there were 67,000 hospital discharges for nontraumatic LEA at a rate of 8.2 per 1,000 persons with diabetes.[9]

CHINESE MEDICAL DISEASE CATEGORIZATION: Acromelic gangrene corresponds to the Chinese medical disease categories of *tuo ju*, knee-side flat abscess, and *lian chuang*, shank sores.

CHINESE DISEASE MECHANISMS:

There are three groups of disease mechanisms which result in diabetic arteriosclerosis obliterans and acromelic gangrene. These are 1) qi and yin dual damage ultimately evolving into yin and yang dual vacuity, 2) static blood obstructing and stagnating, and 3) damp turbidity pouring downward. As we have already seen above, the basic disease mechanism of diabetes is yin-fluid depletion and consumption due to dryness and heat exuberance. However, most diabetics also suffer from spleen vacuity, dampness, and often phlegm. Therefore, most real-life diabetics present a qi and yin vacuity, and, over time, enduring yin vacuity and qi detriment eventually reaches yang, resulting in a yin and yang dual vacuity. In that case, the qi vacuity is mainly a qi vacuity of the heart, lungs, spleen, and kidneys. The yin vacuity is mainly a liver-kidney yin vacuity, and the yang vacuity is a spleen-kidney yang vacuity. Since the heart rules the blood, if the heart qi becomes vacuous and weak, it may not stir the vessels (*i.e.*, propel) the blood with sufficient vigor. Similarly, since the lungs rule downbearing and depurating, if the lung qi becomes vacuous and weak, it may lack the strength to move qi and fluids downward properly.

In addition, most patients with diabetes also present with varying amounts of liver depression. If the liver is depressed and the qi is stagnant, this will eventually give rise to blood stasis, since the qi moves the blood and, if the qi stops, the blood stops. This tendency to blood stasis is all the more likely if dampness and phlegm obstruct the free flow of qi and blood, remembering that blood and fluids flow together and phlegm is nothing other than congealed

dampness. This tendency is also aggravated by blood vacuity due to spleen vacuity, heart qi vacuity due to spleen vacuity, and vacuity cold due to kidney yang vacuity, remembering that cold's nature is constricting and contracting. If the blood becomes static, then the vessels and network vessels will become impeded and obstructed. Thus various areas lose both the warming and shining and the moistening and nourishing of the qi and blood. Instead, the skin becomes somber white in color, it emits a coolness to the touch, the muscles and flesh become atrophied, and the limbs become aching and painful. If the vessels and network vessels in the lower limbs become completely obstructed, this may lead to acromelic gangrene.

At the same time, if dampness due to a damaged spleen and overeating sweet, fatty, greasy foods leads to dampness pouring downward, these damp evils may depress the yang qi transforming dampness into damp heat which then binds and brews heat toxins. This transformation is all the more likely if the person also overeats acrid, hot, peppery foods, drinks alcohol, suffers not only from liver depression but depressive heat, or from yin vacuity with fire effulgence. Since blood and fluids flow together, damp heat and blood stasis may also become mutually binding, thus aggravating each other. Damp heat pouring downward results in the skin becoming dark red, swollen and distended, aching and painful. If severe, damp heat toxins brew and putrefy the blood and fluids, transforming pus and causing erosive sores. Since the righteous qi is vacuous and weak, it may fail to stop leakage from, and constrain and close, these sores. Thus there arise nonhealing sores on the lower limbs which may also lead to necrosis and gangrene.

TREATMENT BASED ON PATTERN DISCRIMINATION:

1. VESSELS & NETWORK VESSELS COLD CONGELATION PATTERN

MAIN SYMPTOMS: The emission of coolness, numbness, soreness, distention, or aching and pain of the extremities, intermittent lameness, decreased warmth in the skin of the affected limb, normal or somber white colored skin, normal or weak pulses in the large and medium arteries, dry mouth, lack of strength, a pale but dark tongue with white fur, and a deep, bowstring, fine pulse

NOTE: This pattern is mainly seen in patients with early stage diabetic arteriosclerosis obliterans.

TREATMENT PRINCIPLES: Warm the channels and free the flow of the network vessels, boost the qi and quicken the blood

RX: *Ji Huang Si Wu Tang Jia Wei* (Milletia & Astragalus Four Materials Decoction with Added Flavors)

INGREDIENTS: Caulis Milletiae Seu Spatholobi (*Ji Xue Teng*), 30g, Radix Astragali Membranacei (*Huang Qi*), 20g, Radix Rubrus Paeoniae Lactiflorae (*Chi Shao*), 15g, Radix Angelicae Sinensis (*Dang Gui*) and Radix Ligustici Wallichii (*Chuan Xiong*), 12g each, Ramulus Cinnamomi Cassiae (*Gui Zhi*), processed Radix Polygoni Multiflori (*He Shou Wu*), and Radix Achyranthis Bidentatae (*Niu Xi*), 9g each, and Flos Carthami Tinctorii (*Hong Hua*), 6g

FORMULA ANALYSIS: *Gui Zhi, Chuan Xiong,* and *Ji Xue Teng* warm the channels and scatter cold, quicken the blood and free the flow of the network vessels, while *Huang Qi, Dang Gui, Chi Shao, Chuan Xiong,* and *Hong Hua* boost the qi and quicken the blood.

ADDITIONS & SUBTRACTIONS: If chilled skin is pronounced, replace *Gui Zhi* with 6-9 grams of Cortex Cinnamomi Cassiae (*Rou Gui*) and nine grams of Radix Lateralis Praeparatus Aconiti Carmichaeli (*Fu Zi*). If pain is severe, add six grams each of processed Resina Olibani (*Ru Xiang*) and Resina Myrrhae (*Mo Yao*). If there is concomitant dry mouth, add nine grams each of Radix Puerariae (*Ge Gen*), Radix Glehniae Littoralis (*Sha Shen*), and Radix Trichosanthis Kirlowii (*Tian Hua Fen*) to engender fluids and stop thirst.

ACUPUNCTURE & MOXIBUSTION: *Xue Hai* (Sp 10), *Zu San Li* (St 36) plus indirectly moxa along the channels of the affected limb with a moxa pole or roll.

FORMULA ANALYSIS: Draining *Xue Hai* quickens the blood and dispels stasis. Draining *Zu San Li* frees the flow of the qi and blood in the lower limb based on this point's being the master or ruling point of the legs. Indirect moxibustion of the channels warms the channels and scatters cold.

ADDITIONS & SUBTRACTIONS: For aching and pain on the anterior aspect of the lower limb, add draining *Jie Xi* (St 41). For aching and pain on the lateral aspect of the lower limb, add draining *Shen Mai* (Bl 62). For aching and pain on the medial aspect of the lower limb, add draining *Zhao Hai* (Ki 6). For aching and pain on the posterior aspect of the lower limb, add draining *Kun Lun* (Bl 60).

EXTERNAL APPLICATION: Decoct 15 grams each of Herba Tougucao (*Tou Gu Cao*), Herba Lycopodii (*Shen Jin Cao*), Folium Artemisiae Argyii (*Ai Ye*), Radix Angelicae Pubescentis (*Du Huo*), and Ramulus Cinnamomi Cassiae (*Gui Zhi*), nine grams each of dry Rhizoma Zingiberis (*Gan Jiang*) and Flos Carthami Tinctorii (*Hong Hua*), and five grams each of Pericarpium Zanthoxyli Bungeani (*Hua Jiao*) and Radix Lateralis Praeparatus Aconiti Carmichaeli (*Fu Zi*) and use the resulting hot medicinal liquid as a fumigant and wash the affected area two times per day.

2. VESSELS & NETWORK VESSELS BLOOD STASIS PATTERN

MAIN SYMPTOMS: Emission of coolness, numbness, soreness, distention, more heaviness, and continuous pain of the affected limb which is even worse at night, more severe intermittent lameness, purplish or dark purple skin, possible purple-brown macules, thickened, hypertrophic, abnormally shaped, slow growing toenails, scanty, sparse hairs on the affected limb, possible muscle and flesh atrophy, weakened or indistinct pulses in the large and medium arteries, dry mouth, lack of strength, a dark, purple tongue or static macules or spots with moist, white fur, and a deep, fine, choppy pulse

NOTE: This pattern is mostly seen in middle stage diabetic arteriosclerosis obliterans.

TREATMENT PRINCIPLES: Quicken the blood and stop pain, warm the channels and free the flow of the network vessels

RX: *Luo Shi Huang Qi Shui Zhi Tang* (Trachelospermum, Astragalus & Leech Decoction)

INGREDIENTS: Caulis Trachelospermi (*Luo Shi Teng*), 30g, mix-fried Radix Astragali Membranacei (*Huang Qi*), 20g, Radix Pseudostellariae Heterophyllae (*Tai Zi Shen*), Radix Rubrus Paeoniae Lactiflorae (*Chi Shao*), and Radix Ligustici Wallichii (*Chuan Xiong*), 15g each, Radix Angelicae Sinensis (*Dang Gui*), 12g, Hirudo Seu Whitmania (*Shui Zhi*), Flos Carthami Tinctorii (*Hong Hua*), and Ramulus Cinnamomi Cassiae (*Gui Zhi*), 9g each, and processed Resina Myrrhae (*Mo Yao*) and Resina Olibani (*Ru Xiang*), 6g each

FORMULA ANALYSIS: *Mo Yao* and *Ru Xiang* free the flow of the network vessels and stop pain. *Shui Zhi* and *Luo Shi Teng* also free the flow of the network vessels and quicken the blood. *Chi Shao, Hong Hua,* and *Chuan Xiong* quicken the blood and transform stasis, while *Dang Gui* both nourishes and quickens the blood. Mix-fried *Huang Qi* boosts the qi and supports the righteous, while *Gui Zhi* warms the channels and scatters cold.

ADDITIONS & SUBTRACTIONS: If the extremities are severely cold replace *Gui Zhi* with 6-9 grams of Cortex Cinnamomi Cassiae (*Rou Gui*) and nine grams of Radix Lateralis Praeparatus Aconiti Carmichaeli (*Fu Zi*). If the pain is severe, add 9-15 grams of Rhizoma Corydalis Yanhusuo (*Yan Hu Suo*).

ACUPUNCTURE & MOXIBUSTION: Same as above

EXTERNAL APPLICATION: Decoct 15 grams each of Herba Tougucao (*Tou Gu Cao*), Herba Lycopodii (*Shen Jin Cao*), Extremitas Radicis Angelicae Sinensis (*Dang Gui Wei*), Radix Achyranthis Bidentatae (*Niu Xi*), Flos Carthami Tinctorii (*Hong Hua*), Radix Rubrus Paeoniae Lactiflorae (*Chi Shao*), Lignum Sappan (*Su Mu*), Radix Rubiae Cordifoliae (*Qian Cao Gen*) and nine grams each of Ramulus Cinnamomi Cassiae (*Gui Zhi*), Resina Olibani (*Ru Xiang*), and Resina Myrrhae (*Mo Yao*) and use the resulting hot medicinal liquid as a fumigant and wash the affected area two times per day.

3. VESSELS & NETWORK VESSELS STASIS & HEAT PATTERN

MAIN SYMPTOMS: Soreness, distention, numbness, and burning hot pain of the extremities, aggravation of pain by exposure to heat but better by exposure to coolness, worse pain at night, dry, scaly, reddish purple skin, possible fissures and cracking of the skin, thickened, abnormally shaped toenails, scanty, sparse hairs on the affected limb or complete shedding of hair, atrophied muscles and flesh, weak or indistinct pulses in the large and medium arteries of the affected limb, dry mouth, polydipsia, a red tongue with yellow fur, and a deep, fine, rapid pulse

TREATMENT PRINCIPLES: Enrich yin and clear heat, quicken the blood and free the flow of the network vessels

RX: *Tian Ren Di Tang* (Trichosanthes, Lonicera & Rehmannia Decoction)

INGREDIENTS: Caulis Lonicerae Japonicae (*Ren Dong Teng*) and Radix Trichosanthis Kirlowii (*Tian Hua Fen*), 30g each, uncooked Radix Rehmanniae (*Sheng Di*) and Radix Scrophulariae Ningpoensis (*Xuan Shen*), 20g each, Radix Albus Paeoniae Lactiflorae (*Bai Shao*), Radix Rubrus Paeoniae Lactiflorae (*Chi Shao*), and Herba Lycopi

Lucidi (*Ze Lan*), 15g each, Herba Dendrobii (*Shi Hu*), Radix Angelicae Sinensis (*Dang Gui*), and Radix Achyranthis Bidentatae (*Niu Xi*), 12g each, Flos Carthami Tinctorii (*Hong Hua*) and Lumbricus (*Di Long*), 9g each, processed Resina Olibani (*Ru Xiang*) and Resina Myrrhae (*Mo Yao*), 6g each, and Scolopendra Subspinipes (*Wu Gong*), 3 strips

FORMULA ANALYSIS: *Sheng Di, Xuan Shen, Shi Hu, Tian Hua Fen,* and *Ren Dong Teng* enrich yin and clear heat. *Dang Gui, Chi Shao, Hong Hua, Ze Lan,* and *Niu Xi* quicken the blood and transform stasis. *Wu Gong, Di Long, Mo Yao,* and *Ru Xiang* free the flow of the network vessels and stop pain.

ADDITIONS & SUBTRACTIONS: If damp heat is marked, add 24 grams of Rhizoma Atractylodis (*Cang Zhu*) and 12 grams of Cortex Phellodendri (*Huang Bai*). If there is concomitant qi vacuity, add 30-60 grams of Radix Astragali Membranacei (*Huang Qi*), 20-30 grams of Radix Codonopsitis Pilosulae (*Dang Shen*), and 15 grams of Rhizoma Atractylodis Macrocephalae (*Bai Zhu*). If there is severe pain, add 9-15 grams of Rhizoma Corydalis Yanhusuo (*Yan Hu Suo*).

ACUPUNCTURE & MOXIBUSTION: *Xue Hai* (Sp 10), *Zu San Li* (St 36), *San Yin Jiao* (Sp 6)

FORMULA ANALYSIS: Draining *Xue Hai* quickens the blood and dispels stasis. Draining *Zu San Li* frees the flow of the qi and blood in the lower limb based on this point's being the master or ruling point of the legs. Supplementing *San Yin Jiao* enriches yin.

ADDITIONS & SUBTRACTIONS: For aching and pain on the anterior aspect of the lower limb, add draining *Jie Xi* (St 41). For aching and pain on the lateral aspect of the lower limb, add draining *Shen Mai* (Bl 62). For aching and pain on the medial aspect of the lower limb, add draining *Zhao Hai* (Ki 6). For aching and pain on the posterior aspect of the lower limb, add draining *Kun Lun* (Bl 60).

4. VESSELS & NETWORK VESSELS STASIS & TOXINS PATTERN

MAIN SYMPTOMS: Purplish black skin in the affected area, ulcerations with pussy, foul-smelling water, erosion and necrosis and absence of new, healthy growth, aching and pain which is difficult to bear and which is worse at night, gradual enlargement of the necrotic area which may even reach the sinews and bones, possible accompanying emission of heat, oral thirst with a liking for chilled drinks, constipation, weak or absent pulses in the large and medium arteries of the affected limb, a crimson red, fissured tongue with dry or slimy, yellow fur, and a bowstring and fine or slippery, rapid pulse

NOTE: This pattern describes diabetic acromelic gangrene with possible secondary infection.

TREATMENT PRINCIPLES: Clear heat and resolve toxins, quicken the blood and stop pain

RX: *Ren Dong Er Ding Jie Du Tang* (Lonicera & Two Dings Resolve Toxins Decoction)[10]

INGREDIENTS: Caulis Lonicerae Japonicae (*Ren Dong Teng*), Herba Violae Yedoensitis Cum Radice (*Zi Hua Di Ding*), Herba Taraxaci Mongolici Cum Radice (*Pu Gong Ying*), and Semen Phaseoli Calcarati (*Chi Xiao Dou*), 30g each, Radix Scrophulariae Ningpoensis (*Xuan Shen*), 20g, Fructus Forsythiae Suspensae (*Lian Qiao*), Radix Angelicae Sinensis (*Dang Gui*), Radix Achyranthis Bidentatae (*Niu Xi*), and Radix Rubrus Paeoniae Lactiflorae (*Chi Shao*), 15g each, and Flos Carthami Tinctorii (*Hong Hua*) and uncooked Radix Glycyrrhizae (*Gan Cao*), 6g each

FORMULA ANALYSIS: *Ren Dong Teng, Zi Hua Di Ding, Pu Gong Ying,* and *Lian Qiao* clear heat and resolve toxins. *Dang Gui, Hong Hua, Chi Shao,* and *Niu Xi* quicken the blood and transform stasis. *Xuan Shen* enriches yin and clears heat, while *Chi Xiao Dou* clears and disinhibits dampness and heat.

ADDITIONS & SUBTRACTIONS: If there is vexatious thirst and polydipsia, one can add 30 grams each of uncooked Gypsum Fibrosum (*Shi Gao*) and Radix Trichosanthis Kirlowii (*Tian Hua Fen*) and nine grams of Rhizoma Anemarrhenae Aspheloidis (*Zhi Mu*) to clear heat, engender fluids, and stop thirst. If there is constipation, one can add 30 grams of uncooked Radix Rehmanniae (*Sheng Di*), 15 grams of Fructus Trichosanthis Kirlowii (*Gua Lou*), and nine grams of wine-processed Radix Et Rhizoma Rhei (*Da Huang*). If there is profuse secretion and suppuration of pussy water with slimy, yellow tongue fur due to damp heat pouring downward, add 30 grams of Semen Coicis Lachyrma-jobi (*Yi Yi Ren*), 15 grams each of Herba Artemisiae Capillaris (*Yin Chen Hao*) and Radix Et Rhizoma Polygoni Cuspidati (*Hu Zhang*), and nine grams each of Cortex Phellodendri (*Huang Bai*) and Semen Plantaginis (*Che Qian Zi*) to clear heat and disinhibit dampness. If blood stasis is marked, add 30 grams each of Radix Salviae Miltiorrhizae (*Dan Shen*) and Caulis Milletiae Seu Spatholobi (*Ji Xue Teng*) and nine grams each of Rhizoma Sparganii (*San Leng*), Rhizoma Curcumae Zedoariae (*E Zhu*), and Hirudo Seu Whitmania (*Shui Zhi*) to quicken the blood and break stasis.

ACUPUNCTURE & MOXIBUSTION: *Xue Hai* (Sp 10), *Zu San Li* (St 36)

FORMULA ANALYSIS: Draining *Xue Hai* quickens the blood and dispels stasis. Draining *Zu San Li* frees the flow of the qi and blood in the lower limb based on this point's being the master or ruling point of the legs.

ADDITIONS & SUBTRACTIONS: Add four corners needling around the periphery of any sores. Add draining *He Gu* (LI 4) and *Qu Chi* (LI 11) for generalized fever. Add draining *Nei Ting* (St 44) for vexatious thirst. Add draining *Nei Ting, Tian Shu* (St 25), *Zhi Gou* (TB 6), and *Da Chang Shu* (Bl 25) for constipation.

EXTERNAL APPLICATION: Decoct 30 grams each of Caulis Lonicerae Japonicae (*Ren Dong Teng*) and Radix Ilicis Pubescentis (*Mao Dong Qing*), 20 grams each of Radix Sophorae Flavescentis (*Ku Shen*), Radix Stemonae (*Bai Bu*), and Rhizoma Smilacis Glabrae (*Tu Fu Ling*), and 15 grams each of Flos Carthami Tinctorii (*Hong Hua*), Cortex Phellodendri (*Huang Bai*), and Rhizoma Atractylodis (*Cang Zhu*) and use the resulting medicinal liquid as a fumigant and wash once per day.

5. QI & BLOOD DEPLETION & VACUITY PATTERN

MAIN SYMPTOMS: Dry skin in the affected area, atrophied muscles and flesh, nonhealing sores with pale grey or dark red halos, suppuration of thin, watery pus, an emaciated body, lack of strength, a pale tongue with white fur, and a deep, fine, forceless pulse

NOTE: This pattern describes diabetic acromelic gangrene which has endured for many days and consumed and damaged the qi and blood.

TREATMENT PRINCIPLES: Boost the qi and nourish the blood

RX: *Yi Qi Fu Zheng Jie Du Tang* (Boost the Qi, Support the Righteous & Resolve Toxins Decoction)

INGREDIENTS: Radix Astragali Membranacei (*Huang*

Qi), 30g, Radix Pseudostellariae Heterophyllae (*Tai Zi Shen*), Radix Albus Paeoniae Lactiflorae (*Bai Shao*), Radix Dioscoreae Oppositae (*Shan Yao*), and Flos Lonicerae Japonicae (*Jin Yin Hua*), 15g each, cooked Radix Rehmanniae (*Shu Di*), 12g, Radix Angelicae Sinensis (*Dang Gui*), Gelatinum Cornu Cervi (*Lu Jiao Jiao*), Pericarpium Citri Reticulatae (*Chen Pi*), and Rhizoma Atractylodis Macrocephalae (*Bai Zhu*), 9g each, and mix-fried Radix Glycyrrhizae (*Gan Cao*), 6g

FORMULA ANALYSIS: *Huang Qi, Shan Yao, Bai Zhu, Tai Zi Shen*, and mix-fried *Gan Cao* supplement the spleen and boost the qi. *Dan Gui, Bai Shao*, and *Shu Di* supplement and nourish blood and yin. *Lu Jiao Jiao* nourishes the blood and invigorates yang, while *Chen Pi* rectifies the qi and transforms dampness. *Jin Yin Hua* clears heat and resolves toxins.

ADDITIONS & SUBTRACTIONS: If emission of coolness is severe in the affected limb, add nine grams of Ramulus Cinnamomi Cassiae (*Gui Zhi*) and 6-9 grams of Radix Lateralis Praeparatus Aconiti Carmichaeli (*Fu Zi*). If there is concomitant torpid intake, add 15 grams of stir-fried Fructus Germinatus Hordei Vulgaris (*Mai Ya*), nine grams each of Massa Medica Fermentata (*Shen Qu*) and scorched Fructus Crataegi (*Shan Zha*), and 3-6 grams of Fructus Amomi (*Sha Ren*). If toxins are more marked, add 15 grams of Flos Chrysanthemi Indici (*Ye Ju Hua*) and Herba Taraxaci Mongolici Cum Radice (*Pu Gong Ying*). If there is concomitant blood stasis, add 30 grams of Radix Salviae Miltiorrhizae (*Dan Shen*) and nine grams each of Radix Rubrus Paeoniae Lactiflorae (*Chi Shao*) and Cortex Radicis Moutan (*Dan Pi*).

ACUPUNCTURE & MOXIBUSTION: *Zu San Li* (St 36), *San Yin Jiao* (Sp 6), *Pi Shu* (Bl 20)

FORMULA ANALYSIS: Even supplementing-even draining *Zu San Li* and *San Yin Jiao* frees the flow of the qi and blood in the lower limb at the same time as it supplements the spleen and boosts the qi. Supplementing *Pi Shu* banks earth and supports the latter heaven source of qi and blood engenderment and transformation.

ADDITIONS & SUBTRACTIONS: Add four corners needling around the periphery of any sores with electroacupuncture.

EXTERNAL APPLICATION: Decoct 30 grams each of Radix Angelicae Sinensis (*Dang Gui*) and Caulis Milletiae Seu Spatholobi (*Ji Xue Teng*), 15 grams each of Radix Codonopsitis Pilosulae (*Dang Shen*), Radix Astragali

Membranacei (*Huang Qi*), and Herba Leonuri Heterophylli (*Yi Mu Cao*), and nine grams each of Radix Polygoni Multiflori (*He Shou Wu*), Semen Cnidii Monnieri (*She Chuang Zi*), and Radix Glycyrrhizae (*Gan Cao*) and use the resulting warm medicinal liquid as a fumigant and wash the affected area once every other day.

ABSTRACTS OF REPRESENTATIVE CHINESE RESEARCH:

Jiang Xi-lin, "The Treatment of 40 Cases of Diabetic Foot with Integrated Chinese-Western Medicine," *Zhe Jiang Zhong Yi Za Zhi* (*Zhejiang Journal of Chinese Medicine*), #9, 2000, p. 388: There were a total of 40 patients in this study, 15 in-patients and 25 out-patients. Among these, 22 were male and 18 were female. Twenty-seven cases had arteriosclerosis obliterans and 13 cases had acromelic gangrene. The oldest patient was 75 and the youngest was 40 years old, with an average age of 48.5 years.

The treatment method consisted of administering the following powdered Chinese medicinals in gelatin capsules: Hirudo Seu Whitmania (*Shui Zhi*), 50g, Semen Coicis Lachryma-jobi (*Yi Yi Ren*), 30g, Cortex Phellodendri (*Huang Bai*) and Tuber Curcumae (*Yu Jin*), 20g each, Rhizoma Atractylodis (*Cang Zhu*), Radix Angelicae Sinensis (*Dang Gui*), Bulbus Shancigu (*Shan Ci Gu*), and Buthus Martensis (*Quan Xie*), 15g each, and Lumbricus (*Di Long*), Sanguis Draconis (*Xue Jie*), and Squama Manitis Pentadactylis (*Chuan Shan Jia*), 12g each. After being powdered and mixed together, these medicinals were put in #0 gelatin capsules each weighing 0.3g. Ten of these capsules were administered orally each time, three times per day. In terms of Western medicine, this consisted of Agkistrodon antithrombotic enzyme, 0.75 units, and 20mg of a medicine identified only as 654-2 added to 300ml of physiologic saline solution and administered as an IV drip once per day. If there was a secondary infection, 5g of cephalosporin was added to 250ml of physiologic saline solution and also administered by IV drip once per day. In addition, the gangrenous wound was surgically debrided. One month of this protocol equaled one course of treatment. At the same time treatment was also given to control the diabetes.

Of the 40 cases treated this way, 23 were judged cured. This meant that their diabetes was under control, their clinical symptoms had disappeared, they were able to return to work, and, there was no recurrence within one year.

Cheng Xin-lu *et al.*, "The Treatment of 72 Cases of Diabetic Foot with Self-composed *Tang Zu Yin* (Diabetic

Foot Drink)," *Si Chuan Zhong Yi (Sichuan Chinese Medicine)*, #12, 1999, p. 30: In this study there were 72 cases, 30 men and 42 women, all between 38-64 years old and all of whom had ulcers on their feet. The largest of these was 10cm x 8cm and the smallest was 2cm x 3cm. The course of these patients' disease was 3-8 months. All had a history of diabetes, lowered temperature in the skin of their feet, dark red colored skin, swelling and distention, aching and pain, or slowing and dulling of sensation. There was difficulty walking and a weakened pulse in the foot. In the worst cases, there was gangrene.

Treatment consisted of a self-composed formula made from: Radix Astragali Membranacei (*Huang Qi*), 60g, Caulis Lonicerae Japonicae (*Ren Dong Teng*), 50g, Herba Violae Yedoensitis Cum Radice (*Zi Hua Di Ding*), 30g, Radix Dioscoreae Oppositae (*Shan Yao*), 25g, Radix Scrophulariae Ningpoensis (*Xuan Shen*), 20g, Radix Achyranthis Bidentatae (*Niu Xi*), 15g, Radix Angelicae Sinensis (*Dang Gui*), 12g, Rhizoma Atractylodis (*Cang Zhu*), 10g, and Flos Carthami Tinctorii (*Hong Hua*), 3g. One *ji* of these medicinals was decocted in water per day and administered internally, with one half month equalling one course of treatment. If the affected area was relatively more red and swollen, 12 grams each of Fructus Chaenomelis Lagenariae (*Mu Gua*) and Radix Salviae Miltiorrhizae (*Dan Shen*) and nine grams of Squama Manitis Pentadactylis (*Chuan Shan Jia*) were added. If aching and pain were severe, nine grams each of processed Resina Olibani (*Ru Xiang*) and Resina Myrrhae (*Mo Yao*) were added. If qi vacuity was severe, the amount of *Huang Qi* was increased even more. Externally, the affected area was fumigated and washed once every other day with a warm decoction of Radix Glycyrrhizae (*Gan Cao*), 30g, and Folium Artemisiae Argyii (*Ai Ye*), 15g. Then a powder made from 10 grams each of Resina Olibani (*Ru Xiang*) and Resina Myrrhae (*Mo Yao*), six grams of Margarita (*Zhen Zhu*), and one gram each of Secretio Moschi Moschiferi (*She Xiang*) and Succinum (*Hu Po*) was applied to the sore.

Cure was defined as disappearance of the aching and pain and swelling and distention in the affected limb, a return of normal skin color and warmth, and closure of the wound. Improvement meant that the aching and pain basically disappeared, the mouth of the sore shrunk, although the patient could still not stand and walk for a long continuous time. No effect meant that, after one course of treatment, there was basically no improvement. The shortest course of treatment was one month, and the longest was four months. Based on the above criteria, 64 patients were judged cured, five improved, and only

three got no effect. Thus the total amelioration rate was 95.8%.

Zhang Cheng-lu & Tan Jin-ling, "The Integrated Chinese-Western Medical Treatment of 16 Cases of Diabetic Foot," *Hu Nan Zhong Yi Za Zhi (Hunan Journal of Chinese Medicine)*, #1, 2000, p. 28: Sixteen patients were treated in this study, all of whom met the WHO criteria for diabetes and all of whom had ulcers on their feet. There were 12 men and four women in this group who ranged from 46-78 years old. These patients had suffered from diabetes for 4.5-22.5 years, and had had diabetic foot from 8-256 days. The Wagner scale was used to rate these ulcers into stages I-IV. Three cases had stage I ulcers, four cases had stage II, six cases had stage III, and three cases had stage IV ulcers. Ten cases had accompanying retinopathy, six cases had accompanying peripheral neuropathy, six cases had hypertension, and four cases had diabetic nephropathy.

All 16 patients were treated with Western hypoglycemic agents to control their blood sugar, which was stabilized at 8.5mmol/L or less, all were treated with antibiotics, and all were treated locally, surgically, and with topical medications. Chinese medical treatment was predicated on the principles of supplementing the qi and enriching yin, freeing the flow of yang and quickening the blood, for which the following self-composed formula was administered: Radix Astragali Membranacei (*Huang Qi*), 30-60g, Caulis Milletiae Seu Spatholobi (*Ji Xue Teng*), 30g, Rhizoma Atractylodis (*Cang Zhu*), 25g, Radix Scrophulariae Ningpoensis (*Xuan Shen*), Radix Achyranthis Bidentatae (*Niu Xi*), and Radix Clematidis Chinensis (*Wei Ling Xian*), 15g each, Semen Pruni Persicae (*Tao Ren*), Radix Angelicae Sinensis (*Dang Gui*), Radix Albus Paeoniae Lactiflorae (*Bai Shao*), Hirudo Seu Whitmania (*Shui Zhi*), and Radix Et Rhizoma Polygoni Cuspidati (*Hu Zhang*), 12g each, Rhizoma Anemarrhenae Aspheloidis (*Zhi Mu*), 10g, and Ramulus Cinnamomi Cassiae (*Gui Zhi*), 6-12g. If qi vacuity was severe, the amount of *Huang Qi* was doubled. If blood stasis was heavy, 30 grams of Squama Manitis Pentadactylis (*Chuan Shan Jia*) and 20 grams of Fructus Liquidambaris Taiwaniae (*Lu Lu Tong*) were added. If there was hypertension, 30 grams of Spica Prunelae Vulgaris (*Xia Ku Cao*) and 15 grams of Ramulus Uncariae Cum Uncis (*Gou Teng*) were added. If there was coronary heart disease, 30 grams of Radix Salviae Miltiorrhizae (*Dan Shen*) and 12 grams of Fructus Trichosanthis Kirlowii (*Gua Lou*) were added. If there was nephropathy, 20 grams of Herba Leonuri Heterophylli (*Yi Mu Cao*) and 12 grams of Radix Dioscoreae Oppositae (*Shan Yao*) were added. If there was retinal bleeding, 12 grams of Cortex Radicis Moutan (*Dan*

Pi) and 10 grams of Radix Pseudoginseng (*San Qi*) were added. One *ji* of these medicinals were decocted in water per day and administered in two divided doses, with 25 days equaling one course of treatment. In addition, all patients were treated externally with ultraviolet light once every five days.

Cure was defined as disappearance of the ulcers. Improvement meant the ulcers shrank more than 25%. No effect meant that the ulcers shrank less than 25% or the limb had to be amputated. Based on these criteria, all three patients with grade I lesions were cured. Three out of four grade II lesions were cured and one improved. Two grade three lesions were cured, three improved, and one got no effect. Of the three grade IV lesions, one improved and two did not. Thus the total amelioration rate using this protocol was 81.25%.

Wang Fan, "The Treatment of 28 Cases of Diabetic Foot with the Methods of Boosting the Qi & Quickening the Blood Combined with the Use of Agkistrodon Antithrombotic Enzyme," *Zhong Yi Za Zhi* (*Journal of Chinese Medicine*), #3, 2001, p. 170: All 28 patients in this study met the WHO criteria for type 2 diabetes. Among these, there were 17 men and 11 women who had had diabetes for 2-24 years, with an average duration of 8.2 years. Eight had skin ulcers (six on a single foot, two on both feet) which had lasted from 2-15 days and an average course of 5.6 days. Twenty had gangrene. Sixteen had dry gangrene, and four had wet gangrene. The duration of gangrene was from 15-60 days, with an average duration of 32.5 days. All the patients had fasting blood sugar during their hospitalization of 9.87-22.8mmol/L, with an average of 15.08mmol/L. Urine glucose was (++⁻+++), and dorsal pedal pulses were absent.

Treatment consisted of administering 1.0-2.0 units of Agkistrodon antithrombotic enzyme intravenously 2-3 times each week. In addition, patients received 2-3 pills each time, three times each day of *Yi Qi Jiao Nang* (Boost the Qi Gelatin Capsules, whose main ingredient was Radix Astragali Membranacei, *Huang Qi*) and *Huo Xue Jiang Tang Jiao Nang* (Quicken the Blood & Lower Sugar Gelatin Capsules, whose main ingredients were Radix Salviae Miltiorrhizae, *Dan Shen*, and Radix Pseudoginseng, *San Qi*). These were administered orally. If there were skin ulcers, the contents of *Yi Qi Jiao Nang* were mixed with alcohol and applied topically once per day. If diet and oral hypoglycemics were not able to control patients' blood sugar satisfactorily, they received subdermal injections of insulin. One month equaled one course of treatment.

Cure was defined as complete healing of the ulcers or complete remission of gangrene with restoration of the dorsal pedal pulse. Marked effect was defined as shrinkage of ulcers by half or more in size, skin which was purplish black in color gradually returning to normal, and restoration of a weak dorsal pedal pulse. Improvement meant that there was new tissue growth or that purplish black skin turned pale red and that there was an indistinct dorsal pedal pulse. No effect meant that there was no improvement in skin lesions or that they got worse and that there was still no dorsal pedal pulse. Based on these criteria, all eight cases of skin ulcers were cured in 10-30 days, with an average length of treatment of 26.2 days. Of the 20 cases of gangrene, one was cured, seven registered a marked effect, 11 improved, and one got no effect, for a total amelioration rate of 96.43%. After treatment, average fasting blood sugar was 8.31mmol/L and urine sugar was (– - ++).

Liang Shao-yong, "The Treatment of 58 Cases of Lower Limb Chronic Ulcers by the Methods of Boosting the Qi & Dispelling Stasis," *Hu Nan Zhong Yi Za Zhi* (*Hunan Journal of Chinese Medicine*), #3, 2001, p. 28: All 58 patients in this study were seen as out-patients. Among them, there were 36 men and 22 women ranging in age from 12-78 years old. Their course of disease had lasted from five months to two years. All were diagnosed with shank sores due to qi vacuity and blood stasis or spleen with dampness gathering based on criteria found in *Zhong Yi Wai Ke Xue* (*A Study of Chinese Medical External Medicine*).

Patients in this study were treated with a combination of internally administered and externally applied Chinese medicinals. The internally administered medicinals consisted of: Caulis Milletiae Seu Spatholobi (*Ji Xue Teng*), 30g, mix-fried Radix Astragali Membranacei (*Huang Qi*), 20g, Sclerotium Poriae Cocos (*Fu Ling*), 15g, Radix Cyathulae (*Chuan Niu Xi*), Radix Codonopsitis Pilosulae (*Dang Shen*), Rhizoma Atractylodis Macrocephalae (*Bai Zhu*), Radix Cynanchi Baiwei (*Bai Wei*), and Flos Lonicerae Japonicae (*Jin Yin Hua*), 10g each, Caulis Akebiae (*Mu Tong*), 6g, and Radix Glycyrrhizae (*Gan Cao*), 5g. One *ji* was decocted in water per day and administered warm in two daily doses, once in the morning and once in the evening. Ten days equaled one course and 3-6 continuous courses were administered. The external medicinals consisted of: Caulis Milletiae Seu Spatholobi (*Ji Xue Teng*), 50g, Radix Cyathulae (*Chuan Niu Xi*), Alum (*Bai Fan*), Ramulus Cinnamomi Cassiae (*Gui Zhi*), uncooked Radix Et Rhizoma Rhei (*Da Huang*), Fructus Chaenomelis Lagenariae (*Mu Gua*), Radix Angelicae

Pubescentis (*Du Huo*), Galla Rhois (*Wu Bei Zi*), and Herba Violae Yedoensitis Cum Radice (*Zi Hua Di Ding*), 20g each, and Resina Olibani (*Ru Xiang*) and Resina Myrrhae (*Mo Yao*), 10g each. One *ji* of these medicinals were decocted in 1000ml of water per day. When the resulting medicinal liquid cooled to 40EC, it was used to wash the affected area once each morning and evening. The course of treatment was the same as for the internally administered medicinals.

Cure meant that the ulcers completely healed. Improvement meant that the ulcers shrank. No effect meant that there was no shrinkage and possibly even enlargement of the ulcers. Based on these criteria, 35 cases were cured, 18 improved, and five got no effect. Thus the total amelioration rate was 91.38%.

Fan Jian-kai & Wang Yao-ping, "A Survey of the Internal & External Treatment of Diabetic Acromelic Gangrene in 33 Cases," *Zhong Yi Za Zhi (Journal of Chinese Medicine)*, #2, 1999, p. 95-97: All the patients in this study were type 2 diabetics. Among these, 20 were male and 13 were female. The youngest was 59 years old and the oldest was 90. The median age was 67.92 ± 20.16 years. The course of diabetes had lasted from six months to 50 years, with a median duration of 16.02 ± 12.55 years. The acromelic gangrene had lasted from seven days to 20 months, with a median duration of 1.14 ± 1.07 months. Based on criteria from the First Chinese Medical Symposium on Diabetes published in *Zhong Guo Tang Niao Bing Za Zhi (The Chinese Diabetes Journal)*, #2, 1996, p. 126, seven of these 33 cases had dry type gangrene, 15 had wet type gangrene, and 11 had mixed gangrene. All cases of gangrene were on the lower extremities. Twenty-six cases were unilateral and seven were bilateral. According to Wagner's staging of diabetic foot disease (as published in *Shi Yong Tang Niao Bing Za Zhi [A Practical Diabetes Journal]*, #2, 1998, p. 45), eight cases were stage II, 10 were stage III, 13 were stage IV, and two were stage V. In terms of causes of gangrene, six cases had developed gangrene after traumatic injury to the skin of the foot or had developed ulceration leading to gangrene after such injury. In the remaining cases, the cause was not clearly apparent. Twenty-six of these 33 patients also had one or more concomitant conditions. Eight cases had simultaneous hypertension, three cases had heart disease, four cases had hypercholesterolemia, and two had kidney disease. Of these, six had both high blood pressure and heart disease, while three had high blood pressure, heart disease, and kidney disease. All these patients had fasting blood sugar levels in excess of 11.1mmol/L. Two cases had fasting blood sugar levels in excess of 20.0mmol/L. Peripheral white blood cell (WBC) counts were less than 9.9×10^9 /L in 16 cases. Amongst these, 11 cases were on antibiotic therapy. Seventeen cases had WBC counts equal to or greater than 10.0×10^9 /L, the highest of which was 27.0×10^9 /L. Neutrophils were less than 0.70 in 14 cases, 0.71-0.80 in 10 cases, and more than 0.80 in nine cases. In 25 cases, an analysis of pus and fluids revealed the presence of a number of different pathological bacteria, such as *E. coli*, *Pseudomonas arugenosa*, and *Staphylococcus pyogenes aureus*.

Internal treatment with Chinese medicinals was based on each patient's pattern discrimination. If there was acute infection with damp heat evil toxins congesting and exuberant with marked local and systemic symptoms, treatment was in order to clear heat and resolve toxins, harmonize the constructive and disinhibit dampness, cool the blood and stop pain. In that case, the formula used was a modification of *Xi Jiao Di Huang Tang* (Rhinoceros Horn & Rehmannia Decoction), *Bi Xie Shen Shi Tang* (Dioscorea Hypoglauca Seep Dampness Decoction), and *Si Miao Yong An Tang* (Four Wonders Resting Hero Decoction). This consisted of: uncooked Radix Rehmanniae (*Sheng Di*), Radix Rubrus Paeoniae Lactiflorae (*Chi Shao*), Cortex Radicis Moutan (*Dan Pi*), Rhizoma Dioscoreae Hypoglaucae (*Bi Xie*), Cortex Phellodendri (*Huang Bai*), Rhizoma Alismatis (*Ze Xie*), Flos Lonicerae Japonicae (*Jin Yin Hua*), Radix Angelicae Sinensis (*Dang Gui*), Radix Scrophulariae Ningpoensis (*Xuan Shen*), Herba Taraxaci Mongolici Cum Radice (*Pu Gong Ying*), etc. Six grams of *Niu Huang Xing Xiao Wan* (Bezoar Arousing & Dispersing Pills) were swallowed with this decoction in divided doses.

If infection was currently under control, the treatment principles were to boost the qi and nourish the blood, harmonize the constructive and free the flow of the network vessels, out-thrust toxins and remove the rotten (or necrotic). The formula used was a modification of *Gu Bu Tang* (Attend to Stepping Decoction) and *Tuo Li Xiao Du San* (Out-thrust the Interior & Disperse Toxins Powder). This consisted of: Radix Astragali Membranacei (*Huang Qi*), Radix Angelicae Sinensis (*Dang Gui*), Herba Dendrobii (*Shi Hu*), Flos Lonicerae Japonicae (*Jin Yin Hua*), Herba Violae Yedoensitis Cum Radice (*Zi Hua Di Ding*), Herba Taraxaci Mongolici Cum Radice (*Pu Gong Ying*), Caulis Milletiae Seu Spatholobi (*Ji Xue Teng*), Radix Ligustici Wallichii (*Chuan Xiong*), Radix Achyranthis Bidentatae (*Niu Xi*), Spina Gleditschiae Chinensis (*Zao Jiao Ci*), Radix Codonopsitis Pilosulae (*Dang Shen*), Rhizoma Atractylodis Macrocephalae (*Bai Zhu*), etc.

During the sores healing stage, treatment was to supplement the qi and nourish the blood, quicken the blood and free the flow of the network vessels, out-thrust the sore and engender muscle (*i.e.*, new skin). The formula used was a modification of *Tao Hong Si Wu Tang* (Persica & Carthamus Four Materials Decoction) and *Ren Shen Yang Rong Tang* (Ginseng Nourish the Constructive Decoction). This consisted of: cooked Radix Rehmanniae (*Shu Di*), Radix Angelicae Sinensis (*Dang Gui*), Radix Albus Paeoniae Lactiflorae (*Bai Shao*), Radix Ligustici Wallichii (*Chuan Xiong*), Semen Pruni Persicae (*Tao Ren*), Flos Carthami Tinctorii (*Hong Hua*), Radix Codonopositis Pilosulae (*Dang Shen*), Radix Astragali Membranacei (*Huang Qi*), Sclerotium Poriae Cocos (*Fu Ling*), Fructus Corni Officinalis (*Shan Zhu Yu*), Rhizoma Atractylodis Macrocephalae (*Bai Zhu*), Pericarpium Citri Reticulatae (*Chen Pi*), etc. One *ji* of the above Chinese medicinals was decocted in water per day and administered orally in two divided doses.

During the acute infectious period, 3.6g of *Shuang Huang Lian Fen Zhen Ji* (Double Coptis Injectable Formula) were administered with 500ml of physiologic saline solution intravenously two times per day until WBC counts were greater than 10.0 x 10^9 /L, neutrophils were greater than 0.70, or the infection in the local area was noticeably improved. In that case, various appropriate antibiotics were administered by either intramuscular injection or orally. At the same time, patients received any one or combination of a variety of blood sugar lowering Western medications. In order to improve the circulation, patients also received 16ml of *Fu Fang Dan Shen Zhu She Ye* (Compound Salvia Injectable Fluid) intravenously with 500ml of physiologic saline solution per day. Fourteen days of this IV treatment equaled one course of treatment. A seven day rest period was given between courses, and 2-3 courses were administered. Orally, patients were also given *Huo Xue Tong Mai Nong Bao* (Quicken the Blood & Free the Flow of the Vessels Capsules). Furthermore, anemia, heart, brain, or kidney disease were also treated with various medications, such as *Ping He Ye* (Balancing Fluid), *Ji Hua Ye* (Extremity Transforming Fluid), and *Huang Qi Zhu She Ye* (Astragalus Injectible Fluid) given by injection.

During the acute infectious stage, various Chinese medicinals were applied locally to the effected area. These included *Jin Huang Gao* (Golden Yellow Ointment), *Yu Lu Gao* (Jade Dew Ointment), *Jin Huang San* (Golden Yellow Powder) and *Yu Lu San* (Jade Dew Powder) mixed with physiologic salt water. If there was ulceration with seepage of foul-smelling liquid, then a 30% solution of hydrogen peroxide was used to clean the lesion followed by the application of a topical antibiotic. Once the seepage was decreased, then *Hong You Gao* (Red Oil Ointment) was applied externally. If the necrotic tissue turned black, *Jiu Yi Dan* (Nine to One Elixir) or *Ba Er Dan* (Eight to Two Elixir) were applied topically to the face of the sore along with *Hong You Gao* (Red Oil Ointment). When the necrotic tissue was sloughed and the margins of the skin were red, *Sheng Ji Gao* (Engender Muscle Ointment) and *Bai Yu Gao* (White Jade Ointment) were applied externally. If the margins of the lesion were white and edematous, *Yu Gan You Lu Mei Su* (Fish Liver Oil Chloramphenicol, a proprietary formula manufactured by the authors' hospital) was applied externally. All these treatments were applied once per day except at the beginning stage when seepage was relatively severe. In that case, treatment was applied two times per day. If the surface of the lesion was large and deep and the necrotic membranes were, therefore, difficult for the body to slough, surgical debridement was done. Physiologic saline solution, hydrogen peroxide, and antibiotic solutions were used to wash the affected area once, or every other day in some cases—for instance, if the necrotic lesion was relatively deep or during the latter stages when the opening of the sore was small but its base had not yet cleared. During the final healing stage after the lesion's opening has closed, the authors also used fumigation therapy with blood-quickening, network vessel-freeing medicinals.

Cure was defined as the healing of the ulcerous lesions, restoration of the function of movement of the effected extremities, and a normal fasting blood sugar level or stable levels at 7.8mmol/L or lower. A good effect meant that the lesions shrank 1/2 or more in size and fasting blood sugar levels were 11.0mmol/L or less. No effect meant that the lesions did not heal, that the gangrenous limb had to be amputated, or the disease led to the patient's death. All 33 patients were hospitalized during this treatment. The shortest period of hospitalization was 15 days and the longest was 120 days. Seventeen patients were judged cured at the time they were discharged from the hospital and another 13 got a good effect. On follow-up after discharge, 10 of these 13 were judged cured and three did not respond. Three cases got no effect. One of these three cases had their leg amputated above their knee, and the other two died of kidney failure.

Thirty days equaled one course of treatment. Twenty-seven patients or 81.8% were cured within four such courses. Of these, 10 cases were cured in a single course (five stage II, two stage III, and three stage IV). Six cases were cured in two courses of treatment (two stage II, two stage III, and two stage IV). Seven cases were cured in three courses of treatment (one stage II, two stage III, four stage IV). And four cases were cured in four courses of treatment (two stage III, two stage IV). Of those who were cured, the shortest was healed in 15 days and the longest in 120 days, with a median time to cure of 60.71 ± 37.31 days. Protection of the tendons and aponeuroses was essential for the preservation of the extremity and lowering the rate of amputation.

Du Ji-hui & Sun Zhi-sheng, "The Treatment of 30 Cases of Diabetic Acromelic Gangrene with External Application of *Xiao Chuang Ye* (Wound Healing Liquid)," *Shan Dong Zhong Yi Za Zhi (Shandong Journal of Chinese Medicine)*, #2, 2000, p. 88: Of the 30 patients seen in this study, 17 were men and 13 were women. Their ages ranged from 44-72 years old, and the duration of their diabetes was from 7-21 years. There were 14 cases of nephropathy and 19 cases of retinopathy. The duration of the symptoms of gangrene was from 15 days to six months. The size of the wounds was from 1.0cm x 1.2cm to 3cm x 4cm. The severity of the wounds was classified in stages from II through IV. Seventeen cases were stage II, nine cases were stage III, and four cases were stage IV. Even though the patients were taking insulin to regulate the blood sugar, their FBG levels were ≤ 7.0 mmol/L, and the PPBG was ≤ 7.8 mmol/L. Antibiotics were administered based upon the results of the bacterial cultures, and 250ml saline solution with 160mg of piperazine extracted from Radix Ligustici Wallichii (*Chuan Xiong*) was also administered as one course of treatment which would normally clear the wound in part. However, when the *Xiao Chuang Ye* (Wound Healing Liquid) was sprayed over the open wound, the wound healed more quickly and smoothly. The primary ingredients of *Xiao Chuang Ye* were: Radix Smilacis Glabrae (*Tu Fu Ling*), Radix Et Rhizoma Rhei (*Da Huang*), Herba Portulacae Oleraceae (*Ma Chi Xian*), and Flos Carthami Tinctorii (*Hong Hua*). For those patients with stage II wound severity, 12 of them had their wounds heal in 15-20 days, five had their wounds heal in 20-30 days. Of the patients with stage III wound severity, six patients had their wounds heal in 30-40 days, two were healed in 40-60 days, and one patient had no results. Of those patients with stage IV severity, one patient had successful wound healing after six months of treatment, and three patients had no results. The amelioration rate was 86.7%.

Fan Guan-jie *et al.*, "Treatment of Diabetic Gangrene by Stage Differentiation," *The Journal of Chinese Medicine*, UK, #65, 2001, p. 50-51: The authors treated 21 cases of diabetic gangrene according to three stages of infection. During the early stage, the patterns were qi and yin vacu-

ity or yang vacuity, both with concomitant blood stasis. For the former pattern, *Zeng Ye Tang Jia Jian* (Increase Humors Decoction with Additions & Subtractions) was prescribed, consisting of: Radix Astragali Membranacei (*Huang Qi*) and uncooked Radix Rehmanniae (*Sheng Di*), 15g each, Radix Codonopsitis Pilosulae (*Dang Shen*), 12g, and Tuber Ophiopogonis Japonici (*Mai Men Dong*), Cortex Radicis Moutan (*Dan Pi*), Radix Rubrus Paeoniae Lactiflorae (*Chi Shao*), Semen Pruni Persicae (*Tao Ren*), and Radix Albus Paeoniae Lactiflorae (*Bai Shao*), 10g each. For the latter pattern, *Si Ni San Jia Jian* (Four Counterflows Powder with Additions & Subtractions) was prescribed, consisting of: Fructus Chaenomelis Lagenariae (*Mu Gua*), 15g, Radix Salviae Miltiorrhizae (*Dan Shen*), 12g, Radix Rubrus Paeoniae Lactiflorae (*Chi Shao*) and Radix Angelicae Sinensis (*Dang Gui*), 10g each, processed Radix Aconiti Carmichaeli (*Chuan Wu*), 9g, processed Radix Aconiti Kusnezoffii (*Cao Wu*) and Ramulus Cinnamomi Cassiae (*Gui Zhi*), 6g each, and Herba Asari Cum Radice (*Xi Xin*), 2g.

The patterns for the middle stage were qi and blood vacuity with accumulation of dampness, accumulation of toxic heat in the intestines, and damp heat in the liver-gallbladder. For qi and blood vacuity with accumulation of dampness pattern, *Dang Gui Bu Xue Tang Jia Jian* (Dang Gui Supplement the Blood Decoction with Additions & Subtractions) was prescribed which consisted of: Radix Smilacis Glabrae (*Tu Fu Ling*), 30g, Radix Astragali Membranacei (*Huang Qi*) and Bulbus Fritillariae (*Tu Bei Mu*), 20g each, Radix Codonopsitis Pilosulae (*Dang Shen*), Semen Coicis Lachryma-jobi (*Yi Yi Ren*), and Radix Trichosanthis Kirlowii (*Tian Hua Fen*), 15g each, Radix Angelicae Sinensis (*Dang Gui*) and Cortex Phellodendri (*Huang Bai*), 10g each, and Spina Gleditschiae Sinensis (*Zao Jiao Ci*), 6g. For the accumulation of toxic heat in the intestines, the prescription was *Si Miao Yong An Tang Jia Jian* (Four Wonders Resting Hero Decoction with Additions & Subtractions) which was composed of: Flos Lonicerae Japonicae (*Jin Yin Hua*), 30g, Radix Angelicae Dahuricae (*Bai Zhi*), 20g, Herba Taraxaci Mongolici Cum Radice (*Pu Gong Ying*) and Herba Patriniae Heterophylae Cum Radice (*Bai Jiang Cao*), 15g each, Radix Scrophulariae Ningpoensis (*Xuan Shen*), Cortex Phellodendri (*Huang Bai*), Fructus Immaturus Citri Aurantii (*Zhi Shi*), and Radix Anemarrhenae Aspheloidis (*Zhi Mu*), 10g each, and Radix Et Rhizoma Rhei (*Da Huang*), 6g. For the damp heat in the liver-gallbladder pattern, the prescription was *Long Dan Xie Gan Tang Jia Jian* (Gentiana Scabra Drain the Liver Decoction with Additions & Subtractions) which consisted of: Radix Smilacis Glabrae (*Tu Fu Ling*), 20g, Radix Gentianae Scabrae (*Long Dan Cao*), 15g, Radix

Scutellariae Baicalensis (*Huang Qin*), Fructus Gardeniae Jasminoidis (*Shan Zhi Zi*), Fructus Immaturus Citri Aurantii (*Zhi Shi*), and Pulvis Indigonis (*Qing Dai*), 10g each, Rhizoma Alismatis (*Ze Xie*), 8g, and Radix Bupleuri (*Chai Hu*), 6g.

The two patterns governing the late stage were liver-kidney yin vacuity with phlegm obstruction and blood stasis and spleen-kidney yang vacuity with blood stasis. For the liver-kidney yin vacuity with phlegm obstruction and blood stasis, the prescription was *Liu Wei Di Huang Wan Jia Jian* (Six Flavors Rehmannia Pills with Additions & Subtractions): cooked Radix Rehmanniae (*Shu Di*), Radix Dioscoreae Oppositae (*Shan Yao*), and Radix Smilacis Glabrae (*Tu Fu Ling*), 20g each, Bulbus Fritillariae (*Tu Bei Mu*) and Semen Coicis Lachryma-jobi (*Yi Yi Ren*), 15g each, Fructus Corni Officinalis (*Shan Zhu Yu*), 10g, powdered Hirudo Seu Whitmania (*Shui Zhi*), 3g, and Radix Pseudoginseng (*San Qi*), 1g. For the spleen-kidney yang vacuity with blood stasis pattern, the prescription was *You Gui Wan Jia Jian* (Restore the Right [Kidney] Pills with Additions & Subtractions): Semen Cuscutae Chinese (*Ti Si Zi*), Fructus Chaenomelis Lagenariae (*Mu Gua*), and Radix Angelicae Dahuricae (*Bai Zhi*), 15g each, Fructus Lycii Chinensis (*Gou Qi Zi*), Cortex Eucommiae Ulmoidis (*Du Zhong*), and Squama Manitis Pentadactylae (*Chuan Shan Jia*), 12g each, Rhizoma Cibotii Barometsis (*Gou Ji*) and Raidx Dipsaci (*Xu Duan*), 10g each, Radix Lateralis Praeparatus Aconiti Carmichaeli (*Fu Zi*), 6g, and powdered Sanguis Draconis, (*Xue Jie*), 0.5g.

The treatment group of 21 cases were divided into three stages: eight cases in the early stage, nine cases in the middle stage, and four cases in the late stage. These were compared to a control group of 18 cases who received vasodilators and anisodamine during the same period of time. Both groups received antibiotics to control infection, followed dietary restrictions, and took insulin. As far as the cure rate, there was no difference between these two groups. However, in vascular clarity and blood flow, the treatment group showed better results.

Hsu Chou-xin & Chen Ze-lin, "Prevention & Treatment of Diabetic Foot," *The International Journal of Oriental Medicine*, #1, 1995, p. 13-16. The authors report on three separate studies for the treatment of diabetic gangrene. The Hunan Medical University study was conducted based on the treatment principles of boosting the qi and nourishing yin, quickening the blood and freeing the flow of the network vessels. Two formulas were prescribed. The first was composed of: Radix Rubrus Paeoniae Lactiflorae (*Chi Shao*), Radix Angelicae Sinensis (*Dang Gui*), Rhizoma Alismatis (*Ze Xie*), Flos Carthami Tinctorii

(*Hong Hua*), Radix Codonopsitis Pilosulae (*Dang Shen*), Herba Dendrobii (*Shi Hu*), Flos Lonicerae Japonicae (*Jin Yin Hua*), Lignum Sappan (*Su Mu*), Semen Euryales Ferocis (*Qian Shi*), Sclerotium Poriae Cocos (*Fu Ling*), Radix Astragali Membranacei (*Huang Qi*), and Concha Ostreae (*Mu Li*). The second formula was composed of: Radix Angelicae Sinensis (*Dang Gui*), Radix Scrophulariae Ningpoensis (*Xuan Shen*), Flos Lonicerae Japonicae (*Jin Yin Hua*), and Radix Glycyrrhizae (*Gan Cao*). Each formula was decocted in water and two doses were administered per day for five days. The formulas were taken alternately for a course of five weeks. Fourteen of the 16 cases in this study got good results, with the return of blood flow throughout the feet enabling the patients to walk. Two cases got no results.

The second study, conducted at the Beijing Xiehe Hospital, concerned two groups of patients, one group of 12 patients with pain in the legs as the major complaint and a second group of six patients with angiopathy, claudication, and gangrene. Both groups remained on insulin and regulated their diets during the study. The treatment principles for the first group were to boost the qi, nourish yin, and quicken the blood. Their prescription was composed of: Radix Astragali Membranacei (*Huang Qi*), uncooked Radix Rehmanniae (*Sheng Di*), Radix Salviae Miltiorrhizae (*Dan Shen*), Herba Leonuri Heterophylli (*Yi Mu Cao*), Radix Scrophulariae Ningpoensis (*Xuan Shen*), Rhizoma Atractylodis (*Cang Zhu*), Radix Puerariae (*Ge Gen*), Radix Rubrus Paeoniae Lactiflorae (*Chi Shao*), Radix Dioscoreae Oppositae (*Shan Yao*), Radix Angelicae Sinensis (*Dang Gui*), Radix Ligustici Wallichii (*Chuan Xiong*), and Radix Auklandiae Lappae (*Mu Xiang*). The pattern for the second group of six patients was yin and yang vacuity with blood stasis. The treatment principles for this group were to supplement the kidneys and quicken the blood, and the formula was composed of: Radix Astragali Membranacei (*Huang Qi*), Semen Litchi Chinensis (*Li Zhi He*), Semen Cuscutae Chinensis (*Tu Si Zi*), Fructus Ligustri Lucidi (*Nu Zhen Zi*), Flos Lonicerae Japonicae (*Jin Yin Hua*), Radix Albus Paeoniae Lactiflorae (*Bai Shao*), Fructus Lycii Chinensis (*Gou Qi Zi*), Fructus Psoraleae Corylifoliae (*Bu Gu Zhi*), Semen Pruni Persicae (*Tao Ren*), Ramulus Cinnamomi Cassiae (*Gui Zhi*), Hirudo Seu Whitmania (*Shui Zhi*), and Buthus Martensis (*Qian Xie*). The first group with leg pain but no angiopathy had more dramatic results, with increased blood flow to the legs, than did the second group, thus indicating that prevention and early treatment of diabetic foot is most important to insure good results.

The third study conducted at the Ruijin Hospital had 30 patients all together, with 14 cases of gangrene in the toes,

14 cases of gengrene in the toes and metatarsals, and two cases which also had gangrene of the heel and instep of the foot. The instep arterial pulse could be felt in only four of the 30 cases. Twenty-six cases were type 2 diabetics and only four were type 1. All patients received good results with no amputations required. The treatment principles were to boost the qi and nourish yin, clear heat, dispel toxins, and quicken the blood. The formula was composed of: Radix Astragali Membranacei (*Huang Qi*), uncooked Radix Rehmanniae (*Sheng Di*), Radix Scrophulariae Ningpoensis (*Xuan Shen*), Radix Pseudostellariae Heterophyllae (*Tai Zi Shen*), Radix Anemarrhenae Aspheloidis (*Zhi Mu*), Radix Trichosanthis Kirlowii (*Tian Hua Fen*), Radix Rubrus Paeoniae Lactiflorae (*Chi Shao*), Cortex Radicis Moutan (*Dan Pi*), Radix Salviae Miltiorrhizae (*Dan Shen*), Ramulus Lonicerae Japonicae (*Ren Dong Teng*), Stylus Zeae Maydis (*Yu Mi Xu*), Herba Violae Yedoensitis Cum Radice (*Zi Hua Di Ding*), Herba Taraxaci Mongolici Cum Radice (*Pu Gong Ying*), and Radix Achyranthis Bidentatae (*Niu Xi*).

For severe dampness with yellow, peeled tongue fur, Herba Agastachis Seu Pogostemi (*Huo Xiang*), Rhizoma Atractylodis (*Cang Zhu*), Cortex Phellodendri (*Huang Bai*), and Flos Lonicerae Japonicae (*Jin Yin Hua*) were added. If the limb was cold, then Radix Lateralis Praeparatus Aconiti Carmichaeli (*Fu Zi*), Radix Angelicae Sinensis (*Dang Gui*), and Ramulus Cinnamomi Cassiae (*Gui Zhi*) were added. For reddening of the skin, a sensation of heat, and aching limbs, Rhizoma Coptidis Chinensis (*Huang Lian*) and Rhizoma Corydalis Yanhusuo (*Yan Hu Suo*) were added. For constipation and tongue sores, Rhizoma Coptidis Chinensis (*Huang Lian*) and Rhizoma Et Radix Rhei (*Da Huang*) were added. When diarrhea was present, then Radix Codonopsitis Pilosulae (*Dang Shen*), Rhizoma Atractylodis Macrocephalae (*Bai Zhu*), Rhizoma Alismatis (*Ze Xie*), and Sclerotium Poriae Cocos (*Fu Ling*) were added. For impotence, Fructus Corni Officinalis (*Shan Zhu Yu*), Semen Cuscutae Chinensis (*Tu Si Zi*), Herba Epimedii (*Yin Yang Huo*), Rhizoma Curculiginis Orchiodis (*Xian Mao*), and Cornu Cervi Parvum (*Lu Rong*) were added. For those patients with arteriosclerosis, Concha Ostreae (*Mu Li*), Tuber Curcumae (*Yu Jin*), and Spica Prunellae Vulgaris (*Xia Ku Cao*) were added.

REPRESENTATIVE CASE HISTORIES:

CASE 1[11]

The patient was a 58 year old male cadre who was first seen on Mar. 16, 1991. The man had been diagnosed with diabetes three years before and he had had polydipsia and blurred vision for the last two years. For the previous half month, he had had a sore on his left large toe which was diagnosed as diabetic foot. The patient had been treated with several different hypoglycemic agents but without marked effect. When admitted to the hospital, he had polydipsia, polyphagia, blurred vision, aversion to cold, cold feet, dark, purple-colored, mottled skin on his feet, and foot pain. The man was emaciated, having lost 10kg of weight in the previous two years. His tongue was dark red with thin, white fur, and his pulse was fine and choppy. At the time of examination, his blood sugar was 14.5mmol/L and his urine glucose was (+++). The presence of ketones in the patient's urine was positive but no proteinuria was detected. Total serum cholesterol was 8mmol/L, triglyceride was 4mmol/L, and blood pressure was 24/14.7kPa.

Based on these signs and symptoms, the man was diagnosed as suffering from type 2 diabetes complicated by hyperlipidemia and gangrene. His Chinese medical pattern was discriminated as qi vacuity with blood stasis obstructing the network vessels and heat toxins internally exuberant. The treatment principles were to supplement the qi and quicken the blood, warm the channels and free the flow of the network vessels, assisted by clearing heat and resolving toxins. Besides being prescribed 2.5mg of glyburide three times per day, one *ji* of the following Chinese medicinals were decocted in water and administered per day: Radix Astragali Membranacei (*Huang Qi*), Radix Salviae Miltiorrhizae (*Dan Shen*), Caulis Milletiae Seu Spatholobi (*Ji Xue Teng*), Flos Lonicerae Japonicae (*Jin Yin Hua*), and Herba Taraxaci Mongolici Cum Radice (*Pu Gong Ying*), 30g each, Radix Albus Paeoniae Lactiflorae (*Bai Shao*) and Radix Ligustici Wallichii (*Chuan Xiong*), 20g each, Fructus Chaenomelis Lagenariae (*Mu Gua*), Radix Puerariae (*Ge Gen*), and Rhizoma Smilacis Glabrae (*Tu Fu Ling*), 15g each, Ramulus Cinnamomi Cassiae (*Gui Zhi*) and Fructus Liquidambaris Taiwaniae (*Lu Lu Tong*), 12g each, Flos Carthami Tinctorii (*Hong Hua*), 10g, and Radix Glycyrrhizae (*Gan Cao*) 6g. In addition, a tincture made from Hirudo Seu Whitmania (*Shui Zhi*) was applied externally to the affected area 3-4 times per day.

After taking the above medicinals for 20 days with various additions and subtractions, the ulcer was healed. At that point, the application of the *Shui Zhi* tincture was replaced by a fumigation and wash with *Huo Xue Zhi Tong San* (Quicken the Blood & Stop Pain Powder)[12] once per day. Fifty-three days later, the color and temperature of the feet had returned to normal and the pain had disappeared. The patient's blood sugar was 9mmol/L, his urine glucose was

(+-++), and he was discharged from the hospital after being instructed to continue treatment for diabetes.

CASE 2 [13]

The patient was a 50 year old male agricultural worker who was first examined on May 11, 1997 and whose main complaint was a ulcer on his left foot which he had had for four months. This patient had a history of diabetes. On examination, the patient's fourth and fifth toes were black and there was an ulcer on the back of his foot which measured 6cm x 4cm through which one could see the sinews and bones. From this ulcer there was a thick, pussy discharge. The skin around this sore was swollen and its color was slightly red. Accompanying signs and symptoms included lack of strength, decreased food intake, difficulty standing and walking, a pale tongue with white fur, and a fine, weak pulse. Blood sugar was 13.7mmol/L, and urine glucose was (+++).

Based on these signs and symptoms, the man was diagnosed with diabetic foot and his Chinese medical pattern was discriminated as blazing and exuberant heat toxins congesting in and obstructing the channels and network vessels with qi and yin depletion and vacuity. The treatment principles were to clear heat and resolve toxins, free the flow of the network vessels and quicken the blood, and boost the qi and nourish yin. Therefore, he was prescribed the following Chinese medicinals: Tuber Ophiopogonis Japonici (*Mai Men Dong*), Radix Scrophulariae Ningpoensis (*Xuan Shen*), and Fructus Chaenomelis Lagenariae (*Mu Gua*), 15g each and Flos Carthami Tinctorii (*Hong Hua*), 3g. Externally, the affected area was fumigated and washed once every other day with a warm decoction of Radix Glycyrrhizae (*Gan Cao*), 30g, and Folium Artemisiae Argyii (*Ai Ye*), 15g. Then a powder made from 10 grams each of Resina Olibani (*Ru Xiang*) and Resina Myrrhae (*Mo Yao*), six grams of Margarita (*Zhen Zhu*), and one gram each of Secretio Moschi Moschiferi (*She Xiang*) and Succinum (*Hu Po*) was applied to the sore. After three months of this treatment, the accompanying signs and symptoms had disappeared, the skin on the fourth and fifth toes had shed, the surface of the lesion had healed nicely, and the man could stand and move about like he had before the ulcer.

CASE 3 [14]

The patient was a 43 year old male who was first hospitalized on Dec. 18, 1998. This man had had diabetes for a number of years and he had always stuck to his treatment regime. Nevertheless, one month before, he had injured his left hand which had become infected. He was treated with antibiotics and the affected area was also treated topically for one month, but no improvement was seen in the wound. Therefore, he was treated with *Huai Ju Xun Xi Fang* (Gangrene Steaming & Washing Formula): Caulis Milletiae Seu Spatholobi (*Ji Xue Teng*), Herba Taraxaci Mongolici Cum Radice (*Pu Gong Ying*), Herba Violae Yedoensitis Cum Radice (*Zi Hua Di Ding*), and Radix Sophorae Flavescentis (*Ku Shen*), 30g each, Radix Salviae Miltiorrhizae (*Dan Shen*), Radix Angelicae Sinensis (*Dang Gui*), Radix Ligustici Wallichii (*Chuan Xiong*), and Ramulus Cinnamomi Cassiae (*Gui Zhi*), 20g each, Radix Lateralis Praeparatus Aconiti Carmichali (*Fu Zi*), Radix Rubrus Paeoniae Lactiflorae (*Chi Shao*), and Radix Albus Paeoniae Lactiflorae (*Bai Shao*), 15g each, Rhizoma Atractylodis (*Cang Zhu*), 12g, and Rhizoma Coptidis Chinensis (*Huang Lian*), 9g. These were boiled for 10-15 minutes in 1000ml of water. While still hot, the resulting medicinal liquid was used as a fumigant for 20 minutes. After this liquid cooled down to 45°C, it was used as a soak, and this was done two times per day. After one week of this treatment, the redness and swelling around the sore gradually disappeared and the aching and pain decreased. New tissue began to grow, and, after two weeks, the ulcer was completely healed.

CASE 4 [15]

The patient was a 68 year old female who entered the hospital on Dec. 28, 1996. The patient had had a dry mouth and polydipsia for three years. During the preceding 10 days her large and small toes on her left foot had turned black and were aching and painful. For the preceding three days there had been an ulcer on her left foot. Accompanying symptoms included emaciation, lassitude of the spirit, lack of strength, a somber white facial complexion, scanty qi, disinclination to talk, a dark, purplish tongue with white fur, and a deep, fine pulse. The skin temperature of her left foot was decreased, and the ulcer was 1cm x 0.5cm in size. Its borders were somber white and there was no seepage. The surrounding skin was purplish and dark, and the dorsal pedal pulse was absent. Fasting blood sugar was 18.92mmol/L and urine glucose was (++++).

Based on the above signs and symptoms, the patient's Chinese medical diagnoses were wasting and thirsting and sloughing flat abscess. Her Chinese medical pattern was categorized as qi vacuity and blood stagnation with stasis obstruction of the vessels and network vessels. Therefore, the treatment principles were to boost the qi and quicken the blood. The patient was prescribed *Yi Qi Jiao Nong* and *Huo Xue Jiang Tang Jiao Nong*, two capsules of each, three times per day, administered orally. She also received 2.0 units of Agkistrodon antithrombotic enzyme intravenously once each time during the second and fifth weeks of treatment. In addition, the contents of *Yi Qi Jiao Nong* were mixed in alcohol and applied to the surface of the ulcer once each day, and the woman received eight, twelve, and then eight units of insulin injected subdermally morning, noon, and night respectively.

After one week of this course of treatment, the ulcer gradually began to shrink. After two weeks, it had closed and the peripheral skin had returned to normal color. After four weeks, the large and small toes on the left foot had returned to normal, the aching and pain had disappeared, and the skin temperature was normal. The left dorsal pedal pulse was now quite pronounced, and the patient was discharged from the hospital after 50 days. At the time of discharge, her fasting blood sugar was 7.82mmol/L and urine glucose was negative.

REMARKS:

1. According to Wang Fan, qi vacuity and blood stasis are the main disease mechanisms of diabetic foot. However, these mechanisms are often complicated by damp heat transforming toxins. According to Hsu Chou-xin and Chen Ze-lin, Radix Salviae Miltiorrhizae (*Dan Shen*), Herba Leonuri Heterophylli (*Yi Mu Cao*), Radix Rubrus Paeoniae Lactiflorae (*Chi Shao*), Radix Ligustici Wallichii (*Chuan Xiong*), and Radix Angelicae Sinensis (*Dang Gui*) are often used in the treatment of diabetic gangrene due to their ability to lower blood viscosity, inhibit platelet aggregation, and prevent thrombosis. The medicinals which increase blood flow in the peripheral arteries and dilate blood vessels are: Radix Rubrus Paeoniae Lactiflorae (*Chi Shao*), Radix Ligustici Wallichii (*Chuan Xiong*), Radix Angelicae Sinensis (*Dang Gui*), Semen Pruni Persicae (*Tao Ren*), and Hirudo Seu Whitmania (*Shui Zhi*). These particular medicinals from the blood-quickening category are highly beneficial for treating gangrene of the limbs and are also useful in those cases of diabetic complications where there is evidence of blood stasis.

2. It is not uncommon to find a combination of heat toxins and cold due to obstruction and possible yang vacuity causing diabetic foot sores. In that case, one typically must combine acrid and warm medicinals, such as Ramulus Cinnamomi Cassiae (*Gui Zhi*) and even Radix Lateralis Praeparatus Aconiti Carmichaeli (*Fu Zi*) with bitter and cold heat-clearing, toxin-resolving medicinals administered internally and applied externally.

3. Externally, *Tong Luo Gao* (Free the Flow of the Network Vessels Ointment) may be used to alleviate redness and swelling. It is composed of: Styrax Liquidis (*Su He Xiang*), Resina Myrrhae (*Mo Yao*), and Resina Olibani (*Ru Xiang*) in an oil and beeswax base. *Mi Tuo Seng Gao* (Lithargyrum Ointment) may be used externally to expel pus, remove the necrotic, and engender the flesh. It is composed of: Lithargyrm (*Mi Tuo Seng*), Minium (*Qian Dan*), and Borneol (*Bing Pian*) in an oil and beeswax base.

4. Acupuncture can be beneficial for relieving spasm of the blood vessels, decreasing pain, and improving the circulation of blood in the affected area in the case of arteriosclerosis obliterans. However, because of the diabetic patient's lowered immunity and susceptibility to infection, one must take care to use proper clean needle technique. Treatment of diabetic gangrene with acupuncture involves using the channels which run through the body areas infected by gangrene, and the use of local points, *e.g.*, *Tai Bai* (Sp 3) and *Tai Chong* (Liv 3) for lesions at the big toe. *Xue Hai* (Sp 10) is also useful for angitis and *Cheng Shan* (Bl 57) for claudication.

5. Indirect moxibustion with a moxa roll at *Yong Quan* (Ki 1) may be done two times per day for 15-30 minutes each time for cold feet.

6. In terms of self-care, it is essential for patients with diabetic arteriosclerosis obliterans to stop smoking since smoking not only hinders the delivery of oxygen to the tissues of the body but also impairs the development of collateral circulation. Adequate exercise should be balanced with rest. Patients are often instructed to walk or use an exercise bicycle for 30 minutes each time, 2-3 times per day, resting if pain or discomfort occurs. In those with diabetes, foot care is especially important. This means wearing comfortable, properly fitting shoes and socks and protecting the feet from injury or infection. The feet should be inspected carefully at least once per day, and prompt medical attention should be sought for corns, calluses, injuries, or signs of infection.

7. The following nutritional supplements are recommended to help prevent and treat arteriosclerosis: Lecithin, two capsules taken with meals. Garlic tablets, taken as directed on the label. Selenium, 200mg per day. Vitamin A, 25,000 IU per day. Vitamin E, 400-1,000 IU per day (increase slowly). Vitamin C (buffered), 6-10g per day in divided doses. Coenzyme Q10, 100mg per day. Germanium, 200mg per day. Calcium (chelate or asporotate), 1,500mg per day. Magnesium, 750mg per day. Vitamin B complex, 100mg, three times per day. Zinc chelate, 50mg per day, and copper chelate, 3mg per day.[16]

ENDNOTES:

[1] www.diabetes.org/DiabetesCare/1997-11/pg1738.htm
[2] According to Hua Zhuan-jin and Quan Xiao-lin, the incidence of gangrene in all diabetic patients in China is 0.9-1.7%, while for that in diabetic patients 60 years old and over, it is 2.8-14.5%. In addition, they report the male to female ratio of the occurrence of this condition to be 3:1. ("Advances in the Chinese Medical Treatment of Diabetic Foot," *Bei Jing Zhong Yi [Beijing Chinese Medicine]*, #3, 2000, p. 54)
[3] Http://healthcentralsympatico.com/mhc/top/000170.cfm
[4] www.egregore.com/diseases/arteriosclerosis.htm
[5] http://healthcentralsympatico.com, op. cit.
[6] *Ibid.*
[7] www.interna.fk.ui.ac.id/referensi/pengukuhans/summarysarwono.htm
[8] www.podiatrynetwork.com/document_disorders2.cfm?ID=204
[9] Http://apha.confex.com/apha/128am/technprogram/paper_17648.htm
[10] "Two Dings" refer to *Zi Hua Di Ding* and *Pu Gong Ying* which is sometimes called *Huang Hua Di Ding*, "Yellow Flower" *Di Ding*.

[11] Chen Jin-ding, *The Treatment of Diabetes with Traditional Chinese Medicine*, Shandong Science & Technology Press, Jinan, 1994, p. 184-185
[12] There are at least three different formulas with this name in the Chinese medical literature. The one that makes the most sense to us as an external wash is from *Gu Qin Yi Jian* (*The Mirror of Ancient & Modern Medicine*): Radix Angelicae Sinensis (*Dang Gui*), uncooked Radix Rehmanniae (*Sheng Di*), and Cortex Radicis Moutan (*Dan Pi*), 15g each, Resina Myrrhae (*Mo Yao*), Resina Olibani (*Ru Xiang*), Radix Rubrus Paeoniae Lactiflorae (*Chi Shao*), Radix Angelicae Dahuricae (*Bai Zhi*), and Radix Ligustici Wallichii (*Chuan Xiong*), 9g each, and Radix Glycyrrhizae (*Gan Cao*), 4.5g.
[13] Cheng Xin-lu *et al.*, "The Treatment of 72 Cases of Diabetic Foot with Self-composed *Tang Zu Yin* (Diabetic Foot Drink)," *Si Chuan Zhong Yi* (*Sichuan Chinese Medicine*), #12, 1999, p. 30
[14] Li Xiu-juan, "The Treatment of Diabetic Gangrene with *Huai Ju Xun Xi Fang* (Gangrene Steaming & Washing Formula)," *Zhe Jiang Zhong Yi Za Zhi* (*Zhejiang Journal of Chinese Medicine*), #3, 2000, p. 103
[15] Wang Fan, "The Treatment of 28 Cases of Diabetic Foot with the Methods of Boosting the Qi & Quickening the Blood Combined with the Use of Agkistrodon Antithrombotic Enzyme," *Zhong Yi Za Zhi* (*Journal of Chinese Medicine*), #3, 2001, p. 170
[16] www.egregore.com, op.cit.

20

DIABETIC DERMATOLOGICAL COMPLICATIONS

A number of skin disorders are more common in people with diabetes. These skin disorders are typically the result of systemic changes associated with hyperglycemia which cause a combination of neurological, vascular, and immune system deficits. As many as one third of all people with diabetes will have a skin disorder either caused or affected by diabetes at some time in their lives.[1] In fact, such dermatological problems are sometimes the first signs of the disease. Some of these dermatological conditions are ones that anyone can have but that people with diabetes get more easily. Others are specific to diabetes patients. The most common dermatological conditions associated with diabetes mellitus include: diabetic dermopathy, necrobiosis lipoidica diabeticorum, diabetic bullae, diabetic anhidrosis, scleroderma diabeticorum, eruptive xanthomatosis, palpebral xanthelasma, disseminated granuloma annulare, diabetic rubeosis of the cheeks and face, carotenemia, pruritus, and bacterial and fungal infections.

DIABETIC DERMOPATHY (DD)

Diabetic dermopathy, a.k.a. pigemented pretibial macules or "shin spots," is the most common diabetic skin lesion, with an incidence of 30-60% of people with diabetes.[2] In fact, diabetic dermopathy is the most common marker of diabetes.[3] Located on the anterior region of the shanks of the legs, it starts as small, pink patches which later transform into oval or circular, scaly, brown or purple pigmented lesions. These lesions are not painful and do not ulcerate or itch. Some people mistake these lesions for "age spots." Occasionally, such lesions may also affect the thighs and arms. Diabetic dermopathy is caused by microangiopathy. Western medicine offers no specific treatment for this condition since it is considered only of cosmetic importance.[4] However, there is a statistically sig-

nificant correlation between the frequency of DD and an increased frequency of diabetic retinopathy, nephropathy, and neuropathy.[5]

NECROBIOSIS LIPOIDICA DIABETICORUM (NLD)

Necrobiosis lipoidica diabeticorum is another disease that may be caused by vasculopathy. It is differentiated from dermopathy in that the spots are fewer but larger and deeper. NLD usually develops on the pretibial area and begins as a dull red, raised area. After some time, this area comes to resemble a shiny scar with a violet border, and the blood vessels under the skin in the center of the lesion may be easier to see, *i.e.*, they have an atrophic telangiectatic center. NLD is sometimes pruritic and painful, and the lesions may sometimes cavitate and ulcerate. NLD is a rare condition and is most commonly found in adult females. Western medicine also offers no specific treatment for this condition, although steroid injections around the borders of the lesion have been suggested.[6]

DIABETIC BULLAE

Also referred to as bullosis diabeticorum, diabetic bullae refer to the spontaneous development of atraumatic, tense, fluid-filled blisters. These blisters usually occur on the distal extremities, such as the backs of the fingers, hands, toes, and feet, and sometimes on the legs or forearms. These sores look like burn blisters and may be quite large (from 0.5-10cm in diameter). However, they are painless and have no associated erythema. Typically, these lesions heal spontaneously without scarring in approximately three weeks, although secondary infection or scarring may occasionally occur. Bullosis diabeticorum tends to develop in patients with long-standing diabetes or those with multiple diabetic complications. A male-to-female ratio of 2:1 is reported in the literature. The Western etiology of diabetic bullae is unknown. Diabetic bullae often occur in people with diabetic neuropathy or nephropathy. Therefore, some authors have hypothesized an etiologic association involving a local, sub-basement membrane, connective tissue alteration.[7] The only Western medical treatment for these blisters is to optimally manage dysglycemia. However, these blistering lesions may be prevented with proper supportive and well fitting shoes and multilayered athletic socks to reduce friction.

DIABETIC ANHIDROSIS

Diabetic anhidrosis is associated with diabetic autonomic neuropathy. It is caused by a lesion within the cutaneous sympathetic plexus. This type of autonomic neuropathy is uncommon, but, when it is found, it is associated with reduced survivability. In such cases, symptoms are not limited to the skin, but also include orthostatic hypotension, pupillary abnormalities, diabetic diarrhea, and Charcot foot.[8]

SCLERODERMA DIABETICORUM

Scleroderma diabeticorum is due to the peripheral vascular disease (PVD) which is commonly associated with diabetes. Skin changes associated with PVD include atrophy, a waxy appearance, loss of hair, and distal digital cooling. People with this condition develop tight, thick, waxy skin on the backs of the hands with obliteration of the transverse grooves over the knuckles. Sometimes the skin on the toes and forehead also becomes thick. The finger joints become stiff and cannot articulate. More rarely, the knees, ankles, or elbows may also stiffen. Eventually, the atrophied skin will develop small fissures, predisposing the patient to infections. This condition occurs mostly in obese adults and more frequently in women. It is found in approximately 5% of all people with diabetes but in 33% of those with type 1 diabetes.[9] It is an excellent predictor for lower extremity amputations. People with abnormal vascular status (ankle-brachial index [ABI] + 40) have a 56% greater likelihood of amputation compared to those with normal ABI.[10] In Western medicine, optimal glycemic control is the only management available.

ERUPTIVE XANTHOMATOSIS & PALPEBRAL XANTHELASMA

Xanthomas are soft or firm, yellow, pea-like skin tumors composed of cholesterol deposits. Each tumor has a red

halo and may itch. Eruptive xanthomas are those which occur suddenly. All patients with eruptive xanthomas have elevated blood triglyceride levels.[11] This condition is correlated to poor glycemic control. Xanthomas are commonly found on the backs of the hands, feet, arms, legs, and buttocks. This disorder usually occurs in young men with type 1 diabetes. In Western medicine, eruptive xanthomas are treated with dietary fat restriction and hypoglycemic agents. Like diabetic bullae, these tumors usually disappear when diabetic control is restored. Palpebral xanthelasma refer to xanthomas specfically located on the eyelids and are usually bilateral. Their pathophysiology is the same as other xanthomas.

DISSEMINATED GRANULOMA ANNULARE

Granuloma annulare is a harmless rash that forms rings on the surface of the skin. It is usually nonpruritic and subtle. Disseminated granuloma annulare consists of sharply defined, ring-shaped or arc-shaped raised areas on the skin. These lesions occur most often on distal areas, such as the fingers or ears. However, on occasion these lesions may also appear on the trunk. They can be red, red-brown, or skin-colored with a yellow center. This condition is relatively rare in those with diabetes. In very widespread cases, certain orally administered Western medicines may be tried. Although these are often successful, the condition tends to relapse as soon as these medications are discontinued.[12] Photochemotherapy (PUVA) can result in long-lasting remission. Sometimes, granuloma annulare responds to topical cortisone, and cortisone injections may be useful. The natural course of granuloma annulare is to spontaneously disappear after several years.[13]

DIABETIC RUBEOSIS OF THE CHEEKS AND FACE

Diabetic rubeosis of the cheeks refers to reddish flushing of the malar region or habitual erythema of the entire face. This condition mostly occurs in middle-aged and older hypertensive males.

CAROTENEMIA

Benign carotenemia manifests as a yellowing of the palms and soles due to inability to convert b-carotene into vitamin A. Although this condition may occur with overeating foods high in carotene as well as in association with other diseases, carotenemia may also be associated with diabetes mellitus. In addition to yellowing, the skin may be dry and cracked. Its only Western medical treatment is to eliminate sources of carotenoids from the diet[14] and to use emollients.

PRURITUS

Pruritus is a very common skin disorder in those with diabetes and may be caused by any of several etiologies, such as yeast infections, dry skin, chronic renal failure, or poor circulation. Itchy skin is a primary symptom of xerosis or dry skin due to a lack of moisture within the tissue. Dry climates and extended periods of low humidity can exacerbate dry skin, as can dry heat at home or at work during the winter. When poor circulation is the cause of the pruritus, the itchiest areas may be the distal parts of the legs. In Western medicine, pruritus due to xerosis is treated by the external application of emollients containing one or more of the following active ingredients: alpha-hydroxy acids, urea, and salicyclic acid.

BACTERIAL & FUNGAL INFECTIONS

People with diabetes tend to have more frequent infections, both bacterial and fungal, due to a combination of decreased cellular immunity (caused by acute hyperglycemia) and circulatory deficits (caused by chronic hyperglycemia). In addition, such infections tend to be more prolonged and severe than nondiabetes sufferers. Peripheral skin infections and oral and vaginal thrush are the most common of these infections. Often, a mycotic infection may be the initial process, leading to wet interdigital lesions, cracks, fissures, and ulcerations that facilitate secondary bacterial infection.

Among bacterial infections, a common condition is a hordoleum or stye. This is a bacterial infection of the glands of the eyelid. Boils or infections of the hair follicles are also common. Carbuncles are deep infections of the skin and underlying tissue. Bacterial infections can also occur around the nails. In the case of bacterial infection, the infected tissue is usually hot, swollen, red, and painful. Although several different organisms can cause infections in people with diabetes, the most common isolate is *Staphylococcus* bacteria. Systemic and/or topical antibiotics and glucose control is the usual Western medical management of these types of infections.

Fungal infections are also more common in people with diabetes. One recently published study from South Africa concludes that, "fungal infections are two and a half times more prevalent in diabetic patients as compared to a healthy individual."[15] Often the culprit in fungal infections is *Candida albicans*. This yeast-like fungus can create itchy, moist, red lesions surrounded by tiny blisters and scales. Such fungal infections tend to occur in warm, moist folds of the skin or intertriginous areas, such as inframammary, axillary, and inguinal areas, around the nails, between the fingers and toes, in the corners of the mouth, under the foreskin in uncircumcised men, and the labia in females. Common fungal infections in people with diabetes include tinea cruris (jock itch), tinea pedis (athlete's foot), ringworm, and vaginitis. Onchomycosis refers to fungal infection of the nails. According to Richard Pollack, MS, of San Antonio, TX, "diabetic patients with fungal nails are three times more likely to have [other] serious foot problems, such as bacterial infections, foot ulcers, and amputations, compared to diabetic patients who aren't affected by fungal nails."[16] The Western medical treatment of fungal infections in patients with diabetes consists of systemic and topical antifungal agents as well as glucose control.

CHINESE DISEASE MECHANISMS:

In China, doctors knew early on that the disease of wasting and thirsting was commonly associated with certain dermatological disorders. For instance, in the Sui dynasty (589-618 CE), Chao Yuan-fang wrote, in his *Zhu Bing Yuan Hou Lun* (*Treatise on the Origin & Symptoms of Various Diseases*) in a chapter titled, "Symptoms of Emission of Sores Secondary to Thirst":

> [If] one with thirst is benefitted and even recovers, heat may [still] harass the tips and ends [of the body], emitting in the skin. The skin first has wind damp. [Then] dampness and heat mutually contend, thus giving rise to sores.

Wang Xue, in a contemporary article titled, "Diabetic Skin Disease Treated by Traditional Chinese Medicine & Relevant Health Care," published on the Internet almost 1,500 years latter, echoes these same beliefs: "According to Chinese medical lore, the treatment of diabetic cutaneous pruritus starts mainly with deficiency, wind, and humid-heat."[17] If one understands the ramifications of the basic diabetic pattern of qi and yin vacuity with both dampness and internal heat, then it is not hard to understand the various disease mechanisms which may result in the dermatological conditions discussed above. As previously explained, qi vacuity means spleen qi vacuity. If the spleen is too vacuous and weak to move and transform body fluids, these may collect and accumulate, transforming into damp evils. These damp evils may spill over into the space between the skin and muscles. For instance, diabetic carotenemia and xanthomatosis is a sign of overflowing dampness due to the spleen's inability to govern fluids, since the spleen, dampness, and the color yellow all correspond to the earth phase. When these damp evils hinder and obstruct the flow of yang qi in the local area, this yang qi may become depressed and transform into heat. If this heat becomes mutually bound with those damp evils, damp heat is engendered. If damp heat steams and brews, it may give rise to sores, ulcers, and putrefaction of the skin. If spleen vacuity fails to engender sufficient blood to nourish and moisten the skin, the skin will become dry and scaly. If blood fails to mother the qi, the qi will counterflow upward and outward, moving frenetically in the skin, manifesting as internally engendered wind and subjectively experienced as itching. If blood vacuity evolves into yin vacuity, dryness, scaling, and itching due to stirring of wind will be even worse. If, due to a combination of dampness, blood vacuity, and emotional stress, liver depression endures and becomes aggravated, it may transform into depressive heat. Since the liver stores the blood, depressive heat in the liver is easily transferred to the blood aspect. When depressive heat is transferred to the blood, it makes the blood move frenetically as well as damages and consumes it. All skin lesions which are red in color involve some sort of evil heat. If dampness, qi stagnation, and blood vacuity endure, eventually this must cause blood stasis in the network vessels. Such blood stasis can be yet another cause of malnourishment of the skin and hair. It may also cause increased pigmentation of brown or purple color, telangiectasis, and/or localized lack of warmth and sensitivity. Further, enduring dampness may congeal into phlegm nodules, especially when dampness is stewed by heat. When qi and yin disease finally reaches yang, yang vacuity failing to warm and move the channels and vessels adds yet another disease mechanism for blood stasis and untransformed fluids.

TREATMENT BASED ON PATTERN DISCRIMINATION:

DIABETIC DERMOPATHY

QI & BLOOD LOSS OF HARMONY PATTERN

MAIN SYMPTOMS: Lower ventrolateral brownish macules whose surfaces are bright and shiny, possible formication, scarring after slight injury, possible spontaneous remission

TREATMENT PRINCIPLES: Quicken the blood and free the flow of the network vessels, boost the qi and engender the flesh

Rx: *Bu Yang Huan Wu Tang Jia Jian* (Supplement Yang &

Restore Five [Tenths] Decoction with Additions & Subtractions)

INGREDIENTS: Radix Astragali Membranacei (*Huang Qi*), 30g, Caulis Milletiae Seu Spatholobi (*Ji Xue Teng*), 15g, and Radix Angelicae Sinensis (*Dang Gui*), Radix Ligustici Wallichii (*Chuan Xiong*), Radix Rubrus Paeoniae Lactiflorae (*Chi Shao*), Semen Pruni Persicae (*Tao Ren*), Flos Carthami Tinctorii (*Hong Hua*), Lumbricus (*Di Long*), and Ramulus Cinnamomi Cassiae (*Gui Zhi*), 9g each

FORMULA ANALYSIS: *Dang Gui, Chuan Xiong, Chi Shao, Tao Ren,* and *Hong Hua* quicken the blood and transform stasis. *Di Long, Ji Xue Tang,* and *Gui Zhi* free the flow of the network vessels. *Huang Qi* boosts the qi and engenders the flesh as well as promotes the movement of blood circulation.

EXTERNAL APPLICATION:[18] Soak 20 grams of Flos Carthami Tinctorii (*Hong Hua*) in 100ml of alcohol for half a month. Then strain out the dregs and reserve the medicinal liquid for use. Use this medicinal liquid to massage the affected area two times per day.

NECROBIOSIS LIPOIDICA DIABETICORUM

QI & BLOOD STASIS & STAGNATION PATTERN

MAIN SYMPTOMS: Pretibial sclerotic macules and lumps which are either yellowish brown or dark red in color and may be accompanied by a dry mouth, polydipsia, numbness in the extremities, lack of strength, frequent, numerous urination, a dark red tongue with white fur, and a deep pulse

TREATMENT PRINCIPLES: Quicken the blood and transform stasis while simultaneously boosting the qi and yin

Rx: *Gui Zhi Fu Ling Wan Jia Wei* (Cinnamon Twig & Poria Pills with Added Flavors)

INGREDIENTS: Radix Salviae Miltiorrhizae (*Dan Shen*), 30g, Caulis Milletiae Seu Spatholobi (*Ji Xue Teng*) and Radix Scrophulariae Ningpoensis (*Xuan Shen*), 15g each, and Ramulus Cinnamomi Cassiae (*Gui Zhi*), Sclerotium Poriae Cocos (*Fu Ling*), Radix Angelicae Sinensis (*Dang Gui*), Radix Rubrus Paeoniae Lactiflorae (*Chi Shao*), Cortex Radicis Moutan (*Dan Pi*), Semen Pruni Persicae (*Tao Ren*), Rhizoma Curcumae Zedoariae (*E Zhu*), and Rhizoma Polygonati (*Huang Jing*), 9g each

FORMULA ANALYSIS: *Gui Zhi* and *Ji Xue Teng* free the

flow of the network vessels and quicken the blood. *Dan Shen* and *Dang Gui* together with *Chi Shao* and *Dan Pi* quicken the blood and transform stasis at the same time as scattering stasis and heat within the blood. *Tao Ren* and *E Zhu* break the blood and soften the hard. *Fu Ling* seeps and disinhibits dampness and moves it downwards, while *Huang Jing* and *Xuan Shen* boost the qi and yin.

ADDITIONS & SUBTRACTIONS: If ulcers have erupted, in order to promote the closing of sores and engenderment of flesh, add 30 grams of uncooked Radix Astragali Membranacei (*Huang Qi*) and nine grams each of processed Resina Olibani (*Ru Xiang*) and Resina Myrrhae (*Mo Yao*).

EXTERNAL APPLICATION: Apply *Sheng Ji Yu Hong Gao* (Engender Flesh Jade Red Ointment)[19] to the affected area one time per day and afterward treat with a TDP lamp for 15 minutes each day.

DIABETIC BULLAE

SPLEEN VACUITY & DAMPNESS BREWING PATTERN

MAIN SYMPTOMS: The spontaneous emission of large water blisters filled with clear liquid and without a red halo accompanied by emaciation, lack of strength, abdominal distention after meals, loose stools, numbness of the extremities, superficial edema, a pale tongue with white, possibly slimy fur, and a soggy, moderate, *i.e.*, relaxed or slightly slow pulse

TREATMENT PRINCIPLES: Fortify the spleen and eliminate dampness

RX: *Chu Shi Wei Ling Tang Jia Jian* (Eliminate Dampness Stomach Poria Decoction with Additions & Subtractions)

INGREDIENTS: Uncooked Radix Astragali Membranacei (*Huang Qi*), Semen Coicis Lachyrma-jobi (*Yi Yi Ren*), Rhizoma Alismatis (*Ze Xie*), Ramulus Cinnamomi Cassiae (*Gui Zhi*), and Caulis Milletiae Seu Spatholobi (*Ji Xue Teng*), 15g each, and Rhizoma Atractylodis Macrocephalae (*Bai Zhu*), Rhizoma Atractylodis (*Cang Zhu*), Sclerotium Poriae Cocos (*Fu Ling*), Talcum (*Hua Shi*), and Cortex Magnoliae Officinalis (*Hou Po*), 9g each

FORMULA ANALYSIS: *Bai Zhu* and uncooked *Huang Qi* fortify the spleen and boost the qi. *Fu Ling, Ze Xie, Hua Shi,* and *Yi Yi Ren* blandly seep and disinhibit dampness. *Cang Zhu* and *Hou Po* dry dampness. *Gui Zhi* and *Ji Xue Teng* quicken the blood and free the flow of the network vessels.

ADDITIONS & SUBTRACTIONS: If there is simultaneous yin vacuity with marked emaciation, a dry mouth, and polydipsia and the fluid within the blisters is thick and scanty in amount, remove *Hou Po, Hua Shi,* and *Yi Yi Ren* and add nine grams each of Radix Glehniae Littoralis (*Sha Shen*), Tuber Ophiopogonis Japonici (*Mai Men Dong*), and Herba Dendrobii (*Shi Hu*).

After the water blisters recede, one may administer *Shen Ling Bai Zhu San* (Ginseng, Poria & Atractylodes Powder) to prevent their recurrence: Semen Coicis Lachyrma-jobi (*Yi Yi Ren*), 20g, Semen Nelumbinis Nuciferae (*Lian Zi*), Radix Dioscoreae Oppositae (*Shan Yao*), and Semen Dolichoris Lablab (*Bai Bian Dou*), 15g each, Rhizoma Atractylodis Macrocephalae (*Bai Zhu*), Sclerotium Poriae Cocos (*Fu Ling*), and Radix Panacis Ginseng (*Ren Shen*), 9g each, Radix Platycodi Grandiflori (*Jie Geng*), 6g, Fructus Amomi (*Sha Ren*), 4.5g, and mix-fried Radix Glycyrrhizae (*Gan Cao*), 3-6g.

EXTERNAL APPLICATION: Disinfect the blister and pop with a sterile needle, discharging the fluid within the blister. Then apply a mixture of *Qing Dai San* (Indigo Powder) and water externally to the affected area. *Qing Dai San* consists of two parts each of powdered Gypsum Fibrosum (*Shi Gao*) and Talcum (*Hua Shi*) to one part each of Indigo Naturalis (*Qing Dai*) and Cortex Phellodendri (*Huang Bai*).

DIABETIC SWEATING ABNORMALITIES

1. YIN VACUITY & FLUID DEPLETION PATTERN

MAIN SYMPTOMS: Anhidrosis or possible scanty sweating, dry skin, burning heat in the skin, a dry mouth and parched throat, heat in the hearts of the hands and feet, a red tongue with scanty fur, and a fine, rapid pulse

TREATMENT PRINCIPLES: Enrich yin and engender fluids, regulate and harmonize the constructive and defensive

RX: *Zeng Ye Tang* (Increase Fluids Decoction) plus *Gui Zhi Tang* (Cinnamon Twig Decoction) with added flavors

INGREDIENTS: Uncooked Radix Rehmanniae (*Sheng Di*), 30g, Radix Scrophulariae Ningpoensis (*Xuan Shen*) and Tuber Ophiopogonis Japonici (*Mai Men Dong*), 15g each, Radix Albus Paeoniae Lactiflorae (*Bai Shao*), 12g, Fructus Lycii Chinensis (*Gou Qi Zi*), Rhizoma Polygoni Odorati (*Yu Zhu*), Cortex Radicis Moutan (*Dan Pi*), and Cortex Radicis Lycii Chinensis (*Di Gu Pi*), 9g each, Ramulus Cinnamomi Cassiae (*Gui Zhi*) and mix-fried Radix Glycyrrhizae (*Gan Cao*), 6g each, Fructus Zizyphi

Jujubae (*Da Zao*), 6 pieces, and uncooked Rhizoma Zingiberis (*Sheng Jiang*), 3 slices

FORMULA ANALYSIS: *Xuan Shen, Mai Men Dong, Sheng Di, Yu Zhu,* and *Gou Qi Zi* enrich yin and engender fluids. *Dan Pi* and *Di Gu Pi* abate vacuity heat. *Gui Zhi, Bai Shao, Sheng Jiang, Gan Cao,* and *Da Zao* harmonize the constructive and defensive. When yin fluids are full and sufficient and the constructive and defensive are regulated and harmonious, then perspiration is emitted normally.

ADDITIONS & SUBTRACTIONS: If there is shortness of breath, lack of strength, and numbness of the extremities due to qi and yin dual vacuity as well as blood stasis, add 30 grams of Radix Salviae Miltiorrhizae (*Dan Shen*) and 15 grams of Radix Pseudostellariae Heterophyllae (*Tai Zi Shen*).

2. STOMACH HEAT & QI VACUITY PATTERN

MAIN SYMPTOMS: Sweating caused by eating, stirring resulting in profuse perspiration, oral thirst, polyphagia, shortness of breath, lack of strength, dry, yellow tongue fur, and a large, forceless pulse

TREATMENT PRINCIPLES: Clear and discharge stomach heat, boost the qi and engender fluids

RX: *Bai Hu Jia Ren Shen Tang Jia Jian* (White Tiger Plus Ginseng Decoction with Additions & Subtractions)

INGREDIENTS: Uncooked Gypsum Fibrosum (*Shi Gao*), decocted first, Radix Pseudostellariae Heterophyllae (*Tai Zi Shen*) and Radix Trichosanthis Kirlowii (*Tian Hua Fen*), 30g each, Radix Glehniae Littoralis (*Sha Shen*) and uncooked Radix Rehmanniae (*Sheng Di*), 15g each, Rhizoma Anemarrhenae Aspheloidis (*Zhi Mu*) and Fructus Schisandrae Chinensis (*Wu Wei Zi*), 9g each, and Radix Glycyrrhizae (*Gan Cao*), 6g

FORMULA ANALYSIS: *Shi Gao, Zhi Mu,* and *Gan Cao* clear and discharge yang ming stomach heat. *Tai Zi Shen, Sha Shen,* and *Wu Wei Zi* boost the qi, engender fluids, and constrain the sweat. *Sheng Di* and *Tian Hua Fen* nourish yin and engender fluids.

ADDITIONS & SUBTRACTIONS: If qi vacuity is pronounced, add 2-3 grams of Radix Panacis Quinquefolii (*Xi Yang Shen*).

EXTERNAL APPLICATION: If there is dry skin and anhidrosis, apply *Gan Cao You* (Licorice Oil). This is made by soaking 50g of Radix Glycyrrhizae (*Gan Cao*) in

two liters of sesame oil. Then cook the oil until the *Gan Cao* turns brown and the oil has a fragrant aroma. Remove the dregs and reserve the medicinal oil for use.

If there is profuse perspiration, grind a suitable amount of Galla Rhois Chinensis (*Wu Bei Zi*) into fine powder. Mix with water into a thick paste, apply to the navel before bed at night, and hold this paste in place with an adhesive plaster. The next morning remove this plaster and paste.

SCLERODERMA DIABETICORUM

1. WIND DAMP IMPEDIMENT & OBSTRUCTION PATTERN

MAIN SYMPTOMS: Thickening and hardening of the skin on the neck, shoulders, and upper back, with swelling and distention, no pitting on pressure, joint aching and pain, bodily fatigue, a pale red tongue with white fur, and a deep pulse

TREATMENT PRINCIPLES: Dispel wind and eliminate dampness, quicken the blood and free the flow of the network vessels

RX: *Qiang Huo Chu Shi Tang* (Notopterygium Eliminate Dampness Decoction) plus *Huang Qi Gui Zhi Wu Wu Tang* (Astragalus & Cinnamon Twig Five Materials Decoction) with additions and subtractions

INGREDIENTS: Radix Et Rhizoma Notopterygii (*Qiang Huo*), Radix Angelicae Pubescentis (*Du Huo*), Radix Et Rhizoma Ligusticum Chinensis (*Gao Ben*), Radix Ledebouriellae Divaricatae (*Fang Feng*), Radix Ligustici Wallichii (*Chuan Xiong*), Fructus Viticis (*Man Jing Zi*), Radix Astragali Membranacei (*Huang Qi*), Ramulus Cinnamomi Cassiae (*Gui Zhi*), Radix Albus Paeoniae Lactiflorae (*Bai Shao*), and Radix Rubrus Paeoniae Lactiflorae (*Chi Shao*), 9g each

FORMULA ANALYSIS: *Qiang Huo* and *Du Huo* scatter wind damp evils from all around the body as well as soothe and disinhibit the joints. *Fang Feng, Gao Ben,* and *Man Jing Zi* scatter wind dampness from the fleshy exterior and upper part of the body. *Huang Qi* boosts the qi and secures the defensive. *Gui Zhi* warms the channels and frees the flow of the network vessels. *Chuan Xiong, Chi Shao,* and *Bai Shao* quicken the blood and harmonize the constructive. It is good if one sweats slightly after taking this formula. A slight amount of sweating opens the interstices and allows wind dampness to be scattered externally.

Then the constructive and defensive and the qi and blood can flow smoothly and easily.

2. YANG VACUITY & COLD CONGELATION PATTERN

MAIN SYMPTOMS: An enduring disease course, sclerotic, hard, swollen skin but no change in skin color, inhibited movement of the extremities, fear of cold, low back chill, a bland affect, a pale tongue with white fur, and a deep pulse

TREATMENT PRINCIPLES: Warm yang and scatter cold, free the flow of the network vessels and disperse swelling

RX: *Yang He Tang Jia Jian* (Yang-harmonizing Decoction with Additions & Subtractions)

INGREDIENTS: Radix Salviae Miltiorrhizae (*Dan Shen*), 15g, cooked Radix Rehmanniae (*Shu Di*) and Radix Angelicae Sinensis (*Dang Gui*), 12g each, Radix Lateralis Praeparatus Aconiti Carmichaeli (*Fu Zi*), Gelatinum Cornu Cervi (*Lu Jiao Jiao*), Ramulus Cinnamomi Cassiae (*Gui Zhi*), Herba Lycopi Lucidi (*Ze Lan*), Rhizoma Curculiginis Orchioidis (*Xian Mao*), Radix Stephaniae Tetrandrae (*Han Fang Ji*), and Radix Clematidis Chinensis (*Wei Ling Xian*), 9g each, and mix-fried Herba Ephedrae (*Ma Huang*), 6g

FORMULA ANALYSIS: *Shu Di, Lu Jiao Jiao, Gui Zhi, Ma Huang, Fu Zi,* and *Xian Mao* warm the kidneys, invigorate yang, and scatter cold. *Dang Gui, Dan Shen, Ze Lan, Han Fang Ji,* and *Wei Ling Xian* quicken the blood and free the flow of the network vessels, disinhibit dampness and disperse swelling.

ADDITIONS & SUBTRACTIONS: If there is concomitant spleen vacuity with lack of strength, torpid intake, abdominal distention, and loose stools, add nine grams each of Radix Codonopsitis Pilosulae (*Dang Shen*) and Rhizoma Atractylodis Macrocephalae (*Bai Zhu*). If there is marked low back soreness and pain, add nine grams each of Cortex Eucommiae Ulmoidis (*Du Zhong*) and Rhizoma Cibotii Barometis (*Gou Ji*).

EXTERNAL APPLICATION (for both the above patterns): Decoct the following medicinals in water and then soak the affected area for 20 minutes each time two times per day: Herba Lycopodii (*Shen Jin Cao*), Folium Artemisiae Argyii (*Ai Ye*), and Ramulus Mori Albi (*Sang Zhi*), 30g each, Herba Tougucao (*Tou Gu Cao*), Radix Angelicae Anomalae (*Liu Ji Nu*), Cortex Cinnamomi Cassiae (*Rou Gui*), and Squama Manitis Pentadactylis (*Chuan Shan Jia*), 15g each, and Lignum Sappan (*Su Mu*) and Flos Carthami Tinctorii (*Hong Hua*), 9g each.

ERUPTIVE XANTHOMATOSIS & PALPEBRAL XANTHELASMA

PHLEGM & DAMPNESS BREWING & BINDING PATTERN

MAIN SYMPTOMS: Yellow-colored papular lesions and small nodulations on the skin accompanied by lack of strength, dizziness, chest oppression, shortness of breath, nausea, abdominal distention, a fat tongue with teeth-marks on its edges and white, slightly slimy fur, and a bow-string pulse

TREATMENT PRINCIPLES: Fortify the spleen and eliminate dampness, transform phlegm and scatter nodulations

RX: *Wu Ling San* (Five [Ingredients] Poria Powder) plus *San Zi Yang Yang Qin Tang* (Three Seeds Nourish [One's] Parents Decoction) with added flavors

INGREDIENTS: Radix Salviae Miltiorrhizae (*Dan Shen*), 20g, Sclerotium Poriae Cocos (*Fu Ling*), Rhizoma Alismatis (*Ze Xie*), and uncooked Fructus Crataegi (*Shan Zha*), 15g each, Sclerotium Polypori Umbellati (*Zhu Ling*), Rhizoma Atractylodis Macrocephalae (*Bai Zhu*), Fructus Perillae Frutescentis (*Zi Su Zi*), and stir-fried Semen Raphani Sativi (*Lai Fu Zi*), 9g each, and Ramulus Cinnamomi Cassiae (*Gui Zhi*) and Semen Sinapis Albae (*Bai Jie Zi*), 6g each

FORMULA ANALYSIS: *Fu Ling, Zhu Ling, Ze Xie, Gui Zhi,* and *Bai Zhu* fortify the spleen and disinhibit dampness. *Bai Jie Zi, Zi Su Zi,* and *Lai Fu Zi* transform phlegm, disperse stagnation, and downbear counterflow. Uncooked *Shan Zha* and *Dan Shen* disperse food, scatter stasis, and lower fat.

ADDITIONS & SUBTRACTIONS: If the body is emaciated, there is polydipsia and polyuria, and the patient's pattern is categorized as qi and yin dual vacuity, remove *Zhu Ling* and *Bai Jie Zi* and add 30 grams of Radix Trichosanthis Kirlowii (*Tian Hua Fen*) and nine grams of Rhizoma Polygonati (*Huang Jing*).

DISSEMINATED GRANULOMA ANNULARE

DAMPNESS & STASIS MUTUALLY BINDING PATTERN

MAIN SYMPTOMS: Pale red or skin-colored, ring or arc-shaped raised area on the skin mostly occurring on the hands and feet, upper back and ears, though possibly occurring on the whole body, which are hard to the touch when pressed but not painful or itchy, and thin, slimy tongue fur

TREATMENT PRINCIPLES: Transform dampness, quicken the blood, and soften the hard

Rx: *Er Zhu Gao* (Two Atractylodes Paste) plus *Tao Hong Si Wu Tang* (Persica & Carthamus Four Materials Decoction) with additions and subtractions

INGREDIENTS: Radix Scrophulariae Ningpoensis (*Xuan Shen*), 15g, and Rhizoma Atractylodis (*Cang Zhu*), Rhizoma Atractylodis Macrocephalae (*Bai Zhu*), Semen Pruni Persicae (*Tao Ren*), Flos Carthami Tinctorii (*Hong Hua*), Radix Ligustici Wallichii (*Chuan Xiong*), Radix Rubrus Paeoniae Lactiflorae (*Chi Shao*), Rhizoma Curcumae Zedoariae (*E Zhu*), Herba Lycopi Lucidi (*Ze Lan*), and Fructus Forsythiae Suspensae (*Lian Qiao*), 9g each

FORMULA ANALYSIS: *Cang Zhu* and *Bai Zhu* fortify the spleen and transform dampness. *Tao Ren, Chuan Xiong, Chi Shao,* and *Ze Lan* quicken the blood and transform stasis. *E Zhu, Xuan Shen,* and *Lian Qiao* soften the hard and scatter nodulation.

ADDITIONS & SUBTRACTIONS: If there is concomitant qi vacuity, add 15 grams each of Radix Pseudostellariae Heterophyllae (*Tai Zi Shen*) and Radix Dioscoreae Oppositae (*Shan Yao*). If there is concomitant yin vacuity and fluid dryness, add 12 grams of Tuber Ophiopogonis Japonici (*Mai Men Dong*) and nine grams of Radix Trichosanthis Kirlowii (*Tian Hua Fen*). If there is concomitant stomach heat with oral thirst, add 15 grams of uncooked Gypsum Fibrosum (*Shi Gao*) and nine grams of Rhizoma Anemarrhenae Aspheloidis (*Zhi Mu*).

EXTERNAL APPLICATION: Apply *Bai Zhi Gang Song Huo Xue Gao* (Angelica Dahurica & Nardostachys Quicken the Blood Ointment) to the affected area several times per day. This ointment consists of 10 grams each of Radix Angelicae Dahuricae (*Bai Zhi*), Rhizoma Nardostachytis (*Gan Song Xiang*), Radix Ligustici Wallichii (*Chuan Xiong*), uncooked Radix Et Rhizoma Rhei (*Da Huang*), Rhizoma Curcumae Longae (*Jiang Huang*), Radix Angelicae Pubescentis (*Du Huo*), Cortex Radicis Acanthopanacis Gracilistylis (*Wu Jia Pi*), Radix Auklandiae Lappae (*Mu Xiang*), Herba Pycnostelmae (*Xi Chang Jing*), and Fructus Gleditschiae Chinensis (*Zao Jiao*) and five grams each of Borneolum (*Bing Pian*) and Camphora (*Zhang Nao*). The first 10 ingredients are

soaked in one liter of vegetable oil for 24-72 hours. Then they are cooked till the herbs turn golden brown. After removing the dregs, and allowing the medicinal oil to cool down a bit, the *Bing Pian, Zhang Nao,* and 100-150 grams of beeswax are stirred in till dissolved. The resulting liquid should be decanted in jars for use, in which the ointment will solidify as it cools.

DIABETIC RUBEOSIS OF THE CHEEKS & FACE

VACUITY FIRE FLAMING UPWARD PATTERN

MAIN SYMPTOMS: Continuous facial redness which does not recede accompanied by red eyes, dizziness, tinnitus, a dry mouth and parched tongue, heat in the heart of the hands and feet, a red tongue with scanty fur, and a fine, rapid pulse

TREATMENT PRINCIPLES: Enrich yin and downbear fire

Rx: *Zhi Bai Di Huang Wan Jia Jian* (Anemarrhena & Phellodendron Rehmannia Pills with Additions & Subtractions)

INGREDIENTS: Uncooked Radix Rehmanniae (*Sheng Di*), 30g, Rhizoma Imperatae Cyclindricae (*Bai Mao Gen*), 15g, Cortex Radicis Moutan (*Dan Pi*), 12g, and Rhizoma Anemarrhenae Aspheloidis (*Zhi Mu*), Cortex Phellodendri (*Huang Bai*), Sclerotium Poriae Cocos (*Fu Ling*), Fructus Corni Officinalis (*Shan Zhu Yu*), Fructus Lycii Chinensis (*Gou Qi Zi*), Rhizoma Alismatis (*Ze Xie*), and Radix Achyranthis Bidentatae (*Niu Xi*), 9g each

FORMULA ANALYSIS: *Sheng Di, Dan Pi, Fu Ling, Shan Zhu Yu,* and *Ze Xie* level and supplement liver-kidney yin. *Zhi Mu* and *Huang Bai* downbear vacuity fire. *Niu Xi* leads the blood to move downward, and *Bai Mao Gen* cools the blood and disinhibits urination. With *Fu Ling* and *Ze Xie*, it helps lead yang downward into the yin tract.

ACUPUNCTURE & MOXIBUSTION: *Tai Xi* (Ki 3), *San Yin Jiao* (Sp 6), *Shen Shu* (Bl 23), *He Gu* (LI 4), *Qu Chi* (LI 11), *Zu San Li* (St 36)

FORMULA ANALYSIS: Supplementing *Tai Xi, San Yin Jiao,* and *Shen Shu* supplements the kidneys and enriches yin. Draining *Zu San Li, He Gu,* and *Qu Chi* clears heat from the face and head region and lowers blood pressure.

EXTERNAL APPLICATION: Decoct 30 grams each of Herba Cephalanoploris Segeti (*Xiao Ji*) and uncooked Flos Immaturus Sophorae Japonicae (*Huai Hua Mi*).

Remove the dregs and allow the medicinal liquid to cool. Then moisten a face cloth in this liquid and apply to the face for 15 minutes each time, two times per day.

CAROTENEMIA

DAMP HEAT DEPRESSION & STEAMING PATTERN

MAIN SYMPTOMS: Yellowing of the face, palms of the hands, and soles of the feet, possible yellowing of the entire body, vexatious heat, oral thirst, reddish yellow urination, a red tongue with slimy, yellow fur, and a bowstring, slippery pulse

TREATMENT PRINCIPLES: Clear heat, disinhibit dampness, and recede yellowing

RX: *Yin Chen Hao Tang Jia Wei* (Artemisia Capillaris Decoction with Added Flavors)

INGREDIENTS: Herba Artemisiae Capillaris (*Yin Chen Hao*), 30g, uncooked Semen Coicis Lachyrma-jobi (*Yi Yi Ren*), Sclerotium Poriae Cocos (*Fu Ling*), and Radix Trichosanthis Kirlowii (*Tian Hua Fen*), 15g each, Fructus Gardeniae Jasminoidis (*Zhi Zi*), Cortex Phellodendri (*Huang Bai*), Rhizoma Alismatis (*Ze Xie*), and uncooked Radix Rehmanniae (*Sheng Di*), 9g each, and Radix Et Rhizoma Rhei (*Da Huang*), 3-6g

FORMULA ANALYSIS: *Yin Chen Hao, Zhi Zi, Huang Bai,* and *Da Huang* clear heat, disinhibit dampness, and recede yellowing. *Fu Ling, Yi Yi Ren,* and *Ze Xie* blandly seep and disinhibit dampness, and *Sheng Di* and *Tian Hua Fen* boost yin and engender fluids.

ADDITIONS & SUBTRACTIONS: If the stools are not dry and bound, consider removing *Da Huang.* If the stools are not crisp but are difficult and loose, add nine grams of Herba Eupatorii Fortunei (*Pei Lan*). If vexatious thirst is pronounced, increase *Tian Hua Fen* up to 30 grams and add 30 grams of uncooked Gypsum Fibrosum (*Shi Gao*). If there is marked liver depression qi stagnation, add nine grams each of Radix Bupleuri (*Chai Hu*), Radix Albus Paeoniae Lactiflorae (*Bai Shao*), Fructus Meliae Toosendan (*Chuan Lian Zi*), and Rhizoma Cyperi Rotundi (*Xiang Fu*).

ACUPUNCTURE & MOXIBUSTION: *Da Zhui* (GV 14), *Zhi Yang* (GV 9), *Gan Shu* (Bl 18), *Dan Shu* (Bl 19), *Yang Ling Quan* (GB 34), *Yin Ling Quan* (Sp 9)

FORMULA ANALYSIS: Draining *Da Zhui* and *Zhi Yang* are the main points in Chinese acupuncture for receding yellowing. Draining *Gan Shu, Dan Shu,* and *Yang Ling Quan* clears heat and eliminates dampness from the liver-gallbladder. Draining *Yin Ling Quan* seeps and disinhibits dampness. *Yang Ling Quan* and *Yin Ling Quan* may be needled through-and-through.

ADDITIONS & SUBTRACTIONS: If there is concomitant spleen vacuity, add supplementing *Pi Shu* (Bl 20) and *Zu San Li* (St 36).

PRURITUS

1. BLOOD VACUITY & LIVER EFFULGENCE PATTERN

MAIN SYMPTOMS: Dry skin, itching which is worse at night, possible scratching causing nail marks or bleeding, heart vexation, tension and agitation, restless sleep at night, a pale red tongue with white fur, and a bowstring, fine pulse

TREATMENT PRINCIPLES: Nourish the blood and moisten dryness, level the liver and extinguish wind

RX: *Dang Gui Yin Zi Jia Jian* (Dang Gui Drink with Additions & Subtractions)

INGREDIENTS: Fructus Tribuli Terrestris (*Bai Ji Li*), 20g, uncooked Radix Rehmanniae (*Sheng Di*), 12g, and Radix Angelicae Sinensis (*Dang Gui*), Radix Ligustici Wallichii (*Chuan Xiong*), Radix Albus Paeoniae Lactiflorae (*Bai Shao*), Radix Polygoni Multiflori (*He Shou Wu*), Cortex Radicis Moutan (*Dan Pi*), Ramulus Uncariae Cum Uncis (*Gou Teng*), and Spina Gleditschiae Chinensis (*Zao Jiao Ci*), 9g each

FORMULA ANALYSIS: *Dang Gui, Bai Shao, Chuan Xiong, Sheng Di,* and *He Shou Wu* nourish the blood and moisten dryness. *Bai Ji Li* and *Gou Teng* level the liver and extinguish wind. *Zao Jiao Ci* dispels wind and stops itching, and *Dan Pi* clears vacuity heat from within the blood.

ADDITIONS & SUBTRACTIONS: If there is liver effulgence and yang hyperactivity with tension, agitation, and easy anger, headache, tinnitus, and insomnia, add 30 grams each of Concha Margaritiferae (*Zhen Zhu Mu*), uncooked Os Draconis (*Long Gu*), uncooked Concha Ostreae (*Mu Li*), and Magnetitum (*Ci Shi*) in order to level the liver and subdue yang, settle, still, and quiet the spirit. If there is recalcitrant itching secondary to eczema or dermatitis, add nine grams each of Radix Sophorae Flavescentis (*Ku Shen*) and Cortex Erythinae (*Hai Tong Pi*) and six grams of Buthus Martensis (*Quan*

Xie) to eliminate dampness, track down wind, and stop itching.

ACUPUNCTURE & MOXIBUSTION: *Ge Shu* (Bl 17), *Gan Shu* (Bl 18), *Qu Chi* (LI 11), *San Yin Jiao* (Sp 6), *Xue Hai* (Sp 10)

FORMULA ANALYSIS: Supplementing *Ge Shu*, *Gan Shu*, and *San Yin Jiao* nourishes the blood. Draining *Qu Chi* dispels wind, and draining *Xue Hai* clears heat from the blood.

ADDITIONS & SUBTRACTIONS: To clear liver heat, add draining *Xing Jian* (Liv 2) and *Yang Ling Quan* (GB 34). For itching in the lower limbs, add draining *Feng Shi* (GB 31). To settle, still, and quiet the spirit, add draining *Bai Hui* (GV 20) and *Yin Tang* (M-HN-3) and even supplementing-even draining *Shen Men* (Ht 7).

EAR ACUPUNCTURE: Lung, Adrenal, Subcortex, *Shen Men*

2. DAMP HEAT POURING DOWNWARD PATTERN

MAIN SYMPTOMS: External genital and perianal dampness and itching, possible lower limb itching, possible nail marks from scratching, worse itching on exposure to heat or when hot, a red tongue with slimy, yellow fur, and a slippery pulse

TREATMENT PRINCIPLES: Clear heat, eliminate dampness, and stop itching

RX: *Long Dan Xie Gan Tang Jia Wei* (Gentiana Drain the Liver Decoction with Added Flavors)

INGREDIENTS: Fructus Kochiae Scopariae (*Di Fu Zi*), Cortex Radicis Dictamni Dasycarpi (*Bai Xian Pi*), and Semen Plantaginis (*Che Qian Zi*), 15g each, and Radix Gentianae Scabrae (*Long Dan Cao*), Radix Scutellariae Baicalensis (*Huang Qin*), Fructus Gardeniae Jasminoidis (*Zhi Zi*), uncooked Radix Rehmanniae (*Sheng Di*), Radix Angelicae Sinensis (*Dang Gui*), and Rhizoma Alismatis (*Ze Xie*), 9g each

FORMULA ANALYSIS: *Long Dan Cao*, *Huang Qi*, and *Zhi Zi* clear heat and dry dampness. *Sheng Di* and *Dang Gui* nourish the blood and protect yin. *Che Qian Zi* and *Ze Xie* blandly seep and disinhibit dampness. *Di Fu Zi* and *Bai Xian Pi* eliminate dampness and stop itching.

ADDITIONS & SUBTRACTIONS: If dampness has damaged the spleen and heat has consumed yin, add 12 grams each of Radix Glehniae Littoralis (*Sha Shen*) and Tuber Ophiopogonis Japonici (*Mai Men Dong*).

ACUPUNCTURE & MOXIBUSTION: *San Yin Jiao* (Sp 6), *Yin Ling Quan* (Sp 9), *Xue Hai* (Sp 10)

FORMULA ANALYSIS: Draining *San Yin Jiao* and *Yin Ling Quan* clears and eliminates dampness and heat. Draining *Xue Hai* clears heat from within the blood aspect.

ADDITIONS & SUBTRACTIONS: For genital itching, add draining *Qu Gu* (CV 2) and *Lou Gu* (Liv 5). For perianal itching, add draining *Chang Qiang* (GV 1) and *Cheng Shan* (Bl 57).

EXTERNAL APPLICATION (for both the above patterns): Apply *Zhi Yang Ding* (Stop Itching Tincture) to the affected area several times per day.[20]

BACTERIAL & FUNGAL INFECTIONS

HORDOLEUM

PHLEGM & FIRE MUTUALLY BINDING PATTERN

MAIN SYMPTOMS: Localized pain, redness, and swelling of the eyelid accompanied by a dry mouth and parched throat, a red tongue, and rapid pulse

TREATMENT PRINCIPLES: Transform phlegm, clear heat, and scatter nodulation

RX: *Qing Wei Tang Jia Wei* (Clear the Stomach Decoction with Added Flavors)

INGREDIENTS: Uncooked Gypsum Fibrosum (*Shi Gao*), 15g, uncooked Radix Rehmanniae (*Sheng Di*), Cortex Radicis Moutan (*Dan Pi*), Radix Scrophulariae Ningpoensis (*Xuan Shen*), Radix Scutellariae Baicalensis (*Huang Qin*), Rhizoma Pinelliae Ternatae (*Ban Xia*), and Bombyx Batryticatus (*Jiang Can*), 9g each, and Rhizoma Coptidis Chinensis (*Huang Lian*) and Rhizoma Cimicifugae (*Sheng Ma*), 6g each

FORMULA ANALYSIS: *Shi Gao*, *Huang Lian*, *Huang Qin*, and *Sheng Ma* clear effulgent heat from the stomach. *Sheng Di* and *Xuan Shen* clear heat and cool the blood as well as nourish and protect yin fluids. In addition, *Xuan Shen* softens the hard and scatters nodulation. *Dan Pi* cools and quickens the blood, while *Ban Xia* and *Jiang Can* transform phlegm and scatter nodulation.

ADDITIONS & SUBTRACTIONS: If there is marked thirst and polydipsia, add nine grams of Rhizoma Anemarrhenae Aspheloidis (*Zhi Mu*). For heat in the large intestine, add 3-6 grams of Radix Et Rhizoma Rhei (*Da Huang*).

EXTERNAL APPLICATION: Apply *Si Huang Gao* (Four Yellows Ointment) over the stye 1-2 times per day.[21] Or make a cold compress from a decoction of 30 grams each of Herba Violae Yedoensitis Cum Radice (*Zi Hua Di Ding*) and Herba Taraxaci Mongolici Cum Radice (*Pu Gong Ying*). Remove the dregs and soak a face cloth in the medicinal liquid. Apply to the affected eyelid for 15-20 minutes each time, two times per day. Or first use this compress and then apply *Si Huang Gao*.

PUSTULOSIS (A.K.A. IMPETIGO)

1. LUNG CHANNEL HEAT & SPLEEN CHANNEL DAMPNESS PATTERN

MAIN SYMPTOMS: Clusters of pustules the size of soybeans or larger or suppurative blisters surrounded by a red halo, very thin-walled blisters which are easily perforated afterwards presenting an ulcerous surface, yellowish scabs when drying, and possible itching, possible emission of heat, aversion to cold, thirst, restlessness, dry stools, yellow urine, a red tongue with thin, yellow or dry, yellow fur, and a fine, rapid pulse if the lesions are widespread

TREATMENT PRINCIPLES: Clear heat, eliminate dampness, and resolve toxins

RX: *Qing Pi Chu Shi Yin* (Clear the Spleen & Eliminate Dampness Drink)

INGREDIENTS: Sclerotium Poriae Cocos (*Fu Ling*), uncooked Radix Rehmanniae (*Sheng Di*), Fructus Forsythiae Suspensae (*Lian Qiao*), and Herba Artemisiae Capillaris (*Yin Chen Hao*), 15g each, Tuber Ophiopogonis Japonici (*Mai Men Dong*), 12g, Rhizoma Atractylodis Macrocephalae (*Bai Zhu*), Rhizoma Atractylodis (*Cang Zhu*), Rhizoma Alismatis (*Ze Xie*), stir-fried Fructus Gardeniae Jasminoidis (*Zhi Zi*), and Rhizoma Cyperi Rotundi (*Xiang Fu*), 9g each, and Radix Astragali Membranacei (*Huang Qi*), 6g

FORMULA ANALYSIS: *Yin Chen Hao* and *Zhi Zi* clear heat and eliminate dampness. *Lian Qiao* clears heat and resolves toxins. *Fu Ling* and *Ze Xie* seep and disinhibit dampness. *Sheng Di* cools the blood and clears heat, while *Mai Men Dong* enriches yin and engenders fluids. *Xiang Fu* rectifies the qi, and *Huang Qi* boosts the qi and secures the exterior, constrains sores and stops leakage.

ADDITIONS & SUBTRACTIONS: If qi and yin vacuity is marked, one can use *Shen Qi Zhi Mu Tang* (Codonopsis, Astragalus & Anemarrhena Decoction): Semen Coicis Lachyrma-jobi (*Yi Yi Ren*), 30g, Cortex Sclerotii Poriae Cocos (*Fu Ling Pi*) and Rhizoma Anemarrhenae Aspheloidis (*Zhi Mu*), 15g each, Tuber Ophiopogonis Japonici (*Mai Men Dong*), Tuber Asparagi Cochinensis (*Tian Men Dong*), Radix Dioscoreae Oppositae (*Shan Yao*), Radix Astragali Membranacei (*Huang Qi*), Radix Codonopsitis Pilosulae (*Dang Shen*), Herba Artemisiae Apiaceae (*Qing Hao*), and Radix Ampelopsis Japonicae (*Bai Lian*), 12g each, and Rhizoma Atractylodis (*Cang Zhu*), Rhizoma Atractylodis Macrocephalae (*Bai Zhu*), uncooked Radix Rehmanniae (*Sheng Di*), cooked Radix Rehmanniae (*Shu Di*), Radix Albus Paeoniae Lactiflorae (*Bai Shao*), and Radix Rubrus Paeoniae Lactiflorae (*Chi Shao*), 9g each.

EXTERNAL APPLICATION: Spread a layer of *Qing Dai Gao* (Indigo Ointment) on a sterile gauze pad and affix to the affected area once or twice per day.[22]

FURUNCULOSIS

DAMP HEAT TOXINS PATTERN

MAIN SYMPTOMS: Red, hot, painful subdermal swellings 5-30mm in diameter on the neck, breast, face, back, and buttocks with possible emission of heat, aversion to cold, thin, yellow tongue fur, and a rapid pulse. As the condition resolves itself, there is central necrosis with discharge of a core of necrotic tissue and yellow, bloody, purulent exudate.

TREATMENT PRINCIPLES: Clear heat, eliminate dampness, and resolve toxins

RX: *Ye Ju Bai Du Tang* (Wild Chrysanthemum Vanquish Toxins Decoction)

INGREDIENTS: Herba Taraxaci Mongolici Cum Radice (*Pu Gong Ying*), 15g, Flos Lonicerae Japonicae (*Jin Yin Hua*), 12g, Flos Chrysanthemi Indici (*Ye Ju Hua*), Radix Scrophulariae Ningpoensis (*Xuan Shen*), Fructus Forsythiae Suspensae (*Lian Qiao*), and Herba Violae Yedoensis Cum Radice (*Zi Hua Di Ding*), 9g each, Bulbus Fritillariae Thunbergii (*Zhe Bei Mu*), 6g, and uncooked Radix Glycyrrhizae (*Gan Cao*), 3g

FORMULA ANALYSIS: *Pu Gong Ying, Jin Yin Hua, Lian Qiao, Zi Hua Di Ding,* and *Ye Ju Hua* all clear heat and resolve toxins. *Xuan Shen* clears heat and resolves toxins, cools the blood and engenders fluids. In addition, it softens the hard and scatters nodulation. *Zhe Bei Mu* transforms phlegm, clears heat, and scatters nodulation, and *Gan Cao* both clears heat and resolves toxins and harmonizes all the other medicinals in this formula.

ADDITIONS & SUBTRACTIONS: For lesions due to contraction of summerheat, add nine grams each of Herba Agastachis Seu Pogostemi (*Huo Xiang*) and Herba Eupatorii Fortunei (*Pei Lan*), 12 grams of Talcum (*Hua Shi*), and 20 grams of Semen Coicis Lachryma-jobi (*Yi Yi Ren*). If heat toxins are especially exuberant, add nine grams each of Radix Scutellariae Baicalensis (*Huang Qin*) and Fructus Gardeniae Jasminoidis (*Zhi Zi*) and 3-6 grams of Rhizoma Coptidis Chinensis (*Huang Lian*). For lesions that are slow to rupture, add nine grams each of Spina Gleditschiae Chinensis (*Zao Jiao Ci*) and Radix Ligustici Wallichii (*Chuan Xiong*). For scanty, reddish yellow urination, add nine grams each of Sclerotium Rubrum Poriae Cocos (*Chi Fu Ling*), Semen Plantaginis (*Che Qian Zi*), and Folium Lophatheri Gracilis (*Dan Zhu Ye*). For dry, bound stools, add six grams each of Radix Et Rhizoma Rhei (*Da Huang*) and Fructus Immaturus Citri Aurantii (*Zhi Shi*) and 3-4.5 grams of Mirabilitum (*Mang Xiao*). For concomitant qi vacuity, add 15 grams of Radix Astragali Membranacei (*Huang Qi*) and nine grams each of Radix Codonopsitis Pilosulae (*Dang Shen*) and Radix Cynanchi Baiwei (*Bai Wei*). For concomitant yin vacuity, add 12 grams each of uncooked Radix Rehmanniae (*Sheng Di*), Tuber Ophiopogonis Japonici (*Mai Men Dong*), and Tuber Asparagi Cochinensis (*Tian Men Dong*).

ACUPUNCTURE & MOXIBUSTION: *Ling Tai* (GV 10) and fire needle into the furuncle itself.

FORMULA ANALYSIS: Draining *Ling Tai* and then squeezing several drops of blood from the point after removing the needle clears heat from both the qi and blood aspects.

ADDITIONS & SUBTRACTIONS: For furuncles on the head and face, add draining *He Gu* (LI 4) and *Qu Chi* (LI 11). For furuncles on the chest and abdomen, add draining *Zu San Li* (St 36) and *San Yin Jiao* (Sp 6). For furuncles on the back, add draining *Wei Zhong* (Bl 40) which may also be bled.

EXTERNAL APPLICATION: Apply *Si Huang Gao* (Four Yellows Ointment) to the affected area 1-3 times per day.[23]

CARBUNCLES

1. BLAZING & EXUBERANT HEAT TOXINS PATTERN

MAIN SYMPTOMS: Millet-sized nodules with pus-filled heads accompanied by pain and itching which eventually become swollen, red, burning hot, and more painful, possibly accompanied by high fever, headache, dry mouth, a red tongue with yellow fur, and a slippery, rapid or surging, rapid pulse

TREATMENT PRINCIPLES: Clear heat, resolve toxins, and cool the constructive

RX: *Wu Wei Xiao Du Yin Jia Jian* (Five Flavors Disperse Toxins Drink with Additions & Subtractions)

INGREDIENTS: Herba Violae Yedoensitis Cum Radice (*Zi Hua Di Ding*) and Herba Taraxaci Mongolici Cum Radice (*Pu Gong Ying*), 15g each, Flos Lonicerae Japonicae (*Jin Yin Hua*), 12g, and Flos Chrysanthemi Indici (*Ye Ju Hua*), Cortex Radicis Moutan (*Dan Pi*), and Radix Rubrus Paeoniae Lactiflorae (*Chi Shao*), 9g each

FORMULA ANALYSIS: *Zi Hua Di Ding*, *Pu Gong Ying*, *Ye Ju Hua*, and *Jin Yin Hua* clear heat and resolve toxins. *Dan Pi* and *Chi Shao* clear heat, cool and quicken the blood.

ADDITIONS & SUBTRACTIONS: If there is constipation, add 3-9 grams of Radix Et Rhizoma Rhei (*Da Huang*) and 6-9 grams of Fructus Immaturus Citri Aurantii (*Zhi Shi*). If there is reddish urination, add nine grams each of Semen Plantaginis (*Che Qian Zi*) and Sclerotium Rubrum Poriae Cocos (*Chi Fu Ling*). If heat is severe, add 9-12 grams of Fructus Forsythiae Suspensae (*Lian Qiao*) and 3-9 grams of Rhizoma Coptidis Chinensis (*Huang Lian*). For severe pain, add six grams each of processed Resina Olibani (*Ru Xiang*) and Resina Myrrhae (*Mo Yao*).

ACUPUNCTURE & MOXIBUSTION: Same as for furunculosis above.

EXTERNAL APPLICATION: Apply *Si Huang Gao* (Four Yellows Ointment) externally 1-3 times per day.[24]

2. EXUBERANT HEAT & DAMAGED FLUIDS PATTERN

MAIN SYMPTOMS: Swollen, red lumps with broad red halos, production of pus but noneruption of the sores, accompanying emission of heat, dry mouth, constipation, a red tongue with flowery, peeled fur, and a rapid pulse

TREATMENT PRINCIPLES: Clear heat, resolve toxins, and engender fluids

RX: *Zhu Ye Shi Gao Tang Jia Jian* (Bamboo Leaves & Gypsum Decoction with Additions & Subtractions)

INGREDIENTS: Uncooked Gypsum Fibrosum (*Shi Gao*), 30g, Tuber Ophiopogonis Japonici (*Mai Men Dong*), 18g, Herba Lophatheri Gracilis (*Dan Zhu Ye*), 15g, Rhizoma Anemarrhenae Aspheloidis (*Zhi Mu*) and Rhizoma Pinelliae Ternatae (*Ban Xia*), 9g each, and Radix Panacis Ginseng (*Ren Shen*), 6g

FORMULA ANALYSIS: *Shi Gao* and *Dan Zhu Ye* drain fire and clear heat. *Zhi Mu* enriches yin and drains fire. *Mai Men Dong* engenders fluids and moistens dryness. *Ban Xia* transforms phlegm and eliminates dampness, and *Ren Shen* supplements the qi and engenders fluids.

ADDITIONS & SUBTRACTIONS: If thirst is severe, add 12 grams of uncooked Radix Rehmanniae (*Sheng Di*) and nine grams of Radix Trichosanthis Kirlowii (*Tian Hua Fen*). If heat toxins are severe, add 15 grams each of Radix Isatidis Seu Baphicacanthi (*Ban Lan Gen*) and Herba Violae Yedoensitis Cum Radice (*Zi Hua Di Ding*) and 3-6 grams of Rhizoma Coptidis Chinensis (*Huang Lian*). If there is constipation, add 12 grams each of Radix Scrophulariae Ningpoensis (*Xuan Shen*) and uncooked Radix Rehmanniae (*Sheng Di*), 3-9 grams of Radix Et Rhizoma Rhei (*Da Huang*), and 6-9 grams of Fructus Immaturus Citri Aurantii (*Zhi Shi*).

ACUPUNCTURE & MOXIBUSTION: Same as above.

EXTERNAL APPLICATION: Grind two parts uncooked Gypsum Fibrosum (*Shi Gao*) to one part Alum (*Bai Fan*), mix the resulting powder together with water and apply to the affected area.

3. YIN VACUITY WITH EXUBERANT HEAT PATTERN

MAIN SYMPTOMS: Flat, dark, purplish sores most commonly seen in the elderly with a broad, diffuse base which do not easily transform and expel pus accompanied by emission of heat, dry mouth, constipation, a red tongue with scanty fur, and a fine, rapid pulse

TREATMENT PRINCIPLES: Enrich yin and engender fluids, clear heat and resolve toxins

RX: *Zhu Ye Huang Qi Tang* (Bamboo Leaves & Astragalus Decoction)

INGREDIENTS: Radix Astragali Membranacei (*Huang Qi*), 12-18g, calcined Gyspum Fibrosum (*Shi Gao*), Herba Lophatheri Gracilis (*Dan Zhu Ye*), Tuber Ophiopogonis Japonici (*Mai Men Dong*), and uncooked Radix

Rehmanniae (*Sheng Di*), 12g each, Radix Albus Paeoniae Lactiflorae (*Bai Shao*), Rhizoma Pinelliae Ternatae (*Ban Xia*), Radix Angelicae Sinensis (*Dang Gui*), Radix Ligustici Wallichii (*Chuan Xiong*), and Radix Scutellariae Baicalensis (*Huang Qin*), 9g each, Radix Panacis Ginseng (*Ren Shen*), 6-9g, and Radix Glycyrrhizae (*Gan Cao*), 3-6g

FORMULA ANALYSIS: *Huang Qi* and *Ren Shen* fortify the spleen and boost the qi. *Dang Gui* and *Bai Shao* nourish the blood to help supplement yin. *Mai Men Dong* enriches yin and engenders fluids. *Ban Xia* transforms phlegm and eliminates dampness. *Shi Gao* and *Dan Zhu Ye* drain fire and clear heat. *Huang Qin* clears heat and eliminates dampness, and *Gan Cao* harmonizes all the other medicinals in the formula at the same time as it clears heat and resolves toxins.

ADDITIONS & SUBTRACTIONS: If the tongue is crimson red with no fur, add nine grams each of Rhizoma Anemarrhenae Aspheloidis (*Zhi Mu*) and Cortex Phellodendri (*Huang Bai*). If pus is difficult to expel, add nine grams each of baked Squama Manitis Pentadactylis (*Chuan Shan Jia*) and Spina Gleditschiae Chinensis (*Zao Jiao Ci*).

ACUPUNCTURE & MOXIBUSTION: Same as above, but add supplementing *Zu San Li* (St 36), *San Yin Jiao* (Sp 6), and *Tai Xi* (Ki 3).

4. QI & BLOOD INSUFFICIENCY PATTERN

MAIN SYMPTOMS: Enduring, flat, erosive, nonhealing sores which discharge clear, thin, watery pus and which refuse to close, a low to medium grade fever, lassitude of the spirit, fatigue, lack of strength, great sweating which dribbles and drips, torpid intake, a fat, enlarged, pale red tongue with white fur, and a fine, forceless, but rapid pulse

TREATMENT PRINCIPLES: Supplement and boost the qi and blood, out-thrust toxins and disperse swelling

RX: *Tuo Li Xiao Du San* (Out-thrust the Interior & Disperse Toxins Powder)

INGREDIENTS: Radix Astragali Membranacei (*Huang Qi*), 15-18g, Flos Lonicerae Japonicae (*Jin Yin Hua*), 12-15g, Rhizoma Atractylodis Macrocephalae (*Bai Zhu*), Radix Angelicae Sinensis (*Dang Gui*), Radix Angelicae Dahuricae (*Bai Zhi*), Radix Ligustici Wallichii (*Chuan Xiong*), Radix Albus Paeoniae Lactiflorae (*Bai Shao*), and Sclerotium Poriae Cocos (*Fu Ling*), 9g each, Radix Panacis Ginseng (*Ren Shen*), 6-9g, Spina Gleditschiae Chinensis

(*Zao Jiao Ci*) and Radix Platycodi Grandiflori (*Jie Geng*), 6g each, and uncooked Radix Glycyrrhizae (*Gan Cao*), 3g

FORMULA ANALYSIS: *Huang Qi, Ren Shen, Bai Zhu,* and *Fu Ling* fortify the spleen and boost the qi. *Dang Gui* and *Bai Shao* nourish the blood. *Chuan Xiong* quickens the blood. *Jin Yin Hua* clears heat and resolves toxins. *Bai Zhi* and *Zao Jiao Ci* ripen and expel pus. *Jie Geng* upbears the qi and transforms phlegm. *Bai Zhi* and *Chuan Xiong* also help in the upbearing of the clear which helps to support the righteous. *Gan Cao* clears heat and resolves toxins and harmonizes all the other medicinals in the formula.

ADDITIONS & SUBTRACTIONS: If there is concomitant yin vacuity, add 12 grams of uncooked Radix Rehmanniae (*Sheng Di*) and nine grams each of Radix Trichosanthis Kirlowii (*Tian Hua Fen*), Radix Dioscoreae Oppositae (*Shan Yao*), and Rhizoma Anemarrhenae Aspheloidis (*Zhi Mu*). If the carbuncles are on the lower extremities, add 21 grams of Semen Coicis Lachryma-jobi (*Yi Yi Ren*) and nine grams each of Radix Achyranthis Bidentatae (*Niu Xi*) and Fructus Chaenomelis Lagenariae (*Mu Gua*). If the urine is turbid, add nine grams each of Rhizoma Dioscoreae Hypoglaucae (*Bie Xie*) and Rhizoma Acori Graminei (*Shi Chang Pu*). If the lower extremities are edematous and swollen, add nine grams each of Radix Stephaniae Tetrandrae (*Han Fang Ji*) and Radix Gentianae Macrophyllae (*Qin Jiao*).

ACUPUNCTURE & MOXIBUSTION: Same as for furunculosis above.

EXTERNAL APPLICATION: Apply *Sheng Ji Yu Hong Gao* (Engender the Flesh Jade Red Ointment) to a sterile gauze and apply 1-2 times per day to the affected area.[25]

5. QI & YIN DUAL VACUITY PATTERN

MAIN SYMPTOMS: Ruptured sores which have discharged their pus but the swelling has not receded, erosive lesions, sores which are slow to close and are dark and purplish around their edges accompanied by low-grade fever, lassitude of the spirit, fatigue, lack of strength, spontaneous perspiration, a low, weak voice and disinclination to speak, a pale red tongue with scanty fur, and a fine, forceless pulse

TREATMENT PRINCIPLES: Supplement the qi and nourish yin

RX: *Sheng Mai San* (Engender the Pulse Powder) plus *Ba Zhen Tang* (Eight Pearls Decoction)

INGREDIENTS: Tuber Ophiopogonis Japonici (*Mai Men Dong*) and uncooked Radix Rehmanniae (*Sheng Di*), 12g each, Radix Angelicae Sinensis (*Dang Gui*), Radix Albus Paeoniae Lactiflorae (*Bai Shao*), Radix Ligustici Wallichii (*Chuan Xiong*), Rhizoma Atractylodis Macrocephalae (*Bai Zhu*), Sclerotium Poriae Cocos (*Fu Ling*), and Fructus Schisandrae Chinensis (*Wu Wei Zi*), 9g each, and Radix Panacis Ginseng (*Ren Shen*) and mix-fried Radix Glycyrrhizae (*Gan Cao*), 6g each

FORMULA ANALYSIS: *Sheng Di* and *Mai Men Dong* supplement yin and engender fluids. *Dang Gui* and *Bai Shao* supplement the blood in order to help supplement yin. *Ren Shen, Bai Zhu, Fu Ling,* and mix-fried *Gan Cao* fortify the spleen and supplement the qi. *Chuan Xiong* quickens the blood, while *Wu Wei Zi* engenders fluids at the same time as it promotes astringing and securing, constraining and containing.

ADDITIONS & SUBTRACTIONS: If there is torpid intake, chest oppression, nausea, and slimy, white tongue fur, add nine grams each of Rhizoma Pinelliae Ternatae (*Ban Xia*), Pericarpium Citri Reticulatae (*Chen Pi*), Caulis Bambusae In Taeniis (*Zhu Ru*), and Fructus Germinatus Hordei Vulgaris (*Mai Ya*). If there is profuse sweating, add 30 grams of Fructus Levis Tritici Aestivi (*Fu Xiao Mai*) and 12 grams of Concha Ostreae (*Mu Li*).

If yin disease has reached yang with reversal chilling of the four extremities, one can use *Fu Gui Shen Qi Wan* (Aconite & Cinnamon Kidney Qi Pills): cooked Radix Rehmanniae (*Shu Di*), Radix Dioscoreae Oppositae (*Shan Yao*), and Fructus Corni Officinalis (*Shan Zhu Yu*), 12g each, Sclerotium Poriae Cocos (*Fu Ling*), Rhizoma Alismatis (*Ze Xie*), and Cortex Radicis Moutan (*Dan Pi*), 9g each, Radix Lateralis Praeparatus Aconiti Carmichaeli (*Fu Zi*), 3-9g, and Cortex Cinnamomi Cassiae (*Rou Gui*), 3-6g

ACUPUNCTURE & MOXIBUSTION: Same as above.

EXTERNAL APPLICATION: Same as above.

CUTANEOUS CANDIDIASIS

EXUBERANT DAMP HEAT TOXINS PATTERN

MAIN SYMPTOMS: Widespread skin lesions, damp, erosive sores, suppuration of white fluid, extreme itching, vexation, agitation, and restlessness, a red tongue with yellow fur, and a slippery, rapid pulse

TREATMENT PRINCIPLES: Clear heat, dry dampness, and resolve toxins

RX: *Dao Chi San* (Abduct the Red Powder) plus *Er Miao San* (Two Wonders Powder) with added flavors

INGREDIENTS: Sclerotium Rubrum Poriae Cocos (*Chi Fu Ling*), Herba Taraxaci Mongolici Cum Radice (*Pu Gong Ying*), and Cortex Radicis Dictamni Dasycarpi (*Bai Xian Pi*), 15g each, uncooked Radix Rehmanniae (*Sheng Di*), Caulis Akebiae (*Mu Tong*), Rhizoma Atractylodis (*Cang Zhu*), Cortex Phellodendri (*Huang Bai*), and Radix Sophorae Flavescentis (*Ku Shen*), 9g each, Folium Lophatheri Gracilis (*Dan Zhu Ye*), 6g, and uncooked Radix Glycyrrhizae (*Gan Cao*), 3g

FORMULA ANALYSIS: *Sheng Di, Dan Zhu Ye, Mu Tong, Gan Cao,* and *Chi Fu Ling* clear the heart and disinhibit water, abduct heat and move it downward. *Cang Zhu, Huang Bai, Ku Shen,* and *Bai Xian Pi* clear heat, dry dampness, and stop itching. *Pu Gong Ying* resolves toxins.

ADDITIONS & SUBTRACTIONS: If there is concomitant qi and yin vacuity, add 12 grams each of Radix Glehniae Littoralis (*Sha Shen*) and Tuber Ophiopogonis Japonici (*Mai Men Dong*). If there is concomitant liver depression, add nine grams each of Fructus Meliae Toosendan (*Chuan Lian Zi*) and Radix Bupleuri (*Chai Hu*). If there is a liver-spleen disharmony, add nine grams each of Fructus Pruni Mume (*Wu Mei*) and Radix Auklandiae Lappae (*Mu Xiang*).

ACUPUNCTURE & MOXIBUSTION: *San Yin Jiao* (Sp 6), *Yin Ling Quan* (Sp 9), *Xue Hai* (Sp 10), *Qu Chi* (LI 11)

FORMULA ANALYSIS: Draining *San Yin Jiao* and *Yin Ling Quan* clears heat and eliminates dampness via urination. Draining *Xue Hai* clears heat from the blood aspect, and draining *Qu Chi* dispels wind and eliminates dampness, clears heat and treats the skin.

ADDITIONS & SUBTRACTIONS: If there is concomitant spleen vacuity, add supplementing *Zu San Li* (St 36) and *Pi Shu* (Bl 20). If there is simultaneous liver heat, add draining *Xing Jian* and/or *Yang Ling Quan* (GB 34).

EXTERNAL APPLICATION: Wash or soak the affected area for 20 minutes each time, two times per day with a cool decoction made from: Radix Sophorae Flavescentis (*Ku Shen*), Fructus Cnidii Monnieri (*She Chuang Zi*), Herba Taraxaci Mongolici Cum Radice (*Pu Gong Ying*), and Cortex Phellodendri (*Huang Bai*), 30g each, and Fructus Kochiae Scopariae (*Di Fu Zi*) and Alum (*Ku Fan*), 20g each. If there are water blisters, first use a sterile needle to poke the blisters and discharge their pus and then wash or soak.

If there are red macules with less suppuration, apply *Qing Dai Gao* (Indigo Ointment) 1-2 times per day to the affected area held in place by cotton gauze and adhesive tape.[26]

TINEA PALMARIS & TINEA PEDIS

EXUBERANT DAMP HEAT TOXINS PATTERN

MAIN SYMPTOMS: Wet, erosive, suppurating skin lesions on the hands and/or feet. If there is a secondary infection, there will also be redness, swelling, and pain of the affected area.

TREATMENT PRINCIPLES: Clear heat, eliminate dampness, and resolve toxins

RX: *Bie Xie Shen Shi Tang* (Dioscorea Hypoglauca Seep Dampness Decoction) plus *Wu Shen Tang* (Five Spirits Decoction) with additions and subtractions

INGREDIENTS: Herba Violae Yedoensitis Cum Radice (*Zi Hua Di Ding*), 30g, uncooked Semen Coicis Lachryma-jobi (*Yi Yi Ren*) and Semen Plantaginis (*Che Qian Zi*), 15g each, Sclerotium Rubrum Poriae Cocos (*Chi Fu Ling*), 12g, and Rhizoma Dioscoreae Hypoglaucae (*Bie Xie*), Cortex Phellodendri (*Huang Bai*), Rhizoma Alismatis (*Ze Xie*), Flos Lonicerae Japonicae (*Jin Yin Hua*), and Radix Achyranthis Bidentatae (*Niu Xi*), 9g each

FORMULA EXPLANATION: *Zi Hua Di Ding* and *Jin Yin Hua* clear heat and resolve toxins. *Huang Bai* clears heat and eliminates dampness, and *Yi Yi Ren, Bie Xie, Che Qian Zi, Chi Fu Ling,* and *Ze Xie* seep and disinhibit dampness. *Niu Xi* is a messenger medicinal that leads the effects of the other medicinals downward to the lower extremities.

EXTERNAL APPLICATION: The external treatment of hand and foot tinea is divided into three stages or types. For the blister type, tincture 20 grams of Flos Caryophylli (*Ding Xiang*) in 100ml of 70% alcohol for seven days and then apply two times per day, morning and night, to the affected area.

For the erosive type, dust the affected area with equal parts of powdered Cortex Phellodendri (*Huang Bai*) and Alum (*Ku Fan*) or use a cold compress made with the medicinal liquid from a decoction of 30 grams each of Radix Sophorae Flavescentis (*Ku Shen*), Fructus Cnidii Monnieri (*She Chuang Zi*), Fructus Xantii Sibirici (*Cang Er Zi*), Herba Agastachis Seu Pogostemi (*Huo Xiang*), and Alum (*Ku Fan*).

For the squamous cornification type, simmer two pieces of Nidus Vespae (*Feng Fang*) in 500ml of white vinegar until the liquid is reduced by half. Cool, strain, and apply externally 2-3 times per day.

ONCHYOMYCOSIS

SPLEEN-STOMACH HEAT DAMAGING THE BLOOD PATTERN

MAIN SYMPTOMS: Atrophic or hypertrophic, greyish, lusterless, possibly fragile finger or toenails which may become separated from the nail bed

TREATMENT PRINCIPLES: Clear heat and eliminate dampness, nourish the blood and kill worms

EXTERNAL APPLICATION: Tincture 30 grams of Herba Agastachis Seu Pogostemi (Huo Xiang) and 12 grams each of Rhizoma Polygonati Odorati (Yu Zhu), Radix Et Rhizoma Rhei (Da Huang), and Melanteritum (Qing Fan) in 500ml of white vinegar for seven days. Remove the dregs and reserve the medicinal liquid. Soak the affected nail(s) in this liquid for 30 minutes per day.

ABSTRACTS OF REPRESENTATIVE CHINESE RESEARCH:

Li Wen-hong, "The Integrated Chinese-Western Medical Treatment of Diabetic Bullosis," *Si Chuan Zhong Yi (Sichuan Journal of Chinese Medicine)*, #7, 1999, p. 44: The author treated 30 cases of diabetic bullosis with both internal and external formulas. In this study, there were 12 men and 18 women, their ages ranged from 51-64 years old, and their median blood sugar was 12.3 ± 6.4mmol/L. There were four cases of septicemia, three cases of renal insufficiency, two cases of retinopathy with blindness in both eyes, and six cases of chronic gastric ulcers. Before the blisters erupted, there was no sensation of pain nor any redness or swelling. The blisters ranged in size from 0.5-10cm and were round or elliptical in appearance. An external wash was prepared for the affected areas consisting of: Radix Sophorae Flavescentis (Ku Shen) and Mirabilitum (Mang Xiao), 30g each, and Herba Lemnae Seu Spirodelae (Fu Ping), 15g. These medicinals were boiled in water and the resulting medicinal liquid was applied externally twice per day. If the blisters did not break, then the patient was advised to soak the infected area with hot water twice per day, for 30 minutes each time. The treatment principles for the internally administered decoction were to course wind and clear heat, resolve toxins and dispel dampness. The prescription was Yin Qiao San Jia Jian (Lonicera & Forsythia Powder with Additions & Subtractions): Flos Lonicerae Japonicae (Jin Yin Hua), Fructus Forsythiae Suspensae (Lian Qiao), Fructus Arctii Lappae (Niu Bang Zi), Herba Menthae Haplocalycis (Bo He), Folium Bambusae (Zhu Ye), Radix Lithospermi Seu Arnebiae (Zi Cao), Radix Glycyrrhizae (Gan Cao), Radix Platycodi Grandiflori (Jie Geng), Talcum (Hua Shi), and Rhizoma Dioscoreae Hypoglaucae (Bie Xie). For more serious conditions, in order to clear heat and cool the blood, resolve toxins and seep dampness, Jia Wei Xiao Du Yin (Added Flavors Disperse Toxins Drink) plus Qing Wei Jie Du Tang (Clear the Stomach & Resolve Toxins Decoction) with additions and subtractions were prescribed: Fructus Forsythiae Suspensae (Lian Qiao), Fructus Arctii Lappae (Niu Bang Zi), Radix Rubrus Paeoniae Lactiflorae (Chi Shao), Radix Scutellariae Baicalensis (Huang Qin), Cortex Radicis Moutan (Dan Pi), Gypsum Fibrosum (Shi Gao, decocted first), Rhizoma Anemarrhenae Aspheloidis (Zhi Mu), uncooked Radix Rehmanniae (Sheng Di), Radix Lithospermi Seu Arnebiae (Zi Cao), Sclerotium Polypori Umbellati (Zhu Ling), Sclerotium Poriae Cocos (Fu Ling), and Semen Coicis Lachryma-jobi (Yi Yi Ren). These medicinals were boiled in water and one *ji* was administered per day. Diet, lifestyle, and insulin were all continued as normal. After four weeks, 22 patients (73.33%) experienced the disappearance of the skin blisters with no new outbreaks of blisters occurring. Five patients (16.67%) showed some moderate improvement, and three patients showed no improvement. Therefore, the total amelioration rate was 90%.

Sun Xue-dong, "The Treatment of 82 Cases of Diabetes-induced Skin Itching with Self-composed *Zhi Yang Tang* (Stop Itching Decoction)," *Bei Jing Zhong Yi (Beijing Chinese Medicine)*, #3, 2000, p. 22: All 82 patients in this study were diagnosed with diabetes according to WHO criteria and all had pruritus. Among these 82, 48 were male and 34 were female. Twenty-one cases were 40-50 years of age, 38 were 51-60, and 23 were 61 years old or older. Nineteen cases had had DM for 1-5 years, 28 had had DM 6-11 years, 22 cases had had DM 12-15 years, and 13 cases had had DM 13 years or more. Forty-two cases had had pruritus for 1-5 years, 29 had had pruritus for 6-10 years, five had had pruritus 11-15 years, and six cases had had pruritus for more than 15 years. Fasting blood glucose was 8-10mmol/L in 38 cases, was 11-12mmol/L in 39 cases, and was more than 12mmol/L in five cases.

Treatment consisted of the following internally administered Chinese medicinals to enrich yin, quicken the blood, and stop itching: Radix Pseudostellariae Heterophyllae (Tai Zi Shen), uncooked Radix Rehmanniae (Sheng Di), and Fructus Lycii Chinensis (Gou Qi Zi), 30g each, Radix

Salviae Miltiorrhizae (*Dan Shen*), 20g, Cortex Radicis Lycii Chinensis (*Di Gu Pi*) and Rhizoma Polygonati (*Huang Jing*), 15g each, Rhizoma Polygonati Odorati (*Yu Zhu*), Radix Trichosanthis Kirlowii (*Tian Hua Fen*), Radix Dioscoreae Oppositae (*Shan Yao*), Bombyx Batryticatus (*Jiang Can*), and Radix Rubrus Paeoniae Lactiflorae (*Chi Shao*), 12g each, Semen Pruni Persicae (*Tao Ren*) and Cortex Radicis Moutan (*Dan Pi*), 10g each, and Radix Glycyrrhizae (*Gan Cao*), 6g. If there was a bitter taste in the mouth and slimy, yellow tongue fur due to severe damp heat, stir-fried Rhizoma Anemarrhenae Aspheloidis (*Zhi Mu*), Cortex Phellodendri (*Huang Bai*), and Radix Gentianae Scabrae (*Long Dan Cao*) were added. If there was tinnitus and low back pain, cooked Radix Rehmanniae (*Shu Di*) was added. If there was fluid depletion constipation, Semen Cannabis Sativae (*Huo Ma Ren*) and Semen Pruni (*Yu Li Ren*) were added. If there were heart palpitations and a dark red tongue, Flos Carthami Tinctorii (*Hong Hua*) and Ramulus Cinnamomi Cassiae (*Gui Zhi*) were added.

Cure was defined as complete disappearance of itching after 30 days of taking the above medicinals with no recurrence within half a year and FBG reduced 2mmol/L from the previous baseline or returned to normal. Marked effect meant that there was marked reduction in the itching after 30 days of treatment, no aggravation within a half year after treatment, and a lowering of FBG. Improvement meant decreased itching after 30 days of treatment with only a slight degree of recurrence after three months, however, full recurrence after half a year. No effect meant that, after 30 days of taking the above Chinese medicinals, there was no improvement in symptoms. Based on these criteria, 43 patients (52.4%) were cured, 28 cases (43.1%) got a marked effect, 10 cases (12.2%) improved, and one case (1.2%) got no effect, for a total amelioration rate of 98.5%.

Gao Hong-mei *et al.*, "The Acupuncture-moxibustion Treatment of 34 Cases of Uremic Pruritus," *Zhong Yi Za Zhi* (*Journal of Chinese Medicine*), #5, 2001, p. 312: Altogether, there were 68 patients in this study. Forty of these were men and 28 were women, ranging in age from 22-72 years, with an average age of 43.6 years. All had either primary or secondary onset kidney disease which had resulted in chronic uremia, all had pruritus for more than one month without rash or ulcer, and, prior to developing uremia, none had had any skin disease. Thirty-four of these patients were assigned to the acupuncture group and the other 34, to the medicine group. The patients in the acupuncture group were needled bilaterally with draining twirling method at *Qu Chi* (LI 11) and with sup-

plementing twirling method at *Zu San Li* (St 36). Each treatment lasted 30 minutes, two treatments were given per week, and four weeks equaled one course of therapy. The patients in the medicine group were administered 4mg of chlorpheniramine maleate orally TID and applied *Pi Yan Ping Rou Gao* (Skin Inflammation Leveling & Softening Ointment) externally to the affected areas. After one course of treatment, the itching had completely disappeared in 24 cases (70.7) out of 34 in the acupuncture group. In another nine cases (26.5%), it had markedly decreased. Only one case (2.9%) in this group failed to experience an effect. In the medicine group, after two weeks of treatment, there were two complete remissions (5.9%), 22 (64.7%) marked improvements, and 10 (29.4%) no effects. The total amelioration rates between these two groups were 97% and 70.6% respectively. In addition, in the medicine group, the itching returned as soon as the treatment was suspended, while the treatment held for one month in 16 cases in the acupuncture group and for three months in another 16 cases. Thus there was a marked difference in outcomes between these two groups (P < 0.01).

REPRESENTATIVE CASE HISTORIES:

CASE 1[27]

The patient was a 57 year old female who was first examined on Jun. 25, 1998. This woman had had upper back sores accompanied by fever for 20 days and she had been diabetic for more than 10 years. Her body temperature was 38.4°C, and the welling abscess on her upper back was 15 x 10cm around and 1-2cm raised above the surface of the back. The center was filled with pus and its periphery was hard to the touch. The skin temperature was elevated, and pressure caused pain. The woman was diagnosed with upper back welling abscess and diabetes. After being admitted to the hospital, she was administered insulin to control her blood sugar and the welling abscess was surgically opened and the pus expelled. After this surgery, the woman was treated with antibiotics in order to prevent secondary infection. However, the wound opening did not heal and the woman continued to have a fever between 37.8-38.5°C. Therefore, she was referred for Chinese medicine.

At this woman's Chinese medical examination, there was lassitude of the spirit, fever in the afternoon, a dark colored sore on her upper back which was flat and exuded relatively copious pale yellow, thin, watery pus at the same time as dark red blood. Inside the mouth of the sore, there was relatively a lot of erosion. The woman's tongue was pale and tender with white, turbid, flowery, peeled fur, and her pulse was fine and rapid. Based on these signs and symptoms, the patient's Chinese medical pattern was categorized as yin vacuity and fire effulgence at the root. Blazing and exuberant fire toxins had consumed her qi and damaged her yin so that her righteous qi had become insufficient and unable to overcome and out-thrust evils externally. Therefore, the treatment principles were to supplement the qi and nourish yin, out-thrust toxins and expel pus. The formula prescribed wasof *Tuo Li Xiao Du Yin Jia Jian* (Out-thrust the Interior & Disperse Toxins Drink with Additions & Subtractions): Radix Codonopsitis Pilosulae (*Dang Shen*) and Tuber Ophiopogonis Japonici (*Mai Men Dong*), 12g each, Rhizoma Atractylodis Macrocephalae (*Bai Zhu*) and Flos Lonicerae Japonicae (*Jin Yin Hua*), 15g each, Radix Angelicae Sinensis (*Dang Gui*) and Radix Angelicae Dahuricae (*Bai Zhi*), 8g each, Radix Astragali Membranacei (*Huang Qi*), 40g, uncooked Radix Glycyrrhizae (*Gan Cao*) and Pericarpium Citri Reticulatae Viride (*Qing Pi*), 6g each, Rhizoma Cimicifugae (*Sheng Ma*), 4g, Spina Gleditschiae Chinensis (*Zao Jiao Ci*) and baked Squama Manitis Pentadactylis (*Chuan Shan Jia*), 10g each, and Sclerotium Poriae Cocos (*Fu Ling*), 30g.

After administering two *ji* of the above medicinals, the fever receded and the woman's affect improved. Her appetite gradually increased, the suppuration from the sore ceased, and the erosion decreased in size. The woman stopped taking the antibiotics and another 10 *ji* of these medicinals were administered with additions and subtractions, after which *Ba Zhen Tang Jia Jian* (Eight Pearls Decoction with Additions & Subtractions) was administered for one month. The erosion was slowly replaced by new tissue growth, the lesion completely healed, and the woman was discharged from the hospital.

CASE 2[28]

The patient was a 45 year old woman who had been diabetic for five years. Even though her blood sugar levels remained normal, she had experienced skin itching for the past year which disturbed her both day and night. Her skin was visibly scarred from scratching, and she was dizzy and fatigued. The woman had no appetite, complained of a bitter taste in her mouth, was both nauseated and constipated, and her urination was yellow and scanty. The color of the patient's skin was dark due to scratching. Her tongue was red with slimy, yellow fur, and her pulses were fine and rapid. The patient's Western medical diagnosis was cutaneous pruritus, and her Chinese medical pattern discrimi-

nation was yin vacuity with internal heat and accumulation of phlegm and dampness in the channels. The treatment principles were to clear heat, nourish yin, and transform phlegm and dampness. The medicinals prescribed were: Sclerotium Poriae Cocos (*Fu Ling*), 15g, Caulis Bambusae in Taeniis (*Zhu Ru*), Cortex Radicis Moutan (*Mu Dan Pi*), Fasciculus Vascularis Luffae (*Si Gua Luo*), Fructus Liquidambaris Taiwaniae (*Lu Lu Tong*), and Fructus Tribuli Terrestris (*Bai Ji Li*), 10g each, Rhizoma Pinelliae Ternatae (*Ban Xia*), wine-processed Radix Et Rhizoma Rhei (*Da Huang*), Pericarpium Citri Reticulatae (*Chen Pi*), Fructus Citri Aurantii (*Zhi Ke*), Periostracum Cicadae (*Chan Tui*), and Exuviae Serpentis (*She Tui*), 6g each, and Rhizoma Coptidis Chinensis (*Huang Lian*), 5g. This formula was decocted in water and administered orally, one *ji* each day for a week. After that, the itching and the other symptoms were much improved. Then an additional seven *ji* were prescribed omitting *Da Huang* and adding 10 grams each of Radix Anemarrhenae Aspheloidis (*Zhi Mu*) and Cortex Phellodendri (*Huang Bai*). After that, the patient's symptoms did not recur and her blood glucose and urine glucose levels remained normal.

CASE 3[29]

The patient was a 50 year old male cadre who was first examined on Jan. 17, 1992 and whose major complaints were polydipsia, polyuria, and emaciation for two years and an upper back abscess for the past three months. This patient had been addicted to drinking alcohol for many years. The abscess had been treated surgically in Oct. 1991 after it had become purulent. At this time, the patient's blood glucose was found to be high. Therefore, he was diagnosed with diabetes accompanied by cellulitis and he was treated by subdermal injections of insulin. However, the abscess did not heal and the man's blood glucose was not satisfactorily controlled. His FBG was 12.4mmol/L (224mg/dL) and urine glucose was (++++). At the time of his examination by Dr. Zhu, there was oral thirst and polydipsia, dryness and heat, sweating, a nonhealing upper back abscess, pruritus, and pricking pain in his four limbs which was difficult to bear and which disturbed his sleep at night. His hands and feet emitted coolness, there was lack of strength, frequent urination, and the man's stools were dry. The patient had a dark red tongue with slimy, white fur, and his pulse was slippery and rapid.

Based on these signs and symptoms, the man's Chinese medical patterns were categorized as qi and yin dual vacuity with dryness and heat entering the blood aspect or division and static blood obstructing the network vessels.

The treatment principles were to boost the qi and nourish yin, clear heat and cool the blood, and quicken the blood and free the flow of the network vessels. Therefore, he was given the following Chinese medicinals: uncooked Radix Astragali Membranacei (*Huang Qi*), 50g, Caulis Milletiae Seu Spatholobi (*Ji Xue Teng*), Herba Leonuri Heterophylli (*Yi Mu Cao*), Radix Scrophulariae Ningpoensis (*Xuan Shen*), uncooked Radix Rehmanniae (*Sheng Di*), and Radix Salviae Miltiorrhizae (*Dan Shen*), 30g each, Ramulus Loranthi Seu Visci (*Sang Ji Sheng*), 20g, Radix Puerariae (*Ge Gen*), 15g, Radix Scutellariae Baicalensis (*Huang Qin*), Fructus Lycii Chinensis (*Gou Qi Zi*), Ramulus Cinnamomi Cassiae (*Gui Zhi*), Radix Clematidis Chinensis (*Wei Ling Xian*), and Lignum Sappan (*Su Mu*), 10g each, and Rhizoma Coptidis Chinensis (*Huang Lian*), 6g. One *ji* of these medicinals was decocted in water and administered per day.

After taking these medicinals for one month, all the patient's symptoms had decreased, the upper back abscess had closed, FBG was 9.99mmol/L, and the amount of insulin the man used was reduced from 54 units to 26 units. However, the patient still had a sensation of piercing pain in the muscles of his four limbs which made it difficult for him to go to sleep. His tongue was pale red with thin, white fur, and his pulse was deep and slippery. Therefore, *Gui Zhi* was removed from his original formula and 15 grams each of Ramulus Uncariae Cum Uncis (*Gou Teng*) and Rhizoma Piperis Hancei (*Hai Feng Teng*) were added. After a month on this prescription, the man completely stopped taking his insulin and only continued with his Chinese herbs. His FBG went up to 14.59mmol/L and his urine glucose was (++++). He still had pricking pain in his four limbs as well as numbness and a cool sensation. At this point, Dr. Zhu increased the strength of the Chinese medicinal formula by adding more ingredients to free the flow of the network vessels but does not follow the case further (perhaps because of the patient's non-compliance with his insulin regime).

REMARKS:

1. For most diabetic skin disorders, external medicinal applications are as or even more important than internally administered medicinals. Except for abnormalities in perspiration and pruritus, acupuncture is not commonly used for these types of dermatological conditions.

2. For diabetic dermopathy, massage of the lower limbs may be used as adjunctive therapy. Likewise, for necrobiosis lipoidica diabeticorum, a warm water soak each evening and/or massage may help quicken the blood and free the flow of the network vessels. However, one should be careful that whatever massage techniques are used, they should not damage the skin.

3. After opening diabetic bullae, it is important to prevent secondary infection.

4. Patients with carotenemia should avoid eating carrots, yellow squash, and other foods with a lot of carotene as well as alcohol, sweet, fatty, and oily foods.

5. Patients with rubeosis of the cheeks and face or pruritus should avoid alcohol and acrid, hot, peppery foods. In addition, they should try to stay calm and not get too excited. The severity of pruritus is commonly closely related to emotional stress. Patients with diabetes and itching should take special care to not scratch their itches for fear of causing a wound which may then easily become infected due to the lowered immunity and slowed wound-healing which are characteristic of diabetes.

6. Patients with fungal infections should be careful to eat a clear, bland diet, avoiding all foods made through fermentation or which mold easily. For more information on the clear, bland diet of Chinese medicine, see Bob Flaws's *The Tao of Healthy Eating* also available from Blue Poppy Press.

ENDNOTES:

[1] www2.sw.org/dnet/manage/skin.htm
[2] www.powerpak.com/ce/skincare_pharm/lesson.cfm
[3] www.diabetic-lifestyle.com/articles/mar99_healt_1.htm
[4] www2.sw.org, *op. cit.*
[5] www.diabetic-lifestyle.com, op. cit.
[6] Perez, M.I. & Kohn, S.R., "Cutaneous Manifestations of Diabetes Mellitus," *Journal of the American Academy of Dermatology*, #30, 1994, p. 519-531
[7] www.emedicine.com/derm/topic62.htm
[8] www2.sw.org, *op. cit.*
[9] *Ibid.*
[10] www.powerpak.com, op. cit.
[11] www.skinsite.com/info_xanthomas.htm
[12] www.dermnet.org.nz/dna.granuloma.annulare/grananu.htm
[13] www.skinsite.com/info_granuloma_annulare.htm
[14] www.pedianet.com/news/illness/diseases/files/hypervit.htm
[15] www.saahip.org.za/conf/2000/d1.htm
[16] www.pslgroup.com/dg/1f69ae.htm
[17] www.colby-usa.com/chinese.htm
[18] For the treatment of dermatological conditions, external applications are usually more effective as adjunctive therapy than acupuncture.
[19] Blue Poppy Herbs' Cut & Sore Ointment is a version of *Sheng Ji Yu Huang Gao*.
[20] Blue Poppy Herbs' Stop Itching Tincture is a version of *Zhi Yang Ding*.
[21] Blue Poppy Herbs' Clear Heat Ointment is a version of *Si Huang Gao*.
[22] Blue Poppy Herbs' Anti-fungal Ointment is a version of *Qing Dai Gao*.
[23] As mentioned above, Blue Poppy Herbs' Clear Heat Ointment is a version of *Si Huang Gao*.
[24] *Ibid.*
[25] Blue Poppy Herbs' Cut & Sore Ointment is a version of *Sheng Ji Yu Huang Gao*.

[26] As mentioned above, Blue Poppy Herbs' Anti-fungal Ointment is a version of *Qing Dai Gao*.

[27] Liao Wei-ku & Lin Chun-yang, "Knowledge Gained from Experience in the Chinese Medical Pattern Discrimination Treatment of Diabetes Complicated by Upper Back Welling Abscesses," *Xin Zhong Yi (New Chinese Medicine)*, #3, 2001, p. 37

[28] Gao Lu-wen, "Regulating Qi and Resolving Phlegm to Treat the Complications of Diabetes," *Journal of Chinese Medicine*, #64, October 2000, p. 20-21

[29] Zhu Chen-zi, anthologized in Dan Shu-jian & Chen Zi-hua's *Xiao Ke Juan (The Wasting & Thirsting Book)*, Chinese National Chinese Medicine & Medicinals Publishing Co., Beijing, 1999, p. 123-125

21

DIABETIC HEART DISEASE

People with diabetes mellitus are 2-4 times more likely to get heart disease than nondiabetics,[1] 76% of deaths in diabetics are due to heart disease,[2] and four out of five patients with type 2 diabetes will die of cardiovascular disease. Diabetes is the most common cause of myocardial infarction (MI) in persons under 30 years of age in the United States.[3] Both insulin-dependent and non-insulin-dependent diabetes mellitus are associated with earlier and more extensive development of atherosclerosis as part of a widespread metabolic derangement including dyslipidemia and glycosylation of the connective tissue. Elevated levels of low density lipoprotein (LDL) and reduced levels of high density lipoprotein (HDL) predispose one to atherosclerosis, and diabetes accelerates the oxidative process. In addition, high levels of insulin in the blood damage the vascular endothelium resulting in vasoconstriction and hypertension. Further, in diabetes, there is an overall procoagulant state with impaired fibrinolysis which promotes the formation of ischemic clots around atherosclerotic plaque. Diabetes mellitus especially puts women at a higher risk of developing coronary artery disease (CAD) and significantly negates the otherwise protective effect of female hormones. Women with diabetes are 3-7 times more likely to develop heart disease than women without diabetes,[4] while men with diabetes are only three times as likely to develop heart disease than men without diabetes.[5]

Although diabetic heart disease may initially be asymptomatic, symptoms of diabetic heart disease may include heart dysrhythmias and chest pain. The discomfort of angina pectoris is highly variable. It is most commonly felt beneath the sternum as a vague ache. However, it may initially manifest as or rapidly become a severe, intense precordial crushing sensation. Pain may radiate to the left shoulder and down the inside of the left arm possibly reaching the fingers. More rarely, this pain may also radiate straight through to the interscapular area. In addition, it sometimes radiates to the throat, jaws, teeth, and even occasionally down the right arm. These variegated manifestations of coronary ischemia are due to the so-called "T2-T12 syndrome" in which different somatic nerve segments intermingle with each other and with visceral nerves. Typical angina pectoris is characteristically triggered by physical activity or emotional intensity and usually lasts only a few minutes, subsiding with rest. It is even more easily triggered by exercise following a meal and is also triggered by exposure to cold causing vasospasm or constriction of a partially blocked vessel. In some patients, angina may occur at night when resting or asleep. Attacks may vary in frequency from several per day to occasional attacks separated by asymptomatic intervals of weeks, months, or even years. Since the symptoms of angina are usually constant for a given individual (due to the constant level of obstruction, provided it is due to stable plaque), any change or worsening in the pattern of these symptoms should be viewed as a poor prognosis.

The Western medical diagnosis of CAD is based on the patient's symptoms, if any, listening to the heart sounds with a stethoscope, an ischemic pattern on serial ECG, exercise tolerance testing, coronary arteriography, and radionuclide studies. Western medical treatment of CAD consists of diet and exercise plus prophylatic and remedial use of nitrate vasodilators, such as sublingual nitroglycerin, beta-adrenergic blocking agents, calcium channel blockers, antiplatelet drugs, such as aspirin, coronary arterial bypass surgery, and angioplasty or, especially in those with diabetes, coronary grafting. Prognosis is determined by age, extent of coronary disease, severity of symptoms, left ventricular function, and the presence of arrhythmia. For instance, men with CAD with angina but no history of myocardial infarction, normal blood pressure, and a normal resting ECG have an annual mortality rate of 1.4%, while men with CAD with systolic hypertension and an abnormal ECG have a 12% annual mortality rate.

RISK FACTORS FOR THE DEVELOPMENT OF DIABETIC CAD

1. Systolic hypertension
2. Obesity (>120 percent desirable body weight); BMI > 28 in women or > 27.3 in men
3. Microalbuminuria
4. Cholesterol >200 mg/dL (5.17mmol/L)
5. LDL cholesterol >130mg/dL (3.36mmol/L)
6. HDL cholesterol <40mg/dL (1.03mmol/L)
7. Triglycerides >250mg/dL (2.82mmol/L)

Kenneth L. Williams, author of the San Antonio Heart Study has devised a point system for the stratification of CAD risk. Since this system is easy to calculate, it is given below.

RISK FACTOR	POINTS
1. Age: 35-44 years	8
45-54 years	18
55 or older	25
2. Parent or sibling with diabetes	4
3. Parent or sibling with myocardial infarction	4
4. Fasting blood sugar of 110mg/dL or more	17
5. Systolic blood pressure 160mm Hg or more or diastolic blood pressure of 90mm Hg or more	10
6. HDL cholesterol of 35mg/dL or less	8
7. Triglycerides above 150mg/dL	10
8. Overweight for height (see below)	10
9. Overweight for height (weight greater than specfied range)	21

SPECIFIED RANGES	
Height	Overweight
5'0"	128-153 pounds
5'2"	136-164 pounds
5'5"	150-180 pounds
5'8"	164-197 pounds
5'11"	179-215 pounds
6'2"	194-233 pounds

SCORE

100 points = 95% risk in 8 years
80 points = 88% risk in 8 years
65 points = 68% risk in 8 years
50 points = 40% risk in 8 years
20 points = 5% risk in 8 years

CHINESE DISEASE MECHANISMS:

In the early stage, most commonly there is a qi and yin vacuity complicated almost universally by liver depression and some sort of heat evils. Because of yin detriment and qi consumption, the heart qi is insufficient, and the heart vessels lose their nourishment. Internal heat or yang hyperactivity may ascend to burn the heart and lungs. Such heat evils may then harass and cause chaos to the heart spirit. Heart qi vacuity and heart loss of nourishment may lead to heart palpitations due to diminished function of the heart in terms of the heart's promoting the stirring and movement of the blood within the vessels. In addition, if heart yang qi is insufficient and qi transformation loses its command, water fluids may not obtain downward movement but rather collect below the heart. This may result in palpitations and stirring below the heart. If the heart qi is insufficient and the movement of the blood is uneasy or unsmooth, the blood vessels may become impeded and obstructed. This may then result in chest oppression, heart palpitations, shortness of breath, spontaneous perspiration, and fearful throbbing. All these symptoms are mostly a reflection of simultaneous lung-kidney qi vacuity with loss of duty of diffusion and depuration and heart-spleen dual vacuity and loss of nourishment of the heart.

In the middle stage, enduring qi and yin vacuity lead to a dual yin and yang vacuity. In that case, qi and yin taxation detriment with heart qi and yang vacuity engender static blood and internal phlegm turbidity which in turn impedes and obstructs the heart vessels. If heart, spleen, and kidney yang qi is insufficient, this must result in the loss of the smooth movement of blood and in the inability of fluids and humors to be transformed. Static blood obstructs internally, while phlegm turbidity collects and gathers. Yin cold congeals and stagnates, and the qi mechanism becomes obstructed and stagnant. Hence the heart vessels are impeded and obstructed, and the symptoms of blood stasis become prominent. In terms of blood stasis, it should be kept in mind that qi vacuity failing to stir the blood may lead to blood stasis. Heat burning the fluids and humors and thus making the blood sticky and stagnant may lead to blood stasis. Qi stagnation not moving the blood may lead to blood stasis. Cold congelation may lead to blood stasis, and phlegm dampness obstructing the network vessels may also lead to blood stasis.

In the late stage, qi and blood and yin and yang are all typically vacuous. Heart yang is vacuous and in decline, and water rheum is harassing the heart and assailing the lungs. With heart yang vacuity and decline, one can see heart palpitations, fearful throbbing, chest oppression, and shortness of breath. If yang vacuity leads to the engenderment of cold internally, cold may congeal the blood vessels. Lack of free flow then leads to pain. Thus one can see heart pain. If there is heart-kidney yang decline, yang may not transform yin and rheum evils may impede and obstruct the heart vessels. This may result in even more severe heart and chest pain as well as lack of warmth in the four extremities. If the kidneys fail to grasp or absorb the qi and the lung qi counterflows upward, this may result in panting respiration and inability to lie horizontally. If this is severe, there may be qi panting, flaring nostrils, gaping mouth, and raised shoulders when breathing, counterflow chilling and cyanosis of the four extremities, scanty urination, water swelling (or edema), and dark lips. If yang qi is on the verge of desertion, one may see massive sweating, reversal chilling of the four extremities, and a faint pulse on the verge of expiry. In the late stage of diabetic heart disease, although one may see many symptoms of a number of different viscera and bowels suffering detriment, heart-kidney yang decline is the primary pattern.

TREATMENT BASED ON PATTERN DISCRIMINATION:

1. YIN VACUITY WITH DRY HEAT AND DISQUIETUDE OF THE HEART SPIRIT PATTERN

MAIN SYMPTOMS: Heart palpitations, easy fright, heart vexation, insomnia, dry mouth, parched throat, dry, bound stools, vexatious heat in the five hearts (or centers), possible vexatious thirst and polydipsia, possible rapid hungering and polyphagia, a red tongue with scanty fur, and a floating, fine or large, rapid pulse

TREATMENT PRINCIPLES: Enrich yin and clear heat, nourish the heart and quiet the spirit

RX: *Tian Wang Bu Xin Dan* (Heavenly Emperor Supplement the Heart Elixir) plus *Xiao Ke Fang* (Wasting Thirst Formula) with additions and subtractions

INGREDIENTS: Radix Salviae Miltiorrhizae (*Dan Shen*), 30g, uncooked Radix Rehmanniae (*Sheng Di*), Radix Scrophulariae Ningpoensis (*Xuan Shen*), Semen Zizyphi Spinosae (*Suan Zao Ren*), and Radix Trichosanthis Kirlowii (*Tian Hua Fen*), 15g each, Tuber Asparagi Cochinensis (*Tian Men Dong*), Tuber Ophiopogonis Japonici (*Mai Men Dong*), Cortex Radicis Moutan (*Dan Pi*), Radix Angelicae Sinensis (*Dang Gui*), Radix Polygalae Tenuifoliae (*Yuan Zhi*), Semen Biotae Oreintalis (*Bai Zi Ren*), and Fructus Schisandrae Chinensis (*Wu Wei Zi*), 9g each, Rhizoma Coptidis Chinensis (*Huang Lian*), 6g

FORMULA ANALYSIS: *Sheng Di, Xuan Shen, Tian Men Dong,* and *Mai Men Dong* enrich and nourish heart yin. *Dang Gui* and *Dan Shen* nourish and quicken the blood. *Dang Gui* primarily nourishes the blood and secondarily quickens it, while *Dan Shen* primarily quickens the blood and secondarily nourishes it. *Suan Zao Ren, Yuan Zhi, Wu Wei Zi,* and *Bai Zi Ren* nourish the heart and quiet the spirit. *Huang Lian* and *Dan Pi* clear the heart and drain heat. *Dan Pi* also helps *Dang Gui* and *Dan Shen* quicken the blood. *Tian Hua Fen* engenders fluids and stops thirst.

ADDITIONS & SUBTRACTIONS: If there is simultaneous shortness of breath, lack of strength, a fat tongue, and other such signs and symptoms of heart qi vacuity, add 15 grams of Radix Astragali Membrancei (*Huang Qi*) and 9-12 grams of mix-fried Radix Glycyrrhizae (*Gan Cao*) to supplement and boost the heart qi. If there is concomitant liver depression qi stagnation, add *Si Ni San* (Four Counterflows Powder) to course the liver and rectify the qi: Radix Bupleuri (*Chai Hu*) and Radix Albus Paeoniae Lactiflorae (*Bai Shao*), 9g each, Fructus Immaturus Citri Aurantii (*Zhi Ke*), 6g, and Radix Glycyrrhizae (*Gan Cao*), 3-6g. If there is constipation, add nine grams of Semen Trichosanthis Kirlowii (*Gua Lou Ren*) and wine-fried Radix Et Rhizoma Rhei (*Da Huang*) to free the flow of the bowels. If there is a dry mouth and polydipsia, add 15 grams of uncooked Gypsum Fibrosum (*Shi Gao*) and nine grams of Rhizoma Anemarrhenae Aspheloidis (*Zhi Mu*).

If there is heart blood debility and vacuity as well as heart qi insufficiency with heart palpitations and a bound or regularly intermittent pulse, use *Zhi Gan Cao Tang* (Mix-fried Licorice Decoction) instead to boost the qi and nourish the blood, enrich yin and recover the pulse: uncooked Radix Rehmanniae (*Sheng Di*), 20g, mix-fried Radix Glycyrrhizae (*Gan Cao*) and Tuber Ophiopogonis Japonici (*Mai Men Dong*), 12g each, Gelatinum Corii Asini (*E Jiao*) and Semen Cannabis Sativae (*Huo Ma Ren*), 9g each, Radix Panacis Ginseng (*Ren Shen*) and Ramulus Cinnamomi Cassiae (*Gui Zhi*), 6g each, uncooked Rhizoma Zingiberis (*Sheng Jiang*), 2-3 slices, and Fructus Zizyphi Jujubae (*Da Zao*), 3-5 pieces.

If there are heart palpitations, shortness of breath, lassitude of the spirit, lack of strength, torpid intake, loose stools, and other such signs and symptoms of heart-spleen dual vacuity, one can use *Gui Pi Tang* (Restore the Spleen Decoction) to fortify the spleen and nourish the heart: Radix Astragali Membranacei (*Huang Qi*), 15g, Semen Zizyphi Spinosae (*Suan Zao Ren*), Arillus Euphoriae Longanae (*Long Yan Rou*), and Sclerotium Poriae Cocos (*Fu Ling*), 12g each, Radix Angelicae Sinensis (*Dang Gui*), Rhizoma Atractylodis Macrocephalae (*Bai Zhu*), and Radix Polygalae Tenuifoliae (*Yuan Zhi*), 9g each, Radix Panacis Ginseng (*Ren Shen*), Radix Auklandiae Lappae (*Mu Xiang*), and mix-fried Radix Glycyrrhizae (*Gan Cao*), 6g each, uncooked Rhizoma Zingiberis (*Sheng Jiang*), 2-3 slices, and Fructus Zizyphi Jujubae (*Da Zao*), 3-5 pieces.

If there is concomitant liver blood-kidney yin vacuity with low back and knee soreness and limpness, dizziness, tinnitus, heart palpitations, and insomnia, one can use *Yi Guan Jian* (One Link Decoction) plus *Suan Zao Ren Tang* (Zizyphus Decoction) to enrich and nourish the liver and kidneys at the same time as nourishing the heart and quieting the spirit: uncooked Radix Rehmanniae (*Sheng Di*) and Semen Zizyphi Spinosae (*Suan Zao Ren*), 15g each, Tuber Ophiopogonis Japonici (*Mai Men Dong*) and Sclerotium Poriae Cocos (*Fu Ling*), 12g each, Radix Glehniae Littoralis (*Sha Shen*), Radix Angelicae Sinensis (*Dang Gui*), Fructus Lycii Chinensis (*Gou Qi Zi*), Fructus Meliae Toosendan (*Chuan Lian Zi*), and Rhizoma Anemarrhenae Aspheloidis (*Zhi Mu*), 9g each, and Radix Glycyrrhizae (*Gan Cao*), 3-6g.

ACUPUNCTURE & MOXIBUSTION: *Tai Xi* (Ki 3), *San Yin Jiao* (Sp 6), *Shen Men* (Ht 7), *Nei Guan* (Per 6), *Dan Zhong* (CV 17), *Jue Yin Shu* (Bl 14), *Xin Shu* (Bl 15), *Nei Ting* (St 44)

FORMULA ANALYSIS: Supplementing *Tai Xi* and *San Yin Jiao* supplements the spleen, liver, and kidneys and enriches yin. Even supplementing-even draining *Shen Men*, *Nei Guan*, *Dan Zhong*, *Jue Yin Shu*, and *Xin Shu* nourishes the heart and quiets the spirit. Draining *Nei Ting* clears heat from the yang ming.

ADDITIONS & SUBTRACTIONS: If there is marked spleen qi vacuity, add supplementing *Tai Bai* (Sp 3) and *Pi Shu* (Bl 20). If there is liver depression qi stagnation, add draining *Tai Chong* (Liv 3) and *He Gu* (LI 4). If there is vexatious thirst, add supplementing *Zhao Hai* (Ki 6) and *Lie Que* (Lu 7).

2. QI & YIN DUAL VACUITY WITH LOSS OF NOURISHMENT OF THE HEART VESSELS PATTERN

MAIN SYMPTOMS: Chest oppression, heart palpitations, shortness of breath, lack of strength, dry mouth, dry stools, possible vexatious heat in the five hearts, possible spontaneous perspiration, a fat, dark tongue with white fur, and a fine, forceless, possibly rapid pulse

NOTE: The difference between this and the previous pattern is that, in pattern #1, symptoms of nonconstruction and malnourishment of the spirit with disquietude are primary, while in this pattern, symptoms of chest oppression, heart palpitations, and shortness of breath are primary.

TREATMENT PRINCIPLES: Boost heart qi and nourish heart yin, loosen the chest and recover the pulse

RX: *Sheng Mai San Jia Jian* (Engender the Pulse Powder with Additions & Subtractions)

INGREDIENTS: Rhizoma Polygonati (*Huang Jing*) and Radix Salviae Miltiorrhizae (*Dan Shen*), 30g each, Radix Trichosanthis Kirlowii (*Tian Hua Fen*), 20g, Radix Pseudostellariae Heterophyllae (*Tai Zi Shen*) and uncooked Radix Rehmanniae (*Sheng Di*), 15g each, Tuber Ophiopogonis Japonici (*Mai Men Dong*), Semen Zizyphi Spinosae (*Suan Zao Ren*), and Polygoni Multiflori (*He Shou Wu*), 12g each, Fructus Schisandrae Chinensis (*Wu Wei Zi*) and Radix Puerariae (*Ge Gen*), 9g each

FORMULA ANALYSIS: *Huang Jing, Tai Zi Shen, Sheng Di, Mai Men Dong, He Shou Wu, Suan Zao Ren*, and *Wu Wei Zi* boost the qi and nourish yin. *Tian Hua Fen* clears heat, engenders fluids, and loosens the chest, while *Ge Gen* upbears the clear and engenders fluids. *Dan Shen* quickens and nourishes the blood.

ADDITIONS & SUBTRACTIONS: If there is qi and yin vacuity with marked liver depression, use *Jie Yu Shu Xin Tang* (Resolve Depression & Soothe the Heart Decoction): Radix Pseudostellariae Heterophyllae (*Tai Zi Shen*) and Tuber Ophiopogonis Japonici (*Mai Men Dong*), 12g each, Fructus Schisdandrae Chinensis (*Wu Wei Zi*), Rhizoma Cyperi Rotundi (*Xiang Fu*), and Radix Salviae Miltiorrhizae (*Dan Shen*), 9g each, Radix Platycodi Grandiflori (*Jie Geng*), Fructus Citri Aurantii (*Zhi Ke*), and Semen Raphani Sativi (*Lai Fu Zi*), 6g each, and Fructus Citri Sacrodactylis (*Fo Shou*) and Flos Rosae Rugosae (*Mei Gui Hua*), 3g each.

ACUPUNCTURE & MOXIBUSTION: Same as for pattern #1 above.

3. QI & YIN DUAL VACUITY WITH QI STAGNATION & BLOOD STASIS PATTERN

MAIN SYMPTOMS: Same as pattern #2 above plus chest and/or stomach duct pain, a dark tongue or possible static macules and/or spots, dark, engorged, tortuous sublingual veins, and a fine, bowstring and/or choppy pulse

TREATMENT PRINCIPLES: Boost the qi and nourish yin, move the qi and quicken the blood

RX: *Huang Dan Tang* (Polygonatum & Salvia Decoction)

INGREDIENTS: Rhizoma Polygonati (*Huang Jing*) and Radix Salviae Miltiorrhizae (*Dan Shen*), 30g each, Radix Astragali Membranacei (*Huang Qi*) and uncooked Radix Rehmanniae (*Sheng Di*), 15g each, Radix Pseudostellariae Heterophyllae (*Tai Zi Shen*) and Radix Scrophulariae Ningpoensis (*Xuan Shen*), 12g each, Semen Pruni Persicae (*Tao Ren*), Radix Ligustici Wallichii (*Chuan Xiong*), Fructus Immaturus Citri Aurantii (*Zhi Shi*), Fructus Citri Sacrodactylis (*Fo Shou*), and Radix Puerariae (*Ge Gen*), 9g each

FORMULA ANALYSIS: *Tai Zi Shen, Huang Jing, Huang Qi, Sheng Di,* and *Xuan Shen* boost the qi and nourish yin. *Dan Shen, Tao Ren,* and *Chuan Xiong* quicken the blood, dispel stasis, and free the flow of the vessels. *Zhi Shi* and *Fo Shou* rectify the qi and stop pain. *Ge Gen* upbears fluids and stops thirst.

ADDITIONS & SUBTRACTIONS: If there is concomitant angina pain, add 15 grams of Rhizoma Corydalis Yanhusuo (*Yan Hu Suo*) and nine grams of Lignum Dalbergiae Odoriferae (*Jiang Xiang*) to rectify the qi, quicken the blood, and stop pain. If qi stagnation is marked, add nine grams each of Fructus Trichosanthis Kirlowii (*Gua Lou*), Flos Rosae Rugosae (*Mei Gui Hua*), and Flos Pruni Mume (*Lu E Mei*). If there is dizziness and heart palpitations, add 12 grams each of uncooked Concha Ostreae (*Mu Li*), Os Draconis (*Long Gu*), Concha Margaritiferae (*Zhen Zhu Mu*), and/or Dens Draconis (*Long Chi*) to settle and subdue. If there are heart palpitations, vexation and agitation, a red tongue, and a fine, rapid pulse, add 3-6 grams of Rhizoma Coptidis Chinensis (*Huang Lian*) and nine grams each of Cortex Radicis Moutan (*Dan Pi*) and Fructus Gardeniae Jasminoidis (*Zhi Zi*) to clear the heart and drain fire. If there is simultaneous bilateral lower limb pain, one can

add nine grams each of Rhizoma Cibotii Barometsis (*Gou Ji*), Radix Achyranthis Bidentae (*Niu Xi*), and Fructus Chaenomelis Lagenariae (*Mu Gua*).

If there is more qi vacuity than yin vacuity as well as marked blood stasis, use *Yi Qi Huo Xue Fang* (Boost the Qi & Quicken the Blood Formula): Radix Astragali Membranacei (*Huang Qi*), 40g, Radix Codonopsitis Pilosulae (*Dang Shen*), 30g, Radix Angelicae Sinensis (*Dang Gui*) and Radix Rubrus Paeoniae Lactiflorae (*Chi Shao*), 20g each, Radix Ligustici Wallichii (*Chuan Xiong*), Radix Salviae Miltiorrhizae (*Dan Shen*), Radix Puerariae (*Ge Gen*), Tuber Ophiopogonis Japonici (*Mai Men Dong*), and Fructus Schisandrae Chinensis (*Wu Wei Zi*), 15g each, and Flos Carthami Tinctorii (*Hong Hua*), 9g. If there is concomitant liver depression qi stagnation, add nine grams each of Fructus Citri Sacrodactylis (*Fo Shou*) and Radix Auklandiae Lappae (*Mu Xiang*).

If there are fire evils and heat binding in the chest and center with burning pain in the heart and/or stomach, dry mouth, vexation and agitation, and constipation, one can use *Xiao Xian Xiong Tang* (Minor Sunken Chest Decoction) plus *Zeng Ye Cheng Qi Tang* (Increase Humors Order the Qi Decoction): Radix Scrophulariae Ningpoensis (*Xuan Shen*), 30g, Tuber Ophiopogonis Japonici (*Mai Men Dong*) and uncooked Radix Rehmanniae (*Sheng Di*), 24g each, Semen Trichosanthis Kirlowii (*Gua Lou Ren*), 12g, Rhizoma Pinelliae Ternatae (*Ban Xia*) and Radix Et Rhizoma Rhei (*Da Huang*), 9g each, Mirabilitum (*Mang Xiao*), 3-6g, and Rhizoma Coptidis Chinensis (*Huang Lian*), 3g.

ACUPUNCTURE & MOXIBUSTION: *Tai Xi* (Ki 3), *Tai Bai* (Sp 3), *San Yin Jiao* (Sp 6), *Pi Shu* (Bl 20), *Shen Shu* (Bl 23), *Tai Chong* (Liv 3), *He Gu* (LI 4), *Xue Hai* (Sp 10)

FORMULA ANALYSIS: Supplementing *Tai Xi* and *Shen Shu* supplements the kidneys and nourishes yin. Supplementing *Tai Bai* and *Pi Shu* fortifies the spleen and boosts the qi. Supplementing *San Yin Jiao* supplements the spleen and kidneys. Draining *Tai Chong* and *He Gu* courses the liver and rectifies the qi, while draining *He Gu* and *Xue Hai* quickens the blood and transforms stasis.

ADDITIONS & SUBTRACTIONS: For chest pain and/or palpitations, add *Nei Guan* (Per 6), *Dan Zhong* (CV 17), *Jue Yin Shu* (Bl 14), and *Xin Shu* (Bl 15). For heat harassing the heart, add *Da Ling* (Per 7). If this heat is depressive heat, drain *Xing Jian* (Liv 2) and omit *Tai Chong*. If this heat is yang ming heat, drain *Nei Ting* (St 44). For heart palpitations, add *Jian Shi* (Per 5). If there is dizziness, drain *Bai Hui* (GV 20) and *Feng Chi* (GB 20).

4. HEART QI YANG VACUITY WITH PHLEGM & STASIS MUTUALLY OBSTRUCTING

MAIN SYMPTOMS: Chest oppression, heart palpitations, precordial pain, fear of cold, chilled limbs, shortness of breath, lack of strength, possible blurred vision, possible numbness and pain of the extremities, possible lower limb edema, a fat, dark tongue with slimy, white fur, and a deep, slippery, possibly bound or regularly intermittent pulse

TREATMENT PRINCIPLES: Supplement the qi and invigorate yang, transform phlegm and dispel stasis

RX: *Sheng Mai San* (Engender the Pulse Powder) plus *Gua Lou Cong Bai Ban Xia Tang* (Trischosanthes, Allium & Pinellia Decoction) with additions and subtractions

INGREDIENTS: Radix Salviae Miltiorrhizae (*Dan Shen*), 30g, Fructus Trichosanthis Kirlowii (*Gua Lou*), 20g, Tuber Ophiopogonis Japonici (*Mai Men Dong*), 12g, Fructus Schisandrae Chinensis (*Wu Wei Zi*), Bulbus Allii (*Cong Bai*), Ramulus Cinnamomi Cassiae (*Gui Zhi*), Pericarpium Citri Reticulatae (*Chen Pi*), Rhizoma Pinelliae Ternatae (*Ban Xia*), Radix Angelicae Sinensis (*Dang Gui*), Fructus Citri Sacrodactylis (*Fo Shou*), 9g each, Radix Panacis Ginseng (*Ren Shen*), 6g

FORMULA ANALYSIS: *Ren Shen, Mai Men Dong,* and *Wu Wei Zi* boost the qi and nourish the heart. *Gui Zhi* and *Cong Bai* free the flow of yang and diffuse impediment. *Gua Lou* and *Ban Xia* transform phlegm. *Chen Pi, Fo Shou, Dang Gui,* and *Dan Shen* rectify the qi and quicken the blood.

ADDITIONS & SUBTRACTIONS: If there is concomitant heart-kidney yang vacuity, combine with *Shen Qi Wan* (Kidney Qi Pills) in order to warm and supplement heart-kidney yang. Practically speaking, this means to add 12 grams of cooked Radix Rehmanniae (*Shu Di*), nine grams each of Radix Dioscoreae Oppositae (*Shan Yao*), Fructus Corni Officinalis (*Shan Zhu Yu*), Sclerotium Poriae Cocos (*Fu Ling*), Cortex Radicis Moutan (*Dan Pi*), and Rhizoma Alismatis (*Ze Xie*), and 3-6 grams of Radix Lateralis Praeparatus Aconiti Carmichaeli (*Fu Zi*). If phlegm turbidity tends to be exuberant, combine with *Di Tan Tang* (Flush Phlegm Decoction) in order to transform phlegm turbidity. Practically speaking, this means to add 12 grams of Caulis Bambusae In Taeniis (*Zhu Ru*), nine grams of Rhizoma Acori Graminei (*Shi Chang Pu*), six grams each of Fructus Immaturus Citri Aurantii (*Zhi Shi*) and bile-treated Rhizoma Arisaematis (*Dan Nan Xing*), and three grams of Radix Glycyrrhizae (*Gan Cao*). Also

substitute Pericarpium Citri Erythrocarpae (*Ju Hong*) for *Chen Pi*. If blood stasis is marked, add nine grams each of Flos Carthami Tinctorii (*Hong Hua*), Radix Rubrus Paeoniae Lactiflorae (*Chi Shao*), and Radix Ligustici Wallichii (*Chuan Xiong*). If there is simultaneous faint swelling in both lower limbs, one can add nine grams each of Herba Leonuri Heterophylli (*Yi Mu Cao*), Herba Lycopi Lucidi (*Ze Lan*), and Sclerotium Polypori Umbellati (*Zhu Ling*) in order to quicken the blood, disinhibit water, and disperse swelling.

If phlegm turbidity transforms heat, *Huang Lian Wen Dan Tang Jia Wei* (Coptis Warm the Gallbladder Decoction with Added Flavors) to clear heat and transform phlegm: Caulis Bambusae In Taeniis (*Zhu Ru*) and Sclerotium Poriae Cocos (*Fu Ling*), 12g each, Rhizoma Pinelliae Ternatae (*Ban Xia*), Pericarpium Citri Reticulatae (*Chen Pi*), Rhizoma Acori Graminei (*Shi Chang Pu*), Tuber Curcumae (*Yu Jin*), 9g each, Fructus Immaturus Citri Aurantii (*Zhi Shi*), Rhizoma Coptidis Chinensis (*Huang Lian*), 3-6g each, Radix Glycyrrhizae (*Gan Cao*), 3g, and Fructus Zizyphi Jujubae (*Da Zao*), 3-5 pieces.

If cold has congealed the heart vessels, one can use *Dang Gui Si Ni Tang* (Dang Gui Four Counterflows Decoction) in order to dispel cold, quicken the blood, and free the flow of the vessels: Radix Albus Paeoniae Lactiflorae (*Bai Shao*), 15g, Radix Angelicae Sinensis (*Dang Gui*) and Ramulus Cinnamomi Cassiae (*Gui Zhi*), 12g each, Caulis Akebiae (*Mu Tong*), 9g, mix-fried Radix Glycyrrhizae (*Gan Cao*), 6g, Herba Asari Cum Radice (*Xi Xin*), 3-6g, and Fructus Zizyphi Jujubae (*Da Zao*), 3-5 pieces.

If there is phlegm and stasis mutually obstructing but no symptoms of cold, use *Guan Tong Tang* (Coronary-freeing Decoction): Fructus Trichosanthis Kirlowii (*Gua Lou*) and Tuber Curcumae (*Yu Jin*), 15g each, Rhizoma Cyperi Rotundi (*Xiang Fu*), 9-15g, Radix Salviae Miltiorrhizae (*Dan Shen*), stir-fried Radix Rubrus Paeoniae Lactiflorae (*Chi Shao*), and Rhizoma Corydalis Yanhusuo (*Yan Hu Suo*), 9g each, Semen Pruni Persicae (*Tao Ren*), 4.5-9g, Radix Polygalae Tenuifoliae (*Yuan Zhi*), 6g, mix-fried Radix Glycyrrhizae (*Gan Cao*) and Lignum Dalbergiae Odoriferae (*Jiang Xiang*), 3g each. If there is concomitant qi vacuity, add 15 grams of Radix Astragali Membranacei (*Huang Qi*) and 12 grams of Radix Codonopsitis Pilosulae (*Dang Shen*). If there is qi and yin dual vacuity, add 12 grams of Tuber Ophiopogonis Japonici (*Mai Men Dong*) and nine grams each of Radix Pseudostellariae Heterophyllae (*Tai Zi Shen*) and Fructus Schisandrae Chinensis (*Wu Wei Zi*). If chest oppression is severe, add nine grams each of

Fructus Citri Sacrodactylis (*Fo Shou*), Bulbus Allii (*Cong Bai*), and Lignum Santali Albi (*Tan Xiang*). If there are heart palpitations, add 12 grams each of Semen Zizyphi Spinosae (*Suan Zao Ren*) and Sclerotium Poriae Cocos (*Fu Ling*). If there is high cholesterol due to damp heat obstructing and stagnating, add 15 grams of Herba Artemisiae Capillaris (*Yin Chen Hao*) and nine grams of Rhizoma Alismatis (*Ze Xie*).

ACUPUNCTURE & MOXIBUSTION: *Zu San Li* (St 36), *Feng Long* (St 40), *Dan Zhong* (CV 17), *Zhong Wan* (CV 12), *Jue Yin Shu* (Bl 14), *Xin Shu* (Bl 15), *He Gu* (LI 4), *San Yin Jiao* (Sp 6)

FORMULA ANALYSIS: Even supplementing-even draining *Zu San Li*, *He Gu*, and *Zhong Wan* rectifies the qi mechanism of the entire body. Even supplementing-even draining *Zu San Li* and *San Yin Jiao* fortifies the spleen and boosts the qi. Even supplementing-even draining *He Gu* and *San Yin Jiao* quickens the blood and transforms stasis. Even supplementing-even draining *Feng Long* and *Zhong Wan* transforms phlegm. Even supplementing-even draining *Dan Zhong*, *Jue Yin Shu*, and *Xin Shu* regulates and rectifies the heart qi.

ADDITIONS & SUBTRACTIONS: If there is heart-kidney yang vacuity, add moxibustion at *Xin Shu* (Bl 15), *Shen Shu* (Bl 23), and *Guan Yuan* (CV 4). If there is phlegm heat, drain *Xing Jian* (Liv 2). If there is concomitant yin vacuity, add supplementing *Tai Xi* (Ki 3). If there is cold congelation, moxa *Dan Zhong* (CV 17). If there is faint swelling in both lower limbs, add draining *Yin Ling Quan* (Sp 9).

5. HEART QI YANG DECLINE WITH WATER RHEUM ATTACKING THE HEART AND ASSAILING THE LUNGS PATTERN

MAIN SYMPTOMS: Heart palpitations, shortness of breath, chest oppression, panting, inability to lie horizontally, fear of cold, chilled limbs, low back and knee soreness and limpness, bilateral lower extremity water swelling, possible blurred vision, possible torpid intake and/or diarrhea, a fat, pale but dark tongue with glossy, white fur, and a deep, fine, rapid pulse

TREATMENT PRINCIPLES: Boost the qi and nourish the heart, depurate the lungs and disinhibit water

RX: *Sheng Mai San* (Engender the Pulse Powder) plus *Ting Li Da Zao Xie Fei Tang* (Lepidium & Red Date Drain the Lungs Decoction) with additions and subtractions

INGREDIENTS: Semen Lepidii Seu Descurainiae (*Ting Li Zi*), Sclerotium Polypori Umbellati (*Zhu Ling*), Sclerotium Poriae Cocos (*Fu Ling*), and Radix Astragali Membranacei (*Huang Qi*), 30g each, Herba Lycopi Lucidi (*Ze Lan*) and Rhizoma Alismatis (*Ze Xie*), 15g each, Cortex Radicis Mori Albi (*Sang Bai Pi*) and Tuber Ophiopogonis Japonici (*Mai Men Dong*), 12g each, Radix Panacis Ginseng (*Ren Shen*), Fructus Schisandrae Chinensis (*Wu Wei Zi*), Ramulus Cinnamomi Cassiae (*Gui Zhi*), Radix Angelicae Sinensis (*Dang Gui*), and Semen Plantaginis (*Che Qian Zi*), 9g each, Fructus Zizyphi Jujubae (*Da Zao*), 5 pieces

FORMULA ANALYSIS: *Ren Shen*, *Huang Qi*, *Wu Wei Zi*, and *Mai Men Dong* boost the qi and nourish the heart. *Ting Li Zi* and *Sang Bai Pi* depurate the lungs and expel rheum, strengthen the heart and disinhibit urination. *Zhu Ling*, *Fu Ling*, *Ze Xie*, *Ze Lan*, *Che Qian Zi*, *Gui Zhi*, and *Dang Gui* warm yang and quicken the blood, disinhibit water and disperse swelling.

ADDITIONS & SUBTRACTIONS: If there is heart-kidney yang vacuity with water rheum attacking above, one can combine with *Zhen Wu Tang* (True Warrior Decoction). Practically speaking, this means adding 9-12 grams of Radix Lateralis Praeparatus Aconiti Carmichaeli (*Fu Zi*), nine grams each of Radix Albus Paeoniae Lactiflorae (*Bai Shao*) and Rhizoma Atractylodis Macrocephalae (*Bai Zhu*), and three slices of uncooked Rhizoma Zingiberis (*Sheng Jiang*).

If there is heart-spleen yang vacuity with scanty appetite, abdominal distention, and loose stools, one can use *Ren Shen Tang* (Ginseng Decoction) plus *Shen Ling Bai Zhu San* (Ginseng, Poria & Atractylodes Powder): Semen Coicis Lachyrma-jobi (*Yi Yi Ren*), 18g, Sclerotium Poriae Cocos (*Fu Ling*), Radix Dioscoreae Oppositae (*Shan Yao*), and Semen Dolichoris Lablab (*Bai Bian Dou*), 12g each, Radix Panacis Ginseng (*Ren Shen*), Rhizoma Atractylodis Macrocephalae (*Bai Zhu*), and Semen Nelumbinis Nuciferae (*Lian Zi*), 9g each, mix-fried Radix Glycyrrhizae (*Gan Cao*), Radix Platycodi Grandiflori (*Jie Geng*), and dried Rhizoma Zingiberis (*Gan Jiang*), 6g each, and Fructus Amomi (*Sha Ren*), 3-6g.

If there is heart-kidney yang vacuity with vacuous yang on the verge of desertion, massive sweating, reversal chilling of the four limbs, and a faint pulse on the verge of expiry, use *Shen Fu Tang* (Ginseng & Aconite Decoction) to rescue yang and stem desertion: Radix Panacis Ginseng (*Ren Shen*), 30g, and Radix Lateralis Praeparatus Aconiti Carmichaeli (*Fu Zi*), 15g.

If there is recalcitrant water swelling, one can use *Wu Ling San* (Five [Ingredients] Poria Powder): Sclerotium Polypori Umbellati (*Zhu Ling*) and Sclerotium Poriae Cocos (*Fu Ling*), 15-30g each, Rhizoma Atractylodis Macrocephalae (*Bai Zhu*), Rhizoma Alismatis (*Ze Xie*), and Ramulus Cinnamomi Cassiae (*Gui Zhi*), 9g each. If there is marked fatigue and lack of strength, add 15-30 grams of Radix Astragali Membranacei (*Huang Qi*). If there is marked edema, add 15 grams of Radix Stephaniae Tetrandrae (*Han Fang Ji*).

ACUPUNCTURE & MOXIBUSTION: *Dan Zhong* (CV 17), *Guan Yuan* (CV 4), *Zhong Ji* (CV 3), *Jue Yin Shu* (Bl 14), *Xin Shu* (Bl 15), *Yin Ling Quan* (Sp 9), *San Yin Jiao* (Sp 6), *Zu San Li* (St 36)

FORMULA ANALYSIS: Even supplementing-even draining *Guan Yuan*, *Zhong Ji*, *Yin Ling Quan*, and *San Yin Jiao* moves water downward and disinhibits urination. Even supplementing-even draining *Zu San Li* and *San Yin Jiao* fortifies the spleen and boosts the qi. Even supplementing-even draining *Dan Zhong*, *Jue Yin Shu*, and *Xin Shu* regulates and rectifies the heart qi.

ADDITIONS & SUBTRACTIONS: If there is concomitant yin vacuity, add supplementing *Tai Xi* (Ki 3). If there is heart-kidney yang vacuity, add moxibustion at *Xin Shu*, *Shen Shu*, and *Guan Yuan*. If there is liver depression, add draining *Tai Chong* (Liv 3) and *He Gu* (LI 4). If there is massive sweating, add *Fu Liu* (Ki 7) and *He Gu* (LI 4). If there are heart palpitations, add *Shen Men* (Ht 7) and *Jian Shi* (Per 5). If there are loose stools, add supplementing *Pi Shu* (Bl 20), *Wei Shu* (Bl 21), and *Da Chang Shu* (Bl 25).

ABSTRACTS OF REPRESENTATIVE CHINESE RESEARCH:

Chen Bao-sheng *et al.*, "Analysis of the Treatment of Diabetic Coronary Heart Disease Using *Xiao Ke An Jiao Nang* (Wasting & Thirsting Calming Capsules)," *Guo Yi Lun Tan* (Chinese Medicine Forum), #3, 1997, p. 33: The authors of this study treated 52 cases of diabetic coronary heart disease with *Xiao Ke An Jiao Nang* (Wasting & Thirsting Calming Capsules). In this group, there were 36 men and 16 women whose ages ranged from 46-65 years old. The course of disease lasted from 5-7 years. Another 25 cases were considered the comparison group, and, of these, 19 were men and six were women. Their ages ranged from 47-66 years, and the course of disease was 1-8 years. The treatment group of 52 patients received *Xiao Ke An Jiao Nang* (Wasting & Thirsting Calming Capsules). Each capsule was composed of 0.5g of Chinese

medicinal granules, and the dosage was four capsules three times per day. The comparison group received gliclazide at 80mg two times per day. All patients were evaluated after three weeks of treatment. The results showed that both groups had lowered blood sugar levels. Before treatment, the group receiving *Xiao Ke An Jiao Nang* had blood sugar levels at 10.06 ± 2.03mmol/L which lowered to 7.12 ± 1.56mmol/L after treatment. The comparison group receiving gliclazide had blood sugar levels at 9.98 ± 1.96mmol/L which lowered to 7.14 ± 1.51mmol/L after treatment. However, concerning the measurement of myocardial ischemia, the treatment group had dramatic results over the comparison group, with amelioration rates of 78.8% over 28%. Although the authors do not specify the entire composition of *Xiao Ke An Jiao Nang*, they do mention the inclusion of Radix Astragali Membranacei (*Huang Qi*), Radix Puerariae (*Ge Gen*), Tuber Ophiopogonis Japonici (*Mai Dong*), and Hirudo Seu Whitmania (*Shui Zhi*).

REPRESENTATIVE CASE HISTORIES:

CASE 1[6]

The patient was a 61 year old male who first entered the hospital in December 1992. He had been a diabetic for four years and, during the last month, had contracted heart palpitations, shortness of breath, pain in the left side of his chest, and lack of bodily strength. The man became easily fatigued by an activity. An electrocardiogram revealed myocardial ischemia. The patient's tongue was dark red with slimy, white fur, and his pulse was fine and weak. His blood sugar level was 9.8mmol/L, and urine sugar was (+++). The electrocardiogram specifically showed myocardial ischemia in the anterior and inferior areas of the patient's heart. The clinical diagnosis was diabetic coronary heart disease. The Chinese medical pattern discrimination was qi and yin dual vacuity complicated by blood stasis. *Xiao Ke An Jiao Nang* (Wasting & Thirsting Calming Capsules) was prescribed at four capsules three times per day. After six days, the palpitations, shortness of breath, and chest pain disappeared, and the man's strength returned to normal. The patient's tongue was red, his pulse was fine and weak, and urine sugar was (++). After continuing for two months with this protocol, the disease disappeared, the tongue became pale red, the pulse remained fine and weak, and urine sugar was still (++). Subsequent electrocardiography was normal. In a follow-up visit three months later, the patient's tongue was still pale red, the pulse was weak, urine sugar was (+), blood sugar was 6.57mmol/L, and the electrocardiogram was normal.

CASE 2[7]

The patient was 53 years old, sex unspecified. They had been diagnosed as suffering from diabetes and coronary heart disease for two years. Symptoms included polydipsia, polyuria, and polyphagia, and a loss of body weight. The patient had not previously used Western medicines. Their fasting blood glucose was 168-298mg/dL, fasting urine glucose was (++++), and postprandial urine glucose was (++++). There was also lack of strength, chest oppression, heart fluster, a dark red tongue with thin, white fur, and a deep, fine pulse. Therefore, the patient's Chinese medical patterns were discriminated as qi and yin dual vacuity with blood stasis. The treatment principles were to quicken the blood and transform stasis, boost the qi and nourish yin, for which the following formula was prescribed: uncooked Radix Astragali Membranacei (*Huang Qi*) and uncooked Concha Ostreae (*Mu Li*), 30g each, Radix Scrophulariae Ningpoensis (*Xuan Shen*), 24g, Radix Dioscoreae Oppositae (*Shan Yao*), Rhizoma Atractylodis (*Cang Zhu*), Radix Salviae Miltiorrhizae (*Dan Shen*), Radix Puerariae (*Ge Gen*), and Sclerotium Poriae Cocos (*Fu Ling*), 15g each, Semen Pruni Persicae (*Tao Ren*), Flos Carthami Tinctorii (*Hong Hua*), Radix Angelicae Sinensis (*Dang Gui*), Radix Ligustici Wallichii (*Chuan Xiong*), Radix Rubrus Paeoniae Lactiflorae (*Chi Shao*), and Lumbricus (*Di Long*), 9g each, and Galla Rhois (*Wu Bei Zi*), 6g. After taking seven *ji* of this formula, the patient's urinary output significantly decreased, urination was 4-5 times per day, and their appetite increased. After another 37 *ji* were administered with additions and subtractions following the symptoms, the "three polys" were markedly decreased as were chest oppression and heart fluster. Fasting blood glucose was 246mg/dL and postprandial urine glucose and fasting urine glucose had decreased to (+).

CASE 3[8]

The patient was a 64 year old retired female cadre who was first examined on Nov. 29, 1993. The patient's main complaints were lack of strength, polydipsia, and polyuria for 10 years and chest oppression for three years. The patient's type 2 diabetes had been diagnosed 10 years before. Her diet was restricted and she was put on Western oral hypoglycemic agents at that time and her symptoms had decreased. However, her blood glucose fluctuated widely. The chest oppression for the past three years was accompanied by discomfort in the left shoulder and upper back. Several ECGs had shown myocardial blood insufficiency. Recent FBG was 12.54mmol/L (226mg/dL), PPBG was 18.09mmol/L (326mg/dL), glycosylation of hemoglo-

bin was 14.25%, and urine glucose was (+++). In terms of Chinese medical signs and symptoms, there was a dry mouth with desire to drink, dry heat, perspiration, heart fluster, low back soreness, lack of strength, numbness of the limbs, blurred vision, nocturia 3-4 times per night, a dark red tongue with thin, white fur, and a deep, bowstring pulse.

Based on these signs and symptoms, the patient's patterns were categorized as qi and yin dual vacuity with heart blood depletion and detriment and static blood obstructing the network vessels. The treatment principles were to boost the qi and nourish yin, nourish the heart and quiet the spirit, quicken the blood and free the flow of the network vessels. Therefore, the following Chinese medicinals were prescribed: Radix Salviae Miltiorrhizae (*Dan Shen*), uncooked Radix Astragali Membranacei (*Huang Qi*), and Caulis Milletiae Seu Spatholobi (*Ji Xue Teng*), 30g each, Radix Trichosanthis Kirlowii (*Tian Hua Fen*) and Ramulus Loranthi Seu Visci (*Sang Ji Sheng*), 20g each, uncooked Radix Rehmanniae (*Sheng Di*), cooked Radix Rehmanniae (*Shu Di*), Radix Glehniae Littoralis (*Sha Shen*), uncooked Fructus Crataegi (*Shan Zha*), and Radix Puerariae (*Ge Gen*), 15g each, and Tuber Ophiopogonis Japonici (*Mai Men Dong*), Fructus Schisandrae Chinensis (*Wu Wei Zi*), Radix Ligustici Wallichii (*Chuan Xiong*), Radix Angelicae Dahuricae (*Bai Zhi*), Flos Chrysanthemi Morifolii (*Jue Hua*), Rhizoma Acori Graminei (*Shi Chang Pu*), Tuber Curcumae (*Yu Jin*), and Fructus Lycii Chinensis (*Gou Qi Zi*), 10g each.

The patient was seen again on Dec. 13. After taking the above medicinals, the nocturia had decreased as had the oral dryness. However, there was still afternoon dizziness, heart fluster, and vacuity sweating. Fasting blood glucose was 8.04mmol/L (145mg/dL) and PPBG was 12.09mmol/L (218mg/dL). The patient's tongue was dark red, and her pulse was fine and bowstring. Therefore, one of her Western hypoglycemic agents was discontinued and *Dan Shen, Ge Gen, Chuan Xiong, Bai Zhi,* and *Ju Hua* were removed from the above formula. Instead, 15 grams each of Radix Dipsaci (*Xu Duan*) and Rhizoma Homalomenae Occultae (*Qian Nian Jian*) and 10 grams of uncooked Radix Dioscoreae Oppositae (*Shan Yao*) were added.

After taking 28 *ji* of this prescription, the patient's symptoms had decreased. However, for the past 10 days she had felt worse lack of strength, lassitude of the spirit, dry mouth, and polydipsia. Fasting blood glucose was 9.04mmol/L (163mg/dL), PPBG was 14.76mmol/L (266mg/dL), and glycosylation of hemoglobin was 10.02%. The patient's tongue was pale but dark, and her pulse fine and bowstring. Now the prescription was changed to: uncooked Radix Astragali Membranacei (*Huang Qi*), Radix Salviae Miltiorrhizae (*Dan Shen*), Radix Scrophulariae Ningpoensis (*Xuan Shen*), and Caulis Milletiae Seu Spatholobi (*Ji Xue Teng*), 30g each, Radix Trichosanthis Kirlowii (*Tian Hua Fen*) and Ramulus Loranthi Seu Visci (*Sang Ji Sheng*), 20g each, cooked Radix Rehmanniae (*Shu Di*), uncooked Radix Rehmanniae (*Sheng Di*), Radix Glehniae Littoralis (*Sha Shen*), uncooked Fructus Crataegi (*Shan Zha*), Radix Puerariae (*Ge Gen*), and Rhizoma Atractylodis (*Cang Zhu*), 15g each, and Tuber Ophiopogonis Japonici (*Mai Men Dong*), Fructus Schisandrae Chinensis (*Wu Wei Zi*), Fructus Lycii Chinensis (*Gou Qi Zi*), Flos Chrysanthemi Morifolii (*Ju Hua*), and Radix Dioscoreae Oppositae (*Shan Yao*), 10g each.

On Feb. 27, 1994, the patient was seen once again. Her condition was stable with a slight degree of lack of strength. Ten days before she had caught a cold with low-grade fever, itchy throat, cough, and a dry mouth. Her FBG was 7.88mmol/L (142mg/dL) and her PPBG was 8.21mmol/L (148mg/dL). The patient's tongue was pale but dark, and her pulse was fine and bowstring. Therefore, *Ju Hua, Tian Hua Fen*, and *Shan Yao* were removed from the formula and 15 grams of Rhizoma Homalomenae Occultae (*Qian Nian Jian*) and 10 grams of Herba Epimedii (*Xian Ling Pi*) were added. In addition, the woman was instructed to drink six *ji* of Ramulus Uncariae Cum Uncis (*Gou Teng*) and Herba Menthae Haplocalycis (*Bo He*), 10g each, as a tea.

On Apr. 18, the patient was seen for the fifth time. There was no chest oppression or heart fluster and the strength had increased in her lower limbs. The mouth was still dry, but there was no more polydipsia. Fasting blood glucose was 9.26mmol/L (167mg/dL) and glycosylated hemoglobin was 7.59%. Tongue and pulse were the same as before. Therefore, the original formula was made into water pills, and the patient was instructed to take 10 grams of these after each meal in order to secure and consolidate the treatment effects. The patient continued taking Chinese medicinals and she was eventually able to discontinue one of her Western hypoglycemic medications and reduce the dose of the other.

CASE 4[9]

The patient was a 62 year old male retired worker who was first examined on May 10, 1993. The patient's main complaints were episodic heart fluster for three years and lack of strength and dry mouth with desire to drink for half a year. The man had developed heart arrhythmia three years before which had been treated and mostly controlled. However, the man still commonly had heart fluster and shortness of breath, especially after taxation or when fatigued. In Nov. 1992, the patient was diagnosed with diabetes based on elevated blood and urine glucose, lack of strength, polydipsia, and polyuria. He was prescribed 25mg of a hypoglycemic medication TID and the "three polys" improved. However, lack of strength continued to be pronounced and his FBG fluctuated around 11.1mmol/L. Other signs and symptoms included low back and knee soreness and limpness, bilateral lower leg soreness, heaviness, pain, and aversion to chill, blurred vision, and frequent, profuse nocturia. The patient's tongue was pale red, and his pulse was fine and bowstring.

Based on these signs and symptoms, the man's Chinese medical patterns were categorized as qi and yin dual vacuity with heart blood insufficiency and liver-kidney depletion and detriment. The treatment principles were to boost the qi and nourish yin, strengthen the heart and return the pulse, enrich and supplement the liver and kidneys. The formula prescribed was *Jiang Tang Sheng Mai Fang Jia Jian* (Lower Sugar & Engender the Pulse Formula with Additions & Subtractions): uncooked Radix Astragali Membranacei (*Huang Qi*) and Caulis Milletiae Seu Spatholobi (*Ji Xue Teng*), Ramulus Loranthi Seu Visci (*Sang Ji Sheng*) and Radix Trichosanthis Kirlowii (*Tian Hua Fen*), 20g, uncooked Radix Rehmanniae (*Sheng Di*), cooked Radix Rehmanniae (*Shu Di*), Radix Glehniae Littoralis (*Sha Shen*), uncooked Fructus Crataegi (*Shan Zha*), and Radix Clematidis Chinensis (*Wei Ling Xian*), 15g each, and Tuber Ophiopogonis Japonici (*Mai Men Dong*), Fructus Schisandrae Chinensis (*Wu Wei Zi*), Fructus Lycii Chinensis (*Gou Qi Zi*), Radix Et Rhizoma Notopterygii (*Qiang Huo*), and Radix Angelicae Pubescentis (*Du Huo*), 10g each.

After taking 20 *ji* of these medicinals, the patient had more strength than before and the lower limb aching and pain had disappeared. However, there was still a dry mouth, dryness and heat, and heart fluster. Fasting blood glucose was 10.6mmol/L and urine glucose was slight. The patient's tongue was pale but dark, and his pulse was deep and bowstring. Therefore, *Gou Qi Zi, Wei Ling Xian, Qiang Huo*, and *Du Huo* were removed and 30 grams of Radix Salviae Miltiorrhizae (*Dan Shen*), 15 grams each of Rhizoma Homalomenae (*Qian Nian Jian*), Radix Dipsaci (*Xu Duan*), Rhizoma Cibotii Barometsis (*Gou Ji*), and Radix Puerariae (*Ge Gen*), 10 grams of Radix Scutellariae Baicalensis (*Huang Qin*), and five grams of Rhizoma Coptidis Chinensis (*Huang Lian*) were added. The patient was seen again on Jul. 5, 1993 when the lower legs had strength, and dryness, heat, and heart fluster had been cured. There was still blurred vision, and FBG was 9.4mmol/L. Therefore, 10 grams of Fructus Tribuli Terrestris (*Bai Ji Li*) was added to the above formula which was continued to be administered. On Sept. 20, 1993, the patient had been taking this formula for two months. All his symptoms were cured, FBG was 7.5mmol/L, and urine glucose was negative. The original formula was made into water pills, and the patient was instructed to take 10 grams of these three times each day in order to secure and consolidate the treatment effects.

CASE 5[10]

The patient was a 66 year old male who was first examined on Aug. 7, 1985. The patient complained of chest pain, dizziness, and vertigo. He had been diagnosed with coronary heart disease and hypertension for 10 years. In the last half year, both lower limbs had become numb and oral thirst and hunger had increased. When examined, the man's blood glucose was 267mg/dL and urine glucose was (+++). When the man took Western hypoglycemic medications, his blood glucose went down. But if he stopped taking these medications, it went back up again. Therefore he had sought out Chinese medical treatment. The man was addicted to alcohol and eating fatty foods, and, therefore, he was quite robust with a pot-belly. His lips were purple and dark and he had extremely bad breath. His mouth was dry and he liked to drink. In addition, his intake of grains was increased. The patient tended to be constipated, only having one bowel movement every three days, while his urine was yellow and turbid. The patient had a red tongue with fissures in the center and scanty fur, and his pulse was fine, rapid, bowstring, and slippery.

Based on the above signs and symptoms, the patient's patterns were discriminated as blazing, exuberant central fire depleting and consuming stomach yin with heat stasis in the blood network vessels. Therefore, the treatment principles were to enrich and moisten dry earth, clear and discharge evil fire, cool the blood and free the flow of the network vessels, for which he was prescribed: Radix Trichosanthis Kirlowii (*Tian Hua Fen*), fresh Rhizoma Imperatae Cylindricae (*Bai Mao Gen*), and Rhizoma Phragmitis Communis (*Lu Gen*), 60g each, uncooked Gypsum Fibrosum (*Shi Gao*), 50g, uncooked Radix Rehmanniae (*Sheng Di*), Radix Scrophulariae Ningpoensis (*Xuan Shen*), Herba Lycopi Lucidi (*Ze Lan*), and Semen Trichosanthis Kirlowii (*Gua Lou Ren*), 30g each, and Cortex Radicis Moutan (*Dan Pi*) and Radix Pseudostellariae Heterophyllae (*Tai Zi Shen*), 10g each.

After taking the above formula for half a month, all the patient's symptoms were greatly decreased. Therefore, *Shi Gao*, *Gua Lou Ren*, and *Dan Pi* were removed from the formula, *Tian Hua Fen*, *Bai Mao Gen*, and *Lu Gen* were decreased to 30 grams each, and 30 grams of Radix Dioscoreae Oppositae (*Shan Yao*) were added. This prescription was continued for three months, after which, blood glucose was normal and urine glucose had turned negative. The man was advised to give up alcohol, prohibited from fats and sweets, and advised to control the amount of carbohydrates he ate, rather increasing his intake of vegetables and bean products.

REMARKS:

1. There are five things that diabetes patients can do to prevent heart disease: 1) control blood glucose levels, 2) stop smoking, 3) eat low-fat foods, 4) avoid high blood pressure, and 5) exercise. According to the American Diabetes Association, "All of these actions will help you keep your large blood vessels wide open for blood to flow to all your vital organs, and you will lower your risk of developing cardiovascular disease dramatically."[11]

2. For the self or home treatment of heart pain, acupressure may be done by the patient or their family at *Zhi Yang* (GV 9), *Nei Guan* (Per 6), *Xin Shu* (Bl 15), *Jue Yin Shu* (Bl 14) and any or all Hua Tuo paravertebral points which are sore to pressure.

3. Auriculotherapy points include: Heart, *Shen Men*, Chest, Lungs, Subcortex, Kidneys, Liver, Internal Secretion, and/or Adrenal. Choose 2-3 points each time alternately.

4. Radix Glycyrrhizae (*Gan Cao*) is one of the main Chinese medicinals for treating heart arrhythmias. However, *Gan Cao* also has a known empirical effect of raising the blood pressure, and many people with diabetes and heart disease also suffer from hypertension. In that case, either *Gan Cao* should be avoided or it should be balanced by other medicinals which seep dampness, such as Sclerotium Poriae Cocos (*Fu Ling*) and Rhizoma Alismatis (*Ze Xie*), and thus tend to reduce blood pressure.

ENDNOTES:

[1] www.cdc.gov/diabetes/pubs/facts98.htm
[2] www.chebutco.ns.ca/Health/Cprc/diabetes.html
[3] www.postgradmed.com/issues/1999/02_99/bohannon.htm
[4] www.karenyontzcenter.org/Information
[5] www.healthyheart.org/Education/diabetes.htm
[6] Chen Bao-sheng, *et.al.* "Analysis of the Treatment of Diabetic Coronary Heart Disease Using *Xiao Ke An Jiao Nang* (Wasting and

Thirsting Calming Capsules)," *Guo Yi Lun Tan* (*Chinese Medicine Forum*), #3, 1997, p. 33

[7] Zhu Chen-zi, anthologized in Shi Yu-guang & Dan Shu-jian, *Xiao Ke Zhuan Zhi* (*Wasting & Thirsting Expertise*), Chinese Medicine Ancient Books Publishing Co., 1997, p. 19

[8] Zhu Chen-zi, anthologized in Dan Shu-jian & Chen Zi-hua's *Xiao Ke Juan* (*The Wasting & Thirsting Book*), Chinese National Chinese Medicine & Medicinals Publishing Co., Beijing, 1999, 129-131

[9] Zhu Chen-zi, anthologized in Dong Zhen-hua *et al.*'s *Zhu Chen Zi Jing An Ji* (*A Collection of Zhu Chen-zi's Experiences*), People's Health & Hygiene Publishing Co., Beijing, 2000

[10] Hu Qiao-zheng, anthologized in Shi Yu-guang & Dan Shu-jian, *op. cit.*, p. 98-99

[11] American Diabetes Association, *Complete Guide to Diabetes*, Bantam Books, NY, 1999, p. 305

22

Diabetic Cerebrovascular Disease

Cerebrovascular disease (CVD) refers to atheroslcerotic or endothelial damage or rupture of the blood vessels in the brain that can result in a cerebral vascular accident (CVA) or "stroke" or death due to lack of circulation in a portion of the brain.[1, 2] The incidence of CVD is 2-4 times higher in persons with diabetes than in those without diabetes.[3] Cerebrovascular disease is one of the macrovascular complications of diabetes (along with coronary artery disease). Other predisposing factors to CVD include hypertension, atherosclerosis, and heart disease (especially dilated cardiomyopathy and rhythm disorders, such as atrial fibrillation), any or all of which are common in middle-aged and elderly patients with diabetes. Premonitory to a full "stroke" or CVA is a transient ischemic attack (TIA). TIAs may manifest as temporary arm or leg paresthesias, facial muscle weakness, difficulty with balance (ataxia), double vision (diplopia) or flash blindness (amaurosis fugax), or speech production problems (dysphasia or dysarthria). The predominance of any of these symptoms or signs depends on which arterial tree is affected and, therefore, which area of the brain is impaired. Attacks often occur on awakening or arising when procoagulant factors, vasoconstriction, and sudden elevation in catecholamines and blood pressure increase. Some authorities also list smoking as a risk factor of diabetic cerebrovascular disease due to smoking's interference with oxygen transport and endothelium health.[4] The pathogenesis of diabetes-associated stroke seems to be linked to excessive glycation and oxidation, endothelial dysfunction, increased platelet aggregation, impaired fibrinolysis, and insulin resistance which precipitates atherogenesis and plasminogen inhibition.[5] It is also possible that *Heliobacter pylori* infection plays an adjuvant vessel inflammatory role in diabetic CVD, since thrombo-occlusive cerebral disease is more prevalent in diabetic patients with *H. pylori* infections than those without such infections.[6]

The Western medical diagnosis of CVD is usually made clinically based on the patient's signs and symptoms, age (usually 50 years or over), and a history of hypertension, diabetes, or atherosclerosis. Diagnosis may be aided or confirmed by CT or MRI scanning of the brain. Intracranial ultrasound and magnetic resonance venous angiography may also be useful in selected cases. Laboratory findings may be useful when procoagulant or antifibrinolytic factors are germane, such as anti-thrombin, fibrinogen, plasminogen activator inhibitor-1, protein C, protein S, etc. In addition, heart monitoring for dysrhythmias and repolarization changes in a 12 lead ECG may provide useful clues. Ultrasound of the heart (echocardiogram) may reveal valvular disease or cardiomyopathy which can lead to an embolus or thrombus. Ultrasound of the carotid arteries may reveal a fixed obstruction or unstable plaque. Arterial angiography is sometimes used to determine the site of arterial occlusion, especially when surgery is contemplated.

The Western medical treatment of this condition mainly revolves around its prevention by treating the disease conditions which predispose one to stroke. After a cerebral vascular accident has occurred, immediate treatment focuses on preventing the spread of the bleeding or aborting further embolization or thrombus formation, *i.e.*, rescuing tissue in jeopardy. Once the patient has stabilized, the emphasis shifts to rehabilitation through physical therapy and nursing aftercare for disabled patients. During the early days of either evolving or completed stroke, neither progression nor ultimate outcome can be easily predicted. Approximately 35% of patients die in the hospital with the mortality rate increasing with age. Any deficits remaining after six months are likely to be permanent. Ten percent of patients with diabetes die due to CVA,[7] and annual hospitalization in Colorado for CVA is nine per 1,000 diabetes patients.[8]

CHINESE DISEASE MECHANISMS:

Overeating fatty, sweet foods and drinking alcohol may lead to the loss of spleen and stomach movement and transformation. Hence the spleen loses its fortification and movement. This results in gathering of dampness which congeals into phlegm, and phlegm depression may transform into heat. Such heat may lead to stirring of liver wind, in which case, wind may draft phlegm upward to impede and obstruct the vessels and network vessels of the brain. As Shen Jin-ao said in the Qing dynasty, "Fat people [are those who] mostly [suffer] windstroke."

If, due to emotional depression and anger, extremes of the five affects transform heat, this may cause stirring of ministerial fire which results in ascendant liver yang hyperactivity and/or internal stirring of liver wind. It is also possible for enduring depressive heat of the liver and stomach or enduring phlegm damp heat to damage and consume liver-kidney yin. In that case, the sinews' vessels may lose their emollient and nourishing and wind yang may also stir internally. Thus in the Ming dynasty, Tai Yuan-li said, "[If] the three wastings endure, the essence and blood must be depleted, and, [therefore,] it is possible that the eyes lose their vision or that the hands and feet [become] hemiplegic."

Other common complications in diabetic CVD include qi vacuity and blood stasis. Qi vacuity is the result of spleen vacuity, while blood stasis may be due to enduring liver depression qi stagnation and/or the presence of phlegm, dampness, and turbidity impeding and obstructing the free flow of the blood.

TREATMENT BASED ON PATTERN DISCRIMINATION:

1. YIN VACUITY WITH WIND STIRRING & STATIC BLOOD OBSTRUCTING THE NETWORK VESSELS PATTERN

MAIN SYMPTOMS: Sudden hemiplegia or possible one-sided numbness, deviated mouth and eyes, a stiff tongue and unclear speech, vexation, agitation, and restlessness, insomnia, dizziness, tinnitus, heat in the heart of the hands and feet, vexatious thirst, polydipsia, easy hungering, reddish urine, dry stools, a red crimson tongue with scanty fluids or a dark red tongue with scanty or no fur, and a fine, rapid or bowstring, fine, rapid pulse

TREATMENT PRINCIPLES: Foster yin and extinguish wind, transform phlegm and free the flow of the network vessels

RX: Unnamed formula

INGREDIENTS: Ramulus Uncariae Cum Uncis (*Gou Teng*) and Ramulus Loranthi Seu Visci (*Sang Ji Sheng*), 30g each, uncooked Radix Rehmanniae (*Sheng Di*) and Radix Trichosanthis Kirlowii (*Tian Hua Fen*), 20g each, Radix Scrophulariae Ningpoensis (*Xuan Shen*), Herba Dendrobii (*Shi Hu*), Fructus Ligustri Lucidi (*Nu Zhen Zi*), Radix Albus Paeoniae Lactiflorae (*Bai Shao*), Radix Rubrus Paeoniae Lactiflorae (*Chi Shao*), Radix Salviae Miltiorrhizae (*Dan Shen*), and Lumbricus (*Di Long*), 15g each, Flos Chrysanthemi Morifolii (*Ju Hua*) and Fructus Lycii Chinensis (*Gou Qi Zi*), 9g each

FORMULA ANALYSIS: *Sheng Di, Xuan Shen, Tian Hua Fen,* and *Shi Hu* enrich yin and clear vacuity heat, engender fluids and stop thirst. *Nu Zhen Zi, Sang Ji Sheng,* and *Gou Qi Zi* enrich the yin of the liver and kidneys so as to enrich water and moisten wood. *Gou Teng* and *Ju Hua* level the liver and extinguish wind as branch treatments. *Chi Shao, Bai Shao, Dan Shen,* and *Di Long* quicken the blood and free the flow of the channels.

ADDITIONS & SUBTRACTIONS: If vacuity heat symptoms are not marked, one can decrease the dosages of the medicinals which enrich yin and clear heat. If signs and symptoms of wind, such as dizziness and tinnitus, are marked, one can increase the dosage of the wind-extinguishing medicinals and add nine grams of Rhizoma Gastrodiae Elatae (*Tian Ma*) and 15 grams each of Fructus Tribuli Terrestris (*Bai Ji Li*) and uncooked Concha Haliotidis (*Shi Jue Ming*). If liver-kidney yin vacuity symptoms are pronounced, such as insomnia, profuse dreams, dry, scratchy eyes, and low back and knee soreness and limpness, one can add nine grams each of Gelatinum Plastri Testudinis (*Gui Ban Jiao*) and Gelatinum Cornu Cervi (*Lu Jiao Jiao*).

ACUPUNCTURE & MOXIBUSTION: The acupuncture treatment of stroke and its sequelae are primarily treated by the severity of the disease and the major symptoms as opposed to the pattern discrimination presented herein. Therefore, please see the section titled, "Treatment with acupuncture & moxibustion," below for a more complete discussion of the treatment of CVD with acupuncture.

2. QI & YIN VACUITY WITH STATIC BLOOD OBSTRUCTING THE NETWORK VESSELS PATTERN

MAIN SYMPTOMS: Hemiplegia, one-sided numbness of the body, possible deviated mouth and eyes, possible stiff tongue and unclear speech, fatigue, lack of strength, shortness of breath, disinclination to speak and/or a weak, faint voice, dry mouth, thirst, spontaneous perspiration and/or night sweats, vexatious heat in the five hearts, heart palpitations, insomnia, yellow or reddish urination, dry stools, a fat tongue body with teeth-marks on its edges and thin, possibly peeled fur, and a bowstring, fine, forceless or bowstring, fine, rapid pulse

TREATMENT PRINCIPLES: Boost the qi and nourish yin, quicken the blood and free the flow of the network vessels

RX: *Bu Yang Huan Wu Tang* (Supplement Yang & Restore Five [Tenths] Decoction) plus *Sheng Mai San* (Engender the Pulse Powder) with additions & subtractions

INGREDIENTS: Caulis Milletiae Seu Spatholobi (*Ji Xue Teng*), 30g, Radix Astragali Membranacei (*Huang Qi*), 25g, Radix Dioscoreae Oppositae (*Shan Yao*), Radix Scrophulariae Ningpoensis (*Xuan Shen*), and Ramulus Loranthi Seu Visci (*Sang Ji Sheng*), 20g each, Radix Codonopositis Pilosulae (*Dang Shen*), Tuber Ophiopogonis Japonici (*Mai Men Dong*), Fructus Schisandrae Chinensis (*Wu Wei Zi*), Radix Angelicae Sinensis (*Dang Gui*), and Radix Ligustici Wallichii (*Chuan Xiong*), 15g each, Radix Puerariae (*Ge Gen*), Semen Pruni Persicae (*Tao Ren*), Flos Carthami Tinctorii (*Hong Hua*), Radix Albus Paeoniae Lactiflorae (*Bai Shao*), Radix Rubrus Paeoniae Lactiflorae (*Chi Shao*), and Radix Achyranthis Bidentatae (*Niu Xi*), 9g each

FORMULA ANALYSIS: *Huang Qi, Dang Shen,* and *Shan Yao* boost the qi and support yang. *Xuan Shen* and *Mai Men Dong* nourish yin and engender fluids. *Ge Gen* boosts the stomach and upbears fluids. *Dang Gui, Chuan Xiong, Tao Ren, Hong Hua, Chi Shao,* and *Bai Shao* quicken the blood and transform stasis. *Ji Xue Teng* and *Dang Gui* nourish the blood, quicken the blood, and free the flow of the channels. *Niu Xi* and *Sang Ji Sheng* enrich and supplement the yin of the liver and kidneys, thus treat the root.

ADDITIONS & SUBTRACTIONS: If qi vacuity is so extreme as to have evolved into yang vacuity, add 1.5 grams of powdered Cornu Parvum Cervi (*Lu Rong*) swallowed with the decoction in order to warm yang and transform the qi. If there is accompanying difficulty speaking, add 12 grams each of Rhizoma Acori Graminei (*Shi Chang Pu*) and Tuber Curcumae (*Yu Jin*). If there is distention of the hands and feet, add 30 grams of Sclerotium Poriae Cocos (*Fu Ling*) and nine grams of Ramulus Cinnamomi Cassiae (*Gui Zhi*) to fortify the spleen, warm yang, and free the flow of the network vessels.

3. WIND, PHLEGM & STATIC BLOOD IMPEDING & OBSTRUCTING THE NETWORK VESSELS PATTERN

MAIN SYMPTOMS: Hemiplegia, one-sided numbness of the body, deviated mouth and, possible stiff tongue and unclear speech, dizziness and vertigo, a dark but pale tongue with thin, white or slimy, white fur, and a bowstring, slippery pulse

TREATMENT PRINCIPLES: Transform phlegm and extinguish wind, quicken the blood and free the flow of the network vessels

RX: *Hua Tan Tong Luo Tang Jia Jian* (Transform Phlegm & Free the Flow of the Network Vessels Decoction with Additions & Subtractions)

INGREDIENTS: Radix Salviae Miltiorrhizae (*Dan Shen*), 30g, Rhizoma Cyperi Rotundi (*Xiang Fu*), 15g, Rhizoma Pinelliae Ternatae (*Ban Xia*), uncooked Rhizoma Atractylodis Macrocephalae (*Bai Zhu*), and Rhizoma Gastrodiae Elatae (*Tian Ma*), 9g each, bile-treated Rhizoma Arisaematis (*Dan Nan Xing*), 6g, and wine-fried Radix Et Rhizoma Rhei (*Da Huang*), 3-6g

FORMULA ANALYSIS: *Ban Xia, Bai Zhu, Dan Nan Xing,* and *Tian Ma* transform phlegm and extinguish wind. *Dan Shen* quickens the blood and frees the flow of the channels, and *Xiang Fu* moves the qi in order to assist the movement of the blood.

ADDITIONS & SUBTRACTIONS: If wind symptoms are pronounced, add 30 grams of Ramulus Uncariae Cum Uncis (*Gou Teng*), 15 grams of Bombyx Batryticatus (*Jiang Can*), and nine grams of Fructus Tribuli Terrestris (*Bai Ji Li*) in order to settle the liver and extinguish wind. If symptoms of phlegm are pronounced, add 20 grams of Sclerotium Poriae Cocos (*Fu Ling*), 15 grams of Caulis Bambusae In Taeniis (*Zhu Ru*), and nine grams of Pericarpium Citri Reticulatae (*Chen Pi*). If symptoms of blood stasis are marked, add 15 grams each of Radix Rubrus Paeoniae Lactiflorae (*Chi Shao*), Radix Albus Paeoniae Lactiflorae (*Bai Shao*), and Radix Ligustici Wallichii (*Chuan Xiong*).

4. PHLEGM HEAT & BOWEL REPLETION WITH WIND & PHLEGM HARASSING ABOVE PATTERN

MAIN SYMPTOMS: Sudden hemiplegia, one-sided numbness of the body, deviated mouth and eyes, unclear speech, possible spirit clouding, aphasia, vexation, agitation and disquietude, dizziness, profuse phlegm, bad breath, rapid, distressed breathing, one bowel movement every three days or more, thick, yellow or yellow-brown and dry tongue fur, and a bowstring, slippery pulse. On the paralyzed side, the pulse is bowstring, slippery, and large.

TREATMENT PRINCIPLES: Free the flow of the bowels and transform phlegm

RX: *Tong Fu Hua Tang Tan Jia Jian* (Free the Flow of the Bowels & Transform Phlegm Decoction with Additions & Subtractions)

INGREDIENTS: Fructus Trichosanthis Kirlowii (*Gua Lou*) and Radix Salviae Miltiorrhizae (*Dan Shen*), 30g each, bile-treated Rhizoma Arisaematis (*Dan Nan Xing*), uncooked Radix Et Rhizoma Rhei (*Da Huang*), and Mirabilitum (*Mang Xiao*), 9g each

FORMULA ANALYSIS: Uncooked *Da Huang* and *Mang Xiao* free the flow of the bowels and abduct stagnation. *Dan Nan Xing* and *Gua Lou* clear and transform phlegm and heat, and *Dan Shen* quickens the blood and transforms stasis.

ADDITIONS & SUBTRACTIONS: Once the patient has had a bowel movement, omit *Mang Xiao* and add 30 grams of Caulis Milletiae Seu Spatholobi (*Ji Xue Teng*) and 15 grams of Radix Rubrus Paeoniae Lactiflorae (*Chi Shao*). If dizziness is severe, add 30 grams of Concha Margaritiferae (*Zhen Zhu Mu*) and 15 grams of Ramulus Uncariae Cum Uncis (*Gou Teng*). If the bowel qi is freely flowing but there is vexation, agitation, restlessness, and insomnia due to phlegm heat internally brewing and yin vacuity, add 30 grams of Caulis Polygoni Multiflori (*Ye Jiao Teng*), 15 grams each of uncooked Radix Rehmanniae (*Sheng Di*) and Tuber Ophiopogonis Japonici (*Mai Men Dong*), and nine grams of Radix Glehniae Littoralis (*Sha Shen*) to foster yin and quiet the spirit.

5. PHLEGM DAMPNESS INTERNALLY BREWING, MISTING & BLOCKING THE HEART SPIRIT PATTERN

MAIN SYMPTOMS: Habitual bodily obesity with profuse dampness and profuse phlegm, spirit clouding, hemiplegia, lack of warmth in the paralyzed limbs, a white facial complexion with dark lips, exuberant phlegm drool and congestion, a pale but dark tongue with thick, slimy, white fur, and a deep, slippery or deep, moderate (*i.e.*, relaxed, slightly slow) pulse

TREATMENT PRINCIPLES: Flush phlegm and transform dampness, open the orifices and arouse the spirit

RX: *Di Dan Tang Jia Jian* (Flush Phlegm Decoction with Additions & Subtractions) plus *Su He Xiang Wan* (Liquid Styrax Pills)

INGREDIENTS: Fructus Trichosanthis Kirlowii (*Gua Lou*), 30g, Pericarpium Citri Rubri (*Ju Hong*) and Sclerotium Poriae Cocos (*Fu Ling*), 15g each, Rhizoma Acori Graminei (*Shi Chang Pu*) and Caulis Bambusae In Taeniis (*Zhu Ru*), 12g each, Rhizoma Pinelliae Ternatae (*Ban Xia*), bile-treated Rhizoma Arisaematis (*Dan Nan Xing*), Fructus Immaturus Citri Aurantii (*Zhi Shi*), and Radix Codonopsitis Pilosulae (*Dang Shen*), 9g each, and Radix Glycyrrhizae (*Gan Cao*), 3-6g. Take one pill of *Su He Xiang Wan* (Liquid Styrax Pills, a ready-made Chinese medicine) swallowed with a decoction made from the foregoing medicinals.

FORMULA ANALYSIS: *Ban Xia, Dan Nan Xing,* and *Ju Hong* dry dampness and transform phlegm turbidity. *Gua Lou* transforms phlegm and clears heat. *Dang Shen, Fu Ling,* and *Gan Cao* fortify the spleen and boost the qi. *Zhu Ru* and *Zhi Shi* harmonize the stomach and downbear turbidity. *Shi Chang Pu* dispels phlegm and opens the orifices. *Su He Xiang Wan* penetratingly and aromatically opens the orifices.

ADDITIONS & SUBTRACTIONS: If the phlegm is thick and yellow, add nine grams each of Radix Scutellariae Baicalensis (*Huang Qin*) and Bulbus Fritillariae Thunbergii (*Zhe Bei Mu*). If wind and phlegm are obstructing internally with a stiff tongue, aphasia, and a bowstring, slippery, rapid pulse, add nine grams each of Rhizoma Gastrodiae Elatae (*Tian Ma*), uncooked Concha Haliotidis (*Shi Jue Ming*), Ramulus Uncariae Cum Uncis (*Gou Teng*), and Buthus Martensis (*Quan Xie*) to dispel phlegm and extinguish wind.

6. QI VACUITY & BLOOD STASIS PATTERN

NOTE: This pattern mainly describes the sequelae of stroke with hemiplegia as the main symptom.

MAIN SYMPTOMS: Hemiplegia, one-sided numbness of the body, deviated mouth and eyes, clear drool flowing from the mouth, unclear speech, a faint voice and disinclination to speak, a bright white facial complexion, shortness of breath, lack of strength, spontaneous perspiration, heart palpitations, loose stools, profuse, long, clear urination, swelling and distention of the hands and feet, a pale but dark tongue with teeth-marks on its edges, dark, purplish sublingual veins, and thin, white or slimy, white fur, and a deep, fine or fine, bowstring pulse

TREATMENT PRINCIPLES: Boost the qi and quicken the blood, free the flow of the channels and quicken the network vessels

RX: *Bu Yang Huan Wu Tang Jia Jian* (Supplement Yang & Restore Five [Tenths] Decoction with Additions & Subtractions)

INGREDIENTS: Uncooked Radix Astragali Membranacei (*Huang Qi*), 45-60g, Caulis Milletiae Seu Spatholobi (*Ji Xue Teng*), 30g, Radix Salviae Miltiorrhizae (*Dan Shen*), Extremitas Radicis Angelicae Sinensis (*Dang Gui Wei*), Lumbricus (*Di Long*), and Radix Rubrus Paeoniae Lactiflorae (*Chi Shao*), 15g each, Radix Cyathulae (*Chuan Niu Xi*), 12g, Radix Ligustici Wallichii (*Chuan Xiong*), Flos Carthami Tinctorii (*Hong Hua*), and Semen Pruni Persicae (*Tao Ren*), 9g each

FORMULA ANALYSIS: *Huang Qi* and *Dang Gui* boost the qi and nourish the blood. *Dan Shen, Chi Shao, Chuan Xiong, Hong Hua, Tao Ren,* and *Di Long* quicken the blood and transform stasis. *Ji Xue Teng* frees the flow of the channels and quickens the blood, and *Chuan Niu Xi* quickens the blood and leads it to move downward.

ADDITIONS & SUBTRACTIONS: If qi vacuity is pronounced, one may add up to 30 grams of Radix Codonopsitis Pilosulae (*Dang Shen*) to increase the strength of qi-boosting. If the disease condition is severe, one may add 0.3 grams of powdered Cornu Parvum Cervi (*Lu Rong*) swallowed with the decoction as well as 15 grams of Radix Polygoni Multiflori (*He Shou Wu*) and nine grams each of Fructus Corni Officinalis (*Shan Zhu Yu*) and Herba Cistanchis Deserticolae (*Rou Cong Rong*) in order to supplement and boost the liver and kidneys, invigorate yang and transform the qi, thus promoting the stirring of qi and the movement of the blood. If there is accompanying difficulty speaking or aphasia, add nine grams each of Rhizoma Acori Graminei (*Shi Chang Pu*), Radix Polygalae Tenuifoliae (*Yuan Zhi*), Tuber Curcumae (*Yu Jin*), and Sclerotium Poriae Cocos (*Fu Ling*) to dispel phlegm and open the orifices. If signs and symptoms of blood stasis are marked, add nine grams each of Scolopendra Subspinipes (*Wu Gong*) and Hirudo Seu Whitmania (*Shui Zhi*) and three grams of powdered Radix Pseudoginseng (*San Qi*) swallowed with the decoction.

TREATMENT WITH ACUPUNCTURE & MOXIBUSTION:

1. For transient ischemic attacks (TIAs), needle *Shang Xing* (GV 23), *Bai Hui* (GV 20), *Yin Tang* (M-HN-3), *Jian Yu* (LI 15), *Qu Chi* (LI 11), *Zu San Li* (St 36), and *Yang Ling Quan* (GB 34) with even supplementing-even draining technique. For dizziness, add *Tou Wei* (St 8) and *Feng Chi* (GB 20). For insomnia, add *Si Shen Cong* (M-HN-1) and *Shen Men* (Ht 7). For vexation and agitation, add *Tai Chong* (Liv 3) and *He Gu* (LI 4).

2. For channel and network vessel stroke,[9] first needle *Nei Guan* (Per 6) with draining technique, then needle *Ren Zhong* (GV 26) with sparrow-pecking hand technique. Follow this with needling *San Yin Jiao* (Sp 6), *Ji Quan* (Ht 1), *Chi Ze* (Lu 5), and *Wei Zhong* (Bl 40) with even supplementing-even draining technique. For inability to extend the upper extremities, add *Qu Chi* (LI 11). For curling of the fingers, add *He Gu* (LI 4) and *Tai Chong* (Liv 3).

3. For viscera and bowel stroke,[10] divide into blockage pattern and desertion pattern. In blockage pattern, the patient suddenly falls down in a faint, unconscious of human affairs. The teeth are tightly closed. The mouth is silent and not open. The two hands are tightly clenched. There is constipation and urinary retention. The limbs are stiff. If blockage pattern is not rescued with force or if the condition of the disease deteriorates, it will develop into desertion pattern. The manifestations of this pattern are blockage of the eyes, open mouth, snoring, faint breathing, hands spread open, chilled limbs, sweat like oil, urinary incontinence, a slack, lolling tongue, and a faint pulse tending to expiry.

For blockage pattern, needle *Nei Guan* (Per 6) and *Ren Zhong* (GV 26) with draining technique. Then bleed the *Shi Xuan* (M-UE-1), exiting 1-2ml of blood from each point.

For desertion pattern, needle *Nei Guan* (Per 6) and *Ren Zhong* (GV 26) with draining technique. Then moxa *Qi Hai* (CV 6), *Guan Yuan* (CV 4), and *Shen Jue* (CV 8) indirectly over Aconite cakes. Also needle *Tai Chong* (Liv 3) and *Nei Ting* (St 44) with supplementing technique.

POST-STROKE SEQUELAE

A. For deviated mouth and eyes, needle *Feng Chi* (GB 20), *Tai Yang* (M-HN-9), *Xia Guan* (St 7), *Di Cang* (St 4) through to *Jia Che* (St 6), and *He Gu* (LI 4) on the healthy or unaffected side.

B. For aphasia, needle *Shang Xing* (GV 23) through to *Bai Hui* (GV 20), *Feng Chi* (GB 20), *Lian Quan* (CV 23), *Tong Li* (Ht 5), and *Tian Zhu* (Bl 10) and bleed *Jin Jin* and *Yu Ye* (M-HN-20).

C. For upper extremity paralysis, needle *Qu Chi* (LI 11), *Feng Chi* (GB 20), *Ji Quan* (Ht 1), *Chi Ze* (Lu 5), *He Gu* (LI 4), *Ba Xie* (M-UE-22), *Jian Yu* (LI 15), and *Wai Guan* (TB 5).

D. For lower extremity paralysis, needle *Wei Zhong* (Bl 40), *San Yin Jiao* (Sp 6), *Huan Tiao* (GB 30), *Yang Ling Quan* (GB 34), and *Kun Lun* (Bl 60).

E. For speech disturbances, needle *Nei Guan* (Per 6), *Ren Zhong* (GV 26), *Feng Chi* (GB 20), and *Lian Quan* (CV 23).

ABSTRACTS OF REPRESENTATIVE CHINESE RESEARCH:

Hua Shi-zuo & Chen Wei-ping, "The Treatment of 24 Cases of Recurrent Transient Ischemic Attacks with *Ling Dan Tang* (Campsis & Salvia Decoction)," *Si Chuan Zhong Yi (Sichuan Chinese Medicine)*, #9, 2000, p. 28: In this report, the authors describe a protocol for the treatment of TIAs using *Ling Dan Tang* (Campsis & Salvia Decoction). In this study, there were 24 males and seven females. Three cases were between 30-39 years of age, five were 40-49, 11 were 50-59, and five were 60 or over. Sixteen had a history of high blood pressure, three had low blood pressure, 21 had arteriosclerosis, three had heart disease, and two had cervical vertebrae disease. Unfortunately, the authors do not state if any of the patients were diabetics. However, given the symptoms and age range, it would not be unlikely that at least some of the patients had diabetes. In terms of clinical manifestations, all 24 suffered from dizziness and nausea. Eleven had bilateral numbness of the extremities, while six had unilateral numbness. In 18 cases, speech was not clear. Eight cases had abnormal sensations in one side of their body, eight cases had double vision, 14 had varying degrees of hemiplegia, and nine had a history of traumatic injury. In terms of frequency of attacks, 17 cases experienced TIAs 1-2 times per day, five cases experienced TIAs once every 2-3 days, and two cases experienced TIAs once a week. CT scans, EEGs, ECGs, brain ultrasonography, and/or brain arteriograms were done on all patients as well as blood lipid analyses. The protocol consisted of administering internally the following Chinese medicinal formula: Flos Campsitis (*Ling Xiao Hua*) and Radix Salviae Miltiorrhizae (*Dan Shen*), 20g each, Semen Pruni Persicae (*Tao Ren*) and Radix

Angelicae Sinensis (*Dang Gui*), 15g each, Flos Carthami Tinctorii (*Huang Hua*) and Radix Ligustici Wallichii (*Chuan Xiong*), 10g each, Ramulus Cinnamomi Cassiae (*Gui Zhi*), 5g, powdered Radix Pseudoginseng (*San Qi*, taken with the strained decoction in two divided doses) and Herba Asari Cum Radice (*Xi Xin*), 2g each, and Radix Astragali Membranacei (*Huang Qi*), 40g. These medicinals were soaked in alcohol and then decocted in water. Each day, one *ji* of this formula was administered orally, with 10 days equaling one course of treatment. This treatment was continued for 60 days. Cure was defined as disappearance of all clinical symptoms with no recurrence within six months. Improvement meant that the clinical symptoms decreased and that the frequency of attacks lessened. No effect meant that there was no improvement in either the symptoms or the frequency of attacks. Based on these criteria, 18 cases were judged cured and six cases improved. Based on the protocol used, it is Hua and Chen's assumption that most TIAs are a combination of blood stasis and qi vacuity.

Zhang Zhan-jun, "Efficacy of Acupuncture in the Treatment of Post-stroke Aphasia," *Journal of Traditional Chinese Medicine*, #9, 1989, p. 87-89: In this report, 150 patients with post-stroke aphasia were treated with acupuncture. Of the 150 patients (75 in each group), 88 were men and 62 were women. Their ages ranged from 21-74 years old. Thirty-eight patients had suffered from aphasia for less then three months, 50 for between three months and one year, 40 for 1-3 years, and 22 for more than three years. Eighty-six cases (57.3%) were classified as having severe speech disorders. These patients presented with no spontaneous speech, inability to articulate or understand verbal communication, deviation of the tongue or limited ability to extend the tongue, inability to raise the soft palate on the paralyzed side, and absence of the pharyngeal reflex. During the acute post-stroke stage, both groups were given conventional Western medical treatment. After they were stabilized, the treatment group received acupuncture at *Yu Men* (Speech Gate, an extra-channel point), while the control group received vasodilators and other symptomatic treatment. The method of needling was to grasp the patient's tongue with one hand, and, while firmly holding the tongue, insert a 28 gauge needle starting about one centimeter from the tip of the tongue on the paralyzed side. The needle was inserted toward the base of the tongue, horizontally and parallel to the veins in the tongue to a depth of 2.5 inches. The needle was then manipulated with even supplementing-even draining method and removed when the qi arrived. This method was applied once every other day for 12 days. If there was no improvement after four courses of treatment, then no further needling was performed. Of the 75 cases in the control group, 38 were considered severe. After acupuncture treatment, nine of these cases were completely cured, seven cases improved and were classified as only slightly impaired, and 15 cases improved and were classified as moderately impaired. Seven cases showed no change. Of the 24 cases considered moderately impaired, eight were restored to normal, and 16 were considered improved. All 13 cases of the slight impairment group were completely cured. According to the author, needling Yu Men causes no pain since there are no large arteries or nerves in the tongue. Local ecchymosis of submucosal vessels did not alter the function or the results of the treatment.

Representative case histories:

Case 1[11]

The patient was a 67 year old male who had had diabetes for six years. The diabetes was complicated by hypertension and high cholesterol, and the patient had been ineffective in controlling his blood sugar. At the time of his visit to the author's clinic, he complained of dizziness and headache, shaking limbs, constipation, and slurred speech for the last two days. Muscle strength in the right lower limb was at stage III and in the left lower limb at stage IV. His post prandial blood sugar level was 13.8mmol/L. CT scan of the man's brain showed many lacunae resulting from cerebral infarction. The patient had little color in his face, his tongue was dull with static macules, and his pulse was choppy and fine.

Based on the above signs and symptoms, the patient's Chinese medical pattern discrimination was qi vacuity and blood stasis, and the treatment principles were to boost the qi and quicken the blood, transform stasis and free the flow of the network vessels. The formula he was administered included: Radix Astragali Membranacei (Huang Qi), 30g, Radix Salviae Miltiorrhizae (Dan Shen), Radix Ligustici Wallichii (Chuan Xiong), and Radix Rubrus Paeoniae Lactiflorae (Chi Shao), 15g each, Radix Angelicae Sinensis (Dang Gui), 12g, and Flos Carthami Tinctorii (Hong Hua) and Lumbricus (Di Long), 10g each. One ji was administered orally per day for one month. After that, the patient's muscle tone was restored to normal, his speech was clear, and his life activities were restored to normal.

Case 2[12]

The patient was a 70 year old female retired worker who

was first examined as an out-patient on Jun. 19, 1994. The patient had had right-sided hemiplegia as the sequela of a stroke for one year. At the time she was hospitalized for the stroke, it was found that her blood and urine glucose were both high, and she was diagnosed with type 2 diabetes. At that time, she was prescribed oral hypoglycemic medications for one month, her symptoms improved, and she was discharged from the hospital. Over the last year, this patient's blood glucose had fluctuated between 7.21-7.99mmol/L (130-144mg/dL). She took 2.5mg of glyburide BID as well as 25mg of Jiang Tang Ling (Lower Sugar Efficacious [Remedy]) BID. However, recovery of the right-sided paralysis had been slow, and the patient was not able to take care of herself. Therefore, she had sought consultation with Dr. Zhu.

When Dr. Zhu examined this woman, he found that both her right hand and foot were swollen and distended, numb, lacked strength, and could not move themselves. There was a dry mouth with a bitter taste, unclear speech, chest oppression, heart fluster, poor appetite, and fluctuating dry or loose stools. Both feet were cool and not warm and there was habitual cramping of the sinews. The woman's tongue was red with thick, slimy, white fur, while her pulse was bowstring and slippery.

Based on the above signs and symptoms, Dr. Zhu's pattern discrimination was qi and yin dual vacuity with blood stasis and non-freely flowing network vessels. Therefore, the treatment principles were to boost the qi and nourish yin, quicken the blood and free the flow of the network vessels using the following medicinals: uncooked Radix Astragali Membranacei (Huang Qi), Caulis Milletiae Seu Spatholobi (Ji Xue Teng), Radix Salviae Miltiorrhizae (Dan Shen), and Radix Scrophulariae Ningpoensis (Xuan Shen), 30g each, Ramulus Loranthi Seu Visci (Sang Ji Sheng) and Herba Siegesbeckiae (Xi Xian Cao), 20g each, Rhizoma Atractylodis (Cang Zhu) and Radix Rubrus Paeoniae Lactiflorae (Chi Shao), 15g each, cooked Radix Rehmanniae (Shu Di), uncooked Radix Rehmanniae (Sheng Di), Radix Angelicae Sinensis (Dang Gui), Radix Ligustici Wallichii (Chuan Xiong), Semen Pruni Persicae (Tao Ren), Flos Carthami Tinctorii (Hong Hua), Lumbricus (Di Long), and Ramulus Cinnamomi Cassiae (Gui Zhi), 10g each, and Rhizoma Coptidis Chinensis (Huang Lian), 5g.

After one month of taking one ji of the above medicinals per day, the swelling and distention in the right hand and foot had disappeared and the numbness had decreased. The right lower limb had more strength. However, the extremities still were not warm and there was still heart fluster, sweating, and a tendency to loose stools. Fasting blood glucose was 7.99mmol/L (144mg/dL), urine glucose was negative, and the pulse was the same as before. Therefore, *Huang Lian*, *Gui Zhi*, and *Sang Ji Sheng* were removed from the above formula and 15 grams of uncooked Fructus Crataegi (*Shan Zha*) and 10 grams each of Rhizoma Atractylodis Macrocephalae (*Bai Zhu*), Semen Coicis Lachryma-jobi (*Yi Yi Ren*), Rhizoma Sparganii (*San Leng*), and Rhizoma Curcumae Zeodariae (*E Zhu*) were added. This formula was then administered for two months.

On Sept. 9, 1994, the patient was re-examined and there was no swelling or numbness of the right foot or hand and skin warmth was normal. Fasting blood glucose was 6.99mmol/L (126mg/dL), the tongue was red, and the pulse was fine and bowstring. Thus the above formula with additions and subtractions was continued for yet another two months, during which time the muscular strength on this woman's right side continued to increase. She could now stand and move on her own, her speech was clear, FBG was 5.99mmol/L (108mg/dL), and urine glucose was negative.

CASE 3[13]

The patient was a 72 year old male who was first examined on Aug. 23, 1993. The patient had had fatigue and polydipsia for more than 30 years and tremors of the hands for 10. In 1962, the man had been diagnosed with diabetes. In 1970, he had begun insulin injections, 44-54 units per day. His FBG was 9.43-12.21mmol/L (170-220mg/dL), two hour PPBG was 9.99-14.42mmol/L (180-260mg/dL), and urine glucose was (++´+++). Tremors of the hands made the patient's grasping difficult. He had already taken a number of types of tremor medication without effect. The patient also had a history of joint disease, cholelithiasis, hypertension, and cerebral infarction. His symptoms at the time of examination included dry mouth and polydipsia, dizziness, tinnitus, lack of strength, limpness of the knees, lower and upper back aching and pain, and inhibited movement. The upper half of the man's body was dry and his feet emitted coolness and were not warm. At night, the patient's urination was frequent. His blood pressure was 25.9/13.3kPa (194/100mmHg), his tongue was dark red with white fur, and his pulse was fine and bowstring.

Based on the above signs and symptoms, this patient's patterns were categorized as liver-kidney insufficiency, yin and yang dual vacuity, and vacuity wind stirring internally. Therefore, the treatment principles were to enrich and

supplement the liver and kidneys, warm yang and foster yin, extinguish wind and free the flow of the network vessels, for which the patient was prescribed: uncooked Radix Astragali Membranacei (*Huang Qi*), uncooked Radix Rehmanniae (*Sheng Di*), Radix Scrophulariae Ningpoensis (*Xuan Shen*), Radix Salviae Miltiorrhizae (*Dan Shen*), uncooked Os Draconis (*Long Gu*) and Concha Ostreae (*Mu Li*), 30g each, Rhizoma Atractylodis (*Cang Zhu*), Radix Puerariae (*Ge Gen*), Sclerotium Poriae Cocos (*Fu Ling*), Rhizoma Alismatis (*Ze Xie*), Ramulus Uncariae Cum Uncis (*Gou Teng*), Rhizoma Cibotii Barometsis (*Gou Ji*), and Rhizoma Homalomenae (*Qian Nian Jian*), 15g each, and Radix Dioscoreae Oppositae (*Shan Yao*), Fructus Corni Officinalis (*Shan Zhu Yu*), Cortex Radicis Moutan (*Dan Pi*), Ramulus Cinnamomi Cassiae (*Gui Zhi*), Radix Albus Paeoniae Lactiflorae (*Bai Shao*), and Fructus Lycii Chinensis (*Gou Qi Zi*), 10g each.

The second examination occurred on Nov. 2 after the patient had taken 50 *ji* of the above formula. The man's affect had improved, his FBG was 7.77mmol/L (140mg/dL), and he took 40 units of insulin per day. However, there was still profuse sweating on one-half of his body, the emission of coolness below the knees, and marked tremor of his hands. His blood pressure was 22.3/9.98kPa (168/75mmHG), his tongue was dark red with white fur, and his pulse was fine and bowstring. Therefore, his patterns were categorized as qi and yin dual vacuity with dryness and heat internally exuberant and liver wind raiding the network vessels, for which the patient was prescribed: uncooked Radix Astragali Membranacei (*Huang Qi*), uncooked Semen Coicis Lachryma-jobi (*Yi Yi Ren*), and Radix Pulsatillae Chinensis (*Bai Tou Weng*), 30g each, cooked Radix Rehmanniae (*Shu Di*), uncooked Radix Rehmanniae (*Sheng Di*), Rhizoma Atractylodis Macrocephalae (*Bai Zhu*), Rhizoma Atractylodis (*Cang Zhu*), and Ramulus Uncariae Cum Uncis (*Gou Teng*), 15g each, Radix Scutellariae Baicalensis (*Huang Qin*), Cortex Phellodendri (*Huang Bai*), Tuber Ophiopogonis Japonici (*Mai Men Dong*), Fructus Schisandrae Chinensis (*Wu Wei Zi*), Radix Angelicae Sinensis (*Dang Gui*), and Fructus Pruni Mume (*Wu Mei*), 10g each, and Rhizoma Coptidis Chinensis (*Huang Lian*), 6g.

The third examination occurred on Dec. 14 after the patient had taken 28 *ji* of the above formula with additions and subtractions. At this time, his sweating was markedly decreased and night-time urination was less frequent. However, there was still tremors of the hands. Blood pressure was normal, and the tongue and pulse were as above. Now the patient's patterns were categorized as yin and yang dual vacuity with liver wind stirring internally. The formula prescribed at this visit included: uncooked Radix Astragali Membranacei (*Huang Qi*), Radix Scrophulariae Ningpoensis (*Xuan Shen*), Radix Salviae Miltiorrhizae (*Dan Shen*), uncooked Os Draconis (*Long Gu*), Concha Ostreae (*Mu Li*), Radix Pulsatillae Chinensis (*Bai Tou Weng*), and Herba Lysimachiae Seu Desmodii (*Jin Qian Cao*), 30g each, cooked Radix Rehmanniae (*Shu Di*), uncooked Radix Rehmanniae (*Sheng Di*), Rhizoma Atractylodis (*Cang Zhu*), Radix Puerariae (*Ge Gen*), Ramulus Uncariae Cum Uncis (*Gou Teng*), and Herba Artemisiae Capillaris (*Yin Chen Hao*), 15g each, and Ramulus Cinnamomi Cassiae (*Gui Zhi*), Radix Albus Paeoniae Lactiflorae (*Bai Shao*), Radix Et Rhizoma Notopterygii (*Qiang Huo*), Radix Angelicae Pubescentis (*Du Huo*), Radix Bupleuri (*Chai Hu*), and Radix Scutellariae Baicalensis (*Huang Qin*), 10g each.

The fourth examination occurred on Jan. 25, 1994. The patient had been taking the above Chinese medicinals for one month. His bodily strength had markedly increased and he was able to walk by himself and climb stairs. In addition, the tremors in his hands were markedly decreased. Fasting blood glucose was 5.94-6.66mmol/L (107-120mg/dL), and his insulin was down to 30 units per day. Because the man's condition was stable, the following medicinals were made into pills in order to secure and consolidate the treatment effects: Caulis Milletiae Seu Spatholobi (*Ji Xue Teng*) and Radix Pulsatillae Chinensis (*Bai Tou Weng*), 90g each, Ramulus Loranthi Seu Visci (*Sang Ji Sheng*), Radix Dipsaci (*Xu Duan*), Ramulus Uncariae Cum Uncis (*Gou Teng*), Rhizoma Cibotii Barometsis (*Gou Ji*), and Rhizoma Homalomenae (*Qian Nian Jian*), 60g each, Fructus Lycii Chinensis (*Gou Qi Zi*) and Herba Siegesbeckiae (*Xi Xian Cao*), 50g each, and Radix Et Rhizoma Notopterygii (*Qiang Huo*), Radix Angelicae Pubescentis (*Du Huo*), Cortex Eucommiae Ulmoidis (*Du Zhong*), Flos Chrysanthemi Morifolii (*Ju Hua*), Radix Angelicae Sinensis (*Dang Gui*), Lignum Sappan (*Su Mu*), Radix Angelicae Anomalae (*Liu Ji Nu*), and Herba Epimedii (*Xian Ling Pi*), 30g each. These medicinals were ground into fine powder, mixed with water, and made into pills. The patient then took 10 grams of these pills after each meal.

REMARKS:

1. While most Chinese authors simply equate CVD with stroke, readers should not forget that TIAs are also a symptom of CVD and may be due to diabetes. Transient ischemic attacks are focal neurological abnormalities of sudden onset and brief duration that reflect dysfunction in the distribution of the internal carotid-middle cerebral or the vertebrobasilar arterial system. Most TIAs are due to cerebral emboli from ulcerated atherosclerotic plaques in the carotid or vertebral arteries in the neck or, less frequently, from mural throbi in a diseased heart. Some TIAs are due to brief reduction in blood flow through stenosed arteries. Predisposing conditions to TIAs include hypertension, atherosclerosis, heart disease, atrial fibrillation, diabetes mellitus, and polycythemia. TIAs are most common in the middle-aged and elderly.

TIAs begin suddenly, last two to 30 minutes or more (but seldom more than 1-2 hours), and then abate without persistent neurologic abnormalities. Consciousness remains throughout the episode. The symptoms of TIAs are identical to stroke but are transient. If there is carotid artery involvement, the symptoms are usually unilateral. Ipsilateral blindness or contralateral hemiparesis, often with paresthesias, are classic but less complete symptoms are, in fact, more common. Aphasia indicates involvement of the dominant hemisphere. Confusion, vertigo, binocular blindness, diplopia, and unilateral or bilateral weakness or paresthesias of the extremities may be present. In addition, slurred speech may occur with carotid or vertebrobasilar involvement.

Patients may have several TIAs per day or only 2-3 over several years. Patients with TIAs are at a markedly increased risk of stroke and should be evaluated for possible causes on an urgent basis. Western medical treatment consists of either surgery (endarterectomy) or internally administered medicinals depending on the degree of arterial obstruction. However, the risk/benefit ratio for endarterectomy is narrow. Antiplatelet drugs or anticoagulants are used when the obstruction is intracranial or vertebrobasilar. Heparin is used initially for recent daily attacks, while warfarin derivatives are used for less frequent attacks. Aspirin is often the antiplatelet drug of choice, but the optimal dosage of aspirin is unknown. Antiplatelet drugs should be continued indefinitely.

The Chinese medical pattern discrimination of diabetic TIAs is the same as for CVD in general as presented above.

2. For the long-term treatment of the sequelae of stroke, ready-made medicines such as *Da Huo Luo Dan* (Major Quicken the Network Vessels Elixir), *Zai Zao Wan* (Renewal Pills), and *Hua Tuo Zai Zao Wan* (Hua Tuo's Renewal Pills) may be used depending on the patient's pattern discrimination.

3. For more information specifically on the acupuncture

treatment of stroke and hemiplegia, see Wu and Han's *Golden Needle Wang Le-ting* also published by Blue Poppy Press.

4. Some Chinese doctors prefer to use head or so-called scalp acupuncture for the treatment of stroke. For information on that acupuncture specialty, please see any of the various books on this subject available in English.

5. Ultimately, in Chinese medicine just as in Western medicine, the best treatment for cerebral vascular accident is prevention. This means appropriate initial treatment of hypertension, atherosclerosis, heart disease, and DM.

ENDNOTES:

[1] Http://pages.prodigy.net/dfan/dfansite/june00.html

[2] In fact, most Chinese sources on diabetic cerebrovascular disease simply equate CVD with stroke. This helps explain the opening symptoms of the patterns below.

[3] www.dotpharmacy.co.uk/updiab.hyml

[4] www.aafp.org/afp/monograph/200001/index.html

[5] www.ssa.gob.mx/actualissate/3/jun00/diab19.htm

[6] Http://vbwg.org/journal_article.cfm?article_id=174

[7] www.pitt.edu/~super1/lectures/lec1921/013.htm

[8] www.coloradohealthnet.org/diabetes/facts_chronic.html

[9] The signs and symptoms of channel and network vessel stroke are deviated mouth and eyes, numbness of the skin, hemiplegia, and impeded speech but no clouding of the spirit or unconsciousness.

[10] This is a more serious form of stroke which is characterized by sudden clouding of the spirit and unconsciousness. When the patient regains consciousness, then they manifest the hemiplegia, etc. of channel and network vessel stroke.

[11] Wang Xiao-hong, "The Treatment of Diabetic Complications Using *Bu Yang Huan Wu Tang* (Supplement Yang Five Returning Decoction)," *Zhejiang Zhong Yi Za Zhi (Zhejiang Journal of Traditional Chinese Medicine)*, 1999, #11, p. 494

[12] Zhu Chen-zi, anthologized in Dan Shu-jian & Chen Zi-hua's *Xiao Ke Juan (The Wasting & Thirsting Book)*, Chinese National Chinese Medicine & Medicinals Publishing Co., Beijing, 1999, p. 131-133

[13] *Ibid.*, p. 146-148

23

DIABETIC NEPHROPATHY

Diabetic nephropathy is a kidney disorder that is a complication of diabetes mellitus. It is characterized by proteinuria and progressive reduction in kidney function culminating in azotemia. Other names for this or subtypes of this condition are Kimmelstiel-Wilson disease, diabetic glomerulosclerosis, and diabetic kidney disease. Kidney damage caused by diabetes most often involves thickening and hardening (sclerosis) of the internal kidney structures, particulary the glomerulus. Kimmelstiel-Wilson disease is a form of diabetic nephropathy in which sclerosis of the glomeruli is accompanied by nodular deposits of hyaline in the afferent arterioles. The glomeruli are the site where blood is filtered and rudimentary urine is formed. As diabetic nephropathy progresses, increasing numbers of glomeruli are destroyed, resulting in impaired kidney functioning. Filtration slows and protein may leak into the urine. Initially, there is intermittent microalbuminuria which progresses to persistent microalbuminuria and, ultimately, to macroalbuminuria. Microalbuminuria is defined as urinary albumin excretion of more than 30mg and less than 300mg per day. Macroalbuminuria is defined as urinary albumin excretion over 550mg per day. Diabetic nephropathy can sometimes cause nephrotic syndrome. Nephrotic syndrome is a severe loss of urinary protein with hypoproteinuria and generalized edema. It may or may not be a terminal event or lead to acute renal failure. The disorder continues to progress rapidly with the appearance of macroproteinuria, with end-stage renal disease (ESRD) typically developing within 2-6 years after the appearance of chronic renal failure or significant hypertension[1,2] and within 12 years after diagnosis of diabetes. Thirty-five to 40% of patients with diabetes eventually develop nephropathy (35% in type 1 DM, 15-60% in type 2 DM depending on genetic predisposition). It is the cause of death of 17% of all those with diabetes[3] and is the leading cause of death in those with diabetes.

The exact mechanisms which cause diabetic nephropathy are unknown. Although probably multifactorial, the cause of nephropathy may be due to accumulation of a reduced sugar product, sorbitol, a tissue toxin that can affect the Na-K-ATP pump. However, in type 2 diabetes, mesangial lymphokine production is associated not only with hyperglycemia but also with insulin resistance and generalized vascular disease. Thus albuminuria may occur even before hyperglycemia develops. Genetic predisposition is also thought to play an important role. Patients who have one or two deletions of the angiotensin-converting enzyme (ACE) gene, a defect in the sodium proton pump, or a family history of hypertension are at increased risk for progression to diabetic nephropathy.[4] A proposed mechanism for the development of nephropathy with type 1 diabetes is elevation of growth hormone levels due to poor glycemic control. This results in hyperperfusion of the glomerulus and glomerular hypertension. Mesangial cells in the glomerulus respond to glomerular hypertension by producing growth factors, especially tumor necrosis factor-A, which results in increased permeability, proliferation of glomerular epithelial cells, and excessive production of the basement membrane and collagen tissue (or hyalinization).

In the early stages of diabetic nephropathy, there are no clinical signs or symptoms of renal disease even though glomerular filtration may be elevated. Glomerular changes are typically first detected during routine urine analysis of a person with diabetes who shows protein in the urine. Although there may be signs but no symptoms for many years, as the condition progresses, clinical disease does manifest (azotemia). This includes edema of the face (especially periorbital) and/or extremities, a foamy appearance of the urine, either unintentional weight gain due to water retention or unintentional weight loss due to actual loss of body mass and protein, poor appetite, nausea and vomiting, general malaise, fatigue, headache, frequent hiccups, and generalized pruritus. Other symptoms which may be associated with this disease are excessive urination, excessive thirst, abnormalities of the nails (*i.e.*, pitting), and hypertension.

Diabetes has become the single, most common cause of end stage renal disease in the U.S. and Europe. This is thought to be due to three factors: 1) diabetes, particularly type 2 diabetes, is increasing in prevalence 2) diabetes patients now live longer, and 3) patients with diabetic ESRD are now being accepted for treatment in ESRD programs who had formerly been excluded. In the U.S., diabetes accounts for 50% of all new cases of ESRD on dialysis.[5] In 1991 in the U.S., the cost for treatment of diabetic patients with ESRD was in excess of $2 billion per year.[6] In 1995, 27,851 people with diabetes developed ESRD. About 20-30% of patients with type 1 or type 2 diabetes develop evidence of nephropathy. In addition, there is considerable racial/ethnic variability in the incidence of ESRD, with Latinos (especially Mexican Americans), Native Americans (especially Pima Indians), and African Americans having much higher risks of developing ESRD than non-Latino whites with type 2 diabetes. Among African Americans, part of this higher risk may be attributable to a greater propensity to develop keloids.

The Western medical prevention of this condition consists of controlling hypertension, hyperlipidemia, and blood glucose levels. Diet should be modified in terms of calories, protein, and fat to help control blood sugar levels and patients should be encouraged to stop smoking. A low protein diet (0.6g/kg of body weight) has the theoretical advantages of decreasing glomerular hypertension, reducing proteinuria, and slowing decline in renal function, while smoking worsens hypertension and albuminuria by increasing catecholamine levels in diabetics. In addition, radiocontrast materials or potentially nephotoxic drugs should be avoided as should overuse of diuretics. If a urinary tract infection develops (and they are common in diabetics), it is typically treated as soon as possible with antibiotics since such infections may damage kidney function. Other preventive measures consist of avoiding dehydration, hypoxia, and the use of antifungal agents and nonsteroidal anti-inflammatory drugs (NSAIDs).

In terms of the Western medical remedial treatment, this consists of oral hypoglycemic agents and/or insulin injections, aggressive treatment of dyslipidemia, and aggressive treatment of hypertension with antihypertensive medica-

tions, particularly ACE inhibitors. ACE inhibitors not only reduce systemic hypertension, they also decrease intraglomerular hypertension. For instance, in patients with diabetic nephropathy, Western physicians attempt to lower blood pressure to below 135/85mmHg and to even lower the systolic level to 100-110mmHg.[7] Some physicians include the use of nondihydropyridine calcium channel blockers to decrease the production of lymphokines. At the microalbuminuria stage, tight glycemic control and protein restriction are still effective. Once macroalbuminuria develops, the course of diabetic nephropathy cannot be reversed. Therefore, it is extremely important to stop this condition's progression before macroalbuminuria develops.

In the early stage of renal failure, dialysis may be used. Unfortunately, dialysis has several disadvantages. It may cause vitreous and other hemorrhages, may result in digital ischemia and gangrene, worsens neuropthy, and accelerates atherosclerosis. Kidney transplant may also be used in the treatment of diabetic nephropathy, with such transplants ideally being performed while the serum creatinine level is still less than 5mg/dL. Renal transplantation is the treatment of choice in younger patients. However, renal transplantation is not an option for almost all patients with type 2 diabetes, and complications with dialysis and transplantation are more common with diabetic nephropathy, with death occurring from such complications twice as often in diabetics than in nondiabetics who require these treatments.[8] In 1995, 98,872 people with diabetes underwent dialysis or kidney transplantation.[9] Experimental treatments include insulin infusion pumps, the use of oral or injected heparin, oral therapy with glycosaminoglycans derived from pig intestines, and danaparoid sodium (Organan).

CHINESE DISEASE MECHANISMS:

Gao Yan-bin, in *Zhong Guo Tang Niao Bing Fang Zhi Tie Se (The Characteristics of the Chinese National Prevention & Treatment of Diabetes)*, divides the disease mechanisms of this condition into early and late stages. In the early or initial stage, Gao says that kidney yin vacuity is the root, while lung-stomach dryness and heat are the branches. The kidneys govern water and command opening and sealing. If diabetes has endured for years, then kidney yin must be depleted and have suffered detriment. In that case, yin detriment consumes the qi, and this results in kidney qi vacuity and detriment. Securing and gathering lose their duty and opening and sealing lose their command. Hence one sees frequent, profuse urination and the urine is turbid and sweet. Because the liver and kidneys share a common source and the essence and blood mutually engender each other, if there is kidney yin depletion and detriment, there will also be a liver yin vacuity. This means the liver and kidneys are both vacuous, and essence and blood are not able to ascend to the eyes. Hence the eyes are dry and scratchy. If yin vacuity results in fire effulgence, this fire may burn and damage the blood vessels in the eyes. Therefore, there is bleeding in the grounds of the eyes accompanied by blurred vision. If liver-kidney yin vacuity leads to ascension of liver yang hyperactivity, there will be dizziness and tinnitus and the blood pressure will tend to be high. If liver-kidney yin vacuity leads to the vessels and network vessels becoming static and obstructed, the sinew vessels will lose their nourishment, and this will result in numbness and pain of the extremities.

In the later stages, yin detriment reaches yang, damaging the heart and spleen and causing spleen-kidney yang vacuity. Water dampness collects and lodges, spilling over into the flesh and skin. Thus there is water swelling of the face and feet. If severe, there will be water in the chest and abdomen. If yang vacuity is not able to warm and shine the four limbs, there will be fear of cold and chilled limbs. In the last stages, qi, blood, yin, and yang are all vacuous. If kidney yang declines and is vanquished, water dampness will spill over and flood and turbid toxins will collect internally. If turbid toxins spill over above, the stomach will lose its harmony and downbearing. This then leads to nausea and vomiting and devitalized eating and drinking. If the spleen and stomach decline and are vanquished, turbid evils will also collect internally and blood and fluids will lose the source of their engenderment and transformation. Hence the facial complexion is sallow yellow and the lips, nails, and tongue are pale. If water dampness and turbid toxins attack the heart and lungs above, there will be heart palpitations, shortness of breath, chest oppression, panting respiration, and inability to lie flat. If the kidney source declines and is exhausted, turbid evils congest and block the three burners and the kidneys bar and do not open. This leads to scanty urination or anuria.

However, while many Chinese authors emphasize the role of kidney vacuity in diabetes and its complications, it is important not to underestimate the role of qi vacuity. In the Ming dynasty, Tai Yuan-li said, "If the three wastings endure and endure and are not treated, qi [must be] extremely vacuous." According to Gao Yan-bin, any of three mechanisms may result in qi vacuity in enduring diabetes: 1) Yin fluid depletion and consumption may result in scattering and consumption of the qi; 2) dry heat evils may damage yin and consume the qi; and 3) if there is a natural endowment insufficiency with habitual bodily qi vacuity on top of which there is an enduring disease which will not recover, this will cause even more detriment and damage to the righteous qi, resulting in even further qi vacuity. However, it is our experience that spleen qi vacuity due to overeating sweets, fats, oils, and alcohol, overtaxation, too much thinking and anxiety, and too little physical exercise precedes or is at least concomitant with any of the above disease mechanisms in the majority of Western diabetics. In any case, it is both our and a number of other Chinese authors' opinion that virtually all cases of diabetic nephropathy are complicated by varying degrees of qi vacuity. This accounts for the fatigue, lack of strength, shortness of breath, and disinclination to speak or a faint, weak voice.

Further, if yin vacuity and fire effulgence cooks and boils the fluids and humors, the blood will become sticky and stagnant. At the same time, if the qi is vacuous, the blood will lack the power to move. Hence, for either or both these reasons, the blood vessels will become static and obstructed. Additionally, damp evils hinder and obstruct the free flow of qi and blood and fluids flow together. This means that water dampness and turbid evils may also result in or aggravate blood stasis. Therefore, blood stasis typically complicates diabetic nephropathy and becomes ever more likely the older the patient and the more serious their condition.

TREATMENT BASED ON PATTERN DISCRIMINATION:

1. LIVER-KIDNEY QI & YIN DUAL VACUITY PATTERN

MAIN SYMPTOMS: Low back and knee soreness and limpness, lassitude of the spirit, lack of strength, shortness of breath, disinclination to speak and/or a faint, weak voice, vexatious heat in the five hearts, a dry mouth and parched throat, bilateral dryness and scratchiness of the eyes, blurred vision, dizziness, tinnitus, possible heart palpitations, possible spontaneous perspiration, dry, bound stools, a dark, fat tongue with white or scanty fur, and a deep, fine, bowstring pulse

NOTE: Although blood stasis is not mentioned in the name of this pattern, nor are there many signs or symptoms of static blood listed above, static blood complicates virtually all cases of diabetic nephropathy.

TREATMENT PRINCIPLES: Enrich and supplement the liver and kidneys, boost the qi and quicken the blood

RX: *Qi Ju Di Huang Wan Jia Jian* (Lycium & Chrysanthemum Rehmannia Pills with Additions & Subtractions)

INGREDIENTS: Uncooked Radix Rehmanniae (*Sheng Di*) and Radix Salviae Miltiorrhizae (*Dan Shen*), 30g each, Radix Scrophulariae Ningpoensis (*Xuan Shen*), 20g, Radix Dioscoreae Oppositae (*Shan Yao*), Radix Trichosanthis Kirlowii (*Tian Hua Fen*), and Rhizoma Polygonati (*Huang Jing*), 15g each, and Fructus Lycii Chinensis (*Gou Qi Zi*), Fructus Corni Officinalis (*Shan Zhu Yu*), Rhizoma Alismatis (*Ze Xie*), Radix Puerariae (*Ge Gen*), and Radix Angelicae Sinensis (*Dang Gui*), 9g each

FORMULA ANALYSIS: *Gou Qi Zi* and *Shan Zhu Yu* enrich and supplement the liver and kidneys. *Huang Jing, Sheng Di,* and *Xuan Shen* boost the qi and nourish yin. *Ge Gen* and *Tian Hua Fen* engender fluids and stop thirst. *Dan Shen* and *Dang Gui* quicken the blood and transform stasis.

ADDITIONS & SUBTRACTIONS: If there is lung-stomach dryness and heat, add 30 grams each of uncooked Gypsum Fibrosum (*Shi Gao*) and Calcitum (*Han Shui Shi*) and nine grams of Rhizoma Anemarrhenae Aspheloidis (*Zhi Mu*) and double the *Tian Hua Fen*. If there is bowel repletion constipation, increase the *Sheng Di* and *Xuan Shen* to 30 grams and add nine grams each of wine-fried Radix Et Rhizoma Rhei (*Da Huang*) and Fructus Immaturus Citri Aurantii (*Zhi Shi*). If there is shortness of breath, lack of strength, heart palpitations, and spontaneous perspiration due to pronounced qi vacuity, add 15 grams each of Radix Astragali Membranacei (*Huang Qi*) and Radix Codonopsitis Pilosulae (*Dang Shen*). If the tongue is purple and dark or if there are static macules or spots showing that blood stasis is more severe, add 15 grams each of Radix Rubrus Paeoniae Lactiflorae (*Chi Shao*) and Radix Ligustici Wallichii (*Chuan Xiong*) and nine grams of Semen Pruni Persicae (*Tao Ren*). If there is bleeding into the eye ground, add nine grams each of carbonized Flos Immaturus Sophorae Japonicae (*Huai Hua Mi*), Cortex Radicis Moutan (*Dan Pi*), and uncooked Pollen Typhae (*Pu Huang*) in order to cool the blood and stop bleeding. If there is yin vacuity and yang hyperactivity with relatively severe dizziness, add 30 grams each of uncooked Concha Ostreae (*Mu Li*) and Os Draconis (*Long Gu*) and 15 grams each of Ramulus Uncariae Cum Uncis (*Gou Teng*) and Radix Achyranthis Bidentatae (*Niu Xi*) to level the liver and subdue yang. If there is low back and knee soreness and limpness and/or numbness and pain of the four extremities, add 30 grams of Fructus Chaenomelis Lagenariae (*Mu Gua*), 15 grams each of Radix Achyranthis Bidentatae (*Niu Xi*) and Rhizoma Cibotii Barometsis (*Gou Ji*), nine grams each of Buthus Martensis (*Quan Xie*) and Zaocys Dhumnades (*Wu Shao She*), and two strips of Scolopendra Subspinipes (*Wu Gong*). If urination is frequent and urgent or there is burning pain with urination and slimy yellow tongue fur indicating urinary bladder damp heat, add 30 grams each of Herba Pyrrosiae (*Shi Wei*), uncooked Radix Sanguisorbae (*Di Yu*), and Semen Plantaginis (*Che Qian Zi*).

ACUPUNCTURE & MOXIBUSTION: *Fei Shu* (Bl 20), *Pi Shu* (Bl 20), *Shen Shu* (Bl 23), *San Yin Jiao* (Sp 6), *Tai Xi* (Ki 3), *Tai Chong* (Liv 3), *Zu San Li* (St 36)

NOTE: Acupuncture is only appropriate in the early stages of diabetic nephropathy when there is as yet no edema. Acupuncture is not appropriate if there is diabetic nephropathy and accompanying edema.

FORMULA ANALYSIS: Even supplementing-even draining *Fei Shu, Pi Shu,* and *Shen Shu* regulates and rectifies the three viscera which are in control of water fluids in the body. Even supplementing-even draining *San Yin Jiao, Shen Shu,* and *Tai Xi* supplements the kidneys and enriches yin, while even supplementing-even draining *San Yin Jiao* and *Tai Chong* courses the liver and rectifies the qi at the same time as it supplements and nourishes the liver. Even supplementing-even draining *Zu San Li* clears dryness and heat from the stomach at the same time as it supplements the spleen qi.

ADDITIONS & SUBTRACTIONS: If there is marked blood stasis, add *Xue Hai* (Sp 10). If there is concomitant urinary bladder damp heat, add *Yin Ling Quan* (Sp 9) and *Zhong Ji* (CV 3). If there is marked liver depression qi stagnation, add *He Gu* (LI 4). If liver depression has transformed heat, add *Xing Jian* (Liv 2) needled through to *Tai Chong*. For lung heat, add *Chi Ze* (Lu 5). For stomach heat, add *Nei Ting* (St 44). For yang hyperactivity and dizziness, add *Feng Chi* (GB 20), *Yi Feng* (TB 17), and *Bai Hui* (GV 20). For numbness and pain in the fingers, add *Ba Xie* (M-UE-22). For numbness and pain in the toes, add *Ba Feng* (M-LE-8). For low back soreness and weakness, add *Yao Yan* (M-BW-24) and *Da Chang Shu* (Bl 25).

2. SPLEEN-KIDNEY QI & YANG DUAL VACUITY PATTERN

MAIN SYMPTOMS: Low back and knee soreness and limpness, lassitude of the spirit, lack of strength, fear of cold, chilled limbs, superficial edema of the face and feet, stomach duct and abdominal distention and fullness, torpid intake, loose stools, profuse nocturia, a dark fat tongue with teeth-marks on its edges, and a deep, fine, forceless pulse

TREATMENT PRINCIPLES: Warm the kidneys and fortify the spleen, boost the qi and quicken the blood

RX: *Er Xian Tang* (Two Immortals Decoction) plus *Wu Ling San* (Five [Ingredients] Poria Powder) with additions and subtractions

INGREDIENTS: Radix Astragali Membranacei (*Huang Qi*), Radix Salviae Miltiorrhizae (*Dan Shen*), Herba Leonuri Heterophylli (*Yi Mu Cao*), Sclerotium Poriae Cocos (*Fu Ling*), Sclerotium Polypori Umbellati (*Zhu Ling*), and Fructus Chaenomelis Lagenariae (*Mu Gua*), 30g each, Herba Epimedii (*Xian Ling Pi*), Semen Euryalis Ferocis (*Qian Shi*), Fructus Rosae Laevigatae (*Jin Ying Zi*), Radix Codonopsitis Pilosulae (*Dang Shen*), Rhizoma Alismatis (*Ze Xie*), and Herba Lycopi Lucidi (*Ze Lan*), 15g each, and Rhizoma Curculiginis Orchioidis (*Xian Mao*), 9g

FORMULA ANALYSIS: *Xian Mao* and *Xian Ling Pi* warm kidney yang. *Qian Shi* and *Jin Ying Zi* supplement the kidneys and secure the essence. *Dang Shen, Huang Qi,* and *Fu Ling* boost the qi and supplement the center, fortify the spleen and seep dampness. *Zhu Ling, Ze Xie, Ze Lan, Yi Mu Cao, Dan Shen,* and *Mu Gua* quicken the blood and transform stasis, disinhibit water and disperse swelling.

ADDITIONS & SUBTRACTIONS: If there is chest oppression, heart palpitations, and a fat tongue with slimy fur due to chest yang impediment and obstruction by phlegm and dampness, add nine grams each of Fructus Trichosanthis Kirlowii (*Gua Lou*), Bulbus Allii (*Cong Bai*), Pericarpium Citri Reticulatae (*Chen Pi*), and Rhizoma Pinelliae Ternatae (*Ban Xia*). If there is diarrhea, fear of cold, and chilled limbs, also administer *Si Shen Wan* (Four Spirits Pills) or *Fu Zi Li Zhong Wan* (Aconite Rectify the Center Pills) to warm and supplement the spleen and kidneys, secure, astringe, and stop diarrhea. If there is sagging and distention in the lower abdomen or difficulty expelling urine, add 30 grams of Herba Pyrrosiae (*Shi Wei*), 15 grams each of Semen Citri Reticulatae (*Ju He*) and Semen Litchi Chinensis (*Li Zhi He*), and nine grams each of Radix Linderae Strychnifoliae (*Wu Yao*) and Rhizoma Acori Graminei (*Shi Chang Pu*). If there is urinary retention due to kidney yang depletion and vacuity with loss of command of qi transformation, also administer *Jin Gui Shen Qi Wan* (*Golden Cabinet* Kidney Qi Pills). If there is low back and knee soreness and limpness, add

30 grams of Fructus Chaenomelis Lagenariae (*Mu Gua*), 15 grams of Rhizoma Cibotii Barometsis (*Gou Ji*), and nine grams each of Radix Dipsaci (*Xu Duan*) and Buthus Martensis (*Quan Xie*).

If edema is pronounced and fear of cold is severe, one can use *Zhen Wu Tang* (True Warrior Decoction) plus *Wu Pi Yin* (Five Skins Drink) with additions and subtractions in order to warm yang and transform the qi, disinhibit water and disperse swelling: Sclerotium Poriae Cocos (*Fu Ling*), 30g, Rhizoma Atractylodis Macrocephalae (*Bai Zhu*), 15g, Pericarpium Arecae Catechu (*Da Fu Pi*) and Cortex Radicis Mori Albi (*Sang Bai Pi*), 12g each, Radix Lateralis Praeparatus Aconiti Carmichaeli (*Fu Zi*), Pericarpium Citri Reticulatae (*Chen Pi*), Rhizoma Alismatis (*Ze Xie*), Ramulus Cinnamomi Cassiae (*Gui Zhi*), and Radix Stephaniae Tetrandrae (*Han Fang Ji*), 9g each, and uncooked Rhizoma Zingiberis (*Sheng Jiang*), 2-3 slices.

ACUPUNCTURE & MOXIBUSTION: *Pi Shu* (Bl 20), *Shen Shu* (Bl 23), *Ming Men* (GV 4), *Qi Hai* (CV 6), *Guan Yuan* (CV 4)

FORMULA ANALYSIS: Moxaing these points fortifies the spleen and warms the kidneys.

3. QI, BLOOD, YIN, & YANG VACUITY PATTERN

MAIN SYMPTOMS: Low back and knee soreness and limpness, shortness of breath, disinclination to speak and/or a faint, weak voice, a blackish facial complexion, pale lips, nails, and tongue, superficial edema of the face and feet, fear of cold, chilled limbs, scanty urination or anuria, either dry or loose stools, a dry mouth but no desire to drink, dread of chill as well as dread of heat, a fat, fissured tongue with white fur, and a deep, fine, forceless pulse

TREATMENT PRINCIPLES: Regulate and supplement yin and yang, boost the qi and quicken the blood

RX: *Dang Gui Bu Xue Tang* (Dang Gui Supplement the Blood Decoction) plus *Ji Sheng Shen Qi Wan* (Aid the Living Kidney Qi Pills) with additions and subtractions

INGREDIENTS: Radix Astragali Membranacei (*Huang Qi*), Radix Salviae Miltiorrhizae (*Dan Shen*), Herba Leonuri Heterophylli (*Yi Mu Cao*), Sclerotium Poriae Cocos (*Fu Ling*), and Sclerotium Polypori Umbellati (*Zhu Ling*), 30g each, Radix Angelicae Sinensis (*Dang Gui*), uncooked Radix Rehmanniae (*Sheng Di*), and Radix Dioscoreae Oppositae (*Shan Yao*), 15g each, Radix Achyranthis Bidentatae (*Niu Xi*), 12g, Fructus Corni

Officinalis (*Shan Zhu Yu*), Rhizoma Alismatis (*Ze Xie*), and Semen Plantaginis (*Che Qian Zi*), 9g each, Radix Lateralis Praeparatus Aconiti Carmichaeli (*Fu Zi*), 6g

FORMULA ANALYSIS: *Sheng Di, Shan Zhu Yu,* and *Fu Zi* enrich yin and warm yang. *Huang Qi* and *Dang Gui* boost the qi and nourish the blood. *Ze Xie, Che Qian Zi, Fu Ling, Zhu Ling,* and *Yi Mu Cao* disinhibit water and disperse swelling. *Dan Shen* and *Dang Gui* quicken the blood and transform stasis.

ADDITIONS & SUBTRACTIONS: For turbid toxins obstructing the center with stomach loss of harmony and downbearing and the symptoms of nausea and vomiting, devitalized eating and drinking, and a fat tongue with thick, slimy fur, add nine grams each of Pericarpium Citri Reticulatae (*Chen Pi*), Rhizoma Pinelliae Ternatae (*Ban Xia*), Caulis Bambusae In Taeniis (*Zhu Ru*), Herba Agastachis Seu Pogostemi (*Huo Xiang*), Herba Eupatorii Fortunei (*Pei Lan*), and wine-fried Radix Et Rhizoma Rhei (*Da Huang*). For stomach and intestine binding and stagnation with bowel repletion constipation, add 15 grams of Fructus Trichosanthis Kirlowii (*Gua Lou*) and nine grams each of Fructus Immaturus Citri Aurantii (*Zhi Shi*) and uncooked Radix Et Rhizoma Rhei (*Da Huang*) to free the flow of the bowels and drain turbidity. If turbid toxins transform heat which then damages and stirs the blood accompanied by symptoms such as nosebleed and bleeding gums, add nine grams of Cortex Radicis Moutan (*Dan Pi*) and three grams of powdered Radix Pseudoginseng (*San Qi*) swallowed with the decoction, to cool the blood and stop bleeding.

For kidney yang decline and vanquishment with retained water dampness, turbid toxins collecting internally, and water dampness ascending to assault the heart and lungs with the symptoms of heart palpitations, chest oppression, panting respiration, inability to lie flat, scanty urination, relatively severe edema and possible water in the chest, abdomen, or pericardium, use *Sheng Mai San* (Engender the Pulse Powder) plus *Ting Li Zi Da Zao Xie Fei Tang* (Lepidium & Red Date Drain the Lungs Decoction) with additions and subtractions: Semen Lepidii Seu Descurainiae (*Ting Li Zi*), Sclerotium Polypori Umbellati (*Zhu Ling*), and Sclerotium Poriae Cocos (*Fu Ling*), 30g each, Tuber Ophiopogonis Japonici (*Mai Men Dong*), Rhizoma Alismatis (*Ze Xie*), and Herba Lycopi Lucidi (*Ze Lan*), 15g each, Radix Panacis Ginseng (*Ren Shen*), Fructus Schisandrae Chinensis (*Wu Wei Zi*), Cortex Radicis Mori Albi (*Sang Bai Pi*), and Semen Plantaginis (*Che Qian Zi*), 9g each, and Fructus Zizyphi Jujubae (*Da Zao*), 5 pieces. For turbid toxins obstructing the center

with stomach loss of harmony and downbearing and the symptoms of nausea and vomiting, devitalized eating and drinking, and a fat tongue with thick, slimy fur, add nine grams each of Pericarpium Citri Reticulatae (*Chen Pi*), Rhizoma Pinelliae Ternatae (*Ban Xia*), Caulis Bambusae In Taeniis (*Zhu Ru*), Herba Agastachis Seu Pogostemi (*Huo Xiang*), Herba Eupatorii Fortunei (*Pei Lan*), and wine-fried Radix Et Rhizoma Rhei (*Da Huang*).

ACUPUNCTURE & MOXIBUSTION: *Ming Men* (GV 4), *Qi Hai* (CV 6), *Guan Yuan* (CV 4)

FORMULA ANALYSIS: Moxaing these points rescues yang and stems desertion.

ABSTRACTS OF REPRESENTATIVE CHINESE RESEARCH:

Shi Ya-hong, "The Treatment of 32 Cases of Diabetic Nephropathy with Integrated Chinese-Western Medicine," *Si Chuan Zhong Yi (Sichuan Chinese Medicine)*, 1999, #4, p. 27: All the patients in this study had diabetes and albuminuria, and all were treated with a combination of modern Western and Chinese medicines. Twenty-five were male and seven were female. The median age was 52 years old. The longest course of disease was 16 years and the shortest was three years. Sixteen cases had accompanying hypertension, six had simultaneous infections, six had either retinopathy or neuropathy, and four had a slight degree of renal insufficiency.

Western medical treatment consisted of blood sugar and hypertension controlling medications combined with 1) antibiotics for infections, 2) supplemental serum albumin for lowering serum albumin, and 3) nerve-nourishing medicines for neurological symptoms. Chinese medicinal treatment consisted of the following basic formula: uncooked Radix Rehmanniae (*Sheng Di*), cooked Radix Rehmanniae (*Shu Di*), Radix Astragali Membranacei (*Bei Qi*), Herba Leonuri Heterophylli (*Yi Mu Cao*), and Fructus Psoraleae Corylifoliae (*Bu Gu Zhi*), 20g each, Sclerotium Poriae Cocos (*Fu Ling*), Cortex Eucommiae Ulmoidis (*Du Zhong*), and Semen Cuscutae Chinensis (*Tu Si Zi*), 25g each, Radix Dioscoreae Oppositae (*Shan Yao*), 18g, Rhizoma Alismatis (*Ze Xie*), Radix Scrophulariae Ningpoensis (*Yuan Shen*), Radix Trichosanthis Kirlowii (*Hua Fen*), Tuber Ophiopogonis Japonici (*Mai Dong*), Fructus Ligustri Lucidi (*Nu Zhen Zi*), Herba Ecliptae Prostratae (*Han Lian Cao*), and Cortex Radicis Moutan (*Dan Pi*), 15g each, Fructus Corni Officinalis (*Shan Zhu Rou*), 12g, and Radix Ligustici Wallichii (*Chuan Xiong*), 10g. In terms of modifications based on pattern discrimination, if there was liver-kidney yin vacuity, 25g of Fructus Lycii Chinensis (*Gou Qi Zi*) and 15g each of Tuber Ophiopogonis Japonici (*Mai Dong*), Fructus Ligustri Lucidi (*Nu Zhen Zi*), and Herba Ecliptae Prostratae (*Han Lian Cao*) were added. If there was kidney yang vacuity, 9g of Radix Lateralis Praeparatus Aconiti Carmichaeli (*Fu Zi*), 25g each of Semen Cuscutae Chinensis (*Tu Si Zi*) and Cortex Eucommiae Ulmoidis (*Du Zhong*), and 20g of Fructus Psoraleae Corylifoliae (*Bu Gu Zhi*) were added. If there was kidney qi vacuity, 20g of Radix Codonopsitis Pilosulae (*Dang Shen*) was added.

If both the clinical symptoms and albuminuria disappeared, this was defined as marked effect. If both improved, this was defined as some effect. If neither improved, this was defined as no effect. Based on these criteria, 16 cases or 50% experienced a marked effect with this protocol. Another 10 cases or 31% experienced some effect. Only six cases or 18.8% experienced no effect. Thus the total amelioration rate was 81%.

Li Hong & Fan Shi-ping, "A Clinical Audit of the Treatment of 42 Cases of Diabetic Nephropathy with Integrated Chinese-Western Medicine," *Fu Jian Zhong Yi Yao (Fujian Chinese Medicine & Medicinals)*, #4, 2000, p. 17-18: There were 42 patients in this study, all of whom were in-patients and all of whom met the WHO criteria for type 2 diabetes as well as Mogensen's criteria for diabetic nephropathy. Among these patients, there were 30 males and 12 females who ranged in age from 35-62 years old, with an average age of 54. Their DM disease course had lasted from 1-23 years, with an average of 10 years, while their nephropathy had lasted from two months to nine years, with an average of 5.6 years. Twenty-seven had early stage diabetic nephropathy (DN), and 15 had clinical stage DN. Nineteen had accompanying hypertension, 25 had retinopathy, 20 had peripheral neuropathy, and seventeen had diabetic heart disease.

Treatment consisted of typical hypoglycemic agents, antihypertensives, diuretics, and a low protein diet. In addition, patients were administered the following Chinese medicinals: uncooked Radix Astragali Membranacei (*Huang Qi*) and Semen Plantaginis (*Che Qian Zi*), 30g each, Radix Salviae Miltiorhizae (*Dan Shen*), 20g, Fructus Corni Officinalis (*Shan Zhu Yu*), Radix Dioscoreae Oppositae (*Shan Yao*), and Sclerotium Poriae Cocos (*Fu Ling*), 15g each, stir-fried Rhizoma Atractylodis Macrocephalae (*Bai Zhu*), Rhizoma Alismatis (*Ze Xie*), and Herba Leonuri Heterophylli (*Yi Mu Cao*), 12g each, and Radix Et Rhizoma Rhei (*Da Huang*), 10g. If there was liver-kidney qi and yin dual vacuity with blood stasis,

cooked Radix Rehmanniae (*Shu Di*), Radix Pseudostellariae Heterophyllae (*Tai Zi Shen*), and Radix Scrophulariae Ningpoensis (*Xuan Shen*) were added. If there was spleen-kidney yang vacuity with blood stasis, Radix Lateralis Praeparatus Aconiti Carmichaeli (*Fu Zi*), Cortex Cinnamomi Cassiae (*Rou Gui*), and Radix Stephaniae Tetrandrae (*Fang Ji*) were added. One *ji* was decocted in water per day and administered orally, and one month equaled one course of treatment.

Marked effect was defined as disappearance of clinical symptoms, 24 hour urine protein less than 0.5g or reduced by more than 2/3, blood creatinine reduced by 1/4, and FBG less than or equal to 7.2mmol/L. Some effect was defined as decrease in clinical symptoms, 24 hour urine protein reduced by 1/3 or more, FBG lowered by 1/3 or more, and marked improvement in kidney function. No effect meant no improvement in clinical symptoms and no improvement in other criteria. Based on these criteria, after 1-2 courses of treatment, 16 patients experienced a marked effect, 21 patients got some effect, and five patients got no effect, for a total amelioration rate of 88.1%.

Fang Lian-shun, "The Treatment of 30 Cases of Diabetic Nephropathy with *Zhen Wu Tang* (True Warrior Decoction)," *Fu Jian Zhong Yi Yao (Fujian Chinese Medicine & Medicinals)*, #3, 2000, p. 34: All 30 patients in this study met WHO criteria for type 2 diabetes and diabetic nephropathy. There were 14 males and 16 females, 14 of whom were 40-50 years old, 11 of whom were 50-60 years old, and five of whom were 60-70 years old. Fifteen patients had early stage DN, 10 had middle stage DN, and five had late stage DN. The main signs and symptoms were bodily emaciation, lassitude of the spirit, lack of strength, heart palpitations, shortness of breath, dizziness, numbness and/or chilling of the hands and feet, inhibited urination, lower extremity superficial edema, blurred vision, impotence, amenorrhea, a pale but dark tongue with possible static macules and white fur, and a deep, fine pulse.

The Chinese medicinals administered consisted of: Radix Lateralis Praeparatus Aconiti Carmichaeli (*Fu Zi*), 10g, Sclerotium Poriae Cocos (*Fu Ling*), Radix Albus Paeoniae Lactiflorae (*Bai Shao*), uncooked Rhizoma Zingiberis (*Sheng Jiang*), and Radix Miltiorrhizae (*Dan Shen*), 9g each, Herba Lycopi Lucidi (*Ze Lan*), 8g, and Rhizoma Atractylodis Macrocephalae (*Bai Zhu*), 6g. If qi vacuity was marked, Radix Codonopsitis Pilosulae (*Dang Shen*) and Radix Astragali Membranacei (*Huang Qi*) were added. If there was qi stagnation and center fullness,

Radix Bupleuri (*Chai Hu*), Fructus Citri Aurantii (*Zhi Ke*), and Cortex Magnoliae Officinalis (*Hou Po*) were added. If blood stasis was relatively severe, Semen Pruni Persicae (*Tao Ren*), Flos Carthami Tinctorii (*Hong Hua*), Rhizoma Sparganii (*San Leng*), and Rhizoma Curcumae Zedoariae (*E Zhu*), were added. If yin vacuity was relatively severe, Tuber Ophiopogonis Japonici (*Mai Men Dong*), Rhizoma Polygonati (*Huang Jing*), and Radix Scrophulariae Ningpoensis (*Xuan Shen*) were added. If there were simultaneous heat toxins, Fructus Forsythiae Suspensae (*Lian Qiao*), Radix Scutellariae Baicalensis (*Huang Qin*), and Rhizoma Coptidis Chinensis (*Huang Lian*) were added and *Sheng Jiang* was removed. If there was vacuity with internal stirring of wind, Fructus Chaenomelis Lagenariae (*Mu Gua*), Ramulus Uncariae Cum Uncis (*Gou Teng*), and Cornu Antelopis Saigatatarici (*Ling Yang Jiao*) were added. If turbid toxins were damaging the spirit, Radix Panacis Ginseng (*Ren Shen*), Concha Margaritiferae (*Zhen Zhu Mu*), and Radix Et Rhizoma Rhei (*Da Huang*) were added. One *ji* of these medicinals was administered orally per day.

Marked effect meant that the clinical symptoms basically disappeared, urine protein decreased by 50% or more, kidney function was normal, HB was normal, and blood glucose and lipids were nearly normal. Improvement meant that clinical symptoms diminished, urine protein decreased, kidney function improved, HB was elevated, and blood glucose and lipids had improved. Some effect meant that the above criteria were all stable or that four of them had improved. No effect meant that none of the preceding criteria had been met. Based on these criteria, four (27%) of the early stage patients were judged to have gotten as marked effect, eight (53%) improved, two (13%) got some effect, and one got no effect, for a total amelioration rate in this subgroup of 93%. In the middle stage patients, six (60%) improved, two (20%) got some effect, one got no effect, and one died, for a total amelioration rate in this subgroup of 80%. In the late stage patients, one (20%) improved, two (40%) got some effect, one got no effect, and one died, for a total amelioration rate in this subgroup of 60%.

Dong Ying *et al.*, "The Treatment of 32 Cases of Diabetic Nephropathy with Integrated Chinese-Western Medicine," *Hu Nan Zhong Yi Za Zhi* (*Hunan Journal of Chinese Medicine*), #2, 2001, p. 45: A total of 62 patients, 23 out-patients and 39 in-patients, were divided into two groups. These patients were 40-72 years of age, with an average age of 55.2 years. They had had diabetes for 3-16 years, with an average duration of 7.2 years. All had had nephropathy for one month to 6.8 years, with an average

duration of 1.7 years. There was no marked statistical difference in sex, age, or disease duration between these two groups. The diagnosis of diabetes was based on WHO criteria. Patients with hypertension and heart failure were excluded as well as those with blood glucose as high as 15.0mmol/L or those taking suflonylureas-type medications which had lost their effect.

Treatment in the so-called comparison group consisted of administering 80-240mg of glyburide per day in two divided doses as well as 25-75mg per day of *Qia Jiang Tuo Pu Ji*, an unidentified Western medication, also in two divided doses. The so-called treatment group received this same treatment plus 40ml of *Dan Shen Zhu She Ye* (Salvia Injectible Liquid) via intravenous drip in 250ml of saline solution one time per day. They also were administered the following Chinese medicinals orally in decoction per day: Radix Astragali Membranacei (*Huang Qi*), Radix Polygoni Multiflori (*He Shou Wu*), and cooked Radix Rehmanniae (*Shu Di*), 30g each, Fructus Corni Officinalis (*Shan Zhu Yu*), Radix Dioscoreae Oppositae (*Shan Yao*), and Herba Leonuri Heterophylli (*Yi Mu Cao*), 20g each, Radix Pseudostellariae Heterophyllae (*Tai Zi Shen*) and Herba Oldenlandiae Diffusae Cum Radice (*Bai Hua She She Cao*), 15g each, and Herba Cistanchis Deserticolae (*Rou Cong Rong*), Semen Cuscutae Chinensis (*Tu Si Zi*), Radix Ligustici Wallichii (*Chuan Xiong*), Flos Carthami Tinctorii (*Hong Hua*), Cortex Phellodendri (*Huang Bai*), Cortex Radicis Moutan (*Dan Pi*), and Rhizoma Alismatis (*Ze Xie*), 10g each. Both groups were treated continuously for two months.

Marked effect was defined as basic disappearance of the symptoms, no proteinuria or protein decreased by more than 2/3. Some effect meant a decrease in symptoms and proteinuria decreased by 1/3 or more. No effect meant that there was no improvement in symptoms and no change or even worsening in proteinuria. Based on these criteria, 12 patients in the treatment group got a marked effect, 17 got some effect, and three got no effect, for a total amelioration rate of 90.63%. In the comparison group, five got a marked effect, 12 got some effect, and 13 got no effect, for a total amelioration rate of 56.67%. This study suggests that the administration of certain Chinese medicinals with glyburide and *Qia Jiang Tuo Pu Ji* is more effective than these Western medicines alone for the treatment of diabetic nephropathy.

Zheng Bi-fang & Zhang Yi, "The Treatment of 21 Cases of Diabetic Nephropathy with Integrated Chinese-Western Medicine," *Shan Xi Zhong Yi* (*Shanxi Chinese Medicine*), #1, 2001, p. 33: All 21 patients in this study suffered from diabetic nephropathy. Among these 21, there were nine men and 12 women, 42-76 years of age who had had diabetes for 4-20 years. Eight cases had stage I DN, 12 had stage II DN, and one case had stage III DN. Stage I meant less than 1.0g of proteinuria per day. Stage II meant more than 1.0g of proteinuria per day, slightly low kidney function, and less than 200umol/L of blood creatine. Stage III meant a marked lowering of kidney function and more than 200umol/L of blood creatinine. Seven patients also had hypertension, two had cerebral sclerosis, 13 had peripheral neuropathy, and six had retinopathy. Treatment consisted of administering the following Chinese medicinals on top of their original hypoglycemic treatments and 20ml of *Fu Fang Dan Shen Zhu She Ye* (Compound Salvia Injectible Fluid) administered as an IV drip per day: Radix Astragali Membranacei (*Huang Qi*), 30g, Radix Angelicae Sinensis (*Dang Gui*), 20g, cooked Radix Rehmanniae (*Shu Di*), 18g, Fructus Corni Officinalis (*Shan Zhu Yu*), Radix Dioscoreae Oppositae (*Shan Yao*), and Radix Salviae Miltiorrhizae (*Dan Shen*), 12g each, Radix Pseudoginseng (*San Qi*), Radix Rubrus Paeoniae Lactiflorae (*Chi Shao*), Cortex Radicis Moutan (*Dan Pi*), Radix Et Rhizoma Rhei (*Da Huang*), and Rhizoma Alismatis (*Ze Xie*), 10g each. One *ji* of these medicinals was decocted in water and administered per day. Treatment continued for four months.

Marked effect was defined as basic disappearance of symptoms, 24 hour proteinuria less than 0.5g or a reduction in proteinuria more than 40%, FBG less than 7.2mmol/L, and lowering of blood creatinine by 1/4. Some effect meant marked improvement in clinical symptoms, reduction in proteinuria 10-39%, FBG reduced by 1/3 or more, and some improvement in blood creatinine. No effect meant that there was no improvement or even possible worsening of symptoms and failure to meet the other criteria described above. Based on these criteria, six cases were judged to have gotten a marked effect, 12 got some effect, and three got no effect, for a total amelioration rate of 85.71%. Mean blood glucose went from 11.70 ± 3.70mmol/L to 8.44 ± 2.24mmol/L, mean proteinuria went from 1.14 ± 1.42g/24hrs to 0.81 ± 1.46g/24hrs, mean blood creatinine went from 124.55 ± 44.10umol/L to 112.49 ± 32.14umol/L, mean total cholesterol went from 7.26 ± 1.98mmol/L to 6.12 ± 0.87mmol/L, and mean triglycerides went from 2.67 ± 0.91mmol/L to 1.95 ± 0.83mmol/L. The P value of all these changes was < 0.05.

Hao Ming-qiang, "The Treatment of 40 Cases of Diabetic Nephropathy with *Jiang Tang Li Shen Fang* (Lower Sugar & Rectify the Kidneys Formula)," *Si Chuan Zhong Yi* (*Sichuan Chinese Medicine*), #10, 2000, p. 21: Seventy-eight patients with DN were divided into two groups, a so-called treatment group and a comparison group. There was no significant statistical difference between these two groups in terms of age, sex, disease duration, etc. The treatment group received self-composed *Jiang Tang Li Shen Fang* which was comprised of: uncooked Radix Astragali Membranacei (*Huang Qi*), 30g, Fructus Corni Officinalis (*Shan Zhu Yu*), Radix Dioscoreae Oppositae (*Shan Yao*), and Herba Agrimoniae Pilosae (*Xian He Cao*), 15g each, and cooked Radix Rehmanniae (*Shu Di*), Galla Rhois (*Wu Bei Zi*), Sclerotium Poriae Cocos (*Fu Ling*), processed Radix Polygoni Multiflori (*He Shou Wu*), Radix Et Rhizoma Rhei (*Da Huang*), added later, Herba Epimedii (*Xian Ling Pi*), and Radix Salviae Miltiorrhizae (*Dan Shen*), 10g each. If there was concomitant coronary artery disease, 10 grams of Radix Ligustici Wallichii (*Chuan Xiong*) and five grams of Lignum Dalbergiae Odoriferae (*Jiang Xiang*) were added. If there was concomitant eye disease, 10 grams each of Fructus Lycii Chinensis (*Gou Qi Zi*) and Flos Chrysanthemi Morifolii (*Ju Hua*) were added. If there was concomitant hyperlipidemia, 10 grams each of Radix Puerariae (*Ge Gen*), stir-fried Rhizoma Atractylodis (*Cang Zhu*), and uncooked Fructus Crataegi (*Shan Zha*) were added. If there was hypertension, 10 grams each of Rhizoma Gastrodiae Elatae (*Tian Ma*), Radix Cyathulae (*Chuan Niu Xi*), and Ramulus Uncariae Cum Uncis (*Gou Teng*) were added. One *ji* of these medicinals was decocted in water and administered per day. The comparison group received 30mg of an oral hypoglycemic agent three times per day as well as 12.5mg of *Qia Jiang Tuo Pu Ji* orally three times per day.

Cure was defined as complete disappearance of proteinuria, urination one time per night, FBG 5.4-6.3mmol/L, and the disease stable for half a year. Marked effect meant that proteinuria was (+), nocturia was two times per night, and FBG was equal to or less than 7.3mmol/L. No effect meant that urinary frequency was not decreased or improved only during the time of treatment and that FBG was equal to or more than 8.5mmol/L. Based on these criteria, 20 of the 40 patients in the treatment group were judged cured, 17 got a marked effect, and three got no effect. Thus the total amelioration rate in the treatment group was 92.5%. In the comparison group, seven patients were judged cured, 13 got a marked effect, and 18 got no effect, for a total amelioration rate of 52.7%.

Gao Ming-song & Xu Jie, "The Treatment of 68 Cases of Type II Diabetic Microalbuminuria with Integrated Chinese-Western Medicine," *He Nan Zhong Yi* (*Henan Chinese Medicine*), #3, 2001, p. 39: All 68 patients in this study had early stage diabetic nephropathy and excreted 30-300mg of albumin in their urine every 24 hours.

Patients with acute or chronic nephritis, urinary tract infections, or ketosis were excluded. These 68 patients were divided into two groups of 34 patients each, a treatment group and a comparison group. In the treatment group, there were 16 men and 18 women aged 39-71 years, with a median age of 53.31 ± 3.13 years. The course of their diabetes had lasted 1-22 years, with a median duration of 10.1 ± 5.2 years. In the comparison group, there were 14 men and 20 women aged 43-72, with a median age of 54.85 ± 2.62 years. These patients had suffered from diabetes for 0.5-20 years, with a median duration of 9.3 ± 7.1 years.

All the patients in both groups were administered 10mg per day of an ACE inhibitor. In addition, those patients in the so-called treatment group also received Yi Qi Yang Yin Gu Shen Tang (Boost the Qi, Nourish Yin & Secure the Kidneys Decoction): uncooked Radix Astragali Membranacei (Huang Qi) and Radix Achyranthis Bidentatae (Niu Xi), 30g each, Sclerotium Poriae Cocos (Fu Ling) and Fructus Lycii Chinensis (Gou Qi Zi), 15g each, stir-fried Rhizoma Atractylodis Macrocephalae (Bai Zhu), Radix Codonopsitis Pilosulae (Dang Shen), uncooked Radix Rehmanniae (Sheng Di), and Sclerotium Polypori Umbellati (Zhu Ling), 12g each, and Tuber Ophiopogonis Japonici (Mai Men Dong), Fructus Schisandrae Chinensis (Wu Wei Zi), Rhizoma Polygonati (Huang Jing), Herba Leonuri Heterophylli (Yi Mu Cao), and Fructus Corni Officinalis (Shan Zhu Yu), 9g each. If there was marked dry mouth, 30 grams each of Cortex Radicis Lycii Chinensis (Di Gu Pi) and Radix Trichosanthis Kirlowii (Tian Hua Fen) were added. If the stools tended to be dry or constipated, 30 grams of Semen Cannabis Sativae (Huo Ma Ren) and nine grams of Semen Pruni Persicae (Tao Ren) were added. One ji of these medicinals was decocted in water per day and administered orally in two divided doses, morning and night. Two months equaled one course of treatment. In the treatment group, microalbuminuria was 153.26 ± 84.3mg/24 hours before treatment and 67.15 ± 51.02mg/24hrs after treatment. In the comparison group, microalbuminuria was 146.54 ± 75.69mg/24hrs before treatment and 86.23 ± 65.27mg/24hrs after treatment. Hence, it was concluded that the administration of these Chinese medicinals with the ACE inhibitor was more effective for reducing albuminuria in patients with early stage diabetic nephropathy than the ACE inhibitor alone.

REPRESENTATIVE CASE HISTORIES:

CASE 1[10]

The patient was a 51 year old female who was first examined on May 15, 1992. The patient had had diabetes for 15 years and hypertension for five. During the last three years, she had had proteinuria (++´++++) and bilateral lower extremity edema. Based on this, she had been diagnosed with DN for three years. In Aug. 1991, the woman had suffered a cerebral infarction which had caused right-sided paralysis. Various Western hypoglycemic and antihypertensive medications had been tried but without stable results. The patient's blood sugar fluctuated between 3.49-14.48mmol/L, and she had been hospitalized three times for hypoglycemic coma. Weekly excretion of protein was 20-40g. At the time of Dr. Zhu's examination, there was a somber white facial complexion, generalized edema which was more severe in the lower extremities, lassitude of the spirit, lack of strength, right-sided hemiplegia, a dry mouth with a desire to drink, poor appetite, fear of cold, chilled limbs, frequent urination, and loose stools. The patient's tongue was pale but dark and the sublingual veins were distended and tortuous. Her pulse was fine and weak. Urine glucose was (++++).

Based on the above signs and symptoms, Dr. Zhu categorized this woman's Chinese patterns as yin and yang dual vacuity with static blood obstructing the network vessels, spleen-kidney insufficiency, and spilling over and flooding of water dampness. Therefore, the treatment principles were to boost the qi and nourish yin, quicken the blood and transform stasis, free the flow of yang and disinhibit water. The formula Dr. Zhu prescribed consisted of: uncooked Radix Astragali Membranacei (Huang Qi), 50g, uncooked Radix Rehmanniae (Sheng Di), Radix Salviae Miltiorrhizae (Dan Shen), and Herba Leonuri Heterophylli (Yi Mu Cao), 30g each, Sclerotium Poriae Cocos (Fu Ling), 20g, Radix Puerariae (Ge Gen) and Radix Dipsaci (Xu Duan), 15g each, and Rhizoma Atractylodis (Cang Zhu), Rhizoma Atractylodis Macrocephalae (Bai Zhu), uncooked Radix Dioscoreae Oppositae (Shan Yao), Fructus Lycii Chinensis (Gou Qi Zi), and Ramulus Cinnamomi Cassiae (Gui Zhi), 10g each.

After taking 40 ji of these medicinals, the patient's blood glucose and blood pressure were both more stable than before. Blood glucose was 5.1-6.99mmol/L (92-126mg/dL), and blood pressure was 20/12kPa (150/90mmHg). Her bodily strength had increased and her appetite had improved. Proteinuria was now (++). Therefore, the same formula with additions and subtractions was prescribed for another eight months. At that point, appetite was extremely good, bodily strength and psyche had both recovered, and the woman could take care of herself within her home. Fasting blood glucose was 4.49mmol/L (81mg/dL), urea nitrogen was 75mg%, creatinine was 2.1mg%, and proteinuria was (+). Except for generalized edema, there were no obvious symptoms. Now the woman's pattern was categorized as simply spleen-kidney yang vacuity not transforming water dampness. Therefore, the prescription was changed to *Gui Fu Di Huang Tang* (Cinnamon & Aconite Rehmannia Decoction) plus *Fang Ji Huang Qi Tang* (Stephania & Astragalus Decoction): uncooked Radix Astragali Membranacei (*Huang Qi*), 50g, Semen Plantaginis (*Che Qian Zi*), 30g, Sclerotium Poriae Cocos (*Fu Ling*), 20g, uncooked Radix Rehmanniae (*Sheng Di*), cooked Radix Rehmanniae (*Shu Di*), Rhizoma Alismatis (*Ze Xie*), Herba Ecliptae Prostratae (*Han Lian Cao*), Rhizoma Dioscoreae Hypoglaucae (*Bie Xie*), and Folium Pyrrosiae (*Shi Wei*), 15g each, and Rhizoma Atractylodis Macrocephalae (*Bai Zhu*), Ramulus Cinnamomi Cassiae (*Gui Zhi*), Radix Lateralis Praeparatus Aconiti Carmichaeli (*Fu Zi*), Fructus Corni Officinalis (*Shan Zhu Yu*), Radix Dioscoreae Oppositae (*Shan Yao*), and Cortex Radicis Moutan (*Dan Pi*), 10g each.

The above Chinese medicinals were administered, one *ji* per day, for one month. At that time, the generalized edema had markedly decreased. However, the patient's appetite had also decreased. Therefore, she was again administered the original formula with additions and subtractions. In Jun. 1993, the patient was re-examined. Fasting blood glucose was 5.99mmol/L (108mg/dL), urea nitrogen was 50mg%, creatinine was 2mg%, urine glucose was (+), proteinuria was (±-+), and the patient's case was basically stable.

CASE 2[11]

The patient was a 60 year old male worker who was first examined in Jul. 1985. The patient's main complaints were polydipsia, polyphagia, and polyuria for 15 years which had gotten worse during the previous half year. When the man was hospitalized, his FBG was 13.66mmol/L. Through proper treatment, the polydipsia, polyphagia, and polyuria were gradually alleviated. However, on Sept. 7, the patient experienced sudden dizziness, headache, and vomiting followed by lassitude of the spirit, listlessness, deviation of the mouth and eye, lower limb edema, a dark yet tender tongue with slimy, white fur, and a deep, fine pulse. Blood urea nitrogen (BUN) was 2.28mmol/L and proteinuria was (+++). Based on these findings, the man was diagnosed as suffering from diabetic nephropathy complicated by chronic uremia, and he was treated with Chinese and Western

medicines to support his life, disinhibit urination, and promote discharge of toxic materials by freeing the flow of the stools. This therapy was carried out for two months, but the man's condition was not controlled and, in fact, deteriorated further. Blood urea nitrogen rose to 37.35mmol/L and serum potassium was 5.5mmol/L.

Based on the fact that the main pathological changes in DN are glomerular atherosclerosis, it was thought that phlegm may be responsible for this man's condition. Therefore, the following medicinals were administered to soften the hard and scatter nodulation, quicken the blood and dispel stasis: Bulbus Fritillariae Thunbergii (*Zhe Bei Mu*), uncooked Concha Ostreae (*Mu Li*) and Sclerotium Poriae Cocos (*Fu Ling*), 30g each, Thallus Algae (*Kun Bu*) and uncooked Rhizoma Zingiberis (*Sheng Jiang*), 20g each, Herba Saragassii (*Hai Zao*) and Semen Pruni Persicae (*Tao Ren*), 15g each, Radix Scrophulariae Ningpoensis (*Xuan Shen*), 12g, and Herba Leonuri Heterophylli (*Yi Mu Cao*), 6g. After 10 *ji* of this formula, headaches, dizziness, and vomiting had all disappeared. After another 20 *ji*, the man's spirit and consciousness were restored to normal, urination increased, and the edema was relieved. Blood urea nitrogen decreased to 21.4mmol/L, electrolytes were normal, and proteinuria was negative. In order to secure and consolidate these therapeutic effects, the man was administered three more months of treatment before being discharged from the hospital.

CASE 3[12]

The patient was a 48 year old male who was first examined on Apr. 25, 1998. This patient had suffered from diabetes for 10 years and from polyuria for six years. In the last half year, this had gotten worse, with urination occurring once per hour during the day and five times per night. This was accompanied by low back and knee soreness and pain, fatigue, lack of strength, a lusterless facial complexion, facial edema, puffy eyelids, and pitting edema of the lower legs. The patient's tongue was purplish and dark and the fur was slimy and white. The man's pulse was fine and weak. Fasting blood glucose was 15.1mmol/L, urine glucose was (+++), proteinuria was (+++), BUN was 10.5mmol/L, creatinine was 191umol/L, triglycerides were 1.7mmol/L, and total cholesterol was 6.9mmol/L. Based on these signs and symptoms, the patient's Chinese patterns were categorized as spleen-kidney dual vacuity with the clear qi falling downward, qi vacuity and blood stasis. Therefore, the patient was administered *Jiang Tang Li Shen Fang* (Lower Sugar & Rectify the Kidneys Formula) described above plus 10 grams each of Radix Puerariae (*Ge Gen*), stir-fried Rhizoma Atractylodis (*Cang Zhu*), and uncooked Fructus Crataegi (*Shan Zha*). After three courses of treatment, *i.e.*, 30 days, all the patient's symptoms had basically disappeared and kidney function and serum examinations were all normal. The man was judged cured and he was discharged from the hospital.

CASE 4[13]

The patient was a 76 year old female who presented with turbid, greasy, profuse urination, thirst, a very dry tongue and throat, a dark facial complexion, low back and knee soreness and pain, cold limbs, and aversion to cold. The patient's blood sugar level was 13.8 mmol/L (248 mg/dL), and her urine glucose was (+). The tongue was small, dark, and pale, and the tongue fur was white and dry. The pulse was deep, fine, and forceless. The Western medical diagnosis was diabetic nephropathy, while the Chinese medical patterns were categorized as insecurity of the lower source with yin exhaustion affecting yang and yin and yang dual depletion. Therefore, the treatment principles were to warm yang and enrich yin, supplement the kidneys and separate the clear from turbid. The prescription included: Radix Dioscoreae Oppositae (*Shan Yao*), Rhizoma Dioscoreae Hypoglaucae (*Bi Xie*), and Semen Plantaginis (*Che Qian Zi*), 15g each, uncooked Radix Rehmanniae (*Sheng Di*), cooked Radix Rehmanniae (*Shu Di*), Fructus Corni Officinalis (*Shan Zhu Yu*), Sclerotium Poriae Cocos (*Fu Ling*), Rhizoma Alismatis (*Ze Xie*), Radix Salviae Miltiorrhizae (*Dan Shen*), Cortex Radicis Moutan (*Dan Pi*), Radix Lateralis Preparatus Aconiti Carmichaeli (*Fu Zi*), Fructus Rubi Chingii (*Fu Pen Zi*), Semen Cuscutae Chinensis (*Tu Si Zi*), Fructus Schisandrae Chinensis (*Wu Wei Zi*), and Rhizoma Polygonati (*Huang Jing*), 10g each, and Cortex Cinnamomi Cassiae (*Rou Gui*), 2g. One *ji* of these medicinals was decocted in water and administered orally per day. After taking seven *ji* of these medicinals, the urination cleared, the white tongue fur became thin, and the thirst was less. The patient remained on this formula until the urination showed no signs of recurring turbidity and the blood glucose levels remained in normal range. She was then switched to *Jin Gui Shen Qi Wan* (*Golden Cabinet* Kidney Qi Pills) for some time following her treatment in order to secure and consolidate the treatment effect.

CASE 5[14]

The patient was a 69 year old male cadre who first entered the hospital on Oct. 8, 1998. The man had been diagnosed with diabetes for eight years and had undergone a number of treatments in the hospital. Currently, the patient was taking unspecified oral hypoglycemic medica-tions. At the time of admittance, the patient's two lower extremities were edematous, his body was cold, and he had low back pain. His abdomen was distended and he had heart palpitations, shortness of breath, torpid intake, and loose stools. His tongue was both dark and pale, while his pulse was deep and fine. Fasting blood glucose was 16.2mmol/L, urine glucose was (+++), albuminuria was (+++), 24 hour urinary albumin was 1.45, BUN was 13.8mmol/L, and creatinine was 289mmol/L. In addition, blood viscosity tended to be high.

Based on the above signs and symptoms, the patient's Chinese medical pattern was categorized as qi vacuity and blood stasis with yang vacuity and water flooding. Therefore, he was administered *Bu Yang Huan Wu Tang Jia Wei* (Supplement Yang & Restore Five [Tenths] Decoction with Added Flavors): Radix Astragali Membranacei (*Huang Qi*) and uncooked Concha Ostreae (*Mu Li*), 30g each, Radix Angelicae Sinensis (*Dang Gui*), Radix Trichosanthis Kirlowii (*Tian Hua Fen*), and Sclerotium Poriae Cocos (*Fu Ling*), 20g each, Rhizoma Atractylodis Macrocephalae (*Bai Zhu*) and Cortex Eucommiae Ulmoidis (*Du Zhong*), 15g each, Radix Ligustici Wallichii (*Chuan Xiong*), Radix Rubrus Paeoniae Lactiflorae (*Chi Shao*), and Semen Arecae Catechu (*Bin Lan*), 12g each, Semen Pruni Persicae (*Tao Ren*), Flos Carthami Tinctorii (*Hong Hua*), and Herba Taraxaci Mongolici Cum Radice (*Pu Gong Ying*), 10g each, and Radix Lateralis Praeparatus Aconiti Carmichaeli (*Fu Zi*), 9g.

After taking 20 *ji* of these medicinals, the edema was markedly decreased, the amount of urine had increased, and the abdominal distention had disappeared. Fasting blood glucose was 9mmol/L, BUN was 9.8mmol/L, and creatinine was 183mmol/L. Therefore, *Bin Lan* was removed from the above formula and 20 grams of Semen Dolichoris Lablab (*Bai Bian Dou*) and 30 grams of Radix Dioscoreae Oppositae (*Shan Yao*) were added. Another 30 *ji* of these medicinals were administered, at which time, the edema had disappeared, the amount of urine was normal, FBG was 7.3mmol/L, BUN was 7.8mmol/L, creatinine was 152mmol/L, and urine albumin was stable at (+). Twenty-four hour albumin excretion was 0.6g, and the patient's blood had returned to normal. *Fu Zi* was removed from the formula and these medicinals were administered continuously for another two months. On follow-up after two years, there had been no recurrence.

REMARKS:

1. The Chinese National Chinese Medical Association Commission on Nephropathy has recently published a

multi-pattern discrimination of this disease.[15] According to this article, there are five patterns: 1) qi, blood, and yin vacuity (also referred to as liver-kidney qi, blood, and yin vacuity) with turbid toxins internally collecting, 2) qi, blood, and yang vacuity (*i.e.*, lung-kidney qi, blood, and yang vacuity) with turbid toxins internally collecting, 3) liver-spleen-kidney qi, blood, yin, and yang vacuity with turbid toxins internally collecting, 4) lung-kidney qi and blood, yin and yang vacuity with turbid toxins internally collecting, and 5) heart-kidney qi and blood, yin and yang vacuity with turbid toxins internally collecting. If one includes the various modifications of the protocols given above, all five of these patterns are accounted for in our three pattern presentation of DN.

2. Jiao Peng is of the opinion that early stage diabetic nephropathy mostly presents as qi and yin vacuity with blood stasis, in which case, blood stasis arises based on the Chinese medical dictum, "[Since] the essence [is] desiccated and blood [is] dry, the vessels and network vessels are static and obstructed." This tallies with our own experience. Although none of the patterns presented above, either our three or the Chinese Medical Association Commission on Nephropathy's five contain the words blood stasis, it is important to note that most Chinese clinicians assume there is an element of blood stasis in all patients with this condition.

3. For uremia, Yan De-xin commonly uses 30 grams each of Folium Eupatorii Chinensis (*Liu Yue Xue*) and uncooked Radix Et Rhizoma Rhei (*Da Huang*). These are decocted in water down to 150ml of liquid and used as a retention enema, one time per day, in order to discharge turbidity through the intestinal tract. According to Dr. Yan, this treatment helps reduce retention of urea nitrogen and creatinine. However, this is a strongly attacking treatment liable to produce strong diarrhea. Therefore, it should be used with care or modified for use in those who are vacuous and weak.

Another enema formula for uremia consists of 30 grams of calcined Concha Ostreae (*Mu Li*), 20 grams of Fructus Forsythiae Suspensae (*Lian Qiao*), and 15 grams of Radix Et Rhizoma Rhei (*Da Huang*). Do once every other day for 14 days with a week's rest between courses.

Yet another Chinese medicinal enema is *Jun Kun Tang* (Army & Feminine Decoction). Here "army" refers to *Da Huang* which is also called *Jun* and "feminine" refers to *Yi Mu Cao* which is also called *Kun Cao*. Ingredients: Radix Et Rhizoma Rhei (*Da Huang*), 40g, Herba Leonuri Heterophylli (*Yi Mu Cao*), 30g, Concha Ostreae (*Mu Li*),

30g, and Radix Lateralis Praeparatus Aconiti Carmichaeli (*Fu Zi*), 15g. Put the medicinals in 500ml of water and decoct until reduced to 200ml. Retain the resulting warm (but not hot) liquid for 20-30 minutes each time. Do one enema per day for 20 days. Then stop for five days before resuming another 20 day's course. If there is concomitant yang vacuity, add three grams of Cortex Cinnamomi Cassiae (*Rou Gui*). If there is yin vacuity, subtract *Fu Zi*. If there is high blood pressure, subtract *Fu Zi* and add 12 grams each of Radix Rubrus Paeoniae Lactiflorae (*Chi Shao*) and Flos Immaturus Sophorae Japonicae (*Huai Hua Mi*). For bloody stools, add 15 grams of Radix Sanguisorbae Officinalis (*Di Yu*). If there are white blood cells in the urine, add 30 grams each of Herba Taraxaci Mongolici Cum Radice (*Pu Gong Ying*) and Cortex Phellodendri (*Huang Bai*).

4. According to recent research, Radix Et Rhizoma Rhei (*Da Huang*), Cordyceps Sinensis (*Dong Chong Xia Cao*), Radix Polygoni Multiflori (*He Shou Wu*), Radix Astragali Membranacei (*Huang Qi*), and Radix Salviae Miltiorrhizae (*Dan Shen*) are particularly good medicinals for treating chronic renal failure. *Huang Qi* and *Dan Shen* imply the common occurrence of qi vacuity and blood stasis respectively as main disease mechanisms of this disease. The fact that qi vacuity and blood stasis are main disease mechanisms of diabetic nephropathy is corroborated by the opinion of Wang Yan-bin.

5. One should avoid prescribing any medicinals for internal use that are nephrotoxic to patients with or who are at risk for diabetic nephropathy. Although there is ongoing debate about this subject, at the time of this writing, the authors suggest that this prohibition should include all members of the Aristolochia family, including Caulis Aristolochiae Manchuriensis which is often sold as Caulis Akebiae (*Mu Tong*), Radix Aristolochiae Fangchi (*Guang Fang Ji*), and Herba Asari Cum Radice (*Xi Xin*).

ENDNOTES:

[1] www.healthcentral.com/mhc/top/000494.cfm
[2] www.aafp.org/afp/971115ap/zoorob.htm
[3] Wang Yan-bin, "The Treatment of 34 Cases of Diabetic Nephropathy by the Methods of Boosting the Qi & Transforming Stasis," *Si Chuan Zhong Yi (Sichuan Chinese Medicine)*, #6, 2001, p. 26
[4] www.postgradmed.com/issues/1999/02_99/bell.htm
[5] www.cdc.gov/diabetes/pubs/facts98.htm
[6] Http://journal.diabetes.org/FullText/Supplements/DiabetesCare/Supplement101/S69.htm
[7] www.postgradmed.com, op. cit.
[8] www.healthcentral.com, op. cit.
[9] www.cdc.gov, op cit.
[10] Zhu Chen-zi, as anthologized in Dan Shu-jian & Chen Zi-hua's *Xiao Ke Juan (The Wasting & Thirsting Book)*, Chinese National Chinese Medicine & Medicinals Publishing Co., Beijing, 1999, p. 133-135

[11] Chen Jin-ding, *The Treatment of Diabetes with Traditional Chinese Medicine*, trans. by Sun Ying-kui & Zhou Shu-hui, Shandong Science & Technology Press, Jinan, 1994, p. 153-154

[12] Hao Ming-qiang, "The Treatment of 40 Cases of Diabetic Nephropathy with *Jiang Tang Li Shen Fang* (Lower Sugar & Rectify the Kidneys Formula)," *Si Chuan Zhong Yi (Sichuan Chinese Medicine)*, #10, 2000, p. 21

[13] Kang Lu-wa, "The Treatment of Diabetes by Pattern Discrimination of the Tongue," *Zhong Yi Za Zhi (Journal of Chinese Medicine)*, #9, 1999, pp. 530-531

[14] Wang Yan-bin, *op. cit.*, p. 26

[15]Chinese National Chinese Medical Association Nephropathy Commission, "Experiences in the Use of Chinese Medicinals & the Chinese Medical Treatment of Diabetic Nephropathy," *Shang Hai Zhong Yi Yao Za Zhi (Shanghai Journal of Chinese Medicine & Medicinals)*, #5, 2001, p. 15-18

24

COMMON OPPORTUNISTIC INFECTIONS IN PATIENTS WITH DIABETES

Because of decreased cellular immunity (impaired leukocyte function) caused by acute hyperglycemia and circulatory deficits caused by chronic hyperglycemia, people with diabetes easily contract opportunistic bacterial and fungal infections. The most common of these are oral and vaginal mycotic infections. However, other common opportunistic infections in persons with diabetes include respiratory tract infections, urinary tract infections, bloodstream infections (septicemia), dermatological infections, biliary tract infections, and periodontal disease. The Western medical treatment of such opportunistic infections in persons with diabetes includes the dietary restriction of sugars and sweets, fats and oils, and alcohol, treatment of the underlying diabetes with oral hypoglycemic agents or insulin, the use of internally administered and externally applied antibiotics and antifungal medications, and possible surgical treatment of gallstones and abscesses. Chinese medicine, including acupuncture and Chinese herbal medicine, may be used as alternatives or complements to antibiotics and antifungal medications.

A. CONCOMITANT RESPIRATORY TRACT INFECTIONS

CHINESE MEDICAL DISEASE CATEGORIZATION: In general, respiratory tract infections correspond to the traditional Chinese medical disease categories of *feng wen*, wind warmth, and *ke sou*, cough.

CHINESE DISEASE MECHANISMS: Due to enduring wasting and thirsting disease, qi is consumed and yin is damaged. Thus the righteous qi is insufficient, and evil toxins may take advantage of this vacuity to enter, attacking the lung defensive. This results in the lungs' losing their diffusion and downbearing. Hence there is coughing, possible profuse phlegm, and possible chest oppression and/or pain.

TREATMENT BASED ON PATTERN DISCRIMINATION:

1. EVILS ASSAILING THE LUNG DEFENSIVE PATTERN

MAIN SYMPTOMS: Aversion to cold, emission of heat (or fever), cough, white or yellow phlegm, chest oppression or pain, a dry mouth and oral thirst, a dry, sore throat, nasal congestion, inhibited respiration, headache, aching bones, a red tongue tip and sides with thin, yellow or thin, white fur and scanty fluids, and a floating rapid pulse

NOTE: This pattern is more commonly referred to as wind heat exterior pattern.

TREATMENT PRINCIPLES: Course wind and clear heat, diffuse the lungs and transform phlegm

RX: *Yin Qiao San Jia Jian* (Lonicera & Forsythia Powder with Additions & Subtractions)

INGREDIENTS: Flos Lonicerae Japonicae (*Jin Yin Hua*), Rhizoma Phragmitis Communis (*Lu Gen*), Cortex Radicis Mori Albi (*Sang Bai Pi*), and Radix Isatidis Seu Baphicacanthi (*Ban Lan Gen*), 15g each, Fructus Forsythiae Suspensae (*Lian Qiao*), 12g, and Herba Lophatheri Gracilis (*Dan Zhu Ye*), Herba Menthae Haplocalycis (*Bo He*), Fructus Arctii Lappae (*Niu Bang Zi*), Spica Seu Flos Schizonepetae Tenuifoliae (*Jing Jie Sui*), Folium Mori Albi (*Sang Ye*), Flos Chrysanthemi Morifolii (*Ju Hua*), Radix Scutellariae Baicalensis (*Huang Qin*), and stir-fried Semen Pruni Armeniacae (*Xing Ren*), 9g each

FORMULA ANALYSIS: *Jin Yin Hua, Lian Qiao, Ban Lan Gen,* and *Huang Qin* clear heat and resolve toxins. *Niu Bang Zi, Lu Gen, Dan Zhu Ye,* and *Bo He* course and scatter wind and heat. *Ju Hua, Sang Ye,* and *Jing Jie Sui* gently diffuse the lung qi.

ADDITIONS & SUBTRACTIONS: If oral thirst is severe, add 30 grams of uncooked Gypsum Fibrosum (*Shi Gao*) and 9-15 grams of Rhizoma Anemarrhenae Aspheloidis (*Zhi Mu*). If cough is severe, double the amount of *Xing Ren* and add 12 grams of Folium Eriobotryae Japonicae (*Pi Pa Ye*). If there is chest pain, add nine grams each of Pericarpium Trichosanthis Kirlowii (*Gua Lou Pi*) and Tuber Curcumae (*Yu Jin*).

If there is contraction of summerheat dampness, use *Xin Jia Xiang Ru Yin* (Newly Augmented Elsholtzia Drink): Semen Dolichoris Lablab (*Bai Bian Dou*) and Flos Lonicerae Japonicae (*Jin Yin Hua*), 15g each, Fructus Forsythiae Suspensae (*Lian Qiao*), 12g, and Herba Elsholtziae Seu Moslae (*Xiang Ru*) and Cortex Magnoliae (*Hou Po*), 9g each. If there is severe dampness, add 9-12 grams of Sclerotium Poriae Cocos (*Fu Ling*). If there is severe heat with thirst and irritability, add 3-6 grams of Rhizoma Coptidis Chinensis (*Huang Lian*).

If there is marked qi vacuity with external contraction, use *Shen Su Yin* (Ginseng & Perilla Drink) plus *Yu Ping Feng San* (Jade Windscreen Powder) with additions and subtractions: Radix Puerariae (*Ge Gen*), 18g, Tuber Ophiopogonis Japonici (*Mai Men Dong*), 12g, Fructus Schisandrae Chinensis (*Wu Wei Zi*), Folium Perillae Frutescentis (*Zi Su Ye*), Radix Codonopsitis Pilosulae (*Dang Shen*), Rhizoma Pinelliae Ternatae (*Ban Xia*), Sclerotium Poriae Cocos (*Fu Ling*), and Radix Peucedani (*Qian Hu*), 9g each, Radix Platycodi Grandiflori (*Jie Geng*), Radix Auklandiae Lappae (*Mu Xiang*), and Radix Glycyrrhizae (*Gan Cao*), 6g each.

If there is yin vacuity and external contraction, use *Wei Ru Tang Jia Jian* (Polygonatum Odoratum Decoction with Additions & Subtractions): Radix Puerariae (*Ge Gen*), 18g, Semen Praeparatum Sojae (*Dan Dou Chi*), 12-15g, Rhizoma Polygonati Odorati (*Yu Zhu*), 12g, Radix Cyanchi Baiwei (*Bai Wei*), Radix Ledebouriellae Divaricatae (*Fang Feng*), and Radix Platycodi Grandiflori (*Jie Geng*), 9g each, Herba Menthae Haplocalycis (*Bo He*) and mix-fried Radix Glycyrrhizae (*Gan Cao*), 6g each, and Fructus Zizyphi Jujubae (*Da Zao*), 3 pieces. If there is sore throat and thick, sticky, hard to expectorate phlegm, add nine grams each of Fructus Arctii Lappae (*Niu Bang Zi*) and Pericarpium

Trichosanthis Kirlowii (*Gua Lou Pi*). For marked thirst and irritability, add nine grams each of Radix Trichosanthis Kirlowii (*Tian Hua Fen*) and Herba Lophatheri Gracilis (*Dan Zhu Ye*).

ACUPUNCTURE & MOXIBUSTION: *He Gu* (LI 4), *Lie Que* (Lu 7), *Wai Guan* (TB 5), *Feng Men* (Bl 12), *Fei Shu* (Bl 13)

FORMULA ANALYSIS: Draining *He Gu* and *Wai Guan* resolves the exterior and clears heat. Draining *Feng Men* resolves the exterior and courses wind. Draining *Lie Que* and *Fei Shu* diffuses the lungs and promotes downbearing and depuration.

ADDITIONS & SUBTRACTIONS: For marked chest pain, add draining *Dan Zhong* (CV 17). For sore throat, add bleeding *Shao Shang* (Lu 11). For high fever, add draining *Qu Chi* (LI 11) and/or bleeding *Da Zhui* (GV 14). For concomitant qi vacuity, add supplementing *Zu San Li* (St 36). For concomitant yin vacuity, add supplementing *Tai Xi* (Ki 3) and *San Yin Jiao* (Sp 6). For oral thirst, add draining *Nei Ting* (St 44) and supplementing *Zhao Hai* (Ki 6) and use even supplementing-even draining at *Lie Que*. For nasal congestion, add draining *Ying Xiang* (LI 20).

2. HEAT EVILS CONGESTING THE LUNGS PATTERN

MAIN SYMPTOMS: Emission of heat, sweating, a dry mouth, oral thirst, cough, chest pain, expectoration of thick, yellow phlegm, panting and rapid breathing, a red facial complexion, vexatious heat, possible constipation and reddish urination, a dry tongue with yellow fur, and a slippery, rapid pulse

TREATMENT PRINCIPLES: Clear the lungs and stop coughing, transform phlegm and level panting

RX: *Sang Bai Pi Tang Jia Jian* (Mulberry Bark Decoction with Additions & Subtractions)

INGREDIENTS: Cortex Radicis Mori Albi (*Sang Bai Pi*), Rhizoma Phragmitis Communis (*Lu Gen*), and Fructus Trichosanthis Kirlowii (*Gua Lou*), 30g each, Flos Lonicerae Japonicae (*Jin Yin Hua*) and Herba Oldenlandiae Diffusae Cum Radice (*Bai Hua She She Cao*), 15g each, Rhizoma Anemarrhenae Aspheloidis (*Zhi Mu*), 12g, and Radix Scutellariae Baicalensis (*Huang Qin*), Rhizoma Coptidis Chinensis (*Huang Lian*), Fructus Perillae Frutescentis (*Zi Su Zi*), Bulbus Fritillariae Thunbergii (*Zhe Bei Mu*), stir-fried Semen Pruni Armeniacae (*Xing Ren*), Cortex Radicis Lycii Chinensis (*Di Gu Pi*), and Radix Platycodi Grandiflori (*Jie Geng*), 9g each

FORMULA ANALYSIS: *Sang Bai Pi, Huang Qin,* and *Huang Lian* clear and discharge lung heat. *Jie Geng, Lu Gen, Zhe Bei Mu, Xing Ren, Zi Su Zi,* and *Gua Lou* diffuse the lungs and transform phlegm. *Jin Yin Hua* and *Bai Hua She She Cao* clear heat and resolve toxins.

ADDITIONS & SUBTRACTIONS: If heat is severe, add 30 grams of uncooked Gypsum Fibrosum (*Shi Gao*) and 12 grams of Radix Trichosanthis Kirlowii (*Tian Hua Fen*). If the stools are dry, add 3-9 grams of Radix Et Rhizoma Rhei (*Da Huang*).

ACUPUNCTURE & MOXIBUSTION: *Qu Chi* (LI 11), *Chi Ze* (Lu 5), *Da Zhui* (GV 14), *Dan Zhong* (CV 17), *Fei Shu* (Bl 13)

FORMULA ANALYSIS: Draining *Qu Chi* and *Da Zhui* clears heat and recedes fever. Draining *Chi Ze, Dan Zhong,* and *Fei Shu* clears the lungs, stops cough, and levels panting.

ADDITIONS & SUBTRACTIONS: If there is constipation and oral thirst, add supplementing *Zhao Hai* (Ki 6) and draining *Nei Ting* (St 44), *Zhi Gou* (TB 6), *Tian Shu* (St 25), and *Da Chang Shu* (Bl 25). If there is reddish urine, add draining *Yin Ling Quan* (Sp 9).

3. HEAT DAMAGING LUNG YIN PATTERN

MAIN SYMPTOMS: Dry cough with scanty phlegm, possible blood-streaked phlegm, possible hacking blood, panting, rapid breathing, chest pain, dry mouth and parched throat, afternoon tidal heat, malar flushing, heat in the hearts of the hands and feet, insomnia, night sweats, emaciated body, a red tongue with scanty fur, and a fine, rapid pulse

TREATMENT PRINCIPLES: Nourish yin and clear heat, transform phlegm and stop cough

RX: *Sha Shen Mai Dong Tang Jia Jian* (Glehnia & Ophiopogon Decoction with Additions & Subtractions)

INGREDIENTS: Radix Trichosanthis Kirlowii (*Tian Hua Fen*), 30g, Radix Glehniae Littoralis (*Sha Shen*), Tuber Ophiopogonis Japonici (*Mai Men Dong*), and Cortex Radicis Lycii Chinensis (*Di Gu Pi*), 15g each, uncooked Radix Rehmanniae (*Sheng Di*), Bulbus Fritillariae Cirrhosae (*Chuan Bei Mu*), and Radix Stemonae (*Bai Bu*), 12g each, Rhizoma Polygonati Odorati (*Yu Zhu*), stir-fried

Semen Pruni Armeniacae (*Xing Ren*), and carbonized Cacumen Biotae Orientalis (*Ce Bai Ye*), 9g each, and powdered Radix Pseudoginseng (*San Qi*), 3g taken with the decocted liquid

FORMULA ANALYSIS: *Sha Shen, Mai Men Dong, Yu Zhu,* and *Sheng Di* enrich and nourish lung yin. *Di Gu Pi* clears vacuity heat. *Bai Bu, Chuan Bei Mu,* and *Xing Ren* moisten the lungs and transform phlegm. *San Qi* and *Ce Bai Ye* quicken the blood and stop bleeding.

ADDITIONS & SUBTRACTIONS: If there is no hacking of blood or blood-streaked phlegm, omit *San Qi* and *Ce Bai Ye*. If there is concomitant constipation, add nine grams each of Semen Pruni Persicae (*Tao Ren*) and Semen Cannabis Sativae (*Huo Ma Ren*). If there is marked thirst, add 12 grams of Rhizoma Anemarrhenae Aspheloidis (*Zhi Mu*). If there is insomnia, add 12 grams each of Semen Zizyphi Spinosae (*Suan Zao Ren*) and Semen Biotae Orientalis (*Bai Zi Ren*). If there are night sweats, add 30 grams of Fructus Levis Tritici Aestivi (*Fu Xiao Mai*) and nine grams of Fructus Schisandrae Chinensis (*Wu Wei Zi*).

ACUPUNCTURE & MOXIBUSTION: *Lie Que* (Lu 7), *Zhao Hai* (Ki 6), *Fei Shu* (Bl 13), *Zhong Fu* (Lu 1)

FORMULA ANALYSIS: Supplementing *Lie Que* and *Zhao Hai* enriches the lungs and clears heat. Supplementing *Fei Shu* and *Zhong Fu* downbears the qi and stops coughing.

ADDITIONS & SUBTRACTIONS: If there is chest pain, add even supplementing-even draining *Dan Zhong* (CV 17). If there is insomnia, add supplementing *Shen Men* (Ht 7) and draining *Feng Chi* (GB 20), *Bai Hui* (GV 20), and *Yin Tang* (M-HN-3). If there are night sweats, add even supplementing-even draining *Yin Xi* (Ht 6). If there is hacking blood, add draining *Xue Hai* (Sp 10).

4. QI & YIN DUAL VACUITY PATTERN

MAIN SYMPTOMS: Forceless cough, shortness of breath, lassitude of the spirit, fatigue, lack of strength, possible blood-streaked phlegm, however the blood is pale red, panting, hasty breathing, disinclination to speak and/or weak voice, afternoon low-grade fever, spontaneous perspiration and/or nights sweats, dry mouth, malar flushing, heat in the hearts of the hands and feet, a tender, red tongue with teeth-marks on its edges and scanty fur, and a fine, rapid, or weak, forceless pulse

TREATMENT PRINCIPLES: Boost the qi and nourish yin, moisten the lungs, stabilize panting, and stop coughing

RX: *Bu Fei Tang Jia Jian* (Supplement the Lungs Decoction with Additions & Subtractions)

INGREDIENTS: Radix Pseudostellariae Heterophyllae (*Tai Zi Shen*), 30g, mix-fried Radix Astragali Membranacei (*Huang Qi*), Tuber Ophiopogonis Japonici (*Mai Men Dong*), and Cortex Radicis Mori Albi (*Sang Bai Pi*), 15g each, Radix Asteris Tatarici (*Zi Wan*), Semen Oroxyli Indici (*Mu Hu Die*), Cortex Radicis Lycii Chinensis (*Di Gu Pi*), Radix Glehniae Littoralis (*Sha Shen*), and cooked Radix Rehmanniae (*Shu Di*), 12g each, Fructus Schisandrae Chinensis (*Wu Wei Zi*), Bulbus Fritillariae Cirrhosae (*Chuan Bei Mu*), and Gelatinum Corii Asini (*E Jiao*), 9g each, and Radix Glycyrrhizae (*Gan Cao*), 6g

FORMULA ANALYSIS: *Tai Zi Shen, Huang Qi*, and *Gan Cao* boost the qi. *Mai Men Dong, Sha Shen, Wu Wei Zi, E Jiao*, and *Shu Di* enrich yin and engender fluids. *Sang Bai Pi, Zi Wan, Mu Hu Die, Di Gu Pi*, and *Chuan Bei Mu* clear heat and transform phlegm, stop coughing and level panting.

ADDITIONS & SUBTRACTIONS: If there is hacking of blood, add nine grams each of Herba Agrimoniae Pilosae (*Xian He Cao*) and Folium Callicarpae (*Zhi Zhu Cao*) and three grams of powdered Radix Pseudoginseng (*San Qi*) taken with the liquid decoction. If there is bone-steaming and night sweats, add 15 grams each of Carapx Amydae Sinensis (*Bie Jia*) and Concha Ostreae (*Mu Li*) and nine grams of Radix Stellariae Dichotomae (*Yin Chai Hu*). If there is abdominal distention and loose stools, add 20 grams of Semen Coicis Lachryma-jobi (*Yi Yi Ren*) and 12 grams each of Semen Dolichoris Lablab (*Bai Bian Dou*) and Semen Nelumbinis Nuciferae (*Lian Zi*).

ACUPUNCTURE & MOXIBUSTION: *Zu San Li* (St 36), *Tai Xi* (Ki 3), *San Yin Jiao* (Sp 6), *Tai Yuan* (Lu 9), *Fei Shu* (Bl 13), *Pi Shu* (Bl 20), *Shen Shu* (Bl 23)

FORMULA ANALYSIS: Supplementing *Zu San Li, San Yin Jiao*, and *Pi Shu* fortifies the spleen and boosts the qi. Supplementing *Tai Xi, San Yin Jiao*, and *Shen Shu* supplements the kidneys and enriches yin. Supplementing *Tai Yuan* and *Fei Shu* moistens the lungs, stabilizes panting, and stops coughing.

ADDITIONS & SUBTRACTIONS: For night sweats, add even supplementing-even draining *Yin Xi* (Ht 6). For abdominal distention and loose stools, add supplementing *Zhong Wan* (CV 12), *Tian Shu* (St 25), *Wei Shu* (Bl 21), and *Da Chang Shu* (Bl 25).

REMARKS:

1. Chinese herbal medicine is typically extremely effective for the treatment of respiratory tract infections.

B. CONCOMITANT URINARY TRACT INFECTIONS

CHINESE MEDICAL DISEASE CATEGORIZATION: Urinary tract infections mostly correspond to the traditional Chinese disease categories of *lin zheng*, strangury conditions.

CHINESE DISEASE MECHANISMS: Acute urinary tract infections concomitant with diabetes are usually species of *re lin* or heat strangury. This heat may be damp heat, depressive heat, or heat toxins. Chronic urinary tract infections typically involve less heat and more vacuity. This vacuity may be liver-kidney yin vacuity, spleen-kidney yang vacuity, or kidney yin and yang vacuity depending on the original disease mechanisms, age of the patient, body constitution, diet, lifestyle, and previous treatment.

TREATMENT BASED ON PATTERN DISCRIMINATION:

1. HEAT TOXIN BLOODY STRANGURY PATTERN

MAIN SYMPTOMS: Emission of heat (*i.e.*, fever), aversion to cold, lower abdominal distention and pain, frequent, urgent urination with hot pain, hematuria and possible pus in the urine, dry, bound stools, low backache, a red tongue with yellow fur, and a bowstring, rapid pulse

NOTE: This pattern mostly presents in diabetic patients with concomitant acute cystitis or acute pyelonephritis.

TREATMENT PRINCIPLES: Clear heat and resolve toxins, cool the blood and stop bleeding

RX: *Jie Di Qing Shen Tang* (Resolve Toxins & Clear the Kidneys Decoction)

INGREDIENTS: Flos Lonicerae Japonicae (*Jin Yin Hua*), Fructus Forsythiae Suspensae (*Lian Qiao*), Herba Cephalanoploris Segeti (*Xiao Ji*), and Folium Pyrrosiae (*Shi Wei*), 30g each, uncooked Radix Rehmanniae (*Sheng Di*), 20g, Nodus Rhizomatis Nelumbinis Nuciferae (*Ou Jie*), 15g, and Radix Scutellariae Baicalensis (*Huang Qin*), Fructus Gardeniae Jasminoidis (*Zhi Zi*), Cortex Radicis

Moutan (*Dan Pi*), uncooked Pollen Typhae (*Pu Huang*), and uncooked Radix Et Rhizoma Rhei (*Da Huang*), 9g each

FORMULA ANALYSIS: *Jin Yin Hua, Lian Qiao, Huang Qin,* and *Zhi Zi* clear heat and resolve toxins. *Sheng Di, Xiao Ji, Ou Jie,* and *Dan Pi* cool the blood and stop bleeding. Uncooked *Da Huang* frees the flow of the bowels and drains turbidity. *Shi Wei* clears and disinhibits dampness and heat.

ADDITIONS & SUBTRACTIONS: If yin is damaged with a red tongue and scanty fur and a fine, rapid pulse, add 15 grams of Radix Scrophulariae Ningpoensis (*Xuan Shen*), 12 grams of Tuber Ophiopogonis Japonici (*Mai Men Dong*), and nine grams of Radix Trichosanthis Kirlowii (*Tian Hua Fen*). If qi stagnation is marked, add nine grams each of Fructus Immaturus Citri Aurantii (*Zhi Shi*) and Cortex Magnoliae Officinalis (*Hou Po*). If damp heat is relatively heavy, add 20 grams of uncooked Semen Coicis Lachryma-jobi (*Yi Yi Ren*) and nine grams each of Rhizoma Atractylodis (*Cang Zhu*) and Cortex Phellodendri (*Huang Bai*). If hematuria is pronounced, add 12 grams each of Rhizoma Imperatae Cyclindricae (*Bai Mao Gen*) and uncooked Radix Sanguisorbae (*Di Yu*) and three grams of powdered Radix Pseudoginseng (*San Qi*) taken with the liquid decoction.

ACUPUNCTURE & MOXIBUSTION: *Qu Chi* (LI 11), *San Yin Jiao* (Sp 6), *Yin Ling Quan* (Sp 9), *Zhong Ji* (CV 3), *Pang Guang Shu* (Bl 28), *Ci Liao* (Bl 32)

FORMULA ANALYSIS: Draining *Qu Chi* clears heat and recedes fever. Draining *San Yin Jiao* and *Yin Ling Quan* clears heat and eliminates dampness. Draining *Zhong Ji, Pang Guang Shu,* and *Ci Liao* clears the bladder and disinhibits urination.

ADDITIONS & SUBTRACTIONS: Add draining *Xue Hai* (Sp 10) for hematuria. If there is damaged yin, use even supplementing-even draining at *San Yin Jiao* and add supplementing *Tai Xi* (Ki 3). For concomitant qi stagnation, add draining *Tai Chong* (Liv 3).

2. DAMP HEAT TURBID STRANGURY PATTERN

MAIN SYMPTOMS: Slight emission of heat, heaviness of the four limbs, frequent, urgent, painful urination, epigastric and abdominal distention and fullness, noncrisp stools, dry mouth but no profuse drinking of water, a red tongue with thick, slimy, yellow fur, and a bowstring, slippery, rapid pulse

TREATMENT PRINCIPLES: Clear and disinhibit dampness and heat, free the flow and disinhibit the two excretions

RX: *Si Miao San Jia Wei* (Four Wonders Powder with Added Flavors)

INGREDIENTS: Uncooked Radix Sanguisorbae (*Di Yu*), Rhizoma Smilacis Glabrae (*Tu Fu Ling*), Folium Pyrrosiae (*Shi Wei*), Sclerotium Rubrum Poriae Cocos (*Chi Fu Ling*), and Semen Coicis Lachryma-jobi (*Yi Yi Ren*), 30g each, Radix Achyranthis Bidentatae (*Niu Xi*), 12g, and Cortex Phellodendri (*Huang Bai*), Rhizoma Atractylodis (*Cang Zhu*), Cortex Magnoliae Officinalis (*Hou Po*), and Radix Auklandiae Lappae (*Mu Xiang*), 9g each

FORMULA ANALYSIS: *Cang Zhu, Huang Bai, Yi Yi Ren, Tu Fu Ling,* and *Chi Fu Ling* clear and disinhibit dampness. *Hou Po* and *Mu Xiang* rectify the qi, fortify the spleen, and harmonize the stomach. *Shi Wei* clears heat and frees the flow of strangury. Uncooked *Di Yu* clears heat and cools the blood, while *Niu Xi* moves the blood downward and guides the other medicinals to the lower burner.

ADDITIONS & SUBTRACTIONS: If there is nausea and scanty intake, add nine grams each of Rhizoma Pinelliae Ternatae (*Ban Xia*), Pericarpium Citri Reticulatae (*Chen Pi*), and Caulis Bambusae In Taeniis (*Zhu Ru*) to harmonize the stomach, downbear counterflow, and stop vomiting. If there is constipation, add nine grams of Fructus Trichosanthis Kirlowii (*Gua Lou*) and 3-9 grams of wine-processed Radix Et Rhizoma Rhei (*Da Huang*).

If dampness is heavier than heat, one can use *Huang Qin Hua Shi Tang* (Scutellaria & Talcum Decoction) plus *San Ren Tang* (Three Seeds Decoction) with additions and subtractions: Talcum (*Hua Shi*) and Semen Coicis Lachryma-jobi (*Yi Yi Ren*), 18g each, Radix Scutellariae Baicalensis (*Huang Qin*), Herba Lophatheri Gracilis (*Dan Zhu Ye*), Rhizoma Pinelliae Ternatae (*Ban Xia*), Cortex Magnoliae Officinalis (*Hou Po*), Sclerotium Poriae Cocos (*Fu Ling*), Sclerotium Polypori Umbellati (*Zhu Ling*), 9g each, and Medulla Tetrapanacis Papyriferi (*Tong Cao*), 6g. If dampness has encumbered the spleen add six grams of Fructus Cardamomi (*Bai Dou Kou*) to arouse the spleen and aromatically transform dampness.

If heat is heavier than dampness, one can use *Ba Zheng San* (Eight [Ingredients] Correcting Powder): Talcum (*Hua Shi*), 15-30g, Semen Plantaginis (*Che Qian Zi*), 15g, Herba Dianthi (*Qu Mai*) and Herba Polygoni Avicularis (*Bian Xu*), 12g each, Fructus Gardeniae Jasminoidis (*Zhi Zi*) and Caulis Akebiae (*Mu Tong*), 9g each, processed Radix Et Rhizoma Rhei (*Da Huang*) and Radix Glycyrrhizae (*Gan*

Cao), 3-9g each, and Medulla Junci Effusi (*Deng Xin Cao*), 3-6g. If there is hematuria, add 15 grams each of Rhizoma Imperatae Cylindricae (*Bai Mao Gen*) and Herba Cephalanoploris Segeti (*Xiao Ji*). For turbid urination, add nine grams each of Rhizoma Acori Graminei (*Shi Chang Pu*) and Rhizoma Dioscoreae Hypoglaucae (*Bie Xie*). If there are sores in the mouth or on the tongue, add 12 grams of uncooked Radix Rehmanniae (*Sheng Di*) and nine grams of Herba Lophatheri Gracilis (*Dan Zhu Ye*).

ACUPUNCTURE & MOXIBUSTION: Same as pattern #1 above minus *Qu Chi*.

3. DEPRESSIVE HEAT QI STRANGURY PATTERN

MAIN SYMPTOMS: Frequent, urgent, painful urination, chest and rib-side fullness and discomfort, lower abdominal distention and pain, neither urination or defecation crisp, a bitter taste in the mouth, dry throat, tension, agitation, and easy anger, possible alternating cold and heat, a darkish tongue with thin, yellow fur, and a bowstring, rapid pulse

TREATMENT PRINCIPLES: Course the liver, resolve depression, and clear heat

RX: *Si Ni San Jia Jian* (Four Counterflows Powder with Additions & Subtractions)

INGREDIENTS: Herba Pyrrosiae (*Shi Wei*), 30g, Radix Rubrus Paeoniae Lactiflorae (*Chi Shao*), Radix Albus Paeoniae Lactiflorae (*Bai Shao*), and Radix Bupleuri (*Chai Hu*), 15g each, Fructus Citri Aurantii (*Zhi Ke*), Fructus Immaturus Citri Aurantii (*Zhi Shi*), Fructus Gardeniae Jasminoidis (*Zhi Zi*), Radix Scutellariae Baicalensis (*Huang Qin*), Rhizoma Cyperi Rotundi (*Xiang Fu*), Radix Linderae Strychnifoliae (*Wu Yao*), and Radix Angelicae Sinensis (*Dang Gui*), 9g each, and Cortex Magnoliae Officinalis (*Hou Po*), 6g

FORMULA ANALYSIS: *Chai Hu, Zhi Ke, Zhi Shi, Xiang Fu, Wu Yao,* and *Hou Po* course the liver and rectify the qi. *Zhi Zi, Shi Wei,* and *Huang Qin* clear and disinhibit dampness and heat. *Dang Gui, Chi Shao,* and *Bai Shao* quicken the blood and transform stasis.

ADDITIONS & SUBTRACTIONS: If lower abdominal distention and pain are pronounced, add 15 grams each of Semen Litchi Chinensis (*Li Zhi He*) and Semen Citri Reticulatae (*Ju He*).

ACUPUNCTURE & MOXIBUSTION: *Tai Chong* (Liv 3), *Xing Jian* (Liv 2), *San Yin Jiao* (Sp 6), *Yin Ling Quan* (Sp 9), *Zhong Ji* (CV 3), *Qi Hai* (CV 6)

FORMULA ANALYSIS: Needling *Tai Chong* through to *Xing Jian* with draining technique courses the liver, resolves depression, and clears heat. Draining *San Yin Jiao, Yin Ling Quan,* and *Zhong Ji* disinhibits and frees the flow of urination. Draining *Qi Hai* rectifies the qi of the lower burner.

ADDITIONS & SUBTRACTIONS: If there is a liver-spleen disharmony, add supplementing *Zu San Li* (St 36) and *Pi Shu* (Bl 20). If there is concomitant blood stasis, add draining *Xue Hai* (Sp 10) and *He Gu* (LI 4).

4. LIVER-KIDNEY YIN VACUITY PATTERN

MAIN SYMPTOMS: Low back and knee soreness and limpness, tension, agitation, easy anger, dizziness or vertigo, vexatious heat in the five hearts, fatigue, lack of strength, taxation may cause the urirnation to be frequent, urgent, hot, and painful, a dark red tongue with white or yellow fur, and a bowstring, fine, rapid pulse

NOTE: Although the name of this pattern does not say so, the symptoms and treatment principles indicate that there is not simply a yin vacuity but a qi and yin vacuity operating here. It is most commonly seen in relapsing-remitting urinary tract infections which will not completely heal.

TREATMENT PRINCIPLES: Enrich and supplement the liver and kidneys, boost the qi and nourish yin

RX: *Yang Yin Qing Shen Tang* (Nourish Yin & Clear the Kidneys Decoction)

INGREDIENTS: Herba Cirsii Japonici (*Da Ji*), Herba Cephalanoploris Segeti (*Xiao Ji*), and Folium Pyrrosiae (*Shi Wei*), 30g each, Radix Scrophulariae Ningpoensis (*Xuan Shen*) and uncooked Radix Rehmanniae (*Sheng Di*), 20g each, Fructus Ligustri Lucidi (*Nu Zhen Zi*), Herba Ecliptae Prostratae (*Han Lian Cao*), and Radix Pseudostellariae Heterophyllae (*Tai Zi Shen*), 15g each, and Radix Scutellariae Baicalensis (*Huang Qin*), 9g

FORMULA ANALYSIS: *Nu Zhen Zi* and *Han Lian Cao* enrich and supplement the liver and kidneys. *Tai Zi Shen, Xuan Shen,* and *Sheng Di* boost the qi and nourish yin. *Shi*

Wei, Huang Qin, Da Ji, and *Xiao Ji* clear heat and disinhibit dampness, cool the blood and stop bleeding.

ADDITIONS & SUBTRACTIONS: If there is concomitant urinary urgency, heat, and pain, add 15 grams each of Herba Violae Yedoensitis Cum Radice (*Zi Hua Di Ding*), Herba Taraxaci Mongolici Cum Radice (*Pu Gong Ying*), and uncooked Radix Sanguisorbae (*Di Yu*) to clear heat and resolve toxins.

ACUPUNCTURE & MOXIBUSTION: *Zu San Li* (St 36), *Tai Xi* (Ki 3), *San Yin Jiao* (Sp 6), *Yin Ling Quan* (Sp 9), *Shen Shu* (Bl 23), *Pang Guang Shu* (Bl 28)

FORMULA ANALYSIS: Supplementing *Zu San Li* and even supplementing-even draining *San Yin Jiao* fortifies the spleen and boosts the qi. Supplementing *Tai Xi* and *Shen Shu* and even supplementing-even draining *San Yin Jiao* supplements the kidneys and nourishes yin. Even supplementing-even draining *San Yin Jiao* and draining *Yin Ling Quan* and *Pang Guang Shu* clears heat and frees the flow of urination.

ADDITIONS & SUBTRACTIONS: If symptoms of liver blood vacuity are marked, add supplementing *Ge Shu* (Bl 17) and *Gan Shu* (Bl 18). If there is concomitant liver depression qi stagnation, add even supplementing-even draining *Tai Chong* (Liv 3). If there is hematuria, add draining *Xue Hai* (Sp 10).

5. SPLEEN-KIDNEY QI VACUITY PATTERN

MAIN SYMPTOMS: Lassitude of the spirit, lack of strength, low back and knee soreness and limpness, fear of cold, chilled limbs, taxation resulting in dribbling and dripping and uneasy urination or urinary incontinence, mild superficial edema, a fat tongue with sticky, slimy, white fur, and a deep, fine, forceless pulse

NOTE: Although the name of the pattern does not indicate it, there are lingering damp heat evils deep-lying in this condition.

TREATMENT PRINCIPLES: Fortify the spleen and boost the kidneys, quicken the blood, clear and disinhibit

RX: *Yi Qi Qing Shen Tang* (Boost the Qi & Clear the Kidneys Decoction)

INGREDIENTS: Uncooked Radix Astragali Membranacei (*Huang Qi*), Rhizoma Smilacis Glabrae (*Tu Fu Ling*), uncooked Radix Sanguisorbae (*Di Yu*), and Folium Pyrrosiae (*Shi Wei*), 30g each, Radix Codonopsitis Pilosulae (*Dang Shen*), 20g, Fructus Rosae Laevigatae (*Jin Ying Zi*), Radix Dipsaci (*Xu Duan*), and Radix Rubrus Paeoniae Lactiflorae (*Chi Shao*), 15g each, Radix Angelicae Sinensis (*Dang Gui*), Semen Euryalis Ferocis (*Qian Shi*), and Cortex Radicis Moutan (*Dan Pi*), 9g each

FORMULA ANALYSIS: *Huang Qi* and *Dang Shen* fortify the spleen and boost the qi. *Qian Shi* and *Jin Ying Zi* supplement the kidneys and secure the essence. *Dang Gui*, *Dan Pi*, and *Chi Shao* cool and quicken the blood. *Tu Fu Ling*, *Shi Wei*, and uncooked *Di Yu* clear and disinhibit dampness and heat.

ADDITIONS & SUBTRACTIONS: To strengthen supplementation of the spleen, add nine grams each of Radix Dioscoreae Oppositae (*Shan Yao*) and Sclerotium Poriae Cocos (*Fu Ling*). To strengthen supplementation of the kidneys, add nine grams each of Fructus Corni Officinalis (*Shan Zhu Yu*) and Semen Cuscutae Chinensis (*Tu Si Zi*). If there is concomitant liver depression qi stagnation, add nine grams each of Fructus Meliae Toosendan (*Chuan Lian Zi*) and Radix Linderae Strychnifoliae (*Wu Yao*).

ACUPUNCTURE & MOXIBUSTION: *Zu San Li* (St 36), *San Yin Jiao* (Sp 6), *Yin Ling Quan* (Sp 9), *Pi Shu* (Bl 20), *Shen Shu* (Bl 23), *Zhi Shi* (Bl 52), *Guan Yuan* (CV 4)

FORMULA ANALYSIS: Supplementing *Zu San Li* and *Pi Shu* and even supplementing-even draining *San Yin Jiao* fortifies the spleen and boosts the qi. Supplementing *Guan Yuan*, *Shen Shu*, and *Zhi Shi*, and even supplementing-even draining *San Yin Jiao* supplements the kidneys and secures the essence. Draining *Yin Ling Quan* and even supplementing-even draining *San Yin Jiao* clears heat and eliminates dampness from the lower burner.

ADDITIONS & SUBTRACTIONS: For concomitant blood stasis, add draining *Xue Hai* (Sp 10) and *He Gu* (LI 4). For concomitant liver depression qi stagnation, add draining *Tai Chong* (Liv 3).

6. KIDNEY YIN & YANG DUAL VACUITY PATTERN

MAIN SYMPTOMS: Dread of both chill and heat, low back and knee soreness and pain, taxation resulting in urination becoming frequent, urgent, hot, and painful, a fat tongue with yellow and white fur simultaneously, and a deep, fine pulse

TREATMENT PRINCIPLES: Regulate and supplement yin and yang assisted by clearing heat

RX: *Tiao Bu Qing Shen Tang* (Regulating, Supplementing & Clearing the Kidneys Decoction)

INGREDIENTS: Folium Pyrrosiae (*Shi Wei*), Rhizoma Smilacis Glabrae (*Tu Fu Ling*), uncooked Radix Sanguisorbae (*Di Yu*), and Radix Salviae Miltiorrhizae (*Dan Shen*), 30g each, cooked Radix Rehmanniae (*Shu Di*) and uncooked Radix Rehmanniae (*Sheng Di*), 12g each, Cortex Phellodendri (*Huang Bai*), Fructus Lycii Chinensis (*Gou Qi Zi*), and Ramulus Cinnamomi Cassiae (*Gui Zhi*), 9g each, and Radix Lateralis Praeparatus Aconiti Carmichaeli (*Fu Zi*), 6g

FORMULA ANALYSIS: *Sheng Di, Shu Di,* and *Gou Qi Zi* enrich and supplement kidney yin, while *Gui Zhi* and *Fu Zi* warm and supplement kidney yang. *Shi Wei, Tu Fu Ling,* and *Huang Bai* clear and disinhibit dampness and heat, while *Dan Shen* and uncooked *Di Yu* cool and quicken the blood.

ADDITIONS & SUBTRACTIONS: If there is liver depression qi stagnation, add nine grams each of Fructus Meliae Toosendan (*Chuan Lian Zi*) and Radix Linderae Strychnifoliae (*Wu Yao*). If there is turbid urination, add nine grams each of Rhizoma Acori Graminei (*Shi Chang Pu*) and Rhizoma Dioscoreae Hypoglaucae (*Bie Xie*). If there is dribbling and dripping or incontinence, add nine grams each of Semen Euryalis Ferocis (*Qian Shi*) and Fructus Rosae Laevigatae (*Jin Ying Zi*). If there is marked low back soreness and pain, add nine grams each of Radix Dipsaci (*Xu Duan*), Cortex Eucommiae Ulmoidis (*Du Zhong*), Radix Achyranthis Bidentatae (*Niu Xi*), and Ramulus Loranthi Seu Visci (*Sang Ji Shen*).

ACUPUNCTURE & MOXIBUSTION: *Tai Xi* (Ki 3), *San Yin Jiao* (Sp 6), *Guan Yuan* (CV 4), *Shen Shu* (Bl 23), *Ming Men* (GV 4)

FORMULA ANALYSIS: Supplementing *Tai Xi* and *San Yin Jiao* supplements the kidneys and enriches yin and treats urogenital disorders in general. Moxaing *Guan Yuan, Shen Shu,* and *Ming Men* supplements the kidneys and invigorates yang.

ADDITIONS & SUBTRACTIONS: When there is urinary frequency, urgency, heat, and/or pain, add draining *Yin Ling Quan* (Sp 9) and use even supplementing-even draining at *San Yin Jiao*.

REMARKS:

1. The first three patterns all describe the acute stage or urinary tract infections. After remedial treatment has caused urine cultures to turn negative, one can administer the above appropriate formula for 10 days each month for half a year in order to prevent an acute urinary tract infection from turning into a chronic one.

2. The second three patterns describe chronic relapsing-remitting urinary tract infections. In treating patients with diabetes with urinary tract infection, particular attention should be paid to the prevention of such relapse. If the infections are recurrent, this means that treatment has been not thorough enough. If one prescribes Chinese medicinals based on the patient's pattern discrimination, one can attain relatively good treatment results.

3. Patients with diabetic UTI typically manifest a root vacuity of qi and yin with a branch repletion of damp heat evils. In this case, it is necessary to boost qi and nourish yin. However, one should avoid enriching medicinals which are also greasy and can obstruct the evil qi from being dispelled. Likewise, in disinhibiting the urine and freeing the flow of strangury, bitter, cold medicinals which can damage qi and yin should be avoided.

4. Due to lowered immunity, diabetic patients easily contract opportunistic infections and especially urinary tract infections. This situation is compounded by the fact that diabetes is often complicated by autonomic neuropathy, in which case the urination is typically inhibited. When retention of urine occurs due to neuropathy, this is called neurogenic bladder. In that case, inhibited urination provides a perfect place for the reproduction of bacteria. To make matters worse, the increase of urine glucose common in those with diabetes only further feeds the reproduction of these bacteria. Therefore, in real life, it is common to find symptoms of neurogenic bladder and UTI simultaneously or one condition transmuting into the other.

5. When the tongue body is dark purple in the center and slightly gray, and the tongue itself is withered and small, the movement of qi is slowed, and spirit qi is lacking. We know that enduring, long-term illness gradually affects the kidneys and enters the network vessels and that, when yin is exhausted, it leads to the exhaustion of yang as well, thus resulting in yin and yang dual depletion. Therefore, formulas that warm and supplement the kidneys, such as *Jin Gui Shen Qi Wan* (*Golden Cabinet* Kidney Qi Pills), and that nourish yin and supplement the blood while securing and astringing the kidneys, such as *Wu Zi Yan Zong Wan* (Five Seeds Increase Progeny Pills), are commonly used guiding formulas for this condition.[1]

C. CONCOMITANT BILIARY TRACT INFECTIONS

CHINESE MEDICAL DISEASE CATEGORIZATION: Biliary tract infections primarily correspond to the traditional Chinese medical disease categories of *xie tong*, rib-side pain, and *huang dan*, jaundice.

CHINESE DISEASE MECHANISMS: Because most cases of diabetes are complicated by qi vacuity, meaning spleen qi vacuity, it is common for the spleen to lose its fortification and movement. In that case, internal brewing of dampness and heat may disturb the liver's coursing and discharging and the gallbladder's free flow and downbearing of the central essence, hence causing stasis and stagnation on top of damp heat.

TREATMENT BASED ON PATTERN DISCRIMINATION:

1. LIVER-GALLBLADDER QI DEPRESSION PATTERN

MAIN SYMPTOMS: Right rib-side distention, fullness, aching, and pain possibly radiating to the upper back with worsening of the pain due to emotional disturbance, chest oppression and discomfort, frequent burping, abdominal distention, a bitter taste in the mouth and dry throat, no marked heat or cold, no jaundice, thin, white or thin, yellow tongue fur, and a bowstring pulse

NOTE: While the name of the pattern only identifies liver-gallbladder qi depression, there is a minor element of damp heat.

TREATMENT PRINCIPLES: Course the liver and disinhibit the gallbladder, move the qi and stop the pain

RX: *Chai Hu Shu Gan San Jia Jian* (Bupleurum Course the Liver Powder with Additions & Subtractions)

INGREDIENTS: Herba Lysimachiae Seu Desmodii (*Jin Qian Cao*), 30g, Radix Albus Paeoniae Lactiflorae (*Bai Shao*), 12g, Radix Bupleuri (*Chai Hu*), Fructus Citri Aurantii (*Zhi Ke*), Fructus Immaturus Citri Aurantii (*Zhi Shi*), Rhizoma Cyperi Rotundi (*Xiang Fu*), Radix

Ligustici Wallichii (*Chuan Xiong*), Fructus Meliae Toosendan (*Chuan Lian Zi*), Radix Auklandiae Lappae (*Mu Xiang*), Radix Scutellariae Baicalensis (*Huang Qin*), Tuber Curcumae (*Yu Jin*), Rhizoma Corydalis Yanhusuo (*Yan Hu Suo*), and Pericarpium Citri Reticulatae Viride (*Qing Pi*), 9g each, and Radix Glycyrrhizae (*Gan Cao*), 6g

FORMULA ANALYSIS: *Chai Hu, Zhi Ke, Zhi Shi, Xiang Fu, Qing Pi*, and *Mu Xiang* course the liver and rectify the qi. *Chuan Xiong* quickens the blood. *Bai Shao* and *Gan Cao* relax cramping and stop pain. *Chuan Lian Zi, Yan Hu Suo*, and *Huang Qin* clear the liver, regulate the qi, and stop pain, and *Jin Qian Cao* disinhibits the gallbladder and expels stones.

ADDITIONS & SUBTRACTIONS: If the stomach has lost its harmony and downbearing with nausea and vomiting, add nine grams each of Flos Inulae Racemosae (*Xuan Fu Hua*) and Rhizoma Pinelliae Ternatae (*Ban Xia*) and two slices of uncooked Rhizoma Zingiberis (*Sheng Jiang*) to harmonize the stomach and stop vomiting. If there is simultaneous stomach dryness and heat with nonfree-flowing stools and abdominal distention and fullness, add 3-9 grams of Radix Et Rhizoma Rhei (*Da Huang*) to discharge heat and free the flow of the stools.

ACUPUNCTURE & MOXIBUSTION: *Dan Nan Xue* (M-LE-23) or *Yang Ling Quan* (GB 34), *Tai Chong* (Liv 3), *Xing Jian* (Liv 2), *Zhang Men* (Liv 13), *Qi Men* (Liv 14), *Dan Shu* (Bl 19)

FORMULA ANALYSIS: Draining the sorest point on the right side between *Yang Ling Quan* and *Dan Nan Xue* as well as *Dan Shu* disinhibits the gallbladder and expels stones. Needling *Tai Chong* through to *Xing Jian* with draining technique courses and drains the liver, clears heat and resolves depression. Draining *He Gu* and *Tai Chong* courses the liver and rectifies the qi. Draining right *Zhang Men* and *Qi Men* frees the flow of the channels and vessels in the rib-side and stops pain.

ADDITIONS & SUBTRACTIONS: If there is constipation, add draining *Zhi Gou* (TB 3), *Nei Ting* (St 44), *Tian Shu* (St 25), and *Da Chang Shu* (Bl 25) and supplementing *Zhao Hai* (Ki 6). If there is nausea and vomiting, add draining *Zhong Wan* (CV 12) and *Nei Guan* (Per 6). If there is concomitant blood stasis, add draining *Xue Hai* (Sp 10). If there is high fever, add draining *Qu Chi* (LI 11).

2. LIVER-GALLBLADDER DAMP HEAT PATTERN

MAIN SYMPTOMS: Right rib-side pain radiating to the upper back and shoulder, alternating heat and cold, a bitter taste in the mouth and dry throat, vexation and agitation, easy anger, nausea and indigestion on eating oily, greasy food, vomiting, abdominal distention, constipation, scanty, yellow-colored urination, possible yellowing of the body and eyes, slimy, yellow tongue fur, and a bowstring, slippery or bowstring, rapid pulse

TREATMENT PRINCIPLES: Clear heat and eliminate dampness, free the flow of the bowels and disinhibit the gallbladder

RX: *Da Chai Hu Tang Jia Jian* (Major Bupleurum Decoction with Additions & Subtractions)

INGREDIENTS: Herba Artemisiae Capillaris (*Yin Chen Hao*) and Herba Lysimachiae Seu Desmodii (*Jin Qian Cao*), 30g each, Radix Et Rhizoma Polygoni Cuspidati (*Hu Zhang*) and Radix Albus Paeoniae Lactiflorae (*Bai Shao*), 15g each, Radix Bupleuri (*Chai Hu*), Radix Scutellariae Baicalensis (*Huang Qin*), Fructus Citri Aurantii (*Zhi Ke*), Fructus Immaturus Citri Aurantii (*Zhi Shi*), stir-fried Fructus Gardeniae Jasminoidis (*Zhi Zi*), and Tuber Curcumae (*Yu Jin*), 9g each, Radix Et Rhizoma Rhei (*Da Huang*), 6-9g, and Mirabilitum (*Mang Xiao*), 3-6g

FORMULA ANALYSIS: *Chai Hu* courses and spreads the liver-gallbladder qi mechanism. *Huang Qin* and *Zhi Zi* clear and drain liver-gallbladder heat. *Zhi Ke, Zhi Shi,* and *Yu Jin* combined with *Da Huang* and *Mang Xiao* move the qi, free the flow of the bowels, and drain heat. *Yin Chen Hao, Jin Qian Cao,* and *Hu Zhang* clear and disinhibit liver-gallbladder damp heat in order to recede yellowing.

ADDITIONS & SUBTRACTIONS: If the tongue is dark and purplish, add 15 grams of Radix Salviae Miltiorrhizae (*Dan Shen*) and nine grams of Semen Pruni Persicae (*Tao Ren*) to quicken the blood and dispel stasis. If rib-side pain is relatively severe, add 12 grams each of Fructus Meliae Toosendan (*Chuan Lian Zi*) and Rhizoma Corydalis Yanhusuo (*Yan Hu Suo*) to course the liver, move the qi, and stop pain.

ACUPUNCTURE & MOXIBUSTION: *Dan Nan Xue* (M-LE-23) or *Yang Ling Quan* (GB 34), *Wai Guan* (TB 5), *Zu Lin Qi* (GB 41), *Yin Ling Quan* (Sp 9), *Zhang Men* (Liv 13), *Qi Men* (Liv 14), *Ling Tai* (GV 10)

FORMULA ANALYSIS: Draining the sorest point on the right side between *Yang Ling Quan* and *Dan Nan Xue* disinhibits the gallbladder and expels stones. Draining right *Wai Guan* and *Zu Lin Qi* moves the qi within and frees the flow of the shao yang channel. Draining *Yin Ling Quan* clears heat and seeps dampness via urination. Draining right *Zhang Men* and *Qi Men* frees the flow of the channels and stops pain in the rib-side.

ADDITIONS & SUBTRACTIONS: If there is constipation, add draining *Zhi Gou* (TB 3), *Nei Ting* (St 44), *Tian Shu* (St 25), and *Da Chang Shu* (Bl 25) and supplementing *Zhao Hai* (Ki 6). If there is nausea and vomiting, add draining *Zhong Wan* (CV 12) and *Nei Guan* (Per 6). If there is concomitant blood stasis, add draining *Xue Hai* (Sp 10).

3. SPLEEN VACUITY & LIVER DEPRESSION PATTERN

MAIN SYMPTOMS: Right rib-side insidious pain, distention, fullness, and discomfort, frequent burping, abdominal distention, torpid intake, nausea and vomiting, fatigue, lack of strength, a bitter taste and sticky, slimy feeling in the mouth, loose stools, slimy tongue fur, and a deep, fine, forceless pulse

NOTE: This pattern mainly presents in chronic conditions with a relatively long disease course.

TREATMENT PRINCIPLES: Fortify the spleen and boost the qi, course the liver and disinhibit the gallbladder

RX: *Xiang Sha Liu Jun Zi Tang* (Auklandia & Amomum Six Gentlemen Decoction) plus *Si Jin San* (Four Golds Powder) with additions and subtractions

INGREDIENTS: Herba Lysimachiae Seu Desmodii (*Jin Qian Cao*), 30g, Radix Codonopsitis Pilosulae (*Dang Shen*), 15g, Rhizoma Atractylodis Macrocephalae (*Bai Zhu*), Sclerotium Poriae Cocos (*Fu Ling*), and Spora Lygodii Japonici (*Hai Jin Sha*), 12g each, and Rhizoma Pinelliae Ternatae (*Ban Xia*), Pericarpium Citri Reticulatae (*Chen Pi*), Fructus Amomi (*Sha Ren*), Endothelium Corneum Gigeriae Galli (*Ji Nei Jin*), Tuber Curcumae (*Yu Jin*), and Radix Auklandiae Lappae (*Mu Xiang*), 9g each

FORMULA ANALYSIS: *Dang Shen, Bai Zhu,* and *Fu Ling* fortify the spleen and boost the qi. *Chen Pi, Sha Ren,* and

Ban Xia penetratingly and aromatically arouse the spleen, harmonize the stomach and stop vomiting. *Yu Jin* and *Mu Xiang* rectify the qi. *Ji Nei Jin* disperses food and transforms stagnation. In addition, when combined with *Jin Qian Cao, Hai Jin Sha,* and *Yu Jin,* it disinhibits the gallbladder and expels stones.

ADDITIONS & SUBTRACTIONS: If there are loose stools, add 12 grams each of Semen Dolichoris Lablab (*Bai Bian Dou*) and Semen Nelumbinis Nuciferae (*Lian Zi*). If there is marked fatigue and lack of strength, add 15-30 grams of Radix Astragali Membranacei (*Huang Qi*). If there is concomitant blood stasis, add 15-30 grams of Radix Salviae Miltiorrhizae (*Dan Shen*). If there is hyperlipidemia, add 15 grams of Fructus Crataegi (*Shan Zha*).

ACUPUNCTURE & MOXIBUSTION: *Dan Nan Xue* (M-LE-23) or *Yang Ling Quan* (GB 34), *Tai Chong* (Liv 3), *He Gu* (LI 4), *Zu San Li* (St 36), *San Yin Jiao* (Sp 6), *Pi Shu* (Bl 20)

FORMULA ANALYSIS: Draining the sorest point between *Yang Ling Quan* and *Dan Nan Xue* on the right side, disinhibits the gallbladder and expels stones. However, only needle if there is an *a shi* point. Draining *Tai Chong* and *He Gu* courses the liver and rectifies the qi. Supplementing *Zu San Li* and *Pi Shu* and even supplementing-even draining *San Yin Jiao* fortifies the spleen and boosts the qi.

ADDITIONS & SUBTRACTIONS: If there is nausea and vomiting, add even supplementing-even draining *Zhong Wan* (CV 12) and draining *Nei Guan* (Per 6). If there are loose stools, add supplementing *Wei Shu* (Bl 21), *Da Chang Shu* (Bl 25), *Zhong Wan* (CV 12), and *Tian Shu* (St 25).

4. LIVER YIN INSUFFICIENCY PATTERN

MAIN SYMPTOMS: Insidious pain in the rib-side area which comes and goes and is worsened by taxation, a dry mouth and parched throat, vexatious heat in the center of the heart, dizziness or vertigo, a red tongue with scanty fur, and a fine, rapid, bowstring pulse

TREATMENT PRINCIPLES: Nourish yin, emolliate the liver, and stop pain

RX: *Yi Guan Jian Jia Wai* (One Link Decoction with Added Flavors)

INGREDIENTS: Uncooked Radix Rehmanniae (*Sheng Di*), Radix Albus Paeoniae Lactiflorae (*Bai Shao*), Radix

Salviae Miltiorrhizae (*Dan Shen*), and Fructus Lycii Chinensis (*Gou Qi Zi*), 15g each, Radix Glehniae Littoralis (*Sha Shen*) and Tuber Ophiopogonis Japonici (*Mai Men Dong*), 12g each, and Radix Angelicae Sinensis (*Dang Gui*), Fructus Meliae Toosendan (*Chuan Lian Zi*), Radix Bupleuri (*Chai Hu*), Fructus Citri Sacrodactylis (*Fo Shou*), and Fructus Citri Medicae (*Xiang Yuan*), 9g each

FORMULA ANALYSIS: *Sheng Di* and *Gou Qi Zi* enrich and supplement the liver and kidneys. *Sha Shen, Mai Men Dong,* and *Dang Gui* nourish yin and emolliate the liver. *Chuan Lian Zi* courses the liver, rectifies the qi, and stops pain. *Chai Hu, Xiang Yuan, Fo Shou,* and *Dan Shen* soothe the liver, regulate the qi, and quicken the blood.

ADDITIONS & SUBTRACTIONS: If there are heart palpitations and insomnia, add 15 grams each of Semen Zizyphi Spinosae (*Suan Zao Ren*), Cortex Albizziae Julibrissinis (*He Huan Pi*), and Caulis Polygoni Multiflori (*Ye Jiao Teng*) to nourish the blood and quiet the spirit. If there is dizziness or vertigo, add 12 grams each of Fructus Ligustri Lucidi (*Nu Zhen Zi*), Herba Ecliptae Prostratae (*Han Lian Cao*), and Fructus Mori Albi (*Sang Shen*) to enrich and supplement the liver and kidneys.

ACUPUNCTURE & MOXIBUSTION: *Tai Xi* (Ki 3), *Qu Quan* (Liv 8), *San Yin Jiao* (Sp 6), *Ge Shu* (Bl 17), *Gan Shu* (Bl 18), *Shen Shu* (Bl 23)

FORMULA ANALYSIS: Supplementing *Qu Quan, San Yin Jiao, Ge Shu,* and *Gan Shu* supplements the liver and nourishes the blood. Supplementing *Tai Xi, San Yin Jiao,* and *Shen Shu* supplements the kidneys and enriches yin.

ADDITIONS & SUBTRACTIONS: If there are heart palpitations and insomnia, add supplementing *Shen Men* (Ht 7) and draining *Bai Hui* (GV 20), *Feng Chi* (GB 20), and *Yin Tang* (M-HN-3). If there is dizziness or vertigo, add even supplementing-even draining *Bai Hui* (GV 20), *Feng Chi* (GB 20), and *Tai Yang* (M-HN-9).

REMARKS:

1. According to modern Western medicine, if there is cholecystitis, there is cholelithiasis. This view has been adopted by most contemporary Chinese medical practitioners and thus the treatment principle of expelling stones above.

2. Acupuncture can be very helpful in helping relieve the pain of acute cholecystitis/cholelithiasis.

D. CONCOMITANT DERMATOLOGICAL INFECTIONS

CHINESE MEDICAL DISEASE CATEGORIZATION: Boils, deep folliculitis, and perifolliculitis are mostly traditionally categorized as *ding* or clove sores in Chinese medicine. Multiple occurring boils are categorized as *jie*, boils. Abscesses and cellulitis are categorized as *yong*, welling abscesses.

CHINESE DISEASE MECHANISMS: Due to the righteous qi insufficiency attendant on qi and yin vacuity, evil toxins may take advantage of this vacuity and attack internally, thus giving rise to brewing of damp heat and fire toxins. These then block and obstruct the channels and network vessels, congealing and binding the qi and blood and hence giving rise to these types of skin lesions.

TREATMENT BASED ON PATTERN DISCRIMINATION:

1. HEAT TOXINS INTERNALLY BLAZING PATTERN

MAIN SYMPTOMS: The initial stage of clove sores and welling abscesses with redness and swelling and burning hot pain of the affected area accompanied by heart vexation, oral thirst, constipation, reddish urination, possible aversion to cold and emission of heat (*i.e.*, fever), a red tongue with yellow fur, and a slippery, rapid, forceful pulse

TREATMENT PRINCIPLES: Clear heat and resolve toxins

RX: *Wu Wei Xiao Du Yin Jia Jian* (Five Flavors Disperse Toxins Drink with Additions & Subtractions)

INGREDIENTS: Flos Lonicerae Japonicae (*Jin Yin Hua*), Herba Taraxaci Mongolici Cum Radice (*Pu Gong Ying*), Radix Trichoisanthis Kirlowii (*Tian Hua Fen*), and uncooked Radix Rehmanniae (*Sheng Di*), 30g each, Flos Chrysanthemi Indici (*Ye Ju Hua*), 20g, Fructus Forsythiae Suspensae (*Lian Qiao*), Herba Violae Yedoensitis Cum Radice (*Zi Hua Di Ding*), and Radix Rubrus Paeoniae Lactiflorae (*Chi Shao*), 15g each, and Cortex Radicis Moutan (*Dan Pi*) and Radix Angelicae Sinensis (*Dang Gui*), 9g each

FORMULA ANALYSIS: *Jin Yin Hua, Lian Qiao, Pu Gong Ying, Zi Hua Di Ding,* and *Ye Ju Hua* clear heat and resolve toxins. *Sheng Di, Dang Gui, Chi Shao,* and *Dan Pi* cool and quicken the blood, disperse swelling and stop pain. *Tian*

Hua Fen clears heat, engenders fluids, and protects yin.

ADDITIONS & SUBTRACTIONS: If there is constipation, add nine grams each of Fructus Trichosanthis Kirlowii (*Gua Lou*) and uncooked Radix Et Rhizoma Rhei (*Da Huang*) to free the flow of the bowels and drain heat. If there is severe pain and the formation of pus, add nine grams each of Radix Angelicae Dahuricae (*Bai Zhi*), Squama Manitis Pentadactylis (*Chuan Shan Jia*), and Spina Gleditschiae Chinensis (*Zao Jiao Ci*) to disperse swelling and expel pus.

EXTERNAL APPLICATION: During the initial stage of clove sores and welling abscesses, apply *Si Huang Gao* (Four Yellows Ointment) to the affected area.[2] If pus ripens, cut open the sore and expel and allow the pus to drain.

2. DAMP HEAT INTERNALLY BREWING PATTERN

MAIN SYMPTOMS: The initial stage of boils and ulcers which are red and swollen, painful, and itchy. Scratching with the fingernails leads to rupture and suppuration. Accompanying signs and symptoms include heart vexation, oral thirst, a red tongue with slimy, yellow fur, and a deep, rapid pulse.

NOTE: This pattern mostly presents in cases of multiple occurring folliculitis and is mostly associated with overeating fatty, sweet foods.

TREATMENT PRINCIPLES: Clear heat, resolve toxins, and disinhibit dampness

RX: *Qing Re Jie Du Li Shi Tang* (Clear Heat, Resolve Toxins & Disinhibit Dampness Decoction)

INGREDIENTS: Flos Lonicerae Japonicae (*Jin Yin Hua*), Herba Taraxaci Mongolici Cum Radice (*Pu Gong Ying*), and Semen Coicis Lachryma-jobi (*Yi Yi Ren*), 30g each, Fructus Forsythiae Suspensae (*Lian Qiao*), Radix Rubrus Paeoniae Lactiflorae (*Chi Shao*), Sclerotium Rubrum Poriae Cocos (*Chi Fu Ling*), Semen Plantaginis (*Che Qian Zi*), and *Liu Yi San* (Six [to] One Powder), 15g each, Radix Angelicae Sinensis (*Dang Gui*), 12g, and Radix Scutellariae Baicalensis (*Huang Qin*), 9g

FORMULA ANALYSIS: *Jin Yin Hua, Lian Qiao, Pu Gong Ying,* and *Huang Qin* clear heat and resolve toxins. *Chi Fu Ling, Yi Yi Ren, Che Qian Zi,* and *Liu Yi San* clear heat and disinhibit dampness. *Dang Gui* and *Chi Shao* quicken the blood and disperse swelling.

EXTERNAL APPLICATION: Make a decoction of Herba Portulacae Oleraceae (*Ma Chi Xian*), Herba Taraxaci Mongolici Cum Radice (*Pu Gong Ying*), and Cortex Phellodendri (*Huang Bai*), 60g each, and Alum (*Bai Fan*), 12g, and wash the affected area with the liquid decoction 2-3 times per day.

3. YIN VACUITY WITH EVILS ATTACHED PATTERN

MAIN SYMPTOMS: Flat sores which are dark and purplish and which are slow to develop pus and ulcerate with thin, watery, possibly bloody pus after ulceration, a dry mouth and oral thirst, an emaciated body, a red tongue with scanty fur, and a fine, rapid pulse

NOTE: From the treatment principles and plan given below, it is clear this is actually a qi and yin vacuity pattern with concomitant lingering heat toxins.

TREATMENT PRINCIPLES: Boost the qi and nourish yin, clear heat and resolve toxins

RX: *Jie Du Yang Yin Tang Jia Jian* (Resolve Toxins & Nourish Yin Decoction with Additions & Subtractions)

INGREDIENTS: Radix Scrophulariae Ningpoensis (*Xuan Shen*), Flos Lonicerae Japonicae (*Jin Yin Hua*), and Herba Taraxaci Mongolici Cum Radice (*Pu Gong Ying*), 30g each, Radix Glehniae Littoralis (*Sha Shen*) and Herba Dendrobii (*Shi Hu*), 15-30g each, uncooked Radix Astragali Membranacei (*Huang Qi*), uncooked Radix Rehmanniae (*Sheng Di*), Rhizoma Polygonati Odorati (*Yu Zhu*), Radix Salviae Miltiorrhizae (*Dan Shen*), and Radix Pseudostellariae Heterophyllae (*Tai Zi Shen*), 15g each, Tuber Ophiopogonis Japonici (*Mai Men Dong*), 12g, and Radix Panacis Quinquefolii (*Xi Yang Shen*), 3-10g decocted and drunk separately

FORMULA ANALYSIS: *Xi Yang Shen, Tai Zi Shen, Sha Shen, Shi Hu, Mai Men Dong, Xuan Shen,* and *Yu Zhu* boost the qi and nourish yin. *Huang Qi* boosts the qi and secures the exterior, while *Dan Shen* supplements the qi and quickens the blood. *Lian Qiao* and *Pu Gong Ying* clear heat and resolve toxins.

4. QI & BLOOD DUAL VACUITY PATTERN

MAIN SYMPTOMS: Scattered, widely diffuse lesions, slow pustulation, after ulceration, difficulty shedding pus and putridity, clear, thin, watery pus, possible open sores which endure and do not heal, slow granulation, lassitude of the spirit, lack of strength, poor appetite, slimy, white tongue fur, and a weak, forceless pulse

TREATMENT PRINCIPLES: Boost the qi and nourish the blood, out-thrust toxins, expel pus, and engender flesh

RX: *Nei Tuo Sheng Ji San Jia Jian* (Out-thrust the Internal & Engender Flesh Powder with Additions & Subtractions)

INGREDIENTS: Mix-fried Radix Astragali Membranacei (*Huang Qi*) and Radix Codonopsitis Pilosulae (*Dang Shen*), 30g each, Radix Trichosanthis Kirlowii (*Tian Hua Fen*), 15g, cooked Radix Rehmanniae (*Shu Di*), 12g, and Radix Albus Paeoniae Lactiflorae (*Bai Shao*), Radix Ligustici Wallichii (*Chuan Xiong*), Radix Angelicae Sinensis (*Dang Gui*), Rhizoma Atractylodis Macrocephalae (*Bai Zhu*), Pericarpium Citri Reticulatae (*Chen Pi*), and uncooked Radix Glycyrrhizae (*Gan Cao*), 9g each

FORMULA ANALYSIS: *Dang Shen* and *Huang Qi* boost the qi, while *Dang Gui, Bai Shao, Chuan Xiong,* and *Shu Di* nourish and quicken the blood. *Tian Hua Fen* protects yin, and *Bai Zhu* and *Chen Pi* fortify the spleen and harmonize the stomach. Uncooked *Gan Cao* harmonizes all the other medicinals in the formula as well as clears heat and resolves toxins.

ADDITIONS & SUBTRACTIONS: If heat toxins are still not finished, add 15 grams each of Herba Taraxaci Mongolici Cum Radice (*Pu Gong Ying*) and Flos Lonicerae Japonicae (*Jin Yin Hua*).

EXTERNAL APPLICATION: Apply *Sheng Ji Yu Hong Gao* (Engender Flesh Jade Red Ointment) externally 1-2 times per day.[3]

E. CONCOMITANT SEPTICEMIA

CHINESE MEDICAL DISEASE CATEGORIZATION: Septicemia occurring in tandem with diabetes is commonly traditionally categorized as *ding du zou huang,* clove toxins going yellow, and *yong du nei xian,* welling abscess toxins falling internally.

CHINESE DISEASE MECHANISMS: Due to righteous qi vacuity, external toxins invade internally. If heat toxins blaze and become exuberant, they may boil and burn the constructive and blood, eventually attacking the heart.

TREATMENT BASED ON PATTERN DISCRIMINATION:

1. HEAT TOXINS BLAZING & EXUBERANT WITH THE QI & CONSTRUCTIVE BOTH BURNT PATTERN

MAIN SYMPTOMS: High fever, vexatious thirst, heart vexation, insomnia, possible deranged speech, dry, bound stools, redness, swelling, heat, and pain in the affected area, dribbling and dripping of watery pus after ulceration, a dry, crimson tongue, and a fine, rapid pulse

NOTE: This pattern describes early stage septicemia due to a skin infection.

TREATMENT PRINCIPLES: Clear the constructive and resolve toxins, cool the blood and protect the heart

RX: *Jie Du Qing Ying Tang* (Resolve Toxins & Clear the Constructive Decoction)

INGREDIENTS: Flos Lonicerae Japonicae (*Jin Yin Hua*), Rhizoma Imperatae Cyclindricae (*Bai Mao Gen*), and Herba Taraxaci Mongolici Cum Radice (*Pu Gong Ying*), 30g each, Fructus Forsythiae Suspensae (*Lian Qiao*), uncooked Radix Rehmanniae (*Sheng Di*), Radix Rubrus Paeoniae Lactiflorae (*Chi Shao*), and Testa Seminis Munginis (*Lu Dou Yi*), 15g each, Radix Rubiae Cordifoliae (*Qian Cao Gen*) and Plumula Nelumbinis Nuciferae (*Lian Zi Xin*), 12g each, uncooked Carapax Amydae Sinensis (*Bie Jia*), 10-15g, Cortex Radicis Moutan (*Dan Pi*) and uncooked Fructus Gardeniae Jasminoidis (*Zhi Zi*), 9g each, and Rhizoma Coptidis Chinensis (*Huang Lian*), 6g

FORMULA ANALYSIS: *Jin Yin Hua, Lian Qiao,* and *Pu Gong Ying* clear heat and resolve toxins. *Zhi Zi* clears heat from the three burners. Combined with *Huang Lian,* it also clears heat from the heart. *Dan Pi, Chi Shao,* and *Qian Cao Gen* clear heat, cool and quicken the blood. *Sheng Di* and *Bai Mao Gen* nourish yin and cool the blood, while *Bie Jia* clears heat and resolves toxins, settles the heart and levels the liver. *Lian Zi Xin* and *Lu Dou Yi* clear heat evils from within the heart.

ADDITIONS & SUBTRACTIONS: If high fever is pronounced, add 15 grams of Cornu Bubali (*Shui Niu Jiao*). If there is constipation, add 3-9 grams of Radix Et Rhizoma Rhei (*Da Huang*).

ACUPUNCTURE & MOXIBUSTION: *He Gu* (LI 4), *Qu Chi* (LI 11), *Da Zhui* (GV 14)

FORMULA ANALYSIS: Draining *He Gu, Qu Chi,* and *Da Zhui* clears heat and recedes fever.

ADDITIONS & SUBTRACTIONS: For vexatious thirst, add supplementing *Zhao Hai* (Ki 6) and draining *Nei Ting* (St 44).

2. HEAT TOXINS BLAZING & EXUBERANT WITH CONSUMPTION & STIRRING OF THE BLOOD PATTERN

MAIN SYMPTOMS: Oral thirst, vexatious heat, generalized fever which is worse at night, dark, purplish skin macules, dimming of the spirit, deranged speech, redness and swelling of the affected area, dribbling and dripping of watery pus after ulceration, a crimson red tongue with scanty fur, and a fine, rapid pulse

TREATMENT PRINCIPLES: Clear heat and resolve toxins, cool and quicken the blood

RX: *Jie Du Liang Xue Tang Jia Jian* (Resolve Toxins & Cool the Blood Decoction with Additions & Subtractions)

INGREDIENTS: Uncooked Gypsum Fibrosum (*Shi Gao*), 60g, carbonized Flos Lonicerae Japonicae (*Jin Yin Hua*), Rhizoma Imperatae Cylindricae (*Bai Mao Gen*), and Radix Trichosanthis Kirlowii (*Tian Hua Fen*), 30g each, carbonized uncooked Radix Rehmanniae (*Sheng Di*), 20g, Cornu Bubali (*Shui Niu Jiao*), Radix Isatidis Seu Baphicacanthi (*Ban Lan Gen*), Herba Violae Yedoensitis Cum Radice (*Zi Hua Di Ding*), and Plumula Nelumbinis Nuciferae (*Lian Zi Xin*), 15g each, Fructus Gardeniae Jasminoidis (*Zhi Zi*), 9g, uncooked Radix Glycyrrhizae (*Gan Cao*), 6g, and Rhizoma Coptidis Chinensis ((*Huang Lian*), 3-6g

FORMULA ANALYSIS: *Shui Niu Jiao* clears heat and cools the blood, resolves toxins and settles fright. Carbonized *Sheng Di* and carbonized *Jin Yin Hua* enter the blood aspect and clear heat toxins within the blood aspect. They are also able to nourish yin and protect the heart. *Zi Hua Di Ding* and *Ban Lan Gen* clear heat and resolve toxins. *Tian Hua Fen, Bai Mao Gen,* and *Lian Zi Xin* nourish yin, cool the blood, and clear the heart. A heavy dose of *Shi Gao* strengthens and increases the function of clearing heat. *Zhi Zi* and *Huang Lian* clear heat toxins from the three burners and strongly clear heat from the heart, and uncooked

Gan Cao clears heat and resolves toxins at the same time that it harmonizes all the other medicinals in the formula.

3. QI & YIN DUAL DAMAGE WITH HEAT TOXINS NOT FINISHED PATTERN

MAIN SYMPTOMS: Lassitude of the spirit, lack of strength, dry mouth with a desire to drink, after rupturing of the lesion, difficult shedding of the pus and putridity, nonclosure of the open sore, low-grade fever at night, a red tongue with scanty fur, and a deep, fine, forceless pulse

---

NOTE: This pattern describes the latter stages of septicemia accompanying diabetes.

TREATMENT PRINCIPLES: Boost the qi and nourish yin, clear heat and resolve toxins

RX: *Jie Du Yang Yin Tang* (Resolve Toxins & Nourish Yin Decoction)

INGREDIENTS: Uncooked Radix Rehmanniae (*Sheng Di*), blackened Radix Scrophulariae Ningpoensis (*Xuan Shen*), and Radix Glehniae Littoralis (*Sha Shen*), 30g each, Flos Lonicerae Japonicae (*Jin Yin Hua*) and Herba Taraxaci Mongolici Cum Radice (*Pu Gong Ying*), 20g each, Herba Dendrobii (*Shi Hu*), Radix Pseudostellariae Heterophyllae (*Tai Zi Shen*), uncooked Radix Astragali Membranacei (*Huang Qi*), and Radix Salviae Miltiorrhizae (*Dan Shen*), 15g each, Tuber Ophiopogonis Japonici (*Mai Men Dong*), 12g, Rhizoma Polygonati Odorati (*Yu Zhu*), 9g, and Radix Panacis Quinquefolii (*Xi Yang Shen*), 6g, decocted and taken separately

FORMULA ANALYSIS: *Sheng Di, Xuan Shen, Sha Shen, Shi Hu, Yu Zhu,* and *Mai Men Dong* nourish yin and engender fluids. *Tai Zi Shen* and *Xi Yang Shen* boost the qi while simultaneously enriching yin and engendering fluids. *Dan Shen* quickens, cools, and nourishes the blood, while *Jin Yin Hua* and *Pu Gong Ying* clear heat and resolve toxins.

REMARKS:

1. This condition is very serious and requires Western medical treatment along with any Chinese medical treatment.

F. CONCOMITANT ORAL CAVITY INFECTIONS

CHINESE MEDICAL DISEASE CATEGORIZATION: Gingivitis and periodontal disease are traditionally categorized as *ya xuan*, gaping gums, in Chinese medicine, while oral thrush is traditionally categorized as *kou chuang*, mouth sores, *kou gan*, mouth *gan*, and *kou fu* and *kou mi*, mouth putrescence or putrefaction in Chinese medicine.

CHINESE DISEASE MECHANISMS: Diabetes is typically associated with dryness and heat. This dryness and heat is primarily in the stomach, although it may eventually spread to the lungs. If stomach heat blazes upward, it may follow the stomach channel to the mouth where it burns and damages the tissues of the mouth and tongue, thus creating sores and ulcers. If this heat is transmitted to the spleen and the heart, this heat may cause sores to arise on the tongue since the tongue is the sprout of the heart, and in the mouth since the spleen opens into the orifice of the mouth. If heat endures, it eventually damages yin. Thus replete heat transforms into vacuity heat. However, heat still floats upward to burn and putrefy the tissues of the tongue and mouth.

TREATMENT BASED ON PATTERN DISCRIMINATION:

1. STOMACH HEAT BLAZING & EXUBERANT PATTERN

MAIN SYMPTOMS: Swelling and pain of the gums, aversion of the teeth to heat and a liking for chilled things, possible gaping gums with discharge of blood, possible ulceration and purulence of the gums, possible swelling and pain of the lip, tongue, and cheeks, a dry mouth and parched tongue, hot mouth odor, dry, bound stools, a red tongue with yellow fur, and a deep, rapid pulse

TREATMENT PRINCIPLES: Clear the stomach and drain heat

RX: *Qing Wei San Jia Jian* (Clear the Stomach Powder with Additions & Subtractions)

INGREDIENTS: Uncooked Gypsum Fibrosum (*Shi Gao*), uncooked Radix Rehmanniae (*Sheng Di*), and Radix Trichosanthis Kirlowii (*Tian Hua Fen*), 30g each, Radix Angelicae Sinensis (*Dang Gui*) and Cortex Radicis Moutan (*Dan Pi*), 9g each, and Rhizoma Coptidis Chinensis (*Huang Lian*) and Rhizoma Cimicifugae (*Sheng Ma*), 6g each

FORMULA ANALYSIS: *Huang Lian* bitterly and coldly clears heat from the stomach. *Sheng Di* and *Dan Pi* cool the blood and clear heat. *Dang Gui* nourishes and quickens the blood, thus helping to disperse swelling and stop pain. *Sheng Ma* scatters fire and resolves toxins, and uncooked *Shi Gao* and *Tian Hua Fen* clear heat, engender fluids, and stop thirst.

ADDITIONS & SUBTRACTIONS: If there is constipation, add nine grams each of Fructus Trichosanthis Kirlowii (*Gua Lou*) and Fructus Immaturus Citri Aurantii (*Zhi Shi*) and 3-9 grams of Radix Et Rhizoma Rhei (*Da Huang*) to free the flow of the bowels and drain heat. If there are bleeding gums, one can add 15 grams of Rhizoma Imperatae Cylindricae (*Bai Mao Gen*) and nine grams each of Radix Achyranthis Bidentatae (*Niu Xi*) and Nodus Rhizomatis Nelumbinis Nuciferae (*Ou Jie*).

ACUPUNCTURE & MOXIBUSTION: *He Gu* (LI 4), *Qu Chi* (LI 11), *Nei Ting* (St 44), *Jia Che* (St 6), *Di Cang* (St 4), *Cheng Jiang* (CV 24)

FORMULA ANALYSIS: Draining *He Gu*, *Qu Chi*, and *Nei Ting* clears heat from the yang ming and the head. Draining *Jia Che*, *Di Cang*, and *Cheng Jiang* drains heat and frees the flow of the network vessels in the area of the mouth and tongue.

ADDITIONS & SUBTRACTIONS: If there is bleeding due to heat in the blood, add draining *Xue Hai* (Sp 10). If there is constipation, add supplementing *Zhao Hai* (Ki 6) and draining *Zhi Gou* (TB 6), *Zhong Wan* (CV 12), *Tian Shu* (St 25), and *Da Chang Shu* (Bl 25). If there is concomitant liver depression transforming heat, add draining *Yang Ling Quan* (GB 34).

2. HEART-SPLEEN ACCUMULATION OF HEAT PATTERN

MAIN SYMPTOMS: Redness, swelling, aching, and pain of the gums, ulceration of the surface of the mouth and tongue which is yellowish red or red in color and like rotten curds, oral thirst, a bitter taste in the mouth, bad breath, short, reddish urination, a red tongue with yellow fur, and a rapid pulse

TREATMENT PRINCIPLES: Clear heat and transform dampness, drain fire and resolve toxins

RX: *Xie Huang San Jia Jian* (Drain the Yellow Powder with Additions & Subtractions)

INGREDIENTS: Uncooked Gypsum Fibrosum (*Shi Gao*),

30g, uncooked Radix Rehmanniae (*Sheng Di*) and Herba Agastachis Seu Pogostemi (*Huo Xiang*), 12g each, Fructus Gardeniae Jasminoidis (*Zhi Zi*), Radix Ledebouriellae Divaricatae (*Fang Feng*), Rhizoma Coptidis Chinensis (*Huang Lian*), Cortex Radicis Moutan (*Dan Pi*), and Rhizoma Cimicifugae (*Sheng Ma*), 9g each, and Radix Glycyrrhizae (*Gan Cao*), 6g

FORMULA ANALYSIS: Uncooked *Shi Gao*, *Zhi Zi*, and *Huang Lian* clear and drain heat from the spleen and stomach. *Huang Lian* combined with *Sheng Di* clears heart fire and cools blood heat. Combined with *Fang Feng*, it scatters deep-lying fire in the spleen and stomach. *Huo Xiang* penetratingly and aromatically transforms dampness, rectifies the qi, and harmonizes the stomach. *Sheng Ma* scatters fire and resolves toxins. *Gan Cao* regulates and harmonizes all the other medicinals in this formula.

ADDITIONS & SUBTRACTIONS: If there is concomitant qi vacuity, add nine grams each of Radix Panacis Ginseng (*Ren Shen*) and Rhizoma Atractylodis Macrocephalae (*Bai Zhu*). If there is marked thirst, add nine grams each of Radix Trichosanthis Kirlowii (*Tian Hua Fen*) and Rhizoma Anemarrhenae Aspheloidis (*Zhi Mu*). If there is concomitant food stagnation, add nine grams each of scorched Massa Medica Fermentata (*Shen Qu*), scorched Fructus Crataegi (*Shan Zha*), and Endothelium Corneum Gigeriae Galli (*Ji Nei Jin*). If there is short, reddish urination, add nine grams each of Sclerotium Poriae Cocos (*Fu Ling*), Rhizoma Alismatis (*Ze Xie*), and Semen Plantaginis (*Che Qian Zi*).

ACUPUNCTURE & MOXIBUSTION: *Yin Ling Quan* (Sp 9), *Lao Gong* (Per 8), *He Gu* (LI 4), *Cheng Jiang* (CV 24), *Jia Che* (St 6), *Di Cang* (St 4)

FORMULA ANALYSIS: Draining *Yin Ling Quan* drains heat and dampness from the spleen. Draining *Lao Gong* clears heat and discharges fire from the heart at the same time as it treats sores in the mouth. Draining *He Gu* clears heat and drains repletions from the head. Draining *Cheng Jiang*, *Jia Che*, and *Di Cang* clears heat and frees the flow of the channels in the area of the mouth.

ADDITIONS & SUBTRACTIONS: For bad breath due to food stagnation, add draining *Nei Ting* (St 44) and *Liang Men* (St 21).

3. YIN VACUITY WITH FIRE EFFULGENCE PATTERN

MAIN SYMPTOMS: Superficial edema and distention of

the gums, insidious pain, loose teeth, if severe, falling teeth, mouth gan, red-colored erosions, a dry mouth and parched throat, dizziness, tinnitus, heat in the hearts of the hands and feet, low back and knee soreness and limpness, a red tongue with scanty fur, and a fine, rapid pulse

TREATMENT PRINCIPLES: Enrich yin and downbear fire

RX: *Liu Wei Di Huang Wan* (Six Flavors Rehmannia Pills) plus *Yu Nu Jian* (Jade Maiden Decoction) with additions and subtractions

INGREDIENTS: Uncooked Gypsum Fibrosum (*Shi Gao*), 30g, cooked Radix Rehmanniae (*Shu Di*) and Radix Scrophulariae Ningpoensis (*Xuan Shen*), 15g each, Radix Achyranthis Bidentatae (*Niu Xi*), Rhizoma Anemarrhenae Aspheloidis (*Zhi Mu*), and Tuber Ophiopogonis Japonici (*Mai Men Dong*), 12g each, and Radix Dioscoreae Oppositae (*Shan Yao*), Fructus Corni Officinalis (*Shan Zhu Yu*), Cortex Radicis Moutan (*Dan Pi*), and Rhizoma Alismatis (*Ze Xie*), 9g each

FORMULA ANALYSIS: *Shu Di, Shan Zhu Yu,* and *Shan Yao* supplement and enrich kidney yin. *Zhi Mu* and *Shi Gao* clear and drain stomach heat. *Xuan Shen* and *Mai Men Dong* enrich yin and clear heat, while *Niu Xi* and *Ze Xie* guide fire to move downward. *Dan Pi* quickens and cools the blood and clears vacuity heat.

ADDITIONS & SUBTRACTIONS: For severe loose teeth, add nine grams of Rhizoma Drynariae (*Gu Sui Bu*). For severe bleeding and spilling over of pus, add six grams of Rhizoma Coptidis Chinensis (*Huang Lian*) and 12 grams each of Herba Violae Yedoensitis Cum Radice (*Zi Hua Di Ding*) and Herba Taraxaci Mongolici Cum Radice (*Pu Gong Ying*). For bad breath, add nine grams each of Fructus Gardeniae Jasminoidis (*Zhi Zi*) and Herba Eupatorei Fortunii (*Pei Lan*). For dizziness, add nine grams each of Fructus Tribuli Terrestris (*Bai Ji Li*) and Rhizoma Gastrodiae Elatae (*Tian Ma*). For tinnitus, add nine grams of Rhizoma Acori Graminei (*Shi Chang Pu*). For low back pain, add 12 grams of Cortex Eucommiae Ulmoidis (*Du Zhong*). For clamoring stomach and abdominal distention after meals, add nine grams each of Rhizoma Acori Graminei (*Shi Chang Pu*), Radix Auklandiae Lappae (*Mu Xiang*), and Rhizoma Atractylodis Macrocephalae (*Bai Zhu*).

ACUPUNCTURE & MOXIBUSTION: *Tai Xi* (Ki 3), *San Yin Jiao* (Sp 6), *He Gu* (LI 4), *Cheng Jiang* (CV 24), *Jia Che* (St 6), *Di Cang* (St 4), *Shen Shu* (Bl 23)

FORMULA ANALYSIS: Supplementing *Tai Xi, San Yin*

Jiao, and *Shen Shu* supplements and enriches kidney yin. Draining *He Gu* clears heat from the head and treats diseases of the head. Draining *Cheng Jiang, Jia Che,* and *Di Cang* clears heat and frees the flow of the channels in the area of the mouth.

ADDITIONS & SUBTRACTIONS: If there is tinnitus, add even supplementing-even draining *Feng Chi* (GB 20), *Ting Gong* (SI 19), and *Yi Geng* (TB 17). For dizziness, add even supplementing-even draining *Feng Chi* (GB 20) and *Bai Hui* (GV 20). For marked dry mouth and parched throat, add supplementing *Zhao Hai* (Ki 6) and *Lie Que* (Lu 7).

REMARKS:

1. For mouth sores associated with the first two patterns above, spray *Xi Gua Shuang* (Watermelon Frost), a Chinese ready-made medicine, on the affected area several times per day.

G. VAGINAL CANDIDIASIS

CHINESE MEDICAL DISEASE CATEGORIZATION: Vaginal candidiasis is traditionally categorized as *yang feng,* itchy wind, and *yin yang,* genital itching, in Chinese medicine.

CHINESE DISEASE MECHANISMS: Vaginal candidiasis in women with diabetes is mainly due to two disease mechanisms. Either spleen vacuity leads to dampness which pours downward and obstructs the free flow of yang qi in the lower burner, thus transforming damp heat, or yin and blood insufficiency fails to nourish the skin. Instead, dryness gives rise to stirring of wind and thus itching.

TREATMENT BASED ON PATTERN DISCRIMINATION:

1. DAMP HEAT POURING DOWNWARD PATTERN

MAIN SYMPTOMS: Female genital itching, swelling, redness, and possible erosion of the affected area, a bitter taste in the mouth, heart vexation, yellow-red urination, yellow, foul-smelling vaginal discharge, slimy, yellow tongue fur, and a soggy, rapid pulse

TREATMENT PRINCIPLES: Clear heat, eliminate dampness, and stop itching

RX: *Long Dan Xie Gan Tang Jia Jian* (Gentiana Scabra

Drain the Liver Decoction with Additions & Subtractions)

INGREDIENTS: Rhizoma Atractylodis (*Cang Zhu*) and Semen Plantaginis (*Che Qian Zi*), 15g each, uncooked Radix Rehmanniae (*Sheng Di*), 12g, Radix Gentianae Scabrae (*Long Dan Cao*), Radix Scutellariae Baicalensis (*Huang Qin*), stir-fried Fructus Gardeniae Jasminoidis (*Zhi Zi*), Rhizoma Alismatis (*Ze Xie*), Radix Bupleuri (*Chai Hu*), Radix Angelicae Sinensis (*Dang Gui*), Cortex Phellodendri (*Huang Bai*), Radix Sophorae Flavescentis (*Ku Shen*), and Fructus Cnidii Monnieri (*She Chuang Zi*), 9g each, and Caulis Akebiae (*Mu Tong*), 6g

FORMULA ANALYSIS: *Long Dan Cao, Huang Qin,* and *Zhi Zi* drain replete fire from the liver-gallbladder and eliminate lower burner damp heat. *Ze Xie, Mu Tong, Che Qian Zi, Huang Bai,* and *Cang Zhu* clear and disinhibit lower burner dampness and heat. *Chai Hu* courses the liver and the liver channel traverses the genitalia. *Sheng Di* and *Dang Gui* nourish, cool, and quicken the blood. *Ku Shen* and *She Chuang Zi* dry dampness and stop itching.

NOTE: Because the bitter, cold medicinals in this formula easily damage the spleen and stomach, it is not appropriate for long-term administration.

ADDITIONS & SUBTRACTIONS: If damp toxins are exuberant with dampness and possible seepage of the affected area relatively profuse, use *Chu Shi Jie Du Tang Jia Jian* (Eliminate Dampness & Resolve Toxins Decoction with Additions & Subtractions): uncooked Semen Coicis Lachryma-jobi (*Yi Yi Ren*) and Rhizoma Smilacis Glabrae (*Tu Fu Ling*), 30g each, Flos Lonicerae Japonicae (*Jin Yin Hua*) and Radix Angelicae Sinensis (*Dang Gui*), 20g each, Cortex Radicis Dictamni Dasycarpi (*Bai Xian Pi*), Talcum (*Hua Shi*), and Fructus Forsythiae Suspensae (*Lian Qiao*), 15g each, Rhizoma Dioscoreae Hypoglaucae (*Bie Xie*) and dry Semen Germinatus Glycinis (*Da Dou Huang Juan*), 12g each, Fructus Gardeniae Jasminoidis (*Zhi Zi*), Cortex Phellodendri (*Huang Bai*), and Cortex Radicis Moutan (*Dan Pi*), 9g each, and Caulis Akebiae (*Mu Tong*) and uncooked Radix Glycyrrhizae (*Gan Cao*), 6g each. If damp heat is due to spleen vacuity, add nine grams each of Radix Codonopsitis Pilosulae (*Dang Shen*) and Rhizoma Atractylodis Macrocephalae (*Bai Zhu*).

EXTERNAL APPLICATION: Wash and douche the affected area with a decoction made from 30 grams of Alum (*Bai Fan*) and 15 grams each of Radix Sophorae Flavescentis (*Ku Shen*), Cortex Phellodendri (*Huang Bai*), and Semen Cnidii Monnieri (*She Chuang Zi*) for 15-20 minutes each time, 1-3 times per day.

ACUPUNCTURE & MOXIBUSTION: *Yin Ling Quan* (Sp 9), *San Yin Jiao* (Sp 6), *Qu Gu* (CV 2)

NOTE: Acupuncture is only an adjunctive treatment for this pattern of this condition.

FORMULA ANALYSIS: Draining *Yin Ling Quan* and *San Yin Jiao* clears dampness and heat from the lower burner and urogenital tract. Draining *Qu Gu* clears heat and frees the flow of the channels in the affected area.

ADDITIONS & SUBTRACTIONS: If damp toxins are relatively exuberant, add draining *Shang Qiu* (Sp 5). If there is concomitant spleen vacuity, add supplementing *Zu San Li* (St 36) and *Pi Shu* (Bl 20) and use even supplementing-even draining at *San Yin Jiao*.

2. YIN-BLOOD INSUFFICIENCY PATTERN

MAIN SYMPTOMS: Female genital itching accompanied by burning heat, pale red, dry skin in the affected area, heart vexation, insomnia, a dry mouth and parched throat, scanty menstruation, a dry red tongue with scanty fur, and a fine, rapid pulse

TREATMENT PRINCIPLES: Enrich yin and nourish the blood, moisten dryness and stop itching

RX: *Si Wu Xiao Feng San Jia Jian* (Four Materials Disperse Wind Powder with Additions & Subtractions)

INGREDIENTS: Uncooked Radix Rehmanniae (*Sheng Di*), 15g, Radix Angelicae Sinensis (*Dang Gui*) and Radix Polygoni Multiflori (*He Shou Wu*), 12g each, and Radix Albus Paeoniae Lactiflorae (*Bai Shao*), Radix Rubrus Paeoniae Lactiflorae (*Chi Shao*), Radix Ligustici Wallichii (*Chuan Xiong*), Spica Seu Flos Schizonepetae Tenuifoliae (*Jing Jie Sui*), Radix Ledebouriellae Divaricatae (*Fang Feng*), Fructus Tribuli Terrestris (*Bai Ji Li*), Cortex Radicis Dictamni Dasycarpi (*Bai Xian Pi*), Radix Lithospermi Seu Arnebiae (*Zi Cao*), Periostracum Cicadae (*Chan Yi*), and Fructus Kochiae Scopariae (*Di Fu Zi*), 9g each

FORMULA ANALYSIS: *Sheng Di, Dang Gui, Bai Shao, Chi Shao, Chuan Xiong, He Shou Wu,* and *Zi Cao* nourish the blood and moisten dryness, quicken the blood and disperse wind. *Jing Jie Sui, Fang Feng,* and *Chan Yi* mildly clear, course, and scatter wind and heat. *Bai Ji Li, Bai Xian Pi,* and *Di Fu Zi* dispel wind and stop itching.

ADDITIONS & SUBTRACTIONS: If there is concomitant spleen qi vacuity, add nine grams each of Radix Pseudostellariae Heterophyllae (*Tai Zi Shen*) and Radix Dioscoreae Oppositae (*Shan Yao*) and 3-6 grams of Radix Panacis Quinquefolii (*Xi Yang Shen*).

EXTERNAL APPLICATION: Wash and douche the affected area with a decoction made from 15 grams each of Fructus Schisandrae Chinensis (*Wu Wei Zi*), Radix Angelicae Dahuricae (*Bai Zhi*), Cortex Phellodendri (*Huang Bai*), Radix Sophorae Flavescentis (*Ku Shen*), and Fructus Cnidii Monnieri (*Shen Chuang Zi*) for 15-20 minutes each time, 1-3 times per day.

ACUPUNCTURE & MOXIBUSTION: *Tai Xi* (Ki 3), *San Yin Jiao* (Sp 6), *Xue Hai* (Sp 10), *Qu Gu* (CV 2) and/or *Hui Yin* (CV 1), *Ge Shu* (Bl 17), *Gan Shu* (Bl 18), *Shen Shu* (Bl 23)

FORMULA ANALYSIS: Supplementing *Tai Xi, San Yin Jiao,* and *Shen Shu* supplements the kidneys and enriches yin. Supplementing *San Yin Jiao, Ge Shu,* and *Gan Shu* supplements the liver and nourishes the blood. Draining *Xue Hai* cools and quickens the blood. Even supplementing-even draining *Qu Gu* and/or *Hui Yin* clears heat and frees the flow of the channels in the affected area.

ADDITIONS & SUBTRACTIONS: For concomitant spleen vacuity, add supplementing *Zu San Li* (St 36) and *Pi Shu* (Bl 20).

REMARKS:

1. Even though the patient may manifest a yin vacuity pattern of vaginitis, externally, one should still wash and douche the affected area in primarily bitter, cold, heat-clearing, dampness-eliminating medicinals, while internally taking sweet and cool, yin-enriching, fluid-engendering medicinals.

2. For a persistent thick, yellow vaginal discharge, place powdered Borax (*Peng Sha*) in an empty gelatin capsule and use as a vaginal suppository once per day.

ABSTRACTS OF REPRESENTATIVE CHINESE RESEARCH:

He Ya-hua, "The Treatment of 30 Cases of Diabetes &

Goose-mouth Sores with *Shen Ling Bai Zhu San* (Ginseng, Poria & Atractylodes Powder)," *Si Chuan Zhong Yi (Sichuan Chinese Medicine),* #9, 1999, p. 19-20: Of the 30 patients in this study, 18 were men and 12 were women aged 50-83 years old. The longest course of diabetes was 30 years and the shortest was one year. All the patients had been diagnosed with DM by WHO criteria, and all had been diagnosed with oral thrush. Treatment consisted of oral administration of the following Chinese medicinals: Radix Dioscoreae Oppositae (*Shan Yao*) and Semen Coicis Lachryma-jobi (*Yi Yi Ren*), 30g each, Sclerotium Poriae Cocos (*Fu Ling*), 20g, Radix Codonopsitis Pilosulae (*Dang Shen*) and Rhizoma Atractylodis Macrocephalae (*Bai Zhu*), 15g each, Semen Dolichoris Lablab (*Bai Bian Dou*), Fructus Amomi (*Sha Ren*), Semen Nelumbinis Nuciferae (*Lian Zi*), and Pericarpium Citri Reticulatae (*Chen Pi*), 10g each, Radix Platycodi Grandiflori (*Jie Geng*), 6g, and mix-fried Radix Glycyrrhizae (*Gan Cao*), 5g. If dampness and turbidity were severe, 15 grams of Rhizoma Atractylodis (*Cang Zhu*) were added. If damp depression had transformed heat, 15 grams of Rhizoma Coptidis Chinensis (*Huang Lian*) and 10 grams each of Radix Scutellariae Baicalensis (*Huang Qin*) and Radix Sophorae Flavescentis (*Ku Shen*) were added. One *ji* was decocted in water and administered per day, and one week equaled one course of treatment. Typically, it required 1-3 courses to achieve a cure.

Cure was defined as disappearance of symptoms with negative fungal oral cavity cultures three successive times. Some effect meant that the symptoms disappeared but as few as one oral cavity culture was negative for fungus. Based on these criteria, 26 cases were cured, three got some effect, and one got no effect, for a total amelioration rate of 96.6%.

Huang Xiao-zhi, "The Treatment of 38 Cases of Diabetic Urinary Tract Infection with *Yi Qi Yu Yin Tong Lin Tang* (Boost the Qi, Foster Yin & Free the Flow of Strangury Decoction)," *Xin Zhong Yi (New Chinese Medicine),* #12, 1998, p. 16-18: Between 1996 and 1998, the author used self-composed *Yi Qi YuYin Tong Lin Tang* to treat type 2 diabetes complicated by urinary tract infection. The patients' urine tests revealed the presence of erythrocytes and leukocytes, and the midstream urine culture resulted in bacterial growth. In the treatment group, there were five males and 33 females. Fifteen of these were between 36-49 years of age, 11 were between 50-59 years of age, nine were between 60-69 years of age, and three were between 70-73 years of age. The shortest duration of disease was two years; the longest duration was 15 years. As for the urinary tract infection, the shortest duration of disease was three months, while the longest was five years. The majority of patients at some time had used antibiotics for the infection, but without any positive results. In this group of patients, 24 also had hypertension, two had neuropathy, 12 had retinitis, and two patients had gangrene. In addition to the symptoms of the diabetes, each patient also had the following symptoms: exhaustion without strength in the limbs, thirst, dry mouth, low back and knee soreness and pain, frequent urination, dribbling and dripping after urination, difficulty stopping the flow of urine, severe fever, and painful urination. Their tongues were red with thin yellow fur, and their pulses were fine and rapid. Fasting blood glucose exceeded 8.2mmol/L (145mg/dL) in all patients, with the highest reading more than 19.6mmol/L (350mg/dL). Urine glucose was (++- ++++), urine leukocyte count was (++- ++++), and urine erythrocyte count was (+- +++).

Yi Qi Yu Yin Tong Lin Tang consisted of: Radix Astragali Membranacei (*Huang Qi*), 30g, uncooked Radix Rehmanniae (*Sheng Di*), Radix Achyranthis Bidentatae (*Niu Xi*), Sclerotium Poriae Cocos (*Fu Ling*), and Semen Plantaginis (*Che Qian Zi*), 15g each, Cortex Phellodendri (*Huang Bai*), Rhizoma Alismatis (*Ze Xie*), Fructus Corni Officinalis (*Shan Zhu Yu*), and Sclerotium Polypori Umbellati (*Zhu Ling*), 12g each, and Radix Glycyrrhizae (*Gan Cao*), 6g. If there was frequent, urgent, and/or painful urination, Fructus Gardeniae Jasminoidis (*Zhi Zi*), Herba Taraxaci Mongolici Cum Radice (*Pu Gong Ying*), and Caulis Akebiae (*Mu Tong*) were added. For dry, bound stools, Radix Et Rhizoma Rhei (*Da Huang*) was added. For hematuria, Rhizoma Imperatae Cylindricae (*Bai Mao Gen*) and Herba Cephalanoploris Segeti (*Xiao Ji*) were added. If there was fever, Flos Lonicerae Japonicae (*Jin Yin Hua*) and Fructus Forsythiae Suspensae (*Lian Qiao*) were added. If there was accompanying peripheral neuritis, Caulis Millettiae Seu Spatholobi (*Ji Xue Teng*) and Ramulus Loranthi Seu Visci (*Sang Ji Sheng*) were added. For accompanying retinitis, Fructus Lycii Chinensis (*Gou Qi Zi*), Flos Chrysanthemi Morifolii (*Ju Hua*), and Semen Prinsepiae (*Rui Ren Rou*) were added. For accompanying gangrene, appropriate external treatments were also used. One *ji* of these medicinals was decocted in water and administered per day, with seven days constituting one course of treatment. The urine was retested once each week. Usually, four courses of treatment were prescribed. During the treatment time period, Chinese and Western drugs were also used to control the diabetes.

Patients were considered cured A) if the symptoms of frequent, urgent, and painful urination disappeared, B) if, after three re-examinations, the urine and urine culture

were negative, and C) if the FBG reading had improved (falling into normal range or falling below 3mmol/L [54mg/dL]). Patients got marked effect if the frequent, urgent, and painful urination symptoms disappeared, and if the urine cultures were approximately normal. Some effect meant that the frequent, urgent, and painful urination improved and the urine culture also improved. No effect meant that the clinical symptoms and urine cultures were unchanged. Based on these criteria, 21 cases were considered cured, seven cases got a marked effect, five cases got some effect, and five cases got no effect. Thus the total amelioration rate was 86.84%. After undergoing this treatment, blood glucose levels in 12 patients were maintained in normal range. Lowering of blood glucose levels in the majority of patients was quite marked.

Shi Xi-zhi *et al.*, "The Chinese Medical Treatment of Chronic Diabetic Pruritus Vulvae," *Ji Lin Zhong Yi Yao* (*Jilin Chinese Medicine & Medicinals*), #2, 1999, p. 31-32: There were 38 women in this study, all of whom had been diagnosed with diabetes. The duration of these patient's disease was 15-20 years. All these women presented with itching of the genital area, profuse white vaginal discharge, burning in the vulvar area, and, because of scratching, the genital area had become red and swollen and the skin had ulcerated. The genitals appeared to have eczema lichenoides, and the skin was chapped.

In terms of treatment, an internal prescription was used together with an external wash. The ingredients of the orally administered prescription were: Radix Trichosanthis Kirlowii (*Tian Hua Fen*), 60g, Tuber Ophiopogonis Japonici (*Mai Men Dong*), uncooked Radix Rehmanniae (*Sheng Di*), and Rhizoma Anemarrhenae Asphelolidis (*Zhi Mu*), 30g each, Cortex Radicis Lycii Chinensis (*Di Gu Pi*), Rhizoma Alismatis (*Ze Xie*), and Radix Scrophulariae Ningpoensis (*Xuan Shen*), 20g each, and Cortex Phellodendri (*Huang Bai*) and Rhizoma Coptidis Chinensis (*Huang Lian*), 10g each. Every day, one *ji* of these medicinals was decocted in water and administered until the blood glucose levels were within normal range. The externally applied formula consisted of: Radix Sophorae Flavescentis (*Ku Shen*) and Cortex Phellodendri (*Huang Bai*), 30g each, Fructus Cnidii Monnieri (*She Chang Zi*), 20g, Radix Ledebouriellae Divaricatae (*Fang Feng*), Rhizoma Atractylodis (*Cang Zhu*), and Herba Seu Flos Schizonepetae Tenuifoliae (*Jing Jie*), 15g each, and Pericarpium Zanthoxyli Bungeani (*Chuan Jiao*), Alumen (*Ming Fan*), and Herba Menthae Haplocalycis (*Bo He*), 10g each. This formula was decocted in water and applied as an external wash twice daily, morning and evening, for 30 minutes each time. One week was one course of treatment. Raw, chilled, and acrid foods were prohibited, and treatment was suspended during menstruation.

If, after three days with the external wash, the genital area no longer itched or burned and the vaginal discharge had lessened, this was considered a markedly good result. Moderately good results meant that, after three days with the external wash, the genital area itching and burning had lessened and the symptoms were completely alleviated after 15-20 days. If there was no change in the symptoms after 20 days, then there were no results. Based on these criteria, 23 cases experienced markedly good results, 12 had gotten moderately good results, and three had gotten no results. Thus, the total amelioration rate was 92.1%.

REPRESENTATIVE CASE HISTORIES:

CASE 1[4]

The patient was a 60 year old female teacher who was first examined on Nov. 20, 1986. Her chief complaint was a recurrent erosive lesion on her buccal membrane for five years which had not healed for the past three months. In addition, the woman had a positive history of diabetes, neurodermatitis, and hypertension. The oral lesion was greyish white with fine reticular striae on both sides of the buccal mucosa and evident hyperemia and erythema. There were also multiple red papules with effusion, scabs, and pigmentation spots on the skin of the extremities. The patient's tongue was slightly red with slimy, yellow fur, and her pulse was fine, bowstring, and slippery.

Based on the above signs and symptoms, the woman was diagnosed with oral ulcer and a liver-kidney yin vacuity with fire effulgence pattern causing blood heat and wind. The treatment principles were to enrich yin and nourish the blood, dispel wind and clear heat, drain liver fire and clear heat from the blood. Based on these principles, the following Chinese medicinals were decocted in water and administered internally along with *Long Dan Xie Gan Wan* (Gentiana Drain the Liver Pills): Concha Haliotidis (*Shi Jue Ming*) and Fructus Kochiae Scopariae (*Di Fu Zi*), 30g each, uncooked Radix Rehmanniae (*Sheng Di*) and uncooked Semen Coicis Lachryma-jobi (*Yi Yi Ren*), 20g each, Cortex Radicis Moutan (*Dan Pi*), Radix Rubrus Paeoniae Lactiflorae (*Chi Shao*), Radix Scutellariae Baicalensis (*Huang Qin*), Herba Lophatheri Gracilis (*Dan Zhu Ye*), Cortex Radicis Dictamni Dasycarpi (*Bai Xian Pi*), Radix Scrophulariae Ningpoensis (*Xuan Shen*), and Fructus Cnidii Monnieri (*She Chuang Zi*), 12g each, and

Fructus Gardeniae Jasminoidis (*Zhi Zi*). Acetonidi unguentum acetatis fluocinoloni was applied locally to the lesions on the extremities.

On the second visit, the patient reported alleviation of most of the symptoms, and no new lesions had appeared on the skin. Therefore, her prescription was switched to: uncooked Radix Rehmanniae (*Sheng Di*), Fructus Forsythiae Suspensae (*Lian Qiao*), uncooked Semen Coicis Lachryma-jobi (*Yi Yi Ren*), Herba Violae Yedeonsitis Cum Radice (*Zi Hua Di Ding*), and Herba Portulacae Oleraceae (*Ma Chi Xian*), 15g each, Radix Rubrus Paeoniae Lactiflorae (*Chi Shao*) and Sclerotium Poriae Cocos (*Fu Ling*), 12g each, Cortex Radicis Moutan (*Dan Pi*), Fructus Citri Aurantii (*Zhi Ke*), and Semen Cnidii Monnieri (*Shen Chuang Zi*), 10g each, and Rhizoma Cyperi Rotundi (*Xiang Fu*), 3g. At the same time, *Fang Feng Tong Shen Wan* (Ledebouriella Flowing from the Spirits Pills) were administered internally as well as vitamin B$_6$ and vitamin B complex.

At the third consultation, the patient's condition had continued to improve. Most of the lesions had disappeared and no new lesions had occured. Therefore she was prescribed: Fructus Kochiae Scopariae (*Di Fu Zi*), 20g, Herba Artemisiae Capillaris (*Yin Chen Hao*) and Semen Coicis Lachryma-jobi (*Yi Yi Ren*), 15g each, Radix Scutellariae Baicalensis (*Huang Qin*), Sclerotium Poriae Cocos (*Fu Ling*), Herba Portulacae Oleraceae (*Ma Chi Xian*), and Herba Lemnae Seu Spirodelae (*Fu Ping Ye*), 12g each, and Herba Lophatheri Gracilis (*Dan Zhu Ye*), 10g, along with *Fang Feng Tong Shen Wan* and the vitamins. By the fourth consultation, most of the lesions on the extremities were healed and the oral mucosa was normal. Only vague striae remained. Therefore, the same prescription was continued. At the fifth consultation, the greyish white striae had disappeared and the woman was judged clinically cured. There was no recurrence of oral or other skin lesions on follow-up after six months.

CASE 2[5]

The patient was a 76 year old male who was first examined on Oct. 16, 1995. The man had entered the hospital due to diabetes accompanied by a pulmonary infection. After treatment in the hospital, the patient's original diseases improved. However, he developed oral thrush. The patient's tongue was slightly red with thick, yellow, geographic fur. If the man ate anything even slightly hot, his tongue was painful. Accompanying symptoms include torpid intake, fatigue, lack of strength, oral thirst, and a fine, weak pulse. The man's patterns were discriminated as spleen-stomach vacuity weakness with damp heat brewing and binding in the middle burner. Therefore, the treatment principles were to fortify the spleen and boost the qi, harmonize the stomach, seep dampness, and clear heat. The formula used was *Shen Ling Bai Zhu San Jia Wei* (Ginseng, Poria & Atractylodes Powder with Added Flavors): Radix Dioscoreae Oppositae (*Shan Yao*) and Semen Coicis Lachryma-jobi (*Yi Yi Ren*), 30g each, Sclerotium Poriae Cocos (*Fu Ling*), 20g, Radix Codonopsitis Pilosulae (*Dang Shen*), Rhizoma Coptidis Chinensis (*Huang Lian*), Rhizoma Atractylodis (*Cang Zhu*), and Rhizoma Atractylodis Macrocephalae (*Bai Zhu*), 15g each, Semen Dolichoris Lablab (*Bai Bian Dou*), Fructus Amomi (*Sha Ren*), Semen Nelumbinis Nuciferae (*Lian Zi*), Radix Scutellariae Baicalensis (*Huang Qin*), Radix Sophorae Flavescentis (*Ku Shen*), and Pericarpium Citri Reticulatae (*Chen Pi*), 10g each, Radix Platycodi Grandiflori (*Jie Geng*), 6g, and mix-fried Radix Glycyrrhizae (*Gan Cao*), 5g.

After taking seven *ji* of the above formula, the white membranes in the mouth receded, the tongue fur was thin and white, but the tongue was still painful if the patient ate anything slightly hot. This suggested that, although dampness and heat had gradually been dispelled, yin fluids had been damaged. Therefore, *Huang Lian* was deleted from the above formula and 10 grams of Herba Dendrobii (*Shi Hu*) was added. After another seven *ji* of this formula, all the symptoms were eliminated. The tongue was pale red with thin, white fur, and three successive oral cavity fungal cultures proved negative. The man was then prescribed *Shen Ling Bai Zhu Wan* (Ginseng, Poria & Atractylodes Pills) in order to secure and consolidate the treatment effects. On follow-up after five years, there had been no recurrence.

CASE 3[6]

The patient was a 50 year old male cadre who was first examined on Jan. 17, 1992 and whose main complaints were polydipsia, polyuria, lack of strength, and emaciation for two years and welling abscesses on his upper back for the past three months. This patient had been addicted to drinking alcohol for many years and had developed the above symptoms in the previous two years. In October of the previous year, a welling abscess had occurred on his upper back which had become purulent. This was surgically excised. At this time, the man's blood glucose was examined and it was found to be high. Therefore, he was diagnosed with diabetes accompanied by cellulitis. The man was treated with subdermal injections of insulin. However, the upper back welling abscess did not close and control of blood glucose was not satisfactory. Fasting blood glucose was 12.4mmol/L (224mg/dL) and urine glucose was (++++). Each day, the man used 54 units of subdermally injected insulin. Other presenting symptoms included dryness and heat, sweating, itchy skin, pricking pain which was difficult to bear in the four extremities and which disturbed his sleep, cold hands and feet, dry stools, a dark red tongue with slimy, white fur, and a slippery, rapid pulse.

Based on these signs and symptoms, the patient's patterns were discriminated as qi and yin dual vacuity with dryness and heat entering the blood aspect or division and static blood obstructing the network vessels. Therefore, the treatment principles were to boost the qi and nourish yin, clear heat and cool the blood, quicken the blood and free the flow of the network vessels. The Chinese medicinals Dr. Zhu initially prescribed to this man included: uncooked Radix Astragali Membranacei (*Huang Qi*), 50g, uncooked Radix Rehmanniae (*Sheng Di*), 30g, Radix Scrophulariae Ningpoensis (*Xuan Shen*), 30g, Rhizoma Atractylodis Macrocephalae (*Bai Zhu*), 15g, Radix Salviae Miltiorrhizae (*Dan Shen*), 30g, Radix Puerariae (*Ge Gen*), 15g, Radix Scutellariae Baicalensis (*Huang Qin*), 6g, Fructus Lycii Chinensis (*Gou Qi Zi*), 10g, Ramulus Loranthi Seu Visci (*Sang Ji Sheng*), 20g, Ramulus Cinnamomi Cassiae (*Gui Zhi*), 10g, Radix Clematidis Chinensis (*Wei Ling Xian*), 10g, Caulis Milletiae Seu Spatholobi (*Ji Xue Teng*), 30g, Herba Leonuri Heterophylli (*Yi Mu Cao*), 30g, and Lignum Sappan (*Su Mu*), 10g. One *ji* of these medicinals was decocted in water and administered per day.

After taking the above medicinals for one month, the man's symptoms had decreased. The sores on his upper back had healed, his fasting blood glucose was 9.99mmol/L (180mg/dL), and the patient was able to decrease the dose of his daily insulin. However, the man still had a sensation of piercing pain in the muscles of his four limbs and he had trouble falling asleep at night. His tongue was pale red with thin, white fur, and his pulse was deep and slippery. Therefore, *Gui Zhi* was deleted from the original formula and 15 grams each of Ramulus Uncariae Cum Uncis (*Gou Teng*) and Rhizoma Piperis Hancei (*Hai Feng Teng*) were added.

The patient then took these Chinese medicinals for one month, after which he completely stopped his insulin. He continued with the Chinese medicinals but there was still some piercing pain in his four limbs, numbness, and a chilly sensation. Therefore, 15 grams of Caulis Trachelospermi (*Luo Shi Teng*) and two strips of large Scolopendra Subspinipes (*Wu Gong*) were added to the preceding formula. After 28 *ji* of this prescription, the pain and other abnormal sensations in this man's extremities were cured.

CASE 4[7]

The patient was a 70 year old female who had had diabetes for 50 years and recurrent urinary tract infections for 40 years. In addition, she had had lower limb paralysis, aching, and pain for 20 years. In the last two years, oral thirst and desire to drink had increased. The patient was also tired and lacked strength, while urination was frequent, painful, and sometimes incontinent. Further, the lower limb paralysis and pain had gotten worse. There was also severe edema in her lower limbs. If the woman drank lots of water, she would vomit, while eating a meal led to distention and pain. At night, the lower limb pain and urinary frequency and pain were so bad that these made it difficult for her to go to sleep. Thus the woman was vexed, agitated, and restless. Previously, she had tried a number of different Chinese and Western medicines, none of which had been markedly effective. At the time of examination, the patient's tongue was tender and red with slimy, yellow fur, and her pulse was bowstring, slippery, and rapid.

Based on these signs and symptoms, Dr. Zhu discriminated this patient's patterns as qi and yin vacuity with phlegm dampness depression and stagnation transforming fire. Thus the treatment principles were to supplement the qi and nourish yin, eliminate dampness and drain fire, and Dr. Zhu prescribed *Qi Mai Di Huang Tang Jia Jian* (Astragalus Pulse Rehmannia Decoction with Additions & Subtractions): Radix Astragali Membranacei (*Huang Qi*) and uncooked Radix Rehmanniae (*Sheng Di*), 15g each, Radix Panacis Ginseng (*Ren Shen*), Tuber Ophiopogonis Japonici (*Mai Men Dong*), Fructus Schisandrae Chinensis (*Wu Wei Zi*), Rhizoma Atractylodis (*Cang Zhu*), Sclerotium Poriae Cocos (*Fu Ling*), Rhizoma Alismatis (*Ze Xie*), and Cortex Radicis Moutan (*Dan Pi*), 10g each, and Radix Angelicae Sinensis (*Dang Gui*), 6g. In addition, the patient was advised to frequently drink a tea made from three grams of Folium Perillae Frutescentis (*Zi Su Ye*) and 10 grams of Massa Medica Fermentata (*Shen Qu*).

After taking 20 *ji* of the above medicinals, the patients appetite and psyche had improved and her pain, paralysis, and urinary frequency and pain were all reduced. Therefore, the above formula was made into pills each weighing nine grams. From then on, the patient was instructed to take one pill TID, which she did for two years. By that time, her urinary urgency, frequency, and

pain as well as the edema had all disappeared, and her lower limb paralysis and pain were greatly reduced. The woman was able to stand and walk and conduct her own affairs. Urine glucose was (+).

CASE 5[8]

The patient was a 35 year old female who had oral thirst and rapid hungering, dizziness and head distention, heart vexation, easy anger, stomach duct glomus and fullness, and severe vaginal itching for three years. The woman was diagnosed with diabetes and vaginitis at Dr. Zhu's hospital, and she was given *Jiang Tang Ling* (Lower Sugar Effective [Remedy]), *Xiao Ke Wan* (Wasting & Thirsting Pills), *Gan Lu Xiao Ke Wan* (Sweet Dew Wasting & Thirsting Pills), and glyburide over a long period of time but without satisfactory effect. She was also prescribed decocted Chinese medicinals to engender fluids, stop thirst, and nourish yin, but these were also not effective. Recently, the woman's vision had become blurred. Her tongue fur was white and slightly slimy, while her pulse was soggy and moderate (*i.e.*, relaxed or slightly slow).

Based on the above signs and symptoms, the patient's patterns were discriminated as dryness above with cold below, damp depression not transforming, and loss of liver wood's spreading and extending. Therefore, Dr. Zhu prescribed *Chai Hu Gui Zhi Gan Jiang Tang Jia Jian* (Bupleurum, Cinnamon Twig & Dry Ginger Decoction with Additions & Subtractions) in order to nourish yin without aggravating dampness or causing further detriment to yang: Radix Scrophulariae Ningpoensis (*Xuan Shen*) and Radix Trichosanthis Kirlowii (*Tian Hua Fen*), 15g each, Radix Bupleuri (*Chai Hu*), Ramulus Cinnamomi Cassiae (*Gui Zhi*), Radix Scutellariae Baicalensis (*Huang Qin*), and Concha Ostreae (*Mu Li*), 10g each, and Radix Glycyrrhizae (*Gan Cao*) and dry Rhizoma Zingiberis (*Gan Jiang*), 6g each. After taking 15 *ji* of these medicinals, the oral thirst and vaginal pruritus had greatly diminished and the woman's psyche had improved. Urine glucose had gone from (++++) to (+). Thus she was given another 15 *ji*. Now her vaginal itching had completely disappeared and urine glucose was (±). At this point, the patient's symptoms were considered cured.

CASE 6[9]

The patient was a 62 year old female who had had frequent, urgent, and painful urination for nearly six months. She had taken antibiotics without results. During the last month, her condition had worsened. She was fatigued and without any strength, short of breath, and had no desire to speak. Her mouth was dry and she was very thirsty. In addition, there was frequent, urgent urination which sometimes was painful, nocturia occurring 3-4 times per night, sagging distention in the lower abdomen, low back and knee soreness and pain, and dizziness. Both lower limbs were mildly edematous. The patient's tongue was pale red with yellowish white fur, and her pulse was deep, fine, and slightly rapid. Urine examination revealed erythrocytes (++), leukocytes (+++), urine glucose (+++), and FBG was 12mmol/L (216mg/dL).

Based on the above signs and symptoms, the Chinese medical disease diagnosis was wasting and thirsting and strangury condition. The patient's pattern was categorized as qi and yin dual vacuity and damp heat in the bladder. The treatment principles were to boost the qi, foster yin, and free the flow of strangury. The formula used was *Yi Qi Yu Yin Tong Lin Tang Jia Wei* (Boost the Qi, Foster Yin & Free the Flow of Strangury Decoction with Added Flavors): Radix Astragali Membranacei (*Huang Qi*), 30g, Rhizoma Imperatae Cylindricae (*Bai Mao Gen*), 20g, uncooked Radix Rehmanniae (*Sheng Di*), Radix Achyranthis Bidentatae (*Niu Xi*), Sclerotium Poriae Cocos (*Fu Ling*), Semen Plantaginis (*Che Qian Zi*), and Semen Cuscutae Chinensis (*Tu Si Zi*), 15g each, Cortex Phellodendri (*Huang Bai*), Rhizoma Alismatis (*Ze Xie*), Fructus Corni Officinalis (*Shan Zhu Yu*), and Sclerotium Polypori Umbellati (*Zhu Ling*), 12g each, and Succinum (*Hu Po*), 3g, mixed with a large amount of water. One *ji* of these medicinals was decocted in water and administered per day for seven days.

After taking this formula, the oral dryness and the dizziness improved and the frequent, urgent urination lessened, as did the nocturia. There was no painful urination, the edema was relieved, and the remaining symptoms improved. Urine examination revealed that erythrocytes were (-), leukocytes were (++), urine glucose was (++), and FBG was 9mmol/L (162mg/dL). Each month, urine testing was done at least once. By the third month, the urine tests remained normal, and the frequent, urgent and painful urination had ceased. In the fourth month, the urine tests were still normal, urine sugar was (- -+), all remaining tests were normal, and FBG was 8.6 mmol/L (155mg/dL). After many successive re-examinations, the urine tests revealed no erythrocytes or leukocytes.

CASE 7[10]

The patient was a 65 year old female who presented with frequent, urgent, and painful urination which she had suf-

fered for one month. Prior treatment with antibiotics had produced no result. Erythrocyte and leukocyte counts were elevated. In addition to painful urination, the patient complained of poor appetite, heaviness in her head, chest oppression, heart palpitations, vomiting, and a cold sensation in her abdomen. She had been diagnosed as suffering from diabetes for 12 years with complications of chronic pelvic inflammation, cystitis, coronary heart disease, and cholecystitis. She also suffered from constipation and oliguria with turbid urine. Her tongue was pink with white, greasy fur, and her pulse was fine, rapid, and forceless. The Chinese medical disease diagnosis was wasting and thirsting and strangury. The patient's pattern was categorized as phlegm dampness and heat in the bladder. The formula prescribed was *Wen Dan Tang Jia Jian* (Warm the Gallbladder Decoction with Additions & Subtractions) which included: Radix Pseudostellariae Heterophyllae (*Tai Zi Shen*), 20g, Sclerotium Poriae Cocos (*Fu Ling*), 15g, Caulis Bambusae In Taeniis (*Zhu Ru*), Herba Plantaginis (*Che Qian Zi*), Radix Linderae Strychnifoliae (*Wu Yao*), Radix Achyranthis Bidentatae (*Niu Xi*), and Semen Pruni Persicae (*Tao Ren*), 10g each, Cortex Phellodendri (*Huang Bai*), 8g, and Fructus Citri Aurantii (*Zhi Ke*), Rhizoma Pinelliae Ternatae (*Ban Xia*), and Pericarpium Citri Reticulatae (*Chen Pi*), 6g each. These medicinals were decocted in water, and, after seven *ji*, the symptoms were alleviated and the patient's tongue fur had improved. The patient recovered after 15 additional *ji*.

ENDNOTES:

[1] Kang Lu-wa, "The Treatment of Diabetes by Pattern Discrimination of the Tongue," *Zhong Yi Za Zhi* (*Journal of Chinese Medicine*), #9, 1999, p. 530-531.
[2] Blue Poppy Herbs' Clear Heat Ointment is a version of *Si Huang Gao*.
[3] Blue Poppy Herbs' Cut & Sore Ointment is a version of *Sheng Ji Yu Hong Gao*.
[4] Chen Ke-ji, *Traditional Chinese Medicine: Clinical Case Studies*, Foreign Languages Press, Beijing, 1994, p. 267-268
[5] He Ya-hua, "The Treatment of 30 Cases of Diabetes & Goose-mouth Sores with *Shen Ling Bai Zhu San* (Ginseng, Poria & Atractylodes Powder)," *Si Chuan Zhong Yi* (*Sichuan Chinese Medicine*), #9, 1999, p. 19-20
[6] Zhu Chen-zi, anthologized in Dan Shu-jian & Chen Zi-hua's *Xiao Ke Juan* (*The Wasting & Thirsting Book*), Chinese National Chinese Medicine & Medicinals Publishing Co., Beijing, 1999, p. 123-125
[7] Zhu Jin-zhong, anthologized in Shi Yu-guang & Dan Shu-jian's, *Xiao Ke Zhuan Zhi* (*Wasting & Thirsting Expertise*), Chinese Medicine Ancient Books Publishing Co., 1997, p. 63-64
[8] *Ibid.*, p. 61
[9] Huang Xiao-zhi, "The Treatment of 38 Cases of Diabetic Urinary Tract Infection with *Yi Qi Yu Yin Tong Lin Tang* (Boost the Qi, Foster Yin & Free the Flow of Strangury Decoction)," *Xin Zhong Yi* (*New Chinese Medicine*), #12, 1998, p. 16-18
[10] Gao Lu-wen, "Regulating Qi and Resolving Phlegm to Treat the Complications of Diabetes", *Journal of Chinese Medicine*, #64, October 2000, p. 19-21

25

DIABETES & OTHER
ENDOCRINE DISORDERS

The endocrine glands form a complex feedback loop system. Therefore, dysfunction of one endocrine gland may lead to dysfunction of one or more other endocrine glands. In addition, if diabetes mellitus is thought to be, at least in part, an autoimmune disease, the same autoimmune response which attacks and damages the islets of Langerhans in the pancreas may, theoretically, attack and damage the cells in other endocrine glands. Concurrent subnormal function of several endocrine glands are, therefore, referred to as polyglandular deficiency syndromes. These are also known as autoimmune polyglandular syndromes and polyendocrine deficiency syndromes. As the authors of *The Merck Manual* state, "Autoimmune disease affecting one gland is frequently followed by impairment of other glands, resulting in multiple endocrine failure."[1] There are three types of polyglandular deficiency syndromes. Type 1 occurs during childhood and is characterized by failure of the adrenals and parathyroid and is seldom associated with diabetes. Type 2 occurs during adulthood and is characterized by failure of the adrenals, thyroid, and islets of Langerhans, thus producing type 1 diabetes. Type 3 also occurs in adulthood and includes at least two of the following: thyroid deficiency, type 1 diabetes, pernicious anemia, vitiligo, and alopecia.[2] In terms of other endocrine disorders commonly occurring with diabetes, acromegaly, Cushing's syndrome, hyperprolactinemia, pheochromocytoma, hyperthyroidism, primary hyperaldosteronism, and glucagonoma of the pancreas may all be associated with increased or decreased secretion of insulin and may either lead to, aggravate, or be aggravated by diabetes.

A. DIABETES & CONCOMITANT HYPERTHYROIDISM

Diabetes and hyperthyroidism are both endocrine dis-

eases, and the onset of both is closely associated to immune factors. A small secretion of thyroid hormone can increase glycogen synthesis, while a large secretion of thyroid hormone can promote glycogen breakdown. In addition, thyroid hormone can promote stomach and intestinal tract glucose uptake. Therefore, although hyperthyroidism does not typically lead to diabetes, it can worsen hyperglycemia. The clinical symptoms of hyperthyroidism include goiter, tachycardia, warm, fine, moist skin, tremor, atrial fibrillation (*i.e.*, heart palpitations), nervousness and increased activity, increased sweating, hypersensitivity to heat, fatigue, increased appetite, weight loss, insomnia, weakness, and frequent bowel movements. Eye signs include staring, lid lag, lid retraction, and a mild degree of conjunctival injection (*i.e.*, bloodshot eyes). In the case of Graves' disease and associated ophthalmopathy, there may be orbital pain, lacrimation, irritation, photophobia, and ocular muscle weakness leading to double vision. Also in Graves' disease, there may be pretibial dermopathy which is often pruritic and erythematous in its early stages and later become brawny. This dermopathy and ophthalmopathy may occur years before or after the onset of hyperthyroidism.

CHINESE DISEASE MECHANISMS: The disease mechanisms of hyperthyroidism are depression and binding of the seven affects giving rise to the liver's loss of coursing and discharge. If qi depression transforms fire, this fire may damage yin fluids and the qi, thus resulting in qi and yin dual vacuity. Similarly, the basic disease mechanism of diabetes is qi and yin depletion and consumption due to exuberance of dryness and heat. When diabetes and hyperthyroidism occur together, their two yangs mutually unite causing dryness and heat to be even more severe. Hence qi and yin are all the more damaged. If the symptoms of diabetes were not obvious before the hyperthyroidism, they will become pronounced after the onset of hyperthyroidism.

TREATMENT BASED ON PATTERN DISCRIMINATION:

1. LIVER DEPRESSION & SPLEEN VACUITY PATTERN

MAIN SYMPTOMS: Shortness of breath, lack of strength, discomfort in the center of the throat, chest and rib-side distention and pain, increased bowel movements, a dry mouth and parched throat, a heavy body, a fat, dark tongue with thin fur, and a bowstring, fine pulse

TREATMENT PRINCIPLES: Course the liver and rectify the qi, fortify the spleen and engender fluids

RX: *Chai Hu Shu Gan San* (Bupleurum Course the Liver Powder) plus *Shen Ling Bai Zhu San* (Ginseng, Poria & Atractylodes Powder) with additions and subtractions

INGREDIENTS: Radix Trichosanthis Kirlowii (*Tian Hua Fen*), 20g, Radix Puerariae (*Ge Gen*), Semen Dolichoris Lablab (*Bai Bian Dou*), Radix Albus Paeoniae Lactiflorae (*Bai Shao*), and Sclerotium Poriae Cocos (*Fu Ling*), 15g each, and Radix Bupleuri (*Chai Hu*), Fructus Citri Aurantii (*Zhi Ke*), Rhizoma Cyperi Rotundi (*Xiang Fu*), Radix Codonopsitis Pilosulae (*Dang Shen*), Rhizoma Atractylodis Macrocephalae (*Bai Zhu*), and Pericarpium Citri Reticulatae (*Chen Pi*), 9g each

FORMULA ANALYSIS: *Chai Hu, Zhi Ke, Xiang Fu,* and *Chen Pi* course the liver and rectify the qi. With *Bai Shao,* these medicinals may also be said to harmonize the liver. *Dang Shen, Bai Zhu, Fu Ling,* and *Bai Bian Dou* fortify the spleen and supplement the qi. *Ge Gen* and *Tian Hua Fen* engender fluids and stop thirst.

ADDITIONS & SUBTRACTIONS: If depression has transformed heat, add nine grams each of Fructus Gardeniae Jasminoidis (*Zhi Zi*) and/or Radix Scutellariae Baicalensis (*Huang Qin*) and/or three grams of Rhizoma Coptidis Chinensis (*Huang Lian*) depending on where the heat is located besides the liver-gallbladder.

ACUPUNCTURE & MOXIBUSTION: *Tai Chong* (Liv 3), *Zu San Li* (St 36), *Pi Shu* (Bl 20), *Nei Ting* (St 44), *Zhao Hai* (Ki 6)

FORMULA ANALYSIS: Draining *Tai Chong* courses and drains the liver. Even supplementing-even draining *Zu*

San Li and supplementing *Pi Shu* fortifies the spleen and supplements the qi. Draining *Nei Ting* and supplementing *Zhao Hai* engenders fluids.

ADDITIONS & SUBTRACTIONS: If there is oral thirst, add draining *Jia Che* (St 6), *Di Cang* (St 4), and *Cheng Jiang* (CV 24). If there are loose stools, add supplementing *Wei Shu* (Bl 21), *Tian Shu* (St 25), and *Da Chang Shu* (Bl 25). To increase the rectification of the qi, add draining *He Gu* (LI 4). If depression has transformed heat, needle *Tai Chong* through to *Xiang Jian* (Liv 2). If heat is severe, add draining *Qu Chi* (LI 11).

2. YIN VACUITY-FIRE EFFULGENCE PATTERN

MAIN SYMPTOMS: Vexation and agitation, easy anger, heart palpitations, insomnia, oral thirst leading to drinking, emaciation, night sweats, increased food intake, trembling hands, quivering tongue, bulging eyes, a staring gaze, enlargement of the neck, a red tongue with scanty fur, and a fine, rapid pulse

NOTE: In this case, yin vacuity and fire effulgence have given rise to the internal engenderment of wind, thus the trembling hands and quivering mouth.

TREATMENT PRINCIPLES: Enrich yin and downbear fire

RX: *Zhi Bai Di Huang Wan Jia Jian* (Anemarrhena & Phellodendron Rehmannia Pills with Additions & Subtractions)

INGREDIENTS: Uncooked Radix Rehmanniae (*Sheng Di*), 20g, Sclerotium Poriae Cocos (*Fu Ling*), Radix Scrophulariae Ningpoensis (*Xuan Shen*), Radix Albus Paeoniae Lactiflorae (*Bai Shao*), and Radix Trichosanthis Kirlowii (*Tian Hua Fen*), 15g each, Tuber Ophiopogonis Japonici (*Mai Men Dong*), 12g, and Rhizoma Anemarrhenae Aspheloidis (*Zhi Mu*), Cortex Phellodendri (*Huang Bai*), Cortex Radicis Moutan (*Dan Pi*), Rhizoma Alismatis (*Ze Xie*), Fructus Corni Officinalis (*Shan Zhu Yu*), and Ramulus Uncariae Cum Uncis (*Gou Teng*), 9g each

FORMULA ANALYSIS: *Shan Zhu Yu, Mai Men Dong, Xuan Shen, Sheng Di,* and *Tian Hua Fen* supplement and enrich liver and kidney yin. *Zhi Mu, Huang Bai, Dan Pi,* and *Ze Xie* clear heat and drain fire. *Bai Shao* and *Gou Teng* emolliate the liver and extinguish wind respectively.

ADDITIONS & SUBTRACTIONS: For night sweats, add

30 grams of Fructus Levis Tritici Aestivi (*Fu Xiao Mai*) and nine grams of Fructus Schisandrae Chinensis (*Wu Wei Zi*). For insomnia, add 12 grams each of Semen Zizyphi Spinosae (*Suan Zao Ren*) and Semen Biotae Orientalis (*Ze Xie*). If liver depression is marked, add 12 grams of Fructus Meliae Toosandan (*Chuan Lian Zi*). If there is constipation, add nine grams of Fructus Trichosanthis Kirlowii (*Quan Gua Lou*). If there is severe thirst, add 30 grams of uncooked Gypsum Fibrosum (*Shi Gao*).

ACUPUNCTURE & MOXIBUSTION: *Tai Xi* (Ki 3), *San Yin Jiao* (Sp 6), *Shen Shu* (Bl 23), *Nei Ting* (St 44), *Qu Chi* (LI 11)

FORMULA ANALYSIS: Supplementing *Tai Xi, San Yin Jiao,* and *Shen Shu* supplements the kidneys and enriches yin. Draining *Nei Ting* and *Qu Chi* clears heat and downbears fire.

ADDITIONS & SUBTRACTIONS: For quivering tongue, add draining *Lian Quan* (CV 23) and *Feng Chi* (GB 20). For insomnia, add draining *Feng Chi* (GB 20) and *An Mian* (N-BW-21). For trembling hands, add draining *Yang Gu* (SI 5), *Yang Chi* (TB 4), and *Yang Xi* (LI 5).

3. QI & YIN DUAL VACUITY PATTERN

MAIN SYMPTOMS: Emaciation, lack of strength, spontaneous perspiration, night sweats, polydipsia, polyuria, heart palpitations, shortness of breath, increased intake of food, diarrhea or loose stools, trembling hands, enlargement of the neck, a red tongue with thin fur, and a fine, rapid pulse

TREATMENT PRINCIPLES: Fortify the spleen and boost the qi, supplement the kidneys and nourish yin

RX: *Bu Zhong Yi Qi Tang* (Supplement the Center & Boost the Qi Decoction) plus *Liu Wei Di Huang Wan* (Six Flavors Rehmannia Pills) with additions and subtractions

INGREDIENTS: Cooked Radix Rehmanniae (*Shu Di*), 30g, Radix Astragali Membranacei (*Huang Qi*), Rhizoma Polygonati (*Huang Jing*), Sclerotium Poriae Cocos (*Fu Ling*), and Radix Dioscoreae Oppositae (*Shan Yao*), 15g each, and Radix Codonopsitis Pilosulae (*Dang Shen*), Rhizoma Atractylodis Macrocephalae (*Bai Zhu*), Radix Angelicae Sinensis (*Dang Gui*), Pericarpium Citri Reticulatae (*Chen Pi*), Radix Bupleuri (*Chai Hu*), Fructus Corni Officinalis (*Shan Zhu Yu*), Cortex Radicis Moutan (*Dan Pi*), and Rhizoma Alismatis (*Ze Xie*), 9g each

FORMULA ANALYSIS: *Huang Qi, Dang Shen, Bai Zhu,* and *Huang Jing* fortify the spleen and boost the qi. *Shu Di, Fu Ling, Shan Yao, Dan Pi, Ze Xie,* and *Shan Zhu Yu,* taken as a whole, supplement and enrich the liver and kidneys. *Chai Hu* and *Chen Pi* rectify the qi and protect the large amounts of qi-boosting, yin-enriching medicinals from obstructing the qi mechanism.

ADDITIONS & SUBTRACTIONS: For diarrhea, add 9-15 grams of Radix Puerariae (*Ge Gen*) and nine grams of Fructus Pruni Mume (*Wu Mei*). For night sweats, add 30 grams of Fructus Levis Tritici Aestivi (*Fu Xiao Mai*) and nine grams of Fructus Schisandrae Chinensis (*Wu Wei Zi*).

ACUPUNCTURE & MOXIBUSTION: *Zu San Li* (St 36), *San Yin Jiao* (Sp 6), *Tai Xi* (Ki 3), *Pi Shu* (Bl 20), *Wei Shu* (Bl 21), *Shen Shu* (Bl 23)

FORMULA ANALYSIS: Supplementing *Zu San Li, San Yin Jiao, Pi Shu,* and *Wei Shu* fortifies the spleen and boosts the qi, while supplementing *Tai Xi, San Yin Jiao,* and *Shen Shu* supplements the kidneys and nourishes yin.

ADDITIONS & SUBTRACTIONS: For night sweats, add draining *Yin Xi* (Ht 6). For spontaneous perspiration, add supplementing *Fu Liu* and draining *He Gu* (LI 4). For shortness of breath, add supplementing *Tai Yuan* (Lu 9).

REMARKS:

1. Hyperthyroidism is treated both medically and surgically in Western medicine. If long-term administration of antithyroid hormone medicines has resulted in leukopenia, add a selection of the following Chinese medicinals based on the patient's pattern discrimination: Cortex Radicis Lycii Chinensis (*Di Gu Pi*), Radix Astragali Membranacei (*Huang Qi*), Radix Et Rhizoma Polygoni Cuspidati (*Hu Zhang*), Radix Polygoni Multiflori (*He Shou Wu*), Squama Manitis Pentadactylis (*Chuan Shan Jia*), Fructus Zizyphi Jujubae (*Da Zao*), Herba Epimedii (*Xian Ling Pi*), Fructus Psoraleae Corylifoliae (*Bu Gu Zhi*), and Gelatinum Cornu Cervi (*Lu Jiao Jiao*). According to Simon Becker, leukopenia may present any of the following patterns: 1) qi and blood insufficiency with nonfortification of the spleen, 2) spleen-stomach vacuity weakness, 3) spleen-kidney dual vacuity, 4) liver-kidney yin vacuity, 5) qi and blood insufficiency with essence depletion and blood stasis, 6) defensive qi vacuity with toxic heat flaming and exuberance, and 7) spleen vacuity with lingering disease evils.[3]

2. Antithyroid drugs may also cause allergic reactions,

nausea, and loss of taste. Typically, Chinese medical treatment, administered on the basis of the patient's pattern discrimination, can decrease or eliminate these adverse reactions when used in tandem with Western medicines. Chinese medicine may also be an alternative to surgery in patients whose disease has recurred after a course of antithyroid drugs, who refuse radioiodine therapy, or who cannot tolerate other drugs because of hypersensitivity.

3. While the main disease mechanism of hyperthyroidism is yin vacuity of the liver and kidneys, a pattern of heart-kidney yin vacuity may sometimes be seen. In addition, if yin disease reaches yang, there may manifest a complex combination of yin vacuity with heart-kidney yang vacuity, a spleen-kidney dual vacuity, or a heart-spleen-kidney yang vacuity. In such cases, appropriate medicinals may be added to the above guiding formulas as indicated by the patient's signs and symptoms.

B. DIABETES & CUSHING'S SYNDROME

Cushing's syndrome refers to a constellation of clinical abnormalities due to chronic exposure to excesses of cortisol, a major adrenocorticoid, or other related corticosteroids. Such excesses of corticosteroids may be due to hypersecretion of ACTH by the pituitary gland or secretion of ACTH by a nonpituitary tumor. The clinical symptoms of this condition include a rounded, "moon" face with a plethoric appearance, truncal obesity with prominent supraclavicular and dorsal cervical fat pads, called "buffalo hump" or "dowager's hump," slender distal extremities and fingers, muscle wasting and weakness, thin, atrophic skin with easy bruising and poor wound healing, possible purple striae on the abdomen, and menstrual irregularities in females. In addition, glucose intolerance is common in patients with Cushing's syndrome, and, due to long-term or heavy administration of glucocorticoids which can raise the blood glucose, this condition may result in the onset or worsening of diabetes.

CHINESE DISEASE MECHANISMS: According to Chinese medicine, the main disease mechanism of this condition is loss of the liver's coursing and discharge. Therefore, the qi mechanism becomes inhibited and the movement of blood becomes uneasy, resulting in the blood vessels becoming static and obstructed. At the same time, the liver invading the spleen results in the spleen's loss of fortification and movement. Thus dampness and turbidity are engendered internally. If dampness, turbidity, and blood stasis endure for some time, they may eventually transform heat. If this heat causes detriment and damage to yin fluids, it may cause or worsen wasting and thirsting disease.

TREATMENT BASED ON PATTERN DISCRIMINATION:

1. SPLEEN LOSS OF FORTIFICATION & MOVEMENT WITH DAMP HEAT INTERNALLY COLLECTING PATTERN

MAIN SYMPTOMS: A red, moist-looking facial complexion, generalized acne, a tendency to high blood pressure, headache as if the head was tightly wrapped or bound, abdominal distention and fullness, constipation, a dry mouth with a predilection for drinking, nausea, torpid intake, a red tongue with slimy, yellow fur, and a bowstring, slippery, rapid pulse

TREATMENT PRINCIPLES: Clear heat, disinhibit dampness, and fortify the spleen

RX: *Si Miao San Jia Wei* (Four Wonders Powder with Added Flavors)

INGREDIENTS: Semen Coicis Lachryma-jobi (*Yi Yi Ren*) and Herba Artemisiae Capillaris (*Yin Chen Hao*), 30g each, Radix Rubrus Paeoniae Lactiflorae (*Chi Shao*), 15g, Radix Achyranthis Bidentatae (*Niu Xi*) and Sclerotium Poriae Cocos (*Fu Ling*), 12g each, Cortex Phellodendri (*Huang Bai*), Fructus Gardeniae Jasminoidis (*Zhi Zi*), Semen Plantaginis (*Che Qian Zi*), Rhizoma Atractylodis (*Cang Zhu*), and Cortex Radicis Moutan (*Dan Pi*), 9g each, and uncooked Radix Et Rhizoma Rhei (*Da Huang*), 6g

FORMULA ANALYSIS: *Huang Bai, Zhi Zi,* and *Da Huang* clear heat and drain fire. *Yin Chen Hao, Yi Yi Ren,* and *Che Qian Zi* clear heat and disinhibit dampness. *Dan Pi, Chi Xiao,* and *Niu Xi* cool and quicken the blood, while *Fu Ling* and *Cang Zhu* fortify the spleen and disinhibit dampness.

ADDITIONS & SUBTRACTIONS: If there is no constipation, omit *Da Huang.* If spleen qi vacuity is more pronounced, add nine grams eavh of Radix Codonopsitis Pilosulae (*Dang Shen*) and Rhizoma Atractylodis Macrocephalae (*Bai Zhu*). If the heat of damp heat has damaged fluids and is accompanied by oral thirst, add 12 grams each of Tuber Ophiopogonis Japonici (*Mai Men Dong*) and Radix Glehniae Littoralis (*Sha Shen*). If there is a headache, add nine grams each of Rhizoma Acori Graminei (*Shi Chang Pu*), Rhizoma Gastrodiae Elatae (*Tian Ma*), and Rhizoma Pinelliae Ternatae (*Ban Xia*).

ACUPUNCTURE & MOXIBUSTION: *Yin Ling Quan* (Sp 9), *Yang Ling Quan* (GB 34), *San Yin Jiao* (Sp 6), *Pi Shu* (Bl 20)

FORMULA ANALYSIS: Draining *Yin Ling Quan* and *Yang Ling Quan* and even supplementing-even draining *San Yin Jiao* clears heat and disinhibits dampness. Supplementing *Pi Shu* and even supplementing-even draining *San Yin Jiao* fortifies the spleen and supplements the qi.

ADDITIONS & SUBTRACTIONS: If there is concomitant heat stasis, add draining *Xue Hai* (Sp 10). For headache, add draining *Tai Yang* (M-HN-9) and *Feng Chi* (GB 20). If there is oral thirst, add draining *Jia Che* (St 6), *Di Cang* (St 4), and *Cheng Jiang* (CV 23). If there is constipation, add draining *Zhi Gou* (TB 6), *Zhong Wan* (CV 12), *Tian Shu* (St 25), and *Da Chang Shu* (Bl 25). For nausea and torpid intake, add draining *Nei Guan* (Per 6) and even supplementing-even draining *Zu San Li* (St 36) and *Zhong Wan* (CV 12).

2. QI & YIN DUAL VACUITY WITH BLOOD VESSEL STASIS & OBSTRUCTION PATTERN

MAIN SYMPTOMS: Shortness of breath, lack of strength, abdominal distention, constipation, scanty menstruation in females, a dry mouth but no desire to drink, dizziness, heart palpitations, a fat, dark tongue, and a bowstring, choppy pulse

TREATMENT PRINCIPLES: Boost the qi, nourish yin, and quicken the blood

RX: *Bu Zhong Yi Qi Tang* (Supplement the Center & Boost the Qi Decoction) plus *Tao Hong Si Wu Tang* (Persica & Carthamus Four Materials Decoction) with additions and subtractions

INGREDIENTS: Radix Astragali Membranacei (*Huang Qi*), Radix Codonopsitis Pilosulae (*Dang Shen*), and Radix Scrophulariae Ningpoensis (*Xuan Shen*), 15g each, uncooked Radix Rehmanniae (*Sheng Di*), Tuber Ophiopogonis Japonici (*Mai Men Dong*), and Radix Rubrus Paeoniae Lactiflorae (*Chi Shao*), 12g each, and Rhizoma Atractylodis Macrocephalae (*Bai Zhu*), Radix Angelicae Sinensis (*Dang Gui*), Radix Bupleuri (*Chai Hu*), Pericarpium Citri Reticulatae (*Chen Pi*), Semen Pruni Persicae (*Tao Ren*), Flos Carthami Tinctorii (*Hong Hua*), and Radix Ligustici Wallichii (*Chuan Xiong*), 9g each

FORMULA ANALYSIS: *Huang Qi*, *Dang Shen*, and *Bai Zhu* fortify the spleen and supplement the qi. *Chai Hu* and *Chen Pi* rectify the qi and disinhibit the qi mechanism. *Sheng Di*, *Xuan Shen*, and *Mai Men Dong* enrich yin and engender fluids, while *Dang Gui*, *Chi Shao*, *Tao Ren*, *Hong Hua*, and *Chuan Xiong* quicken the blood and dispel stasis.

ACUPUNCTURE & MOXIBUSTION: *Zu San Li* (St 36), *Tai Xi* (Ki 3), *San Yin Jiao* (Sp 6), *Xue Hai* (Sp 10), *Pi Shu* (Bl 20), *Shen Shu* (Bl 23)

FORMULA ANALYSIS: Supplementing *Zu San Li* and *Pi Shu* and even supplementing-even draining *San Yin Jiao* fortifies the spleen and supplements the qi. Supplementing *Tai Xi* and *Shen Shu* and even supplementing-even draining *San Yin Jiao* supplements the kidneys and enriches yin. Even supplementing-even draining *San Yin Jiao* and draining *Xue Hai* quickens the blood and dispels stasis.

ADDITIONS & SUBTRACTIONS: For abdominal distention and constipation, add draining *Zhi Gou* (TB 6), *Tian Shu* (St 25), and *Da Chang Shu* (Bl 25) and even supplementing-even draining *Zhong Wan* (CV 12). For heart palpitations, add even supplementing-even draining *Shen Men* (Ht 7), *Nei Guan* (Per 6), and *Xin Shu* (Bl 15). For dizziness, add draining *Bai Hui* (GV 20) and *Feng Chi* (GB 20). For dry mouth and parched throat, add supplementing *Zhao Hai* (Ki 6) and *Lie Que* (Lu 7) and draining *Jia Che* (St 6), *Di Cang* (St 4), and *Cheng Jiang* (CV 23).

REMARKS:

1. The Western medical treatment of this condition consists of surgical excision if there is a pituitary tumor. This operation is successful in 70% of cases, but works best with microadenomas under 1cm in diameter. About 20% of tumors recur. If no tumor is found, the next step is usually supervoltage irradiation of the pituitary. However, response to radiation may require several months. Bilateral adrenalectomy is reserved for patients with pituitary hyperadrenalcorticism who do not respond to both surgery and irradiation. Adrenalectomy requires steroid replacement therapy for the remainder of the patient's life.[4] Therefore, Chinese medicine can be used for those in whom surgery is contraindicated, to prevent recurrence of tumor growth, in those whom surgery has been unsuccessful, as an option to irradiation, while waiting for irradiation to take effect, and for those who have not responded to either surgery or irradiation.

C. DIABETES & ACROMEGALY

Acromegaly is a form of hyperpituitarism nearly always due to a pituitary adenoma of the somatotrophis resulting in excessive secretion of growth hormone (GH). If GH hypersecretion begins in childhood before closure of the epiphyses, this leads to exaggerated skeletal growth. However, GH excess most commonly begins between the third and fifth decades of life. When GH hypersecretion begins after epiphyseal closure, the earliest clinical symptoms are coarsening of the facial features and soft tissue swelling of the hands and feet. The increase in dimension of the acral parts is responsible for the name, acromegaly. In adults, coarse body hair increases, and the skin thickens and frequently darkens. The size and function of sebaceous and sweat glands increases, leading to both excessive perspiration and body odor. Overgrowth of the mandible leads to protrusion of the jaw and malocclusion of the teeth. Cartilaginous proliferation of the larynx leads to deepening of the voice and costal growth leads to a barrel chest. Articular cartilaginous proliferation may lead to necrosis and erosion and/or crippling degenerative arthritis. Peripheral neuropathies are common, as are headaches. In addition, the tongue is frequently enlarged and furrowed. In terms of diabetes, increased growth hormone can result in insulin resistance. Therefore, one quarter of patients with acromegaly also have diabetes.[5]

CHINESE DISEASE MECHANISMS: The disease mechanisms of this condition when present with diabetes are essentially the same as for Cushing's syndrome above: spleen loss of fortification and movement plus damp heat internally collecting, with enduring heat leading to eventual qi and yin vacuity.

TREATMENT BASED ON PATTERN DISCRIMINATION:

1. SPLEEN LOSS OF FORTIFICATION & MOVEMENT WITH DAMP HEAT INTERNALLY COLLECTING PATTERN

MAIN SYMPTOMS: Coarsening of the facial features and enlargement of the four extremities, shortness of breath, lack of strength, spontaneous perspiration, headache and heavy-headedness, the sound of phlegm in the throat, oral thirst but no desire to drink excessively, a fat, red tongue with slimy, yellow fur, and a bowstring, slippery, rapid pulse

TREATMENT PRINCIPLES: Clear heat, disinhibit dampness, and fortify the spleen

RX: Huang Lian Wen Dan Tang Jia Jian (Coptis Warm the Gallbladder Decoction with Additions & Subtractions)

INGREDIENTS: Semen Coicis Lachryma-jobi (Yi Yi Ren), 30g, Sclerotium Poriae Cocos (Fu Ling) and Semen Dolichoris Lablab (Bai Bian Dou), 15g each, Rhizoma Pinelliae Ternatae (Ban Xia), Pericarpium Citri Reticulatae (Chen Pi), Fructus Immaturus Citri Aurantii

(Zhi Shi), Radix Bupleuri (Chai Hu), and Radix Scutellariae Baicalensis (Huang Qin), 9g each, and Rhizoma Coptidis Chinensis (Huang Lian), 6g

FORMULA ANALYSIS: Ban Xia, Chen Pi, Huang Lian, Huang Qin, and Yi Yi Ren clear heat, transform phlegm, and eliminate dampness. Chen Pi, Zhi Shi, and Chai Hu rectify the qi, and Fu Ling and Bai Bian Dou fortify the spleen and disinhibit dampness.

ADDITIONS & SUBTRACTIONS: For dry mouth and oral thirst, add 12 grams of Tuber Ophiopogonis Japonici (Mai Men Dong) and nine grams of Radix Trichosanthis Kirlowii (Tian Hua Fen). For shortness of breath, lack of strength, and spontaneous perspiration, add 15 grams of Radix Astragali Membranacei (Huang Qi) and nine grams each of Fructus Schisandrae Chinensis (Wu Wei Zi) and Rhizoma Atractylodis Macrocephalae (Bai Zhu). For headache and heavy-headedness, add nine grams each of Radix Ligustici Wallichii (Chuan Xiong), Rhizoma Gastrodiae Elatae (Tian Ma), and Rhizoma Acori Graminei (Shi Chang Pu).

ACUPUNCTURE & MOXIBUSTION: Same as for this pattern under Cushing's syndrome above. However, if there is marked qi vacuity, add supplementing Zu San Li. If there is spontaneous perspiration, add supplementing He Gu (LI 4).

2. LIVER-KIDNEY YIN VACUITY WITH SPLEEN QI INSUFFICIENCY PATTERN

MAIN SYMPTOMS: Coarsening of the facial features, enlargement of the four extremities, a dark facial complexion, spontaneous perspiration and night sweats, shortness of breath, lack of strength, numbness of the limbs, low back soreness and lower leg limpness, oral thirst with no desire to drink, amenorrhea in females, impotence in males, a fat, red tongue with scanty fur, and a bowstring, fine, forceless pulse

TREATMENT PRINCIPLES: Boost the qi and nourish yin

RX: Si Jun Zi Tang (Four Gentlemen Decoction) plus You Gui Yin (Return the Right [Kidney] Drink) with additions and subtractions

INGREDIENTS: Cooked Radix Rehmanniae (Shu Di), Radix Albus Paeoniae Lactiflorae (Bai Shao), Sclerotium Poriae Cocos (Fu Ling), and Rhizoma Cibotii Barometsis (Gou Ji), 15g each, and Radix Dioscoreae Oppositae (Shan Yao), Fructus Corni Officinalis (Shan Zhu Yu),

Semen Cuscutae Chinensis (*Tu Si Zi*), Fructus Lycii Chinensis (*Gou Qi Zi*), Radix Achyranthis Bidentatae (*Niu Xi*), Gelatinum Cornu Cervi (*Lu Jiao Jiao*), Gelatinum Plastri Testudinis (*Gui Ban Jiao*), Radix Codonopsitis Pilosulae (*Dang Shen*), Rhizoma Atractylodis Macrocephalae (*Bai Zhu*), and Radix Angelicae Sinensis (*Dang Gui*), 9g each

FORMULA ANALYSIS: *Shan Yao, Dang Shen, Bai Zhu,* and *Fu Ling* fortify the spleen and boost the qi. *Shu Di, Shan Zhu Yu, Tu Si Zi, Gou Qi Zi,* and *Gui Ban Jiao* nourish yin and supplement the kidneys. *Dang Gui* and *Bai Shao* nourish the blood and emolliate the liver, while *Gou Ji, Tu Si Zi,* and *Niu Xi* supplement and strengthen the low back. *Lu Jiao Jiao* nourishes the blood and supplements yang in order to help foster the essence.

ADDITIONS & SUBTRACTIONS: For marked thirst, add 12 grams of Tuber Ophiopogonis Japonici (*Mai Men Dong*) and nine grams each of Radix Trichosanthis Kirlowii (*Tian Hua Fen*) and Rhizoma Anemarrhenae Aspheloidis (*Zhi Mu*). For spontaneous perspiration, add 15 grams of Radix Astragali Membranacei (*Huang Qi*) and nine grams of Fructus Schisandrae Chinensis (*Wu Wei Zi*). For yin vacuity giving rise to vacuity heat or fire effulgence, add nine grams each of Rhizoma Anemarrhenae Aspheloidis (*Zhi Mu*) and Cortex Phellodendri (*Huang Bai*). For impotence, add nine grams each of Herba Epimedii (*Xian Ling Pi*) and Rhizoma Curculiginis Orchioidis (*Xian Mao*).

ACUPUNCTURE & MOXIBUSTION: Same as for qi and yin vacuity under Cushing's syndrome above. However, if there is no blood stasis, omit *Xue Hai* and use supplementing technique at *San Yin Jiao*.

ADDITIONS & SUBTRACTIONS: For numbness of the extremities, add even supplementing-even draining *Ge Shu* (Bl 17) and *Gan Shu* (Bl 18,) and *Bai Xie* (M-UE-22) for the upper extremities and *Ba Feng* (M-LE-8) for the lower extremities. For low back pain, add supplementing *Yao Shu* (GV 2), *Yang Yang Guan* (GV 3), and *Yao Yan* (M-BW-24).

REMARKS:

1. The Western medical treatment of pituitary tumors is ablative via surgery or radiation. However, if surgery and radiotherapy are contraindicated or have failed to provide a cure, medical therapy, including Chinese medical therapy, is indicated. Chinese medicine can also be used while waiting for radiation to take effect.

2. Bob Flaws's teacher, Dr. Yu Min, working at the Yue Yang Hospital affiliated with the Shanghai University of Chinese Medicine, is a *zhong liu ke* or tumor specialist. She believes that pituitary tumors should be treated radically under the traditional Chinese rubric of wind and phlegm headache. Dr. Yu treated 16 patients with pituitary tumors with the following self-composed formula and, in all cases, the patients' clinical symptoms decreased or were completely eliminated: Herba Salviae Chinensis Cum Radice (*Shi Jian Chuan*) and uncooked Concha Ostreae (*Mu Li*), 30g each, Bombyx Batryticatus (*Jiang Can*), Sclerotium Poriae Cocos (*Fu Ling*), and Sclerotium Polypori Umbellati (*Zhu Ling*), 15g each, Rhizoma Arisaematis (*Nan Xing*), Rhizoma Pinelliae Ternatae (*Ban Xia*), Spica Prunellae Vulgaris (*Xia Ku Cao*), and Rhizoma Acori Graminei (*Shi Chang Pu*), 10g each, Yu Nai Wan (Taro Pills), 9g wrapped, Sclopendra Subspinipes (*Wu Gong*), 2 strips, and Gecko (*Ge Jie*), 2 strips. These medicinals were decocted in water and administered internally.

If headache was severe, Rhizoma Dioscoreae Bulberiferae (*Huang Yao Zi*) and Buthus Martensis (*Quan Xie*) were added. If the vision was blurred, Semen Cassiae Torae (*Jue Ming Zi*), Semen Celosiae (*Qing Xiang Zi*), Fructus Lycii Chinensis (*Gou Qi Zi*), and Flos Chrysanthemi Morifolii (*Ju Hua*) were added. If there was ductal oppression and torpid intake, Pericarpium Citri Reticulatae (*Chen Pi*), uncooked Semen Coicis Lachyrma-jobi (*Yi Yi Ren*), Endothelium Corneum Gigeriae Galli (*Ji Nei Jin*), and scorched Massa Medica Fermentata (*Shen Qu*) were added. If there was liver-kidney insufficiency, Radix Angelicae Sinensis (*Dang Gui*), uncooked Radix Rehmanniae (*Sheng Di*), Radix Glehniae Littoralis (*Sha Shen*), Tuber Ophiopogonis Japonici (*Mai Men Dong*), and Fructus Lycii Chinensis (*Gou Qi Zi*) were added. If there was amenorrhea, Radix Angelicae Sinensis (*Dang Gui*) and Radix Ligustici Wallichii (*Chuan Xiong*) were added. If there was vomiting of acid, Radix Auklandiae Lappae (*Mu Xiang*), Caulis Bambusae In Taeniis (*Zhu Ru*), Pericarpium Citri Reticulatae (*Chen Pi*), Flos Inulae Racemosae (*Xuan Fu Hua*), and Aspongopus (*JiuXiang Chong*) were added. If there was impotence, Semen Cuscutae Chinensis (*Tu Si Zi*), Herba Epimedii (*Xian Ling Pi*), and Rhizoma Curculiginis Orchioidis (*Xian Mao*) were added. If there was qi vacuity, Radix Astragali Membranacei (*Huang Qi*) and Radix Pseudostellariae Heterophyllae (*Tai Zi Shen*) were added. And if there was insomnia, Medulla Junci Effusi (*Deng Xin Cao*), Radix Polygalae Tenuifoliae (*Yuan Zhi*), and Cinnabar (*Zhu Sha*) were added.

According to Dr. Yu, recalcitrant phlegm should be treated by warm, drying medicinals since "phlegm is a yin evil which, without warmth, cannot be got rid of." Therefore, one must take care to prevent damage to yin and consumption of fluids using this formula. However, Dr. Yu does give modifications for yin vacuity above.

D. DIABETES & PHEOCHROMOCYTOMA

Pheochromocytoma is a tumor of the chromaffin cells that secretes catecholamines, thus causing hypertension. In about 80% of cases, pheochromocytomas are found in the adrenal medulla but may also be found in other tissues derived from neural crest cells. Those in the adrenal medulla appear equally in both sexes, are bilateral in 10% of cases (20% in children), and are usually benign (95%). Extra-adrenal tumors are more often malignant (30%). Although pheochromocytomas may occur at any age, their maximum incidence is between 30-50 years of age.[6] The most prominent feature of pheochromocytomas is hypertension. This is paroxysmal in 45% of cases, persistent in 50% of cases and is rarely absent (5%). Common clinical signs and symptoms include tachycardia, diaphoresis, postural hypotension, dyspnea, tachypnea, angina, flushing, cold, clammy skin, severe headache, heart palpitations, nausea, vomiting, epigastric pain, visual disturbances, paresthesias, constipation, and an impending sense of doom. Paroxsymal attacks may be provoked by palpation of the tumor, postural changes, abdominal compression or massage, induction of anesthesia, emotional trauma, administration of beta-blockers, and urination if the tumor is in the bladder. If not treated in a timely manner, death typically occurs in 5-10 years due to a combination of heart arrhythmia, heart failure, and hypertension. Hyperglycemia, glycosuria, and overt diabetes may be present with a pheochromocytoma, with elevated fasting levels of plasma free fatty acid and glycerol.

CHINESE DISEASE MECHANISMS: There are two main mechanisms for pheochromocytomas in Chinese medicine. The first of these is heart-spleen dual vacuity. Due to excessive worry, thinking, taxation, and/or fatigue or to an unregulated diet, the spleen and stomach may suffer detriment and damage. Hence the source of qi and blood engenderment and transformation become insufficient. This may then result in a heart blood and spleen qi dual vacuity. The second Chinese disease mechanism of this condition is liver-kidney yin depletion. This may be due to a former heaven natural endowment insufficiency, excessive bedroom taxation, overtaxation and fatigue in general, and internal injury by the seven affects consuming the essence and blood. Thus liver-kidney yin becomes depleted, yin cannot control yang, and yang ascends and becomes hyperactive.

TREATMENT BASED ON PATTERN DISCRIMINATION:

1. HEART-SPLEEN DUAL VACUITY WITH QI & YIN DUAL VACUITY PATTERN

MAIN SYMPTOMS: Dizziness, possible syncope, a somber white facial complexion, heart palpitations, shortness of breath, faint, weak breathing, spontaneous perspiration, chilled skin, a pale tongue with white fur, and a deep, fine, weak pulse

TREATMENT PRINCIPLES: Boost the qi and secure desertion

RX: Sheng Mai San Jia Wei (Engender the Pulse Powder with Added Flavors)

INGREDIENTS: Uncooked Os Draconis (Long Gu) and Concha Ostreae (Mu Li), 30g each, Radix Astragali Membranacei (Huang Qi), 20g, Tuber Ophiopogonis Japonici (Mai Men Dong) and Fructus Corni Officinalis (Shan Zhu Yu), 12g each, and Fructus Schisandrae Chinensis (Wu Wei Zi) and Radix Panacis Ginseng (Ren Shen), 9g each

FORMULA ANALYSIS: Ren Shen and Huang Qi boost the qi and secure desertion. Shan Zhu Yu, Mai Men Dong, and Wu Wei Zi enrich yin and constrain and restrain consumption and scattering of the qi. Uncooked Long Gu and Mu Li settle the heart and quiet the spirit.

ADDITIONS & SUBTRACTIONS: If there is marked oral dryness, add 12 grams of Radix Glehniae Littoralis (She Shen). If there is marked qi vacuity, add 15 grams of Radix Pseudostellariae Heterophyllae (Tai Zi Shen).

ACUPUNCTURE & MOXIBUSTION: Zu San Li (St 36), Bai Hui (GV 20)

FORMULA ANALYSIS: Moxibustion at Zu San Li and Bai Hui strongly supplements the qi, upbears yang, and secures desertion.[7]

2. LIVER-KIDNEY INSUFFICIENCY WITH YIN VACUITY-YANG HYPERACTIVITY PATTERN

MAIN SYMPTOMS: Dizziness, headache, tinnitus, numbness of the extremities, generalized heat, excessive sweating, emaciation of the body, a red tongue with scanty fur, and a bowstring, fine, rapid pulse

TREATMENT PRINCIPLES: Supplement and enrich the liver and kidneys, level the liver and subdue yang

Rx: *Yi Guan Jian* (One Link Decoction) plus *Qi Ju Di Huang Wan* (Lycium & Chrysanthemum Rehmannia Pills) with additions and subtractions

INGREDIENTS: Uncooked Radix Rehmanniae (*Sheng Di*), 20g, Radix Albus Paeoniae Lactiflorae (*Bai Shao*) and Sclerotium Poriae Cocos (*Fu Ling*), 15g each, Tuber Ophiopogonis Japonici (*Mai Men Dong*), 12g, and Radix Glehniae Littoralis (*Sha Shen*), Radix Angelicae Sinensis (*Dang Gui*), Fructus Lycii Chinensis (*Gou Qi Zi*), Fructus Meliae Toosendan (*Chuan Lian Zi*), Flos Chrysanthemi Morifolii (*Ju Hua*), Cortex Radicis Moutan (*Dan Pi*), Rhizoma Gastrodiae Elatae (*Tian Ma*), and Ramulus Uncariae Cum Uncis (*Gou Teng*), 9g each

FORMULA ANALYSIS: *Sheng Di, Sha Shen, Mai Men Dong,* and *Gou Qi Zi* nourish yin and enrich and supplement the liver and kidneys. *Ju Hua* and *Dan Pi* clear heat and cool the blood. *Dang Gui* and *Bai Shao* nourish the blood and emolliate the liver. *Tian Ma* and *Gou Teng* level the liver and extinguish wind. *Chuan Lian Zi* courses the liver and rectifies the qi without plundering yin.

ADDITIONS & SUBTRACTIONS: For tinnitus, add nine grams each of Magnetitum (*Ci Shi*) and Rhizoma Acori Graminei (*Shi Chang Pu*). For headache, add 15 grams of Radix Ligustici Wallichii (*Chuan Xiong*). For numbness of the extremities, add 18 grams of Caulis Milletiae Seu Spatholobi (*Ji Xue Teng*) and 15 grams of Radix Salviae Miltiorrhizae (*Dan Shen*).

ACUPUNCTURE & MOXIBUSTION: *Tai Xi* (Ki 3), *Tai Chong* (Liv 3), *San Yin Jiao* (Sp 6), *He Gu* (LI 4), *Qu Chi* (LI 11), *Zu San Li* (St 36), *Feng Chi* (GB 20)

FORMULA ANALYSIS: Supplementing *Tai Xi* and even supplementing-even draining *San Yin Jiao* supplements the kidneys and enriches yin. Even supplementing-even draining *Tai Chong* and *San Yin Jiao* nourishes the liver at the same time as it drains liver repletion. Draining *He Gu*, *Zu San Li*, and *Qu Chi* subdues yang, while draining *Feng Chi* levels the liver and extinguishes wind.

ADDITIONS & SUBTRACTIONS: If there is vexation, agitation, and restlessness, heart palpitations, or insomnia, add even supplementing-even draining *Shen Men* (Ht 7), *Nei Guan* (Per 6), *Dan Zhong* (CV 17), and *Xin Shu* (Bl 15). If there is dizziness or to increase the effects of quieting the spirit and subduing yang, add draining *Bai Hui* (GV 20). If there is headache, add *Tai Yang* (M-HN-9).

REMARKS:

1. The Western medical treatment of pheochromocytomas consists of surgical excision of the neoplasm. However, this operation is usually delayed until the patient is restored to optimal physical condition. This may be accomplished via the administration of alpha and beta-blockers and/or the use of Chinese medicine, including acupuncture and internally administered Chinese medicinals. The authors have not found any published evidence to date that Chinese medicine alone is capable of radically curing this condition.

ABSTRACTS OF REPRESENTATIVE CHINESE RESEARCH:

Lu Yuan-zhong & Wu Yu-ning, "Clinical Observations on the Treatment of 50 Cases of Menopausal Diabetes with *Bu Shen Fang* (Supplement the Kidneys Formula)," *Shan Xi Zhong Yi (Shanxi Chinese Medicine),* #3, 2001, p. 16-18: Altogether, there were 80 female patients in this study, all of whom met the WHO criteria for type 2 diabetes. Twenty were seen as in-patients and 60 as out-patients. Fifty of these patients were assigned to a so-called treatment group and 30 were assigned to a comparison group. In the treatment group the youngest patient was 53 and the oldest was 70 years old, with an average age of 63. The shortest course of disease was one year and the longest was 13 years, with an average duration of seven years. In the comparison group, the youngest patient was 50, the oldest was 68, and the average age was 61 years old. The shortest duration was nine months, the longest was 11 years, and the average was five years. In addition, there was also another comparison group made up of 25 healthy women who ranged in age from 50-70 years, with an average age of 62. The diagnosis of diabetes and the pattern discrimination of kidney vacuity pattern were both based on criteria published in 1993 as a result of a national Chinese medical conference on diabetes. Low back and knee soreness and pain, tinnitus, deafness, falling or loose teeth, and decreased libido were the main symptoms of kidney vacuity, and all patients had to have two of these.

The treatment group received *Bu Shen Fang* which consisted of: Fructus Ligustri Lucidi (*Nu Zhen Zi*), 30g, uncooked Radix Rehmanniae (*Sheng Di*), Fructus Corni Officinalis (*Shan Zhu Yu*), Radix Dioscoreae Oppositae (*Shan Yao*), and Semen Cuscutae Chinensis (*Tu Si Zi*), 15g each, and Radix Scrophulariae Ningpoensis (*Xuan Shen*), Fructus Lycii Chinensis (*Gou Qi Zi*), and Rhizoma Atractylodis (*Cang Zhu*), 10g each. The comparison group received *Yi Qi Yang Yin Qing Re Fang* (Boost the Qi, Nourish Yin & Clear Heat Formula) which consisted of: Tuber Ophiopogonis Japonici (*Mai Men Dong*) and Radix Trichosanthis Kirlowii (*Tian Hua Fen*), 30g each, uncooked Radix Rehmanniae (*Sheng Di*), Radix Pseudostellariae Heterophyllae (*Tai Zi Shen*), and Radix Astragali Membranacei (*Huang Qi*), 20g each, Radix Dioscoreae Oppositae (*Shan Yao*) and Cortex Radicis Lycii Chinensis (*Di Gu Pi*), 15g each, and Rhizoma Anemarrhenae Aspheloidis (*Zhi Mu*), 10g. One *ji* of either of these two formulas was decocted in water and administered TID on an empty stomach. Three months equaled one course of treatment for both groups.

Before treatment, the difference in indices between the treatment and comparison groups was not statistically significant, but the differences in C peptide, insulin, E_2, and testosterone (T) between the treatment group and the comparison group were significant (P < 0.05). The differences in FBG, PPBG, HbA1C, insulin, E_2, T, and E_2 to T ratio from before to after treatment in the treatment group were significant, while, in the comparison group, these differences were not significant. For instance, FBG went from a mean of 10.35 ± 2.33mmol/L before treatment to 7.86 ± 3.12mmol/L after treatment in the treatment group and from 11.45 ± 3.98mmol/L before treatment to 9.22 ± 6.21mmol/L after treatment in the comparison group. Two hour PPBG went from a mean of 16.38 ± 8.51mmol/L before treatment to 12.01 ± 3.56mmol/L after treatment in the treatment group, while it went from 14.24 ± 6.68mmol/L before treatment to 16.99 ± 5.89mmol/L after treatment in the comparison group. HbA1C went from 10.55 ± 2.98% before treatment to 8.56 ± 3.46% after treatment in the treatment group, and from 12.45 ± 3.16% to 11.21 ± 2.68% in the comparison group. E_2 went from 13.86 ± 5.63pg/ml before treatment to 20.28 ± 6.35pg/ml after treatment in the treatment group, and only from 12.98 ± 5.55pg/ml to 13.32 ± 5.88pg/ml in the comparison group. Testosterone went from 1.02 ± 0.52ng/ml to 0.96 ± 0.42ng/ml in the treatment group, and from 1.13 ± 0.56ng/ml to 1.01 ± 0.52ng/ml in the comparison group. And the ratio of E_2 to T went from 12.22 ± 5.32 to 21.23 ± 8.38 in the treatment group, while it went from 10.38 ± 3.63 to 12.98 ± 5.01 in the comparison group. Thus *Bu Shen Fang* was better able to regulate hormone levels, boost the secretion of insulin from the islets of Langerhans, and lower blood glucose levels in those with kidney vacuity pattern type 2 DM than was *Yi Qi Yang Yin Qing Re Fang*.

REPRESENTATIVE CASE HISTORIES:

CASE 1[8]

The patient was a 25 year old female who had a history of diabetes for five years and amenorrhea for one year. Five years before, for no apparent reason, the patient developed the symptoms of oral thirst, polydipsia, polyphagia, polyuria, emaciation, and loss of strength. Subsequent to glucose tolerance and insulin release tests, the diagnosis was type 1 diabetes. After continuous insulin treatments, fasting blood glucose stabilized at 7.8 mmol/L. However, three years later, the woman's menstruation became irregular, with increasingly delayed menstruation. During this time, the menses typically arrived only once every 2-3 months, and the amount of flow was comparatively less than before. Then amenorrhea occurred which continued for one year. This was accompanied by a lusterless facial complexion, a dry mouth and throat, dizziness, tinnitus, low back and knee aching and weakness, fatigue, loss of strength, vexatious heat, night sweats, blurred vision, a pale red tongue with scanty fur, and a fine, weak pulse.

Based on the above, the Chinese medical pattern was categorized as liver-kidney yin vacuity with loss of nourishment of the chong and ren. The treatment was to enrich and supplement the liver and kidneys, fortify the spleen and engender blood, and moisten and nourish the chong and ren. The formula prescribed was *Zuo Gui Wan* (Restore the Left [Kidney] Pills) in combination with *Si Wu Tang* (Four Materials Decoction) with additions and subtractions: Fructus Lycii Chinensis (*Gou Qi Zi*), Radix Dioscoreae Oppositae (*Shan Yao*), processed Radix Polygoni Multiflori (*He Shou Wu*), Fructus Ligustri Lucidi (*Nu Zhen Zi*), and Radix Astragali Membranacei (*Huang Qi*), 30g each, uncooked Radix Rehmanniae (*Sheng Di Huang*), Plastrum Testudinis (*Gui Ban*), Fructus Corni Officinalis (*Shan Zhu Yu*), Semen Cuscutae Chinensis (*Tu Si Zi*), Herba Cistanchis Deserticolae (*Rou Cong Rong*), Radix Ligustici Wallichii (*Chuan Xiong*), and Radix Rubrus Paeoniae Lactiflorae (*Chi Shao*), 15g each, and Radix Angelicae Sinensis (*Dang Gui*), 12g.

After taking 12 *ji* of these medicinals, the patient's low back and knee aching and weakness were alleviated and so were her fatigue and loss of strength. After taking 12 more *ji*, her vision was clearer than before and all the above symptoms markedly improved. She continued taking another 24 *ji*, and the only symptoms remaining were a distended, full feeling in her lower abdomen and a dull pain just before the onset of her menstrual flow. Therefore, 12 grams each of Flos Carthami Tinctorii (*Hong Hua*) and Semen Pruni Persicae (*Tao Ren*) and 15 grams of Radix Cyathulae (*Chuan Niu Xi*) were added to the original formula. These were in order to quicken the blood and free the flow of the network vessels so as to assist the movement of blood. After the patient had taken five *ji*, the menstrual flow came like a tide. The color was dull red, the amount was scanty, and the flow lasted one day. With similar such variations to the original formula, the patient recuperated within six months. Her menstruation came monthly with a normal color and amount.

CASE 2[9]

The patient was a 24 year old female who had a history of diabetes for six years and amenorrhea for one and a half years. Six years before, after contracting a high fever, she began to suffer from insulin-dependent diabetes. Although the patient used insulin over a long period of time, her FBG still fluctuated between 8.3-13.6 mmol/L. Her menses had become scanty and their color had become pale. Three years later, the menstrual cycle became irregular and the menstrual periods became gradually more delayed, leading to menstrual block or amenorrhea. Examination revealed a somber white facial complexion, lassitude of the spirit, loss of strength, low back and knee aching and weakness, fear of cold, chilled limbs, decreased eating, loose stools, frequent, profuse nocturia, a pale yet dark or dull tongue with teeth-marks on the edges and scanty fur, and a deep, fine pulse.

Based on the above signs and symptoms, the Chinese medical pattern was categorized as spleen-kidney yang vacuity with chong and ren loss of regulation and nourishment. The treatment principles were to warm the kidneys and fortify the spleen, regulate and supplement the chong and ren. The formula prescribed was *You Gui Wan* (Restore the Right [Kidney] Pills) combined with *Si Wu Tang* (Four Materials Decoction) with additions and subtractions: Fructus Lycii Chinensis (*Gou Qi Zi*), Radix Dioscoreae Oppositae (*Shan Yao*), processed Radix Polygoni Multiflorae (*He Shou Wu*), and Radix Astragali Membranacei (*Huang Qi*), 30g each, Fructus Corni Officinalis (*Shan Zhu Yu*), Gelatinum Cornu Cervi (*Lu Jiao Jiao*), Semen Cuscutae Chinensis (*Tu Si Zi*), uncooked Radix Rehmanniae (*Sheng Di*), Radix Angelicae Sinensis (*Dang Gui*), and Rhizoma Atractylodis Macrocephalae (*Bai Zhu*), 15g each, Radix

Ligustici Wallichii (*Chuan Xiong*) and Herba Epimedii (*Yin Yang Huo*), 12g each, and Cortex Cinnamomi Cassiae (*Rou Gui*), 9g.

After 12 *ji* of this prescription, the low back and knee aching and weakness, the fear of cold, and chilled limbs had taken an obvious turn for the better. When another 12 *ji* were taken, the nocturia was reduced and her strength increased. Fifteen grams each of Radix Cyathulae (*Chuan Niu Xi*) and Radix Achyranthis Bidentatae (*Huai Niu Xi*) were added to the formula. After 24 *ji* of this modified formula were taken, all the symptoms were greatly reduced. At the same time, the lower abdomen felt slightly distended and full. After 12 more *ji* of the same formula, lower abdomen distention and pain were very noticeable, indicating that the menstrual flow was about to arrive. Therefore, 12 grams each of Semen Pruni Persicae (*Tao Ren*) and Flos Carthami Tinctorii (*Hong Hua*) were added to the formula. After three *ji* of this formula were taken, the menstrual flow came like a tide. The color was dull, it was profuse in amount, and ended after half a day. For the next six months, this modified formula was given regularly. All the symptoms recovered, FBG stabilized at 7mmol/L, and the menstrual flow came on schedule. After these changes had taken place, *Jin Gui Shen Qi Wan* (*Golden Cabinet* Kidney Qi Pills) and *Ren Shen Gui Pi Wan* (Ginseng Restore the Spleen Pills) were given in order to consolidate the treatment effect. At a follow-up visit one year later, menstruation was normal.

ENDNOTES:

[1] *The Merck Manual*, 17th edition, ed. by Mark H. Beers & Robert Berkow, Merck Research Laboratories, Whitehouse Station, NJ, 1999, p. 119

[2] www.ahealthyadvantage.com/topic/topic100587321

[3] Becker, Simon, *A Handbook of Chinese Hematology*, Blue Poppy Press, Boulder, CO, 2000, p. 145-152

[4] *The Merck Manual*, op. cit., p. 108

[5] Gao Yan-bin, *Zhong Guo Tang Niao Bing Fang Zhi Tie Se (The Characteristics of the Chinese National Prevention & Treatment of Diabetes)*, Heilongjiang Science & Technology Publishing Co., Harbin, 1995, p. 780

[6] *The Merck Manual*, op. cit., p. 111

[7] It is important to understand that upbearing yang in this situation will not aggravate the hypertension. Although hypertension is commonly associated with ascendant yang hyperactivity, not all cases of hypertension are. In addition, lack of upbearing of the clear can cause depression which then leads to the engenderment of internal heat which, over time, may lead to yin vacuity and ascendant hyperactivity of yang.

[8] Xu Yun-sheng & Cheng Yi-chun, "Experiences in the Treatment of Two Cases of Diabetes & Amenorrhea," *Zhong Yi Za Zhi (Journal of Chinese Medicine)*, # 6, 1997, p. 338

[9] *Ibid.*

26

DIABETIC PSYCHOLOGICAL DISTURBANCES

Since blood glucose levels affect the brain and central nervous system directly, it is common to see psychological disturbances in patients with diabetes. Both hyper- and especially hypoglycemic states may cause the patient to experience a variety of psychoemotional disorders. For instance, a drop in blood sugar below certain levels may result in neuroglycopenia and central nervous system depression. In addition, the diagnosis of diabetes and the stresses of dealing with a chronic, potentially life-threatening disease also commonly cause their own psychological reactions. Some common negative emotional responses experienced by those who have just learned they have diabetes include shock, fear, anger, anxiety, grief, guilt, and depression.[1] For instance, depression is more common in people with diabetes, recurs more frequently, and lasts longer compared with the general population.[2] Symptoms of depression include loss of pleasure in previously enjoyed activities, trouble falling and/or staying asleep at night, fatigue, loss of pleasure in eating, loss of appetite or increased food consumption, weight gain or loss, difficulty concentrating, difficulty sitting still, difficulty making decisions, feelings of guilt or lack of self-worth, and/or thoughts about suicide or self-injury. Patients with diabetes have shown higher scores on the Strait Trait Anger Expression Inventory.[3] Patients with diabetes have also shown higher scores on the Strait Trait Anxiety Inventory (STAI).[4] Feelings of anxiety may exist independently or coexist with depression. Symptoms of anxiety include restlessness, irritability, difficulty concentrating, excessive worry, fatigue, difficulty sleeping, frequent headaches, and muscular tension. For some patients, abnormal psychoemotional states are most pronounced in the weeks and months following initial diagnosis, after which these patients make certain psychological adjustments.[5] However, in others, abnormal psychological symptoms or behaviors increase in severity as the disease progresses or fluctuate depending on their other intercurrent illness, familial predisposition, and stressors in their life.

CHINESE MEDICAL DISEASE CATEGORIZATION: In Chinese medicine, depression is called *yu zheng*, depressive condition, while *kong jing*, fear and fright, cover a variety of anxiety disorders. However, most of the various symptoms which make up both depression and anxiety are disease categories in their own right, such as *pi juan*, fatigue, *shi mian*, loss of sleep, *xin ji*, heart palpitations, *jian wang*, impaired memory, *huang hu*, abstraction, *yi nu*, easy anger or irritability, and *tou tong*, headache.

CHINESE DISEASE MECHANISMS: In general, psychological disturbances associated with diabetes tend to fall into two categories depending on stage of disease and bodily constitution. During the early stages, there tends to be a combination of liver depression and spleen vacuity. This liver depression results in irritability and depression, while the spleen vacuity results in nonengenderment of the qi and blood and nontransformation of water fluids. If qi and blood engenderment and transformation are insufficient, this may lead to nonconstruction and malnourishment of the heart spirit. Because of this nonconstruction and malnourishment, the spirit is disquieted and easily agitated. At the same time, nontransportation and nontransformation of water fluids in the body may lead to the accumulation of phlegm turbidity. Once phlegm turbidity is engendered internally, it will aggravate both liver depression qi stagnation and spleen vacuity weakness. It may also ascend to confound the orifices of the heart. If qi depression and phlegm bind, they may transform depressive heat which then further harasses the heart spirit.

During the middle and latter stages, depressive heat has damaged yin fluids and spleen qi vacuity has given rise to spleen-kidney qi vacuity. Yin is no longer able to control yang, thus giving rise to hyperactivity of yang and the engenderment of internal heat or fire. Since heat is yang in nature, it has an inherent tendency to rise. Thus heat tends to accumulate in the heart all the more harassing and disquieting the spirit. Therefore, in the latter stages, there are often more prominent agitation, restlessness, insomnia, and other such yin vacuity-fire effulgence symptoms.

TREATMENT BASED ON PATTERN DISCRIMINATION

1. HEART-GALLBLADDER QI TIMIDITY PATTERN

MAIN SYMPTOMS: Psychoemotional depression and despondency, apathy, agitated emotions, heart palpitations, fearfulness, insomnia, impaired memory, sorrowful, excessive crying, chest oppression, deep sighing, lack of strength in the limbs, confusion of dreams with reality, a pale tongue with white, slimy fur, and a fine, forceless pulse

NOTE: The name of this pattern is short hand for the complicated combination of patterns of liver depression with spleen vacuity giving rise to nonconstruction and malnourishment of the heart spirit and phlegm turbidity.

TREATMENT PRINCIPLES: Enrich yin and nourish the heart, boost the qi and resolve depression

Rx: Er Yin Jian Jia Wei (Two Yins Drink with Added Flavors)

INGREDIENTS: Radix Astragali Membrancei (Huang Qi), 9-18g, uncooked Radix Rehmanniae (Sheng Di), 12-15g, Tuber Ophiopogonis Japonici (Mai Men Dong), Semen Biotae Orientalis (Bai Zi Ren), and Semen Zizyphi Spinosae (Suan Zao Ren), 12g each, Caulis Akebiae (Mu Tong), Tuber Curcumae (Yu Jin), Sclerotium Poriae Cocos (Fu Ling), Radix Polygalae Tenuifoliae (Yuan Zhi), and Herba Leonuri Heterophylli (Yi Mu Cao), 9g each, and Radix Panacis Ginseng (Ren Shen), 6-9g

FORMULA ANALYSIS: Huang Qi and Ren Shen fortify the spleen and boost the qi, while Sheng Di, Mai Men Dong, Bai Zi Ren, and Suan Zao Ren enrich yin and nourish the heart. Mu Tong drains fire from the heart via urination. Yu Jin and Yuan Zhi both rectify the qi and resolve depression. Fu Ling both aids Huang Qi and Ren Shen in fortifying the spleen and Mu Tong in leading yang downward into the

yin tract. Yi Mu Cao quickens the blood and transforms stasis without damaging the blood and/or yin. In addition, Bai Zi Ren, Suan Zao Ren, Fu Ling, Yuan Zhi, and Ren Shen all quiet the spirit.

ADDITIONS & SUBTRACTIONS: If the limbs are heavy and the tongue fur tends to be slimy, add nine grams each of Rhizoma Acori Graminei (Shi Chang Pu), Cortex Magnoliae Officinalis (Hou Po), Pericarpium Citri Reticulatae (Chen Pi), and Rhizoma Pinelliae Ternatae (Ban Xia) to transform phlegm and eliminate turbidity. If there is a red tongue tip, possible red tongue sides, a bitter taste in the mouth, and a possibly rapid pulse, add 3-6 grams of Rhizoma Coptidis Chinensis (Huang Lian) to clear depressive heat from the heart and liver.

ACUPUNCTURE & MOXIBUSTION: Shen Men (Ht 7), Dan Zhong (CV 17), Xin Shu (Bl 15), Zu San Li (St 36), Feng Long (St 40), San Yin Jiao (Sp 6), Zhang Men (Liv 13)

FORMULA ANALYSIS: Even supplementing-even draining Shen Men, Dan Zhong, and Xin Shu supplements and clears the heart and quiets the spirit. Even supplementing-even draining Zhang Men, Zu San Li, and San Yin Jiao supplements the spleen at the same time as it courses the liver and rectifies the qi. Draining Feng Long transforms phlegm and downbears turbidity.

ADDITIONS & SUBTRACTIONS: If there are severe signs of upper wasting, add draining Fei Shu (Bl 13), Nei Guan (Per 6), and Yu Ji (Lu 10). For blurred vision, add even supplementing-even draining Guang Ming (GB 37). For dizziness, add draining Shang Xing (GV 23) and Feng Chi (GB 20). To quiet the spirit more, add draining Yin Tang (M-HN-3) and Bai Hui (GV 20).

2. YIN VACUITY-FIRE EFFULGENCE PATTERN

MAIN SYMPTOMS: Dry mouth, heart vexation, irritability, easy anger, incessant speech, easy fright, heart palpitations, insomnia, rib-side fullness and oppression, easy sweating, frequent, urgent urination, a red tongue, and a fine, bowstring, rapid pulse

TREATMENT PRINCIPLES: Enrich yin and clear the liver, drain fire and calm the spirit

Rx: Zi Shui Qing Gan Yin Jia Jian (Enrich Water & Clear the Liver Drink with Additions & Subtractions)

INGREDIENTS: Uncooked Radix Rehmanniae (Sheng Di) and Radix Dioscoreae Oppositae (Shan Yao), 15-18g each,

Semen Zizyphi Spinosae (*Suan Zao Ren*), Concha Margaritiferae (*Zhen Zhu Mu*), and Magnetitum (*Ci Shi*), 12g each, and Sclerotium Poriae Cocos (*Fu Ling*), Radix Angelicae Sinensis (*Dang Gui*), Cortex Radicis Moutan (*Dan Pi*), Rhizoma Alismatis (*Ze Xie*), Radix Albus Paeoniae Lactiflorae (*Bai Shao*), Fructus Corni Officinalis (*Shan Zhu Yu*), Radix Bupleuri (*Chai Hu*), and Fructus Gardeniae Jasminoidis (*Zhi Zi*), 9g each

FORMULA ANALYSIS: *Sheng Di, Suan Zao Ren, Shan Zhu Yu, Dang Gui,* and *Bai Shao* enrich and nourish the blood and yin. *Chai Hu* courses the liver and resolves depression, while *Zhi Zi* clears heat from the liver-gallbladder. *Zhen Zhu Mu* and *Ci Shi* heavily subdue yang and downbear counterflow, while *Fu Ling* and *Ze Xie* lead yang downward into the yin tract. *Shan Yao* supplements both the spleen and kidney qi, while *Fu Ling* helps fortify the spleen, and *Shan Zhu Yu* helps secure the kidneys. *Dan Pi* both clears heat from the blood as well as quickens the blood and transforms stasis. It aids *Fu Ling* and *Ze Xie* keep ministerial fire level in its lower source.

ADDITIONS & SUBTRACTIONS: If yin vacuity insomnia is severe, add 12-15 grams each of Plastrum Testudinis (*Gui Ban*) and Concha Ostreae (*Mu Li*) and 9-12 grams of Rhizoma Anemarrhenae Aspheloidis (*Zhi Mu*). For low back weakness and frequent urination, increase the dosage of *Shan Zhu Yu* and add 9-12 grams of Cortex Eucommiae Ulmoidis (*Du Zhong*). For profuse sweating, add 9-12 grams of Herba Agrimoniae Pilosae (*Xian He Cao*). For menstrual irregularities due to qi stagnation leading to blood stasis, add 9-12 grams of Herba Leonuri Heterophylli (*Yi Mu Cao*).

ACUPUNCTURE & MOXIBUSTION: *Shen Men* (Ht 7), *Nei Guan* (Per 6), *Xin Shu* (Bl 15), *Tai Xi* (Ki 3), *San Yin Jiao* (Sp 6), *Shen Men* (Bl 23), *Guan Yuan* (CV 4)

FORMULA ANALYSIS: Even supplementing-even draining *Shen Men, Nei Guan,* and *Xin Shu* clears and supplements the heart as it quiets the spirit. Supplementing *Tai Xi, San Yin Jiao,* and *Shen Shu* supplements the kidneys and enriches yin so that yin can control hyperactive yang. *Guan Yuan* supplements the kidneys and banks the root, thus leading yang back down to its lower source as well as securing the essence and controlling urination.

ADDITIONS & SUBTRACTIONS: To quiet the spirit more, add draining *Yin Tang* (M-HN-3) and *Bai Hui* (GV 20). To drain heart fire more, add draining *Da Ling* (Per 7) and/or *Lao Gong* (Per 8). If there is concomitant liver depression, add draining *Tai Chong* (Liv 3). If there is liver fire or depressive heat, add draining *Xing Jian* (Liv 2). For insomnia, add draining *An Mian* (N-HN-22a &/or b) and *Si Shen Cong* (M-HN-1). For heart palpitations, switch *Nei Guan* to *Jian Shi* (Per 5). If there are night sweats, add draining *Yin Xi* (Ht 6).

REPRESENTATIVE CASE HISTORIES:

CASE 1[6]

The patient was a 59 year old female who was slightly obese and who had suffered from diabetes for 12 years. This woman had tried many medicines, both Chinese and Western, to control her glucose levels but none of these had been successful. The patient's diabetes was severe, and, in the last two months, her emotional state had gradually worsened. This worsening of her emotional state was accompanied by insomnia and forgetfulness. In addition, she was easily frightened and experienced heart palpitations, chest oppression, deep sighing, and lack of strength in her limbs. The woman's tongue was pale with white fur, and her pulse was fine and forceless. Her blood pressure was 17/11.5kPa, FBG was 9.8mmol/L, two-hour PPBG was 13.6mmol/L, and glycosuria was (+++). There were no other remarkable symptoms. In terms of her current Western medications, the woman continued taking gliclazide, 80mg BID, and dimethylguanidine, 50mg BID.

Based on the above signs and symptoms, the patient's Chinese medical pattern discrimination was qi and yin vacuity with liver depression and malnourishment of the heart spirit. Therefore, the treatment principles were to enrich yin and nourish the heart, boost the qi and resolve depression. The formula prescribed was *Er Yin Jian Jia Wei* (Two Yins Drink with Added Flavors): uncooked Radix Rehmanniae (*Sheng Di*), Tuber Ophiopogonis Japonici (*Mai Men Dong*), Tuber Curcumae (*Yu Jin*), and Herba Leonuri Heterophylli (*Yi Mu Cao*), 20g each, Radix Panacis Ginseng (*Ren Shen*), Radix Astragali Membranacei (*Huang Qi*), Sclerotium Poriae Cocos (*Fu Ling*), Semen Biotae Orientalis (*Bai Zi Ren*), and uncooked and stir-fried Semen Zizyphi Spinosae (*Suan Zao Ren*), 15g each, Radix Polygalae Tenuifoliae (*Yuan Zhi*), 12g, Radix Bupleuri (*Chai Hu*), 10g, Caulis Akebiae (*Mu Tong*), 6g, and Rhizoma Coptidis Chinensis (*Huang Lian*), 4.5g. One *ji* was decocted in water and administered each day for 10 days. At the follow-up visit after taking these medicinals, the patient's emotions had calmed, her insomnia had abated, her FBG was 8.2mmol/L, and the glycosuria was (++). At that time, 10 more *ji* were prescribed, and, on the next return visit, all the patient's symptoms had been alleviated. Her blood and urine glucose tests were now within normal ranges. Then *Bai Zi Yang Xin Wan* (Biota Seed Nourish the Heart Pills) and *Chai Hu Shu Gan San* (Bupleurum Course the Liver Powder) were prescribed. On follow-up after two years, there had been no recurrence of the above symptoms.

CASE 2[7]

The patient was a 58 year old male who had had diabetes for eight years. He was taking 80mg of gliclazide twice a day. He had tried hypoglycemic medicines with no result, and his blood glucose levels fluctuated unstably. The patient was usually irritable, had a dry mouth, heart vexation, and irritability, was easily angered, had profuse dreams, and was easily frightened. In addition, there was profuse sweating, frequent urination, a red tongue, and a fine, rapid pulse. His blood pressure was 17/11kPa, FBG was 12.5mmol/L, and glycosuria was (+++). There were no other remarkable symptoms.

Based on these signs and symptoms, the patient's Chinese medical pattern was categorized as yin vacuity with fire effulgence. Therefore, the treatment principles were to enrich yin and clear the liver, drain fire and quiet the spirit. The formula prescribed was *Zi Shui Qing Gan Yin Jia Jian* (Enrich Water & Clear the Liver Drink with Additions & Subtractions): Magnetitum (*Ci Shi*), 30g decocted first, uncooked Radix Rehmanniae (*Sheng Di*), Plastrum Testudinis (*Gui Ban*), and Rhizoma Anemarrhenae Aspheloidis (*Zhi Mu*), 20g each, Concha Ostreae (*Mu Li*), 18g, decocted first, Concha Margaritiferae (*Zhen Zhu Mu*), also decocted first, Radix Dioscoreae Oppositae (*Shan Yao*), and Radix Albus Paeoniae Lactiflorae (*Bai Shao*), 15g each, Sclerotium Poriae Cocos (*Fu Ling*), Cortex Radicis Moutan (*Dan Pi*), and Fructus Gardeniae Jasminoidis (*Zhi Zi*), 12g each, and Rhizoma Alismatis (*Ze Xie*), 10g. One *ji* was decocted in water and administered each day for 10 days. After taking these medicinals, the patient's vexation and dry mouth had considerably improved and only the profuse sweating persisted. At that time, Herba Agrimoniae Pilosae (*Xian He Cao*), Fructus Corni Officinalis (*Shan Zhu Yu*), and

Cortex Eucommiae Ulmoidis (*Du Zhong*) were added to the formula and another 10 *ji* were prescribed. After that, the FBG was reduced to 8.1mmol/L. Still another 10 *ji* were prescribed and then the symptoms were finally alleviated. For the next two months, the patient took the basic formula without *Ci Shi*, and the anxiety was alleviated, while blood glucose levels remained normal.

REMARKS:

1. If negative emotions last a long time or are intense, patients should be referred to a mental health professional.

2. Support groups are often quite useful in dealing with the negative emotions often associated with a diagnosis of diabetes.

3. The above pattern discrimination is only a broad, general discussion of the Chinese medical treatment of psychological disturbances in patients with diabetes. Depending on the patient's age, sex, constitution, diet, lifestyle, and treatment, there are a number of other patterns individual patients may display. Therefore, for a more complete discussion of the Chinese medical treatment of psychological disturbances in general, the reader is referred to Bob Flaws and James Lake's *Chinese Medical Psychiatry*, also published by Blue Poppy Press.

4. Acupuncture can be especially effective for immediately resolving depression and quieting the spirit.

ENDNOTES:

[1] www.womenshealthmatters.ca/centres/diabetes/emotions/common.htm
[2] American Diabetes Association, *Complete Guide to Diabetes*, Bantam Books, NY, 1999, p. 373
[3] www.theime.de/ppmp/03_00/169.htm
[4] *Ibid.*
[5] www.womenshealthmatters.ca/*op./cit.*
[6] Qu Li-qing, "A Discussion of Pattern Discrimination in the Treatment of Diabetic Psychological Disturbance," *Shan Dong Zhong Yi Za Zhi* (*Shandong Journal of Chinese Medicine*), #11, 1999, p. 496-497
[7] *Ibid.*, p. 496-497

27
SYNDROME X

In 1988, Dr. Gerald Reaven, in an acceptance speech for the Banting Award from the American Diabetes Association, first described a constellation of six metabolic abnormalities he labeled syndrome X. These metabolic changes include glucose intolerance, insulin resistance, hyperinsulinemia, hypertriglyceridemia, low high-density lipoprotein (HDL), and hypertension. Today, some doctors and researchers also include blood-clotting or dysfibrinoloysis.[1] All these abnormalities increase the risk of heart attack. Although patients with syndrome X do not have diabetes, this syndrome is associated with blood sugar metabolism abnormalities or dysglycemia and, in many cases, does lead to eventual diabetes. Therefore, we have chosen to include a short discussion of syndrome X in this work. Other names for syndrome X include insulin resistance syndrome, polymetabolic syndrome, cardiovascular dysmetabolic syndrome, and visceral fat syndrome. This syndrome is primarily found in developed countries. It is estimated that one in every 3-4 Americans (i.e., 60-75 million persons) is at risk for developing syndrome X. Other sources say that two-thirds of all Americans have syndrome X,[2] and half or more heart attacks occur because of syndrome X.[3]

In terms of the causes of syndrome X, it is a multifactorial condition which develops as a result of the interaction between one's lifestyle (including diet) and genes. Insulin resistance occurs when the normal amount of insulin secreted by the pancreas is not able to unlock the doors to the cells for the transport of serum glucose into the cells. When this occurs, the pancreas secretes additional insulin. This results in hyperinsulinemia. If the cells continue to resist or do not respond to even high levels of plasma insulin, glucose builds up in the blood, thus leading to hyperglycemia and eventual type 2 diabetes. However, if this additional secretion of insulin is able to push the glucose into the cells, the person's blood glucose

levels may be normal or only slightly elevated. The complex process whereby insulin facilitates the transportation of serum glucose into the cells depends on many genes, and it is currently believed that insulin resistance is a combination of genetic flaws rather than the fault of a single gene. It is now known that persons of non-European ancestry are more likely to be insulin resistant than those of European ancestry.[4]

However, genetic predisposition is only responsible for half the causes of syndrome X. The other half is attributable to lifestyle. The specific lifestyle characteristics that have been identified as risk factors for syndrome X are: excessive body weight, insufficient physical exercise, tobacco smoke inhalation, alcohol intake, and diet. The more overweight one is, the greater degree of insulin resistance. In particular, it is central obesity, i.e., obesity of the central trunk (or gut), that is particularly at fault, and increased physical exercise is able to reduce body weight. In terms of diet, insulin resistance is caused, in large part, by over consumption of refined carbohydrates, such as breads, pastas, and sugary foods. In addition, eating too many saturated fats (found in beef), omega-6 fatty acids (found in vegetable oils), and trans-fatty acids (found in margarine and foods containing partially hydrogenated oils) also increases the risk of insulin resistance.[5] One explanation for this is that, when a person eats a lot of refined carbohydrates year after year, a dangerous cascade occurs. Insulin levels remain chronically high, and the cells become less responsive and thus resistant to the insulin. As a consequence, relatively little glucose gets burned and levels in the blood remain high. If the glucose levels in the blood are chronically elevated, insulin resistance evolves into diabetes.

When blood glucose is steadily higher than normal

(above 120mg/dL), it auto-oxidizes and spins off free radicals. Free radicals are molecules with an unpaired electron which can react pathologically with normal molecules in the body. These free radicals oxidize cholesterol. This is called lipid peroxidation and sets the stage for coronary heart disease.[6] Excessive free radical burden and oxidation, which can be measured in the urine and/or serum, is called oxidative stress. In addition, insulin helps convert calories into triglycerides and cholesterol, thus further setting the stage for atherosclerosis and coronary heart disease.[7] According to our coauthor, Dr. Robert Casañas, there are four mechanisms by which insulin resistance leads to hypertension:

1. Excessive renal sodium reabsorption
2. Activation of the sympathetic nervous system
3. Altered vascular function
     a. Endothelial cell dysfunction
     b. Smooth muscle cell dysfunction
     c. Altered cation fluxes
4. Atherosclerosis

Almost all individuals with type 2 diabetes and many with hypertension, cardiovascular disease, and obesity are insulin resistant. In the U.S., these diseases and conditions are among the leading contributors to morbidity and mortality.[8]

There are no outward physical signs of insulin resistance *per se*, and it is estimated that 20-25% of the healthy population may be insulin resistant.[9] A definitive diagnosis of insulin resistance as of this writing requires complicated, unpleasant, and expensive serum analysis. However, some of the early nonspecific signs and symptoms include feeling mentally and physically sluggish, especially after eating, and a steady upward creep of weight, blood pressure, blood sugar, cholesterol, and triglycerides year by year after 35. Optimally, blood pressure should be less than 130/85, while fasting blood sugar should be under 110 (under 100 even better). According to researcher Jean-Pierre Despres, Ph.D., a waistline over 39 inches in both men and women usually indicates the presence of syndrome X. Despres says, "The best correlate of the insulin resistance syndrome is too much abdominal-visceral fat."[10] Another indication is the ratio of total cholesterol to high-density lipoprotein, the so-called "good cholesterol." When one divides the HDL number into the total cholesterol number, 4 or over places one at risk for heart disease in general, while a ratio over 5 points specifically to syndrome X. This is even if the total cholesterol is under 200. In one study, people with total cholesterol under 200 but a high ratio between total cholesterol and

HDL accounted for one-third of heart attacks.[11] Another suggestor of syndrome X according to Dr. William Castelli, *Prevention* medical advisor, are triglycerides above 150mg/dL.[12]

The Western medical treatment of syndrome X consists primarily of increased exercise and reduction of total calories to lose weight plus a diet low in saturated fat (less than 10% of total calories) and moderate in total fat content (40% of total calories). According to Dr. Reaven, the remaining calories should be divided into 15% protein and 45% carbohydrates.[13] In addition, cessation of smoking and lowering of or moderation in alcohol consumption are also suggested. This diet plan can reduce elevated insulin levels, lower elevated triglycerides, and raise HDL. If there is hypertension which has not responded to these diet and lifestyle changes, this should be treated by ACE inhibitors followed, as needed, by calcium channel blockers. Thiazide diuretics and beta-blockers may increase insulin resistance and, therefore, should not be used in patients with syndrome X. In terms of nutritional supplements, research suggests that daily supplementation of at least 600mg of alpha-lipoic acid may stimulate insulin activity and, hence, lower and stabilize glucose levels. Other supplements capable of lowering and/or stabilizing glucose levels include vanadium, chromium, omega-3 fatty acids (found in fish oils), and vitamin E (400 IU or more per day).

Chinese medicine & syndrome X

As yet, the authors have failed to find any Chinese medical articles specifically on syndrome X. However, there are a number of published Chinese articles on insulin resistance. One of these articles is on insulin resistance and hypertension. Since these are two of the salient features of syndrome X, we believe this article and the study it describes does shed some light on the Chinese medical patterns most commonly associated with this syndrome. The article was written by Zhang Yu-jin and Zhang Wen-zhi and its title is, "An Exploration of the Pattern Discrimination of Hypertension & Insulin Resistance."[14] There were a total of 65 patients in this study, all of whom were diagnosed with hypertension according to 1978 WHO criteria. Forty-five of these patients were seen as in-patients and 20 as out-patients. Thirty-six were men and 29 were women. Their ages ranged from 45-67 years, with a median age of 54.1 ± 7.2 years. Their course of disease (*i.e.*, hypertension) had lasted from 1-21 years, with a mean duration of 11.7 ± 6.8 years. Sixteen patients had first degree hypertension, 42 had second degree hypertension, and eight had third degree hypertension. Four cases had coronary artery disease, four had concomitant cerebral sclerosis and coronary artery disease, and three simply had concomitant cerebral sclerosis. Patients with secondary hypertension, diabetes, or liver or kidney disease were excluded from this study.

The patterns of the patients in this study were discriminated according to Chinese medical theory into four basic patterns: 1) phlegm dampness congestion and exuberance pattern, 2) ascendant liver yang hyperactivity pattern, 3) liver-kidney yin vacuity pattern, and 4) yin and yang dual vacuity pattern. The ratio of male to female patients manifesting the first two patterns was 23:12, while for the second two patterns, it was 13:17. Patients with patterns #1 and 2 had the highest body mass indices (BMI), being $24.60 \pm 1.71 kg/m^2$ and $22.88 \pm 1.34 kg/m^2$ respectively. The BMI of the latter two groups was 21.78 ± 0.90 and 22.90 ± 1.31 respectively, and the median BMI of the control group was 22.15 ± 1.23. Although the yin and yang vacuity pattern patients had the highest mean systolic pressures, the patients with pattern #2 and 1 had the second and third highest mean systolic pressures *and* the two highest diastolic pressures. In addition, the average age of patients with pattern #1 was 48.7, while the average age of patients with pattern #4 was 62.3. Further, the disease course of patients with pattern #1 was the shortest, averaging 7.9 years, and the disease course of patients with pattern #4 was the longest, averaging 14.8 years. The disease course of patients with pattern #3 averaged 12.2 years.

Blood glucose, insulin, and C-peptide reactivity were tested on an empty stomach and two hours after a meal to compare the insulin resistance in the hypertensive group to a normotensive group of 15 subjects of similar age and sex. Results showed no statistically significant difference (P>0.05) in fasting blood glucose between these two groups. However, two hours after eating, there was a statistically marked difference between blood glucose, insulin, and C-peptides between the comparison group and patients with patterns #1 and 2 (P<0.01), while there was no marked difference in these parameters between the control group and patients with patterns #3 and 4 (P>0.05). Based on these findings, Zhang and Zhang concluded that a high BMI, insulin resistance, and hypertension are associated with the two patterns of phlegm dampness congestion and exuberance and ascendant liver yang hyperactivity.

While this is only one study, it does suggest that patients with syndrome X should first be examined for the presence of either phlegm dampness or yang hyperactivity. The diagnostic criteria Zhang and Zhang give for phlegm dampness are: dizziness, headache, chest oppression, ductal distention, a bland taste in the mouth, reduced appetite, a fat tongue with slimy, white fur, and a slippery pulse. The diagnostic criteria they give for yang hyperactivity include: headache, head distention, dizziness, tinnitus, tenseness, agitation, easy anger, a red tongue with thin fur, and a bowstring pulse. Of course, in real life, phlegm dampness may complicate yang hyperactivity. In Chinese medicine, adipose tissue is seen as nothing other than an accumulation of phlegm, dampness, and turbidity. This study also suggests, at least to us, that it is the point at which repletion transforms into vacuity that separates syndrome X from diabetes.

As for the Chinese medical treatment of syndrome X, this should be based on each patient's personal pattern discrimination. However, since patients with syndrome X do have hypertension and hyperlipidemia, one should be able to find an appropriate Chinese medicinal and/or acupuncture treatment plan under the patterns of phlegm dampness or yang hyperactivity in the chapters on diabetic hypertension and diabetic hyperlipoproteinemia. For instance, ascendant liver yang hyperactivity is the first pattern in the chapter on diabetic hypertension, and phlegm dampness obstructing the center is the third. According to Zhang and Zhang, medicinals given on the basis of pattern discrimination can improve the therapeutic effects in the treatment of insulin resistance and hypertension.

ENDNOTES:

[1] www.syndromexweb.com/sxwhat.htm
[2] www.healthwell.com/delicious-online/D_Backs/Jan_01/syndrome.cfm
[3] www.syndromexweb.com, *op. cit.*
[4] www.syndromexweb.com/learncauses.htm
[5] www.syndrome-x.com
[6] *Ibib.*
[7] *Ibid.*
[8] http://syndromex.standford.edu/InsulinResistance.htm
[9] *Ibid.*
[10] www.prevention.com/healing/living/synx.htm
[11] *Ibid.*
[12] *Ibid.*
[13] www.syndromexweb.com/preventsteps.htm
[14] Zhang Yu-jin & Zhang Wen-zhi, "An Exploration of the Pattern Discrimination of Hypertension & Insulin Resistance," *He Nan Zhong Yi (Henan Chinese Medicine)*, #1, 2001, p. 35-36

28

PATIENT ADHERENCE
& PRACTITIONER MONITORING

The Chinese medical treatment of diabetes is a long-term affair. While some patients diagnosed with type 2 DM may be cured in 6-12 weeks with acupuncture, dietary therapy, exercise therapy, and/or Chinese medicinals,[1] many patients with type 2 diabetes and virtually all type 1 DM patients require treatment over years or even tens of years. In such patients, adherence or compliance to the treatment regime may become an issue as well as monitoring the patient and periodically changing the treatment plan.

PATIENT ADHERENCE

Patient adherence[2] means the patient's willingness and ability to stick to the treatment plan as envisaged by the prescribing practitioner. In order to achieve optimal patient adherence, the practitioner should begin by assessing the patient's knowledge about their condition and about the process of Chinese medicine. For instance, it must be explained to the patient that their Chinese medical treatment is directed at rebalancing the imbalance implied by the name of their Chinese medical pattern(s). It is not predicated on their disease diagnosis alone or even primarily. Therefore, they should report any change in their signs and symptoms to the prescribing practitioner. If signs and symptoms change, that means their pattern probably has as well, and that typically means they need a new acupuncture and/or Chinese medical prescription. It is important to explain to patients that any major change in their signs and symptoms may require a new Chinese prescription. Blindly taking the old prescription will not achieve its desired effect and may even have a negative effect. The more patients understand about their Chinese pattern discrimination and the Chinese rationale for their treatment plan, the more likely they are to adhere to that treatment plan correctly.

Secondly, the practitioner should also do everything possible to empower the patient. This means explaining to the patient all he or she can do for themselves. This includes dietary and exercise therapies as well as other self-treatments, such as Chinese self-massage or acupressure. The more the patient feels they are in control of their situation, the better they will feel about their situation, including their medical treatment. Therefore, although discussions about Chinese dietary therapy, etc. may seem time-consuming and tedious to the practitioner, they typically pay off in the long run with better, more enthusiastic adherence. One of the benefits of the Chinese medical methodology of basing treatment on pattern discrimination as opposed to solely on disease diagnosis is that the terminology of Chinese medicine is based on everyday consensual reality in the phenomenal world. Although concepts such as qi, yin, and yang may initially sound foreign and have to be explained, everyone can immediately understand concepts such as dryness, dampness, and heat. Likewise, the concepts of qi stagnation, blood stasis, and phlegm are not that difficult to understand. Once one knows their condition is too hot and too dry, then it is easy to understand what one can do to keep from aggravating that heat and dryness. In comparison, being told that one is insulin resistant or glucose intolerant leaves most patients feeling powerless. One of Chinese medicine's greatest gifts to patients is its ability to empower patients with everyday explanations based on metaphors from the natural world, and we believe that every practitioner should make maximum conscious use of this ability of Chinese medicine.

ADDRESSING PHYSICAL & TEMPORAL LIMITATIONS

Practitioners should address any physical and temporal

limitations which may adversely affect the patient's adherence to their treatment plan. For instance, patients with advanced retinopathy may not be able to come frequently for in-office acupuncture treatment if they cannot drive themself. In that case, patients may be better served by internally administered Chinese medicinals and Chinese self-massage which they can do in the confines of their own home. Similarly, patients on long-term Chinese medicinal therapy may find the decocting of bulk-dispensed medicinals time-consuming and, therefore, their adherence may falter. In that case, convenient ready-made pills or desiccated extracts should be used instead. Although these forms of administration may not be as potent in terms of dosages delivered as decoctions nor as easily modified, regular, long-term adherence may be more important in the long run.

EVALUATING FINANCIAL RESOURCES

Not all people have health care insurance and, even among those that do, not all health care insurance policies pay for acupuncture and Chinese medicine. To make matters worse, diabetes tends to be a disease of the elderly, and many of the elderly are on fixed incomes with only so much they can spend on health care. While Chinese medicine is often cheaper than modern Western medicine, most patients with diabetes in the West will probably be on a combination of Chinese and Western medicine if they are using Chinese medicine at all. In general, internally administered Chinese medicinals are cheaper than acupuncture treatments when compared month by month. Therefore, practitioners should evaluate the relative costs and benefits of the various therapies they have to offer any given patient keeping in mind the patient's typically finite resources. There is little value in initiating a long-term course of acupuncture which the patient does not stick with because it simply costs too much. Thus, if the practitioner chooses to administer acupuncture either instead of or in addition to internally administered Chinese medicinals, there should be a sound medical reason for this decision. For instance, a course of electroacupuncture might be used specifically to treat a lower leg ulcer. However, as soon as that ulcer has healed, acupuncture might be terminated and the patient may return to only taking their internally administered Chinese medicinals.

EVALUATING SOCIAL SUPPORTS

As mentioned above, some of the complications of diabetes may require the assistance of friends or family members for transportation or even the administration of home therapies. An example would be doing skin-needling on the back transport points. This therapy needs to be done daily in order to achieve much of a result. However, people cannot tap the points on their own backs. Therefore, there has to be a friend or family member willing and capable to do this for the patient. Slightly different is the patient's family's attitude toward Chinese medicine. For instance, if a husband or wife objects to the smell of decocting bulk-dispensed Chinese medicinals, this may affect the patient's adherence. This means that the practitioner may not only have to explain their therapy to the patient but also the patient's spouse or other caretaker, helping to ensure that they are also willing to participate wholeheartedly in the patient's treatment plan.

COMPETING FACTORS

Health is only one of the valuables in life. For many people, the self-esteem that comes from successfully fulfilling their ambitions are also just as or even more valuable than health. Therefore, the practitioner needs to be clear about any competing factors that may affect the patient's adherence to their treatment plan. For some patients, some treatments may just not be worth it. For instance, some patients may say they do not have the time to exercise or they do not have the time to come for acupuncture. Others may say they cannot live without this or that "comfort" food. Yet others may be afraid of certain therapies, for instance, acupuncture. The more patient and practitioner are clear about such competing factors, the more realistic everyone's expectations will be about treatment outcomes. The practitioner is, ultimately, simply a resource person. The patient must choose whether to use that resource or not to its fullest potential. The practitioner should explain the probable outcomes of choosing not to adhere to a particular treatment plan, but it is the patient, after all, who must make that choice.

SETTING REALISTIC GOALS

When dealing with diabetes, results are not just measured in the severity of clinical symptoms. Much of the progress or lack of it in the treatment of patients with diabetes is monitored by tests such as blood glucose, urine glucose, glycosylated hemoglobin, and blood pressure. Because people are people and life is not perfect, patient and practitioner need to set realistic goals in terms of the outcomes of these various tests. When patients set realistic goals and then achieve those goals, they are more likely to stick with their treatment plan. This may mean that the patient sets a goal that is less than what the practitioner believes is theoretically ideal. While the practitioner may wish for tight glycemic control, the patient may be willing to settle for less once he or she understands both the short- and long-term costs involved. In other words, although ideal goals are ideal, neither we or our patients live in an ideal world, and everyone should try to keep a realistic view of what is and is not possible in terms of treatment outcomes. As the reader has already seen, in the overwhelming majority of clinical audits reported in this book, only a percentage of patients in a given study were cured, while most experienced varying degrees of partial improvement.

MONITORING CLOSELY

As should by now be clear, the diagnosis and tracking of diabetes is closely related to various numerical test indices. While these tests cannot be used by themselves to establish a Chinese medical pattern discrimination, they are important and useful tools in tracking the patient's response to treatment. Therefore, practitioners of Chinese medicine should encourage their diabetes patients to adhere to the schedule of monitoring these indices established by their Western medical practitioner and they should take these indices into account in their own treatment planning. In general, if blood glucose is stable, monitoring should be carried out by the patient 2-3 times per week. However, if blood glucose is unstable or the patient is on insulin, monitoring should be done 2-3 times per day. Ideal fasting blood glucose should be between 80-120mg/dL. Ideal bedtime blood glucose should be between 100-140mg/dL, and ideal glycosylated hemoglobin should be less than seven percent and should be measured every three months.

CHANGING THE TREATMENT PLAN

When changing the patient's Chinese medicinal treatment plan, the best rule is to "go slow and low." This means not making radical changes over a short period of time (except, of course, in an emergency situation) and starting out with low doses and increasing these doses as necessary. As the reader will have seen, it is not uncommon for Chinese doctors to use quite high doses of certain Chinese medicinals in the treatment of diabetes and its complications. Frequently, these high doses are necessary to achieve the desired results. This is typical of many difficult to treat, knotty diseases. Nevertheless, it is always best to use the lowest possible dose which gets the desired effect, rather than overdosing, creating adverse reactions, and then having to lower the dose.

One should consider changing the patient's Chinese med-

ical treatment plan if FBG is over 140mg/dL or PPBG is over 180mg/dL. These levels suggest that more optimal levels of blood glucose might be striven for. However, one may accept higher blood glucose levels in the elderly in order to avoid hypoglycemia, since the elderly are at risk for the complications of hypoglycemia. On the other hand, glycosylated hemoglobin (HbA1c) below seven percent suggests that the treatment plan is working well and that a change to a less aggressive plan may be in order. This may mean lowering doses of Chinese medicinals and/or switching to pills or desiccated extracts. Likewise, improvements in other comorbidities, lipids, blood pressure, or smoking may suggest that the patient's treatment plan may need to be adjusted downward or relaxed.

ALLOWING THE PATIENT PERIODIC RESTS

It is common in Chinese medicine to allow patients a 3-5 day to one week rest between successive courses of treatment in those with chronic conditions requiring long-term care. These periodic rests allow the patient's system to dehabituate to the Chinese medicinals. Typically, after such a rest, the patient and practitioner may see a noticeable leap forward even though the dose and composition of the formula may remain unchanged. Similar periodic rests are also allowed to those undergoing long-term courses of acupuncture.

DIABETES & DENIAL

Denial is a psychological process that is learned and used as a defense mechanism. The process of denial is an unconscious reaction that offers protection to the self from stressful situations. Sometimes denial serves a purpose. It is a way of coping with bad news. It can keep the patient from becoming overwhelmed and depressed. It lets them accept news little by little and in their own time, when they are ready. However, denial is commonly met in patients with diabetes and seriously affects the prognosis of this disease. For instance, denying that diabetes is serious allows the patient to avoid self-care. It insulates them from the fact that diabetes is a lifelong, chronic illness which, if left untreated, can result in potentially life-threatening or at least disabling complications. Denial also allows the patient's family and friends to pretend that "nothing is wrong." Most people go through at least some level of denial when they are first diagnosed with diabetes. This first reaction is not the real problem. In fact, it is so common that some doctors think it is part of the process of or stage in accepting the diagnosis of diabetes mellitus. The real trouble comes when the patient continues to deny their diabetes. Long-term denial prevents them from learning what they need to know to keep themselves healthy.

In our personal experience as clinicians, many patients with diabetes are angry at the diabetes itself for changing their lives. They see the world as unfair because they have diabetes. Ironically, they feel worse and take care of themselves less as their anger continues to grow. The demands of diabetes self-management are relentless. Those with diabetes must perform a number of life-altering tasks every day, day in and day out, to control their glucose levels. There can be no departure from the schedule, and many patients with diabetes do not have the patience necessary to perform this kind of discipline. Instead, they may become angry at their physician or health care provider for advising them to adhere to such a program, and, in the end, may not be willing even to see their physician since they do not want to be reminded of their failure to meet this responsibility.

Anger also manifests in those patients with diabetes who are very dedicated to their treatment programs but who do not experience as good results as either they were told they would or they would like. As a result, they not only feel anger but also guilt and blame for doing something wrong even though it is not their fault. Since treatment plans for diabetes work differently for every patient, each patient reacts differently to their treatment regime. Therefore, practitioners should not hold those with diabetes to impossible treatment plans. Otherwise, patients will be overwhelmed by their self-care duties and finally deny that they must self-care at all.

Because denial plays a role in any or all aspects of diabetes self-care, it can be very dangerous. Any denial sabotages the diabetes patient's health care. Patients may not bother to check their blood glucose regularly. They may claim that, since they feel all right, there is no need to check these levels. Patients may ignore their meal plans. Changing life-long eating habits and food preferences is difficult. In addition, the diabetes patient may think that their families will not accept such changes in diet and meal times, that it is too expensive to eat properly, or that

there is no healthy food accessible at their workplace. Diabetes patients may also not care for their feet daily, often continue to smoke, and often ignore advice on exercise and lifestyle changes. The stress of daily diabetes management can build. The patient may feel alone or set apart from friends and family because of this extra burden. If the patient faces diabetes complications, such as neuropathy, or if they are having trouble controlling blood glucose levels, they may feel as though they are losing the battle against diabetes. Even tension between the patient and the doctor may result in frustration and sadness. If the patient is depressed and has no energy, then even the task of regular blood glucose testing may become too much. Likewise, if they feel so anxious they cannot think straight, it will be difficult to maintain a good diet. The patient may even not feel like eating at all which, in turn, will affect their glucose levels.

In our experience, the best antidote to denial in patients with diabetes is education. Practitioners must be aware that patients with diabetes easily fall through the loopholes in their care and maintenance. Partly, this is due to their non-adherence to such programs, and, partly, it is due to their denial that treatment plans are important. Follow-up care and continued monitoring should be at the forefront of the management of every case of diabetes, and practitioners should seek to involve the patient's family and close friends in this care. In addition, treatment plans should be designed with the patient in mind and should not be prescribed as "one size fits all," theoretical programs without flexibility and adaptability. Since each diabetes patient's experience with this disease is unique, each treatment program for such patients should reflect that uniqueness.

ENDNOTES:

[1] Although some Western authorities believe that diabetes mellitus cannot be cured, it is the position and the experience of many Chinese doctors that it can. Therefore, our use of this controversial word is based on the Chinese medical usage of its Chinese equivalent, yu (愈).

[2] Adherence is also called compliance. However, recently some have argued that the term compliance is too passive and implies a top-down hierarchical relationship with the patient.

29

INTEGRATING CHINESE & WESTERN MEDICINES

In the course of day-to-day clinical practice in the West, acupuncturists and practitioners of Chinese medicine are often asked to treat patients who are currently taking one or more Western prescription drugs, and this is especially the case when it comes to diabetes mellitus and its many complications. In addition, many of these patients would prefer not to be on those Western drugs. Therefore, Western practitioners of Chinese medicine frequently have two questions: 1) Should they start administering Chinese medicinals while the patient is concurrently taking Western medications, and 2), if so, how should they adjust or discontinue Western medications for patients making this request?

HERB-DRUG INTERACTIONS

The first concern has to do with the question of the established safety or inherent risk involved in combining Western pharmaceuticals with Chinese medicinals. Unfortunately, at this time, this is largely *terra incognita*, as all the potential interactions between Western and Chinese medicinals have not been clearly established. Conversely, we know of no published Chinese sources suggesting that certain specific Chinese medicinals should not be taken with certain specific Western medicinals.[1] However, a number of anecdotal reports of toxic or lethal interactions suggest that a conservative approach should be followed when Chinese medicinals and Western pharmaceuticals are used concurrently. For example, several deaths have been reported among chronic hepatitis patients in Japan taking *Xiao Chai Hu Tang* (Minor Bupleurum Decoction) along with interferon.[2]

In spite of many newly formed information services or initiatives to monitor and improve quality control of Chinese medicinal herbs, at present there is no definitive database detailing reported or potential medicinal interactions. This situation is made even more complex due to the fact that Chinese doctors prescribe multivalent doses of multi-ingredient formulas. Therefore, our conservative recommendation to Western Chinese medical practitioners is to do what they do in China: proceed cautiously, prescribing only small initial doses for a few days in order to monitor for any unwanted or potentially dangerous drug side effects or interactions. This conservative approach can be extended to the recommendation that doses should be increased only in the absence of unwanted effects. In view of the paucity of published studies documenting the safety of combining specific Chinese and Western medicines, many Western physicians may be reluctant to assume the risk of advising or even permitting their patients to take Chinese medicinals concurrently with Western synthetic medicines. However, it is our hope that the extensive case histories and research abstracts included throughout this book will serve to allay such fears. In the People's Republic of China, Chinese medicinals are routinely prescribed with such oral hypoglycemics as glyburide and biguanide as well as with insulin, and we have failed to find a single published article that describes an adverse reaction from such a combination.

Happily, the Center for Complementary and Alternative Medicine at the U.S. National Institutes of Health (NIH) has acknowledged the inherent difficulties in the clinical study of compound Chinese herbal formulas, and, recently, the NIH waived a previous requirement for studies verifying that every possible combination of Chinese medicinal and Western pharmaceutical is safe. Subsequently, the NIH has given permission to the Food and Drug Administration (FDA) to register such formulas as "safe for investigational purposes." We believe this cautious but progressive attitude is an appropriate stance to take when dealing with clinical issues related to lack of knowledge and evolving standards of practice surrounding uses of Chinese medicines in Western countries. Chinese medicine has been used safely in China by millions of people for thousands of years. A recent poll in the People's Republic of China confirmed that a majority of Chinese citizens who use Chinese medicines report few, minor, or no side effects. The results of this survey suggest that the majority of Chinese believe that Chinese medicines can cure diseases in cases where Western medicine offers little help.[3] The authors feel strongly that it would be unreasonable to not take advantage of the vast body of accumulated Chinese medical knowledge because contemporary Western scientific approaches to verification of efficacy or mechanism of action have not yet strongly endorsed many uses of Chinese medicine. Only by employing Chinese medical therapeutics in a Western milieu can clinicians and researchers begin to more completely understand fundamental aspects of Chinese medicine.

STICKING TO ONE'S SCOPE OF PRACTICE

The progress of therapy in those with diabetes can be and typically is monitored by a number of different objective tests, such as blood glucose, urine glucose, and glycolated hemoglobin tests. Since many patients with diabetes monitor themselves on a regular basis, if they see improvement in these tests due to taking Chinese medicinals in addition to their Western drugs, it is not uncommon for them to ask their Chinese medical practitioner if and how they can reduce the doses of those Western drugs, many of which have the potential for a number of short- and long-term side effects. However, all three authors feel strongly that all questions of changing or discontinuing Western medications brought to the attention of a Chinese medical practitioner should be referred to the patient's Western physician. At this point in time, Chinese medical practitioners are not trained in Western medical pharmacology and are, therefore, not in a position to provide competent or safe advice to patients. The only exception to this general rule are Chinese medical practitioners who have been dually trained *and licensed* to practice Western medicine. The patient's Western physician is the legally licensed prescribing physician and, therefore, the clinician with *sole* authority to recommend dosing changes, alternative Western medications, or discontinuation of Western medications. Further, in most if not all states in the United States, it is illegal for Chinese medical practitioners to offer specific advice concerning dosage or discontinuation of Western medications being used by patients under their care.

Therefore, it follows that, in cases when a patient is taking Western medications while undergoing Chinese medical treatment and reports signs or symptoms suggesting a need for re-evaluation of current medications, the patient should be referred back to his or her prescribing Western physician for consultation. Subsequently, the question of deciding whether, when, or how to discontinue Western medications will be addressed between the patient and his or her Western physician. The authors feel strongly that it is the Chinese medical practitioner's ethical responsibility to contact the patient's Western physician or other medical providers in order to explain Chinese medical treatments being provided and the rationale for such treatments.[4] However, the authors can think of no instance in which it is or should be the Chinese medical practitioner's responsibility or role to adjust Western medications or advise patients about Western medical care, other than to refer the patient back to their prescribing physician. Hopefully, by sharing the research included in this book, the patient's Western MD will be able to make a more informed decision regarding such adjustments.

MAINTAINING A BROAD-MINDED POINT OF VIEW

Westerners, both patients and practitioners, are recent converts to Chinese medicine, and, like converts the world over, there is a tendency to be even more stringent and orthodox in our beliefs than those who have grown up within a system of belief. Regrettably, some Western practitioners of Chinese medicine are just as dogmatic in their anti-Western medical stance as are some ultraconservative MDs in their dismissal of Chinese medicine. Similarly, some Western patients distrust everything manufactured by Western pharamceutical companies. However, we believe there is no ontological difference between Western and Chinese medicinals. Ultimately, both are composed of chemicals which react biochemically within the patient's body. While it may be argued that phytochemicals may be more "rounded" or buffered in their effect, they are, nevertheless, chemicals. Therefore, rather than arguing over such amorphous concepts as "natural," we believe we would be better served by recognizing that the true worth of any medicinal, no matter what its source, is whether or not it achieves its intended therapeutic effects without causing any short- or long-term adverse reactions. If a medicinal achieves its intended effects in a particular patient without any short- or long-term adverse reactions, than that medicinal is a good one in that instance.

Medicinals are tools and, as such, are neither good or bad

in and of themselves. When a medicinal causes a side effect, it means that that dose of that medicinal was inappropriate for that patient at that time. It is our belief that prescribing Western medicinals according to Chinese medical pattern discrimination would help in minimizing their side effects. In that case, we have no *a priori* objection to their use, and we hope that our Western Chinese medical colleagues may also come to the same conclusion. According to Prof. Zhang Su-qing of Xian, in the early stage of diabetes, orally administered Chinese medicines alone, even ready-made Chinese medicines such as *Xiao Tang Pian* (Disperse Sugar Tablets), are sufficient to markedly reduce glucose levels. However, in the middle and late stages, small amounts of Western antidiabetic drugs plus Chinese medicinals get significantly better results than Western medicines alone and can A) reduce the adverse reactions of those Western medicines, and B) markedly prevent cardiac, cerebral, and nephrotic complications.[5] As the many case histories and clinical audits included in this book show, Chinese and Western medicines are routinely integrated in the People's Republic of China. Although such integration can be done shoddily and in such a way as to be detrimental to the long-term evolution of Chinese medicine, it does not have to be done poorly. It is our personal experience that such an integration can be done in such a way that both medicines

are enriched and enhanced, impoverishing neither. It is also our experience that such an integration is more effective for treating such typically complex geriatric conditions as diabetes mellitus than either system alone. Therefore we encourage both Chinese and Western medical practitioners to remain as broad-minded and collegial as possible—if not for our own benefit, then for our patients' sakes.

ENDNOTES:

[1] John Chen has made some suggestions along these lines (all using the verb "may"), but these suggestions seem to be based on theory as opposed to real-life case histories or clinical studies. See Chen, John, "Recognition & Prevention of Herb-Drug Interactions," *Clinical Manual of Oriental Medicine*, Lotus Herbs, La Puente, CA, 1998, p. 4/25-4/27

[2] *California Journal of Oriental Medicine*, #1, 1999, p. 48

[3] "Chinese Medicine Preferred," News, News, News, *The Journal of Chinese Medicine*, May, 1999, p. 4

[4] Practitioners should obtain written permission from their patient before contacting other health care providers and discussing the patient's care with these providers. Interestingly, 80% of "crossover" patients, *i.e.*, those simultaneously using both modern Western and alternative medicines, do not tell their Western MD about any complementary therapies they are concurrently receiving. We believe this is not only a procedural mistake but also a great wasted opportunity.

[5] Zhao Kun *et al.*, "Professor Zhang Su-qing's Experience of the Diagnosis & Treatment of Diabetes," *Xin Zhong Yi (New Chinese Medicine)*, #5, 2001, p. 15

APPENDIX A

AN ANALYSIS OF CHINESE MEDICINALS USED IN ANCIENT FORMULAS FOR THE TREATMENT OF WASTING & THIRSTING

In 1998, Zhang Hong-ying published an analysis of Chinese medicinals used in ancient formulas for the treatment of wasting and thirsting.[1] Zhang looked at nine premodern texts covering five dynasties, tabulating the frequency of use of individual medicinals in formulas indicated for wasting and thirsting. From the Tang dynasty, there were three books: *Qian Jin Yao Fang (Essential Formulas [Worth] A Thousand [Pieces of] Gold)*, *Qian Jin Yi Fang (Supplement to Formulas [Worth] A Thousand [Pieces of] Gold)*, and *Wai Tai Bi Yao (Secret Essentials of the External Platform)*. From the Song dynasty there were two books: *Tai Ping Sheng Hui Fang (Tai Ping [Era] Imperial Grace Formulary)* and *Sheng Ji Zong Lu (Imperial Aid Assembled Records)*. From the Yuan dynasty there was one book: *Shi Yi De Xiao Fang (Effective Formulas from Generations of Physicians)*. From the Ming dynasty there was one book: *Pu Ji Fang (Universal Aid Formulas)*, and from the Qing dynasty there were two books: *Yi Bu Jin Lu (Golden Medical Records)* and *Lin Zheng Zhi Nan Yi An (Clinical Symptoms & Medical Reference)*. From these books, Zhang selected 275 medicinals from a principle group of 1282 formulas. The single medicinals with the highest frequency of use in traditional formulas for the treatment of wasting and thirsting were as follows:

MEDICINAL NAME	NUMBER OF TIMES USED	FREQUENCY
Radix Puerariae (*Ge Gen*)	564	44%
Radix Glycyrrhizae (*Gan Cao*)	415	32%
Tuber Ophiopogonis Japonici (*Mai Men Dong*)	275	21%
Radix Trichosanthis Kirlowii (*Tian Hua Fen*)	230	18%
Radix Panacis Ginseng (*Ren Shen*)	224	17%
Sclerotium Poriae Cocos (*Fu Ling*)	222	17%
Rhizoma Coptidis Chinensis (*Huang Lian*)	204	16%
Radix Scutellariae Baicalensis (*Huang Qin*)	194	15%
uncooked Gypsum Fibrosum (*Shi Gao*)	157	12%
uncooked Radix Rehmanniae (*Sheng Di*)	125	10%
Radix Et Rhizoma Rhei (*Da Huang*)	119	9%
Fructus Crataegi (*Shan Zha*)	101	8%
Radix Bupleuri (*Chai Hu*)	100	8%
Radix Astragali Membranacei (*Huang Qi*)	96	7%
Cortex Cinnamomi Cassiae (*Rou Gui*)	94	7%
Fructus Citri Aurantii (*Zhi Ke*)	90	7%
Cortex Radicis Lycii Chinensis (*Di Gu Pi*)	89	7%

Other medicinals mentioned in order of frequency were: Fructus Schisandrae Chinensis (*Wu Wei Zi*), Radix Rubrus Paeoniae Lactiflorae (*Chi Shao*), Radix Sophorae Flavescentis (*Ku Shen*), Radix Angelicae Sinensis (*Dang Gui*), Concha Ostreae (*Mu Li*), Cornu Rhinocerotis (*Xi Jiao*), Pericarpium Citri Reticulatae (*Chen Pi*), Semen Pruni Armeniacae (*Xing Ren*), Rhizoma Phragmitis Communis (*Lu Gen*), Carapax Amydae Sinensis (*Bie Jia*), Cortex Radicis Mori Albi (*Sang Bai Pi*), Mirabilitum (*Mang Xiao*), Fructus Pruni Mume (*Wu Mei*), Rhizoma Alismatis (*Ze Xie*), Herba Lophatheri Gracilis (*Dan Zhu Ye*), Radix Albus Paeoniae Lactiflorae (*Bai Shao*), Radix Platycodi Grandiflori (*Jie Geng*), and Fructus Trichosanthis Kirlowii (*Gua Lou*).

Of the 13 most commonly prescribed medicinals (more than 7% frequency), four primarily nourish yin and engender fluids: *Ge Gen*, *Mai Men Dong*, *Tian Hua Fen*, and *Sheng Di*. Three medicinals primarily boost the qi and fortify the spleen: *Gan Cao*, *Ren Shen*, and *Fu Ling*. Three are bitter, cold medicinals that clear heat: *Huang Lian*, *Huang Qin*, and uncooked *Shi Gao*. In addition, *Shan Zha* disperses food and moves stagnation, *Chai Hu* courses the liver and rectifies the qi, and *Da Huang* precipitates and frees the flow of the stools. According to Zhang, the choice of these medicinals reflects attention to both the root and branches of this disease. Interestingly, these ancient formulas for the treatment of wasting and thirsting do not include medicinals which quicken the blood and transform stasis as frequently as do Chinese medicinal formulas for diabetes today. As we have seen above, contemporary Chinese formulas for the treatment of diabetes and its complications commonly include one or more blood-quickening medicinals, such as Radix Salviae Miltiorrhizae (*Dan Shen*), Semen Pruni Persicae (*Tao Ren*), and/or Radix Rubrus Paeoniae Lactiflorae (*Chi Shao*).

Zhang also classifies these 275 medicinals according to their functions. Below, these categories are presented in descending order according to the frequency of their use:

1. Heat-clearing medicinals
2. Qi-supplementing medicinals
3. Wind heat scattering medicinals
4. Yin-supplementing medicinals
5. Heat-clearing, dampness-drying medicinals
6. Spleen-fortifying, dampness-disinhibiting medicinals
7. Qi-moving medicinals
8. Wind cold scattering medicinals
9. Heat-clearing, phlegm-transforming medicinals
10. Moistening & precipitating medicinals
11. Lung-diffusing, phlegm-transforming medicinals
12. Liver-settling, yang-subduing medicinals
13. Interior-warming medicinals
14. Blood-supplementing medicinals
15. Yang -supplementing medicinals
16. Astringing & securing medicinals
17. Urine-disinhibiting, strangury-freeing medicinals
18. Blood-quickening, stasis-dispelling medicinals
19. Vacuity heat clearing medicinals
20. Aromatic, phlegm-transforming medicinals
21. Spirit-quieting medicinals
22. Externally applied medicinals

The main roots and branches of wasting and thirsting, *i.e.*, qi and yin vacuities as roots and heat as branch, are treated by the first four categories above. The reason that wind heat scattering medicinals are used so frequently in these premodern formulas for wasting and thirsting is because *Ge Gen* and *Chai Hu* fall under this category. Although *Ge Gen* is categorized as an acrid, cool exterior-resolver, it also engenders fluids and upbears yang, thus aiding in the supplementation of both qi and yin. Likewise, although *Chai Hu* is an acrid, cool exterior-resolver, it is primarily used in the context of wasting and thirsting in order to course the liver, rectify the qi, and out-thrust depressive heat.

The authors feel that the above analysis is useful for identifying not only the main traditional Chinese medicinals used for wasting and thirsting or diabetes but also for emphasizing the main principles in the treatment of this condition. This analysis firmly underscores the primary importance of qi and yin vacuities accompanied by dryness and heat as the main disease mechanisms of this disease.

ENDNOTES:

[1] Zhang Hong-ying, "Characteristic Analysis of Medicinals Used in Ancient Formulas to Treat Wasting & Thirsting Disease," *Bei Jing Zhong Yi (Beijing Chinese Medicine)*, #3, 1998, p. 49-51

APPENDIX B

WESTERN DIABETES MEDICATIONS & THEIR POSSIBLE SIDE EFFECTS

The following are the main Western medicines currently used for the treatment of diabetes mellitus.

1. SULFONYLUREAS

Suflonylureas are a class of orally administered medications which simulate the pancreatic production of insulin and help the body utilize the insulin it makes, thus lowering blood glucose. For these medications to be effective, the pancreas must still be producing insulin on its own.

GENERIC NAMES	BRAND NAMES
acetohexamide	Dymelor
chlorpropamide	Diabinese
glimepiride	Amaryl
glipizide	Glucotrol, Glucotrol XL
glyburide	DiaBeta, Glynase PreTab, Micronase
tolazamide	Tolinase
tolbutamide	Orinase

Possible side effects from sulfonylureas include hypoglycemia, upset stomach, skin rashes and/or itching, and weight gain. Tolazamide and tolbutamide have been especially associated with atherogenesis leading to coronary artery disease.

2. BIGUANIDES

Biguanides are orally administered medications which decrease the amount of sugar made by the liver and increase the peripheral uptake of glucose. They also help correct insulin resistance and decrease lipids. They are the drug of choice for "prediabetics."

GENERIC NAMES	BRAND NAMES
metformin	Glucophage

Possible side effects from biguanides include nausea, vomiting, and diarrhea initially, fatigue, weakness, trouble breathing, a metallic taste in the mouth, aggravation of kidney problems, and lactic acidosis.

3. ALPHA-GLUCOSIDASE INHIBITORS

Alpha-glucosidase inhibitors are orally administered medications which slow the absorption of starches consumed.

GENERIC NAMES	BRAND NAMES
acarbose	Precose
miglitol	Glyset

Possible side effects of alpha-glucosidase inhibitors include stomach problems and flatulence.

4. THIAZOLIDINEDIONES

Thiazolidinediones are orally administered medications which make one more sensitive to insulin. Therefore, insulin can move more easily from the blood into the cells for energy. They also increase high density lipids, preserve B cell function, and protect vascular function.

GENERIC NAMES	BRAND NAMES
pioglitazone	Actos
rosiglitazone	Avandia

Possible side effects of thiazolidinediones include nausea, vomiting, stomach pain, lack of appetite, fatigue, yellowing of the skin and/or whites of the eyes, or dark-colored urine, possible hypoglycemia, infertility, weight gain, and edema of the lower limbs. Liver monitoring is required during use of this class of medications.

5. MEGLITINIDES

Meglitinides are orally administered medications which stimulate the pancreas to make more insulin.

GENERIC NAMES	BRAND NAMES
repaglinide	Prandin

Possible side effects of meglitinides include hypoglycemia and weight gain. Meglitinides are contraindicated in sulfa-sensitive patients, and should be used cautiously in those with hepatic and renal problems.

6. INSULINS

Insulins are, as of this writing, primarily injectable medications. They are also used in insulin pumps. However, oral and inhalable insulins are currently being developed. Insulin is used for patients whose pancreases no longer make their own insulin (type 1 DM) or for type 2 DM patients under stress, during intercurrent illness, undergoing surgery, and for gestational diabetes. Insulin lowers blood glucose by moving sugar from the blood into the cells to provide energy for life activities.

TYPES	BRAND NAMES
quick-acting	Humalog
short-acting	Regular (R) insulin
intermediate-acting	NPH(N), Lente(L), Humulin-N
long-acting	Ultralente
mixed	NPH & Regular insulin mixture

Intermediate-acting is the most frequently used of these types of insulin.

Possible side effects of insulin include hypoglycemia, insulin allergy, fat atrophy, and fat hypertrophy.

GLOSSARY

ACETONE: A chemical substance produced during the breakdown of body fat and checked in the urine when poorly controlled

ACIDOSIS: The abnormal state of too much acid in the blood. This condition can be a serious complication of type 1 diabetes or treatment with metformin.

ALBUMIN: A type of water soluble blood protein that may appear in the urine when the kidneys are damaged

ALBUMINURIA: The presence of albumin in the urine

ALPHA CELLS: A type of cell found in the islets of Langerhans which produce and secrete a hormone called glucagon (the main counter-regulatory hormone) which raises the level of glucose in the blood

AMAUROSIS DIABETICA: Complete loss of vision, especially when there is no known pathology of the eye

ARTHROPATHY: Any joint disease with or without pain (arthralgia)

ATHEROSCLEROSIS: A chronic disease in which excessive amounts of fats and cholesterol remaining in the bloodstream collect on the inside walls of the arteries, forming plaque that gradually thickens and hardens the arterial walls, thus slowing down and interfering with the circulation of blood until a blockage occurs.

ATHLETE'S FOOT: A fungal infection of the feet, also called tinea pedis and Hong Kong foot

AUTOIMMUNE PROCESS: A process where the body's immune system attacks and destroys the body's own tissue, mistaking it for foreign matter based on molecular mimicry

AUTONOMIC NEUROPATHY: Dysfunction of the nerves of the autonomic nervous system, including those that affect the function of the stomach, intestines, esophagus, bladder, genitalia, sweat glands, and even the heart and other organs which regulate the blood pressure

BACKGROUND DIABETIC RETINOPATHY (A.K.A. NONPROLIFERATIVE RETINOPATHY): The earliest stage of diabetic retinopathy in its mildest form. In this condition, the fine blood vessels and capillaries within the retina become narrowed, clogged, and swollen and form balloon-like sacs. These altered vessels leak blood and fluid, causing the retina to swell or form deposits called exudates in the center of the retina or macula.

BALANITIS DIABETICA: Inflammation of the glans penis and under the prepuce with the presence of a purulent discharge

BETA CELLS: Insulin-producing and secreting cells in the islets of Langerhans

BLOOD GLUCOSE: The main sugar in the blood that the body makes from food and is used by the cells for energy or stored as glycogen for future energy needs. However, cells cannot make use of this sugar without the help of insulin.

BLOOD LIPID: Fat present in the blood, including triglycerides and cholesterol

BLOOD PRESSURE: The force of the blood against the artery walls

BLOOD UREA NITROGEN (BUN): A common blood test that can determine the level of urea in the blood which, in turn, is a rough measure of hydration and kidney function

BRITTLE DIABETES (A.K.A. LABILE OR UNSTABLE DIABETES): Marked fluctuations in blood glucose concentrations which are difficult to control, causing frequent episodes of insulin reactions or coma despite good therapy for management and medical supervision

CALORIE: Unit used to express the heat or energy value of food

CARBOHYDRATE: One of three major sources of calories in the diet. Carbohydrate is broken down into glucose during digestion and is the main nutrient that raises blood glucose levels. Carbohydrates come primarily from sugar (*i.e.*, simple carbohydrate) and starch (*i.e.*, complex carbohydrate).

CARDIOVASCULAR DISEASE: Disease processes affecting the peripheral circulation and the heart muscle

CEREBROVASCULAR DISEASE: Disease processes affecting the blood supply to the brain, particularly with reference to pathologic changes such as stroke and other cognitive defects

CEREBRAL VASCULAR ACCIDENT (*I.E.,* STROKE): Impaired cerebral blood supply

CHOLESTEROL: A wax-like fatty substance found in foods and manufactured internally by the liver. Found in blood, muscle, the liver, brain, and other tissues. Cholesterol is a form of lipid. In the correct amount, it performs important functions as a building block for cells and certain hormones. When its levels in the blood become too high, it causes atherosclerosis.

CHRONIC HYPERGLYCEMIA: Excessively high blood glucose that is slowly progressing and long continuing and may result in diabetic ketoacidosis or nonketotic hyperosmolar coma

CLAUDICATION: A condition caused by local temporary deficiency of blood to the muscles due to atherosclerosis of the arteries (peripheral vascular disease) and characterized by attacks of tightness or pain in the affected thigh, calf, or other muscles brought on by walking or other exercise and always associated with the same amount of effort

COMA: Loss of consciousness

CORONARY ARTERY DISEASE: Atherosclerosis of the large blood vessels leading to the heart resulting in decreased blood supply to the heart muscle. Its symptoms include arrhythmias, fatigue, congestive heart failure, enlarged heart, syncope or collapse, angina, dyspnea, myocardial infarction, or thrombosis. It is the most common form of heart disease.

CREATININE CLEARANCE: A proportional test using a 24 hour urine sample and a blood sample showing how well the kidneys are working to cleanse the blood

CRYSTALLINE INSULIN: Regular insulin

CYSTITIS: Inflammation of the bladder

DIABETES: Either diabetes insipidus or diabetes mellitus; diseases having the symptoms of polyuria in common. However, when used without qualification and by common usage, this term refers to diabetes mellitus characterized by high glucose levels.

DIABETES COMPLICATIONS: Either short-term (acute) or long-term (chronic) impairments which affect the microvascular or macrovascular blood vessels in persons with diabetes, such as (acute) hypoglycemia, hyperglycemia, diabetic ketoacidosis, and nonketotic hyperosmolar coma; and (chronic) visual impairments, diabetic nephropathy, cardiovascular and cerebrovascular disease, and diabetic neuropathy

DIABETES EDUCATION: Approved American Diabetes Association patient and family education for self-management and treatment of diabetes by 1) diet, 2) exercise, 3) self-monitoring of glucose levels, and 4) taking diabetes medications as prescribed

DIABETES INSIPIDUS: Chronic excretion of very large amounts of urine causing dehydration and extreme thirst ordinarily resulting from pituitary dysfunction, damage, or injury

DIABETES MELLITUS: A disorder which prevents the body from converting digested food into the energy needed for daily activities. It is caused by either an absolute or relative deficiency of insulin; either the body cannot make enough insulin or it cannot use the insulin it does produce properly. Diabetes is a metabolic disorder of fat metabolism which changes the way our bodies break down and use starches and glucose. It is a disease of the pancreas characterized by excessive thirst, hunger, urination, weakness, acidosis, and, without treatment, coma and death.

DIABETIC: Relating to or suffering from diabetes

DIABETIC COMA: Loss of consciousness due to brain edema developing when insulin and blood glucose are so out of balance that ketones accumulate in the blood. It is marked by high blood glucose levels and ketones in the urine and occurs almost exclusively in persons with type 1 diabetes.

DIABETIC KETOACIDOSIS (DKA): A life-threatening metabolic emergency resulting from either an absolute deficiency of insulin or acute resistance to insulin developing when absolute insulin deficiency and excess counter-regulatory hormones increase liver glucose production, decrease peripheral glucose utilization, and stimulate release of fatty acids from fat cells and the production of ketones by the liver. These changes cause hyperglycemia, osmotic diuresis, volume depletion, and acidosis.

DIABETIC NEUROPATHY: Damage to the nervous system which affects either or both the peripheral and autonomic nervous systems. Damage to the peripheral nervous system causes impairment of the motor nerve affecting voluntary movement and sensory nerves affecting touch and feeling sensations, especially the ability to feel pain impulses.

DIABETIC RETINITIS: Inflammation of the retina of the eye caused or complicated by diabetes

DIABETIC RETINOPATHY: A progressive disorder of the retina damaging the receptor cells and small blood vessels in the eye that can lead to vision changes and, eventually, complete blindness

DIABETOLOGIST: A physician specializing in the study and treatment of diabetes, an internist/endocrinologist

DIALYSIS: A method of removing waste from the body and maintaining the chemical balance of the blood when the kidneys have become damaged and are no longer functioning properly. There are two basic types: hemodialysis and peritoneal dialysis. In hemodialysis, the person is connected to an artificial kidney blood filtering machine three times per week. Peritoneal dialysis enables people to do dialysis without an articifial kidney blood filtering machine practically anywhere clean.

DIPLOPIA: Double vision. This can occur with cerebral

vascular accident (CVA) affecting posterior (vertebral) circulation.

EMERGENCY MEASURES (EMERGENCY DIABETIC ASSISTANCE): The regimen of treatment for the rapid onset of hypoglycemia. There are three degrees of hypoglycemia requiring such emergency measures: 1) a mild range of severity requiring emergency self-treatment, 2) a moderate range of severity which may require assistance in treatment, and 3) a severe range which usually requires immediate attention and assistance by someone else.

ENDOCRINOLOGIST: A internal medicine physician subspecializing in the study and treatment of the endocrine glands and their pathologies, including the pancreas and diabetes mellitus

FASTING BLOOD SUGAR (FBG): A laboratory test taken after at least eight hours of fasting; useful in making a diagnosis of diabetes

FAT: One of the three groups of nutrients which supply energy to the body. Fat in the blood is measured as triglycerides and cholesterol.

FIBER: The indigestible portion of plant foods such as fruit, vegetables, cereals, and grains

FOOD EXCHANGE: Foods grouped together due to similarities in nutritional value. Food exchanging is a way to help people stay on special food plans by letting them replace items from one food group with items from another food group.

FOOT ULCERATION: A wound with superficial loss of tissue from trauma which may become ulcerated if infection occurs. Such a foot ulceration may go undetected in persons with diabetes who have diabetic neuropathy because of loss of sensation and inability to feel the pain normally associated with such wounds and ulcers.

FRUCTOSE: A carbohydrate sugar found in fruits and candy

GANGRENE: The death of body tissue, often caused by loss of blood flow, as in arteriosclerosis or peripheral vascular disease

GESTATIONAL DIABETES MELLITUS (GDM): Diabetes mellitus that develops during pregnancy and usually goes away spontaneously after delivery. However, 60% of women experiencing GDM will eventually develop type 1 diabetes.

GLAUCOMA: A disease of the eye characterized by high intraocular pressure, damaged optic disk, atrophy of the optic nerve, and hardening of the eyeball resulting in partial defect in the field of or complete loss of vision. Glaucoma is associated with high blood pressure, diabetes, atherosclerosis, and optic nerve damage.

GLOMERULOPATHY: Any disease of the glomerulus of the kidney

GLOMERULOSCLEROSIS DIABETICA: Fibrosis of the renal glomeruli seen in some cases of diabetes

GLUCAGON: A hormone produced by the alpha cells which stimulates release of glycogen stored in the liver and muscles, thus raising the level of blood glucose when the blood glucose falls to levels below normal. Glucagon is available as an injectible preparation for very severe low blood glucose reactions.

GLUCOSE: A simple form of sugar that acts as the body's fuel. It is produced when foods are metabolized in the digestive system and carried by the blood to the cells for energy. The amount of glucose in the blood is known as the blood glucose level or glycemia.

GLUCOSE TOLERANCE TEST: A blood test utilizing 4-5 specimens over 3-4 hours; used to make the diagnosis of diabetes, including gestational diabetes

GLYCOGEN: The stored form of glucose found in the liver and muscles

GLYCOSURIA: The urinary secretion of glucose, usually in enhanced quantities

GLYCOSYLATED HEMOGLOBIN (HBA1C): A test administered to review average blood glucose control for the past 3-4 months

HEMODIALYSIS: The most common form of treatment for end stage renal failure. After surgically implanting a piece of graft material tubing, an artificial kidney is used to remove waste from the person's blood.

HEMOGLOBIN: A substance in red blood cells that picks up oxygen in the lungs and supplies oxygen to the cells of the body

HIGH DENSITY LIPOPROTEIN (HDL): Called the "good" cholesterol, high density lipoprotein removes cholesterol from the blood stream, thus preventing it from accumulating in the blood vessels

HORMONE: A chemical substance produced in tiny quantities by the body's endocrine glands and circulated by the blood

HYPERGLYCEMIA: A high blood glucose level

HYPERGLYCEMIC EPISODE OR REACTION: Refers to slow onset of severe elevation in blood glucose levels causing acute complications, such as stupor, lethargy, blurred vision, disorientation, slow responses, weakness, diabetic ketoacidosis, and nonketotic hyperosmolar coma

HYPERINSULINISM (HYPERINSULINEMIA): Increased levels of insulin in the plasma due to increased secretion of insulin by the beta cells of the pancreatic islets and decreased liver removal of insulin or insulin resistance. This condition is most commonly found in obese persons with hyperglycemia.

HYPERLIPIDEMIA: The presence of abnormally large amounts of lipids or fats in the circulating blood

HYPERTENSION: High blood pressure

HYPERTRIGLYCERIDEMIA: High levels of triglycerides in the blood

HYPOGLYCEMIA (GLUCOPENIA): A condition in which blood glucose drops too low and which can occur slowly (CNS symptoms) or rapidly (sympathetic symptoms). Hypoglycemia may cause cognitive dysfunction and loss of consciousness if untreated.

HYPOGLYCEMIA UNAWARENESS: The lack of ability to recognize warning signs of hypoglycemia, such as weakness, nervousness, sweating, increased heart rate, and irritability. This condition is found in the elderly, long-term diabetes patients, and those using beta-blockers.

HYPOGLYCEMIC COMA: Loss of consciousness resulting from excessive doses of exogenous insulin or oral hypoglycemic agents

HYPONATREMIA: Low blood sodium

IMPAIRED GLUCOSE TOLERANCE: A condition in which blood sugar levels are higher than normal but are not high enough to be classified as diabetes. However, this is a risk factor for type 2 diabetes.

IMPOTENCE: Inability to achieve and/or sustain an erection

INSULIN: A hormone manufactured by the pancreas in the beta cells of the islets of Langerhans which facilitates the entry of glucose into the cells of the body. This hormone is needed to convert glucose, starches, and other food into energy needed for daily life.

INSULIN DELIVERY (INSULIN INJECTIONS): The method of injecting exogenous insulin into the body's bloodstream

INSULIN-DEPENDENT DIABETES MELLITUS (IDDM, TYPE 1 DIABETES): A chronic condition in which a person is unable to properly metabolize glucose leading to severe hyperglycemia. Persons with this type of diabetes must take exogenous insulin to prevent the development of ketoacidosis.

INSULIN REACTIONS: (DIABETIC SHOCK OR HYPO-GLYCEMIC REACTION): Severe hypoglycemia produced by administration of insulin, manifested by sweating, tremor, anxiety, vertigo, and diplopia, followed by delirium, convulsions, and collapse

INSULIN RECEPTORS: Proteins that extend through the cell membranes that bind insulin which then transports glucose into the cell

INSULIN RESISTANCE: A partial blocking of the effect of insulin thus preventing the glucose in the blood from entering the cells for use as energy or storage for future use

ISLETS OF LANGERHANS: Clusters of alpha, beta, delta, and polypeptide cells throughout the pancreas

JUVENILE DIABETES: An old term for type 1 or insulin-dependent diabetes. While the onset of type 1 diabetes is typically detected in children, it may also occur in adults.

KETOACIDOSIS: Acidosis due to an excess of ketone bodies

KETONES: Acids produced when the body breaks down fat for fuel. This occurs when there is not enough insulin to permit glucose to enter the cells.

KETONEMIA: The presence of recognizable concentrations of ketone bodies in the plasma

KETONURIA: The presence of ketones in the urine

KETOSIS: An enhanced production of ketone bodies secondary to the breakdown of fat

KETO-STIX: A test for ketones in the urine

KIDNEY THRESHOLD: The level at which sugar spills over into the urine. This level varies among individuals.

KUSSMAUL BREATHING: Deep, rapid breathing seen in diabetic acidosis

LABILE DIABETES: A term used to indicate that a person's blood glucose often swings quickly from high to low and from low to high. This is also known as brittle diabetes.

LABORED BREATHING: Kussmaul breathing

LACTIC ACIDOSIS: The accumulation of excessive lactic acid in the blood resulting from the muscles burning glucose in anaerobic conditions. It is characterized by bicarbonate levels less than 10mmol/L and normal plasma ketones.

LACTOSE: Milk sugar

LATENT DIABETES (CHEMICAL DIABETES): A mild form of diabetes mellitus in which the person displays no overt symptoms but does display certain abnormal responses to diagnostic procedures, such as elevated fasting blood glucose concentration or reduced glucose tolerance. A diet high in glucose and simple carbohydrates may cause latent diabetes to become evident.

LIPID: A term for fat. There are many types of lipids in the body.

LIPOATROPHY: Dents or depressions in the skin that may form when insulin is constantly injected into the same place. This can cause problems with absorption of insulin.

LIPODYSTROPHY: Lumps or depressions in the skin that may develop when insulin is constantly injected into the same place

LIPOHYPERTROPHY: Lumps in the skin that may develop when insulin is constantly injected into the same place

LOW DENSITY LIPOPROTEIN (LDL): Called the "bad" cholesterol because it carries most of the cholesterol in the blood

MACULOPATHY (MACULAR EDEMA): Clogging and swelling of the retinal capillaries causing leaking of fluid into the retina where it pools in the center of the retina or macula

MACROSOMIA: Literally, this term means "large body." It refers to a baby who is considered larger than normal due to the mother's higher than normal blood sugar levels during pregnancy.

MATURITY ONSET DIABETES IN YOUTH (MODY): Type 2 or noninsulin-dependent diabetes occurring in children and young people

MELITURIA: The presence of sugar in the urine

METABOLISM: The complex physical breakdown and synthesis of chemical changes occurring in the tissues of the body and especially the conversion of food substances into energy

MG/DL: Abbreviation for milligrams per deciliters, the unit of measurement used in the U.S. when referring to blood glucose levels

MMOL/L: Abbreviation for millimoles per liter, the unit of measurement used in Europe and the People's Republic of China when referring to blood glucose levels. Diabetes is diagnosed when the level of glucose in the blood is greater than 7.0mmol/L (fasting) or greater than 11.1mmol/L (random).

MONILIASIS (CANDIDIASIS): A fungal infection common in people with diabetes, frequently in the vagina

NEOVASCULARIZATION: Growth of tiny new abnormal blood vessels in areas where circulation is impaired, *e.g.*, the retina of the eye in diabetic retinopathy. This condition leads to loss of vision.

NEPHROPATHY: Damage to the nephrons or filtering portions of the kidneys, a degenerative kidney disease that may occur in long-term diabetes

NEUROPATHY: Damage to nerve tissue causing loss of sensation and reflexes and/or burning or stabbing pain, especially at night. Neuropathy can affect many parts of the body and is one of the common long-term complications of diabetes.

NONINSULIN-DEPENDENT DIABETES MELLITUS (NIDDM): Type 2 diabetes

NPH INSULIN: Intermediate-acting insulin

OBESITY: The condition of being more than 20% in excess of ideal body weight

ORAL GLUCOSE TOLERANCE TEST (OGTT): A three hour test used to diagnose diabetes mellitus which includes glucose loading after fasting for eight hours and then determining blood glucose levels every hour afterwards for three hours

ORAL HYPOGLYCEMIC: Any orally administered medication meant to lower blood glucose in patients with type 2 diabetes. Such oral hypoglycemic agents are not insulin or a substitute for insulin.

OVERWEIGHT: The condition of being less than 20% in excess of ideal body weight

PANCREAS: The endocrine gland located in the abdomen behind the stomach that produces insulin and digestive enzymes

PERIPHERAL ARTERY DISEASE: Blockage of the arteries of the extremities (mostly the lower extremities) by atherosclerotic plaques causing intermittent claudication and leading to infections, gangrene, and possible amputation

PERIPHERAL NEUROPATHY: Neuropathy affecting the peripheral nervous system. It is further subdivided into: 1) distal symmetrical polyneuropathy, 2) mononeuropathy, 3) cranial mononeuropathy, 4) truncal mononeuropathy, 5) proximal motor neuropathy, and 6) focal neuropathy depending on which nerves are affected in which areas of the body.

PHTHISIS: Any wasting or atrophic disease

POLYDIPSIA: Excessive thirst, due in turn to excessive urination with subsequent dehydration, leading to excessive drinking that is relatively chronic

POLYPHAGIA: Excessive appetite, literally "numerous eating"

POLYURIA (HYDRURIA): Excessive urination

POSTPRANDIAL BLOOD GLUCOSE (PPBG): A blood test performed 1-2 hours after a meal to detect blood glucose levels

PREDIABETES: The condition prior to the development of clinical diabetes

PROLIFERATIVE RETINOPATHY: A disease of the small blood vessels of the retina of the eye caused by retinal neovascularization. These new vessels are quite fragile and may break and bleed into the clear fluid that fills the center of the eye causing vision changes.

PROTEIN: One of the three major food substances which is used to build body tissues

PRURITUS: Itching

REBOUND HYPERGLYCEMIA (SOMOGYI EFFECT): An abnormally high rise in blood glucose after an episode of low blood glucose that may result from overtreatment of hypoglycemia or from secretion of counter-regulatory hormones that raise the blood glucose level in reactive hypoglycemia

REGULAR INSULIN: Fast-acting insulin

RENAL FAILURE: As a result of excessive glucose in the bloodstream, the capillary walls overwork in filtering the waste products and build up scar-like material that eventually collapse the glomeruli filtering process, causing kidney damage. The kidneys almost completely stop cleaning wastes from the blood. Therefore, wastes build up to poisonous levels and can cause death. When creatinine and blood urea nitrogen levels in the blood are high, kidney failure will likely progress more rapidly unless treated. The two choices for renal failure are dialysis or transplant.

RENAL THRESHOLD: The concentration of plasma substance above which the substance appears in the urine

REST PAIN: An unpleasant sensation associated with actual or potential tissue damage usually occurring in the extremities during bodily inactivity, such as sitting or lying down

RETINOPATHY: Disorder of the retina or nerve tissue in the eye often seen in diabetes

SECONDARY DIABETES: A type of diabetes caused by another disease or damage to the pancreas from chemicals, certain medicines, or disease of the pancreas, such as pancreatic cancer. Secondary diabetes may occur as a consequence of acromegaly, Cushing's syndrome, hyperthyroidism, or surgical removal of the pancreas.

SEMI-LENTE INSULIN: Rapid-acting insulin

SENILE DIABETES: Also known as adult onset diabetes, this is an old term for type 2 or noninsulin-dependent diabetes

SERUM CREATININE: A test to determine the amount of creatinine in the blood. Increases may signal renal failure, urinary obstruction, dehydration, and/or hyperthyroidism.

STROKE: Damage to part of the brain that happens when the blood vessels supplying that part of the brain are blocked, as occurs with atherosclerosis and thrombus/embolus (dry stroke) or as a result of vessel rupture (wet stroke)

STUPOR: Marked cessation of mental activity or feeling, often produced by sleepiness, illness, or the effects of alcohol or narcotics

SUCROSE: Ordinary table sugar which breaks down to glucose and fructose in the body

SULFONYLUREAS: A class of oral medications for type 2 diabetes, also known as oral hypoglycemic agents. They lower blood sugar primarily by improving insulin production and tissue sensitivity to insulin.

SYNCOPE: A brief loss of consciousness from a transient deficiency in the oxygen-carrying capacity of the blood to the brain due to brainstem dysfunction, cardiac valve disease, or heart block dysrhythmia (Stokes-Adams syndrome)

SYNDROME X: A combination of central obesity, high blood pressure, insulin resistance, and a high HDL to total cholesterol ratio predisposing a person to heart disease

TABES: A gradual, progressive wasting in any chronic disease

TABES DIABETICA: Peripheral neuritis affecting the spinal cord

TEMPORARY PRECIPITATING FACTOR: A transient, unforseen or unknown event that contributes to or results in insulin reaction episodes in spite of conscious efforts by a person with diabetes and their health care team

TES-TAPE: A test for sugar in the urine

TIGHT MANAGEMENT: A treatment regimen suggested by the American Diabetes Association as a way to delay the onset and dramatically slow the progression of microvascular complications from diabetes. This consists of intensive insulin therapy, strict monitoring of blood glucose levels, lifestyle changes, exercise, and healthier diet.

TISSUE DAMAGE: Impairment of the usefulness of the four basic tissues in the body: 1) epithelium, 2) connective tissue, including blood, bone, and cartilage, 3) muscle tissue, and 4) nerve tissue, any of which may be affected as a result of diabetes

TRIGLYCERIDE: A type of blood fat which requires insulin to remove it from the bloodstream

TYPE 1 DIABETES: A condition in which the pancreas makes so little insulin that the body cannot use blood glucose as energy and which must be controlled by daily injections of insulin

TYPE 2 DIABETES: A condition in which the body either makes too little insulin or cannot use the insulin it does make to convert blood glucose into energy. This type of diabetes can often be controlled through proper meal plans, exercise, and either oral hypoglycemic agents or insulin.

ULCER: A break or deep sore in the skin

ULTRALENTE: Long-acting insulin

URINE TEST (URINANALYSIS): The analysis of the fluid and dissolved substances excreted by the kidneys and found in the urine. Urine tests for ketones are the only test for measuring ketones and are important in preventing ketoacidosis.

VASCULAR CHANGES: Complications relating to or consisting of the thickening of the blood vessel linings causing decreased blood flow of nutrients through narrowed arteries (atherosclerosis) to the heart (cardiovascular), brain (cerebrovascular), and extremities (peripheral vascular)

VISUAL CHANGES: Diabetes-induced alteration from normal vision due to pathological changes in the small arteries that provide blood to the retina. Diabetic vision complications include: 1) cataracts, 2) background retinopathy, 3) macular edema, 4) retinitis, 5) proliferative retinopathy, 6) glaucoma, 7) retinal detachment, and 8) blindness.

VITRECTOMY: A surgical operation to remove blood that sometimes collects at the back of the eyes when a person has eye disease

XANTHOMA DIABETICA: Cutaneous tumorous disease associated with uncontrolled diabetes mellitus

BIBLIOGRAPHY

CHINESE LANGUAGE BIBLIOGRAPHY

BOOKS

Chen Ao-zong, *Qian Fang Zhi Bai Bing* (*Thousands of Prescriptions to Treat Hundreds of Diseases*), People's Army Medical Press, Beijing, 1994

Chen Bao-ming & Zhao Jin-xi, *Gu Fang Miao Yong* (*Ancient Formulas, Wondrous Uses*), Beijing Science & Technology Publishing Co., Beijing, 1994

Cheng Bao-shu et al., *Zhen Jiu Da Ci Dian* (*The Great Dictionary of Acupuncture & Moxibustion*), Beijing Science & Technology Publishing Co., Beijing, 1988

Chen Jia-yang, *Shi Yong Zhong Yi Shen Jing Bing Xue* (*A Study of Practical Chinese Medical Neurology*), Gansu Science & Technology Publishing Co., Lanzhou, 1989

Chen Kang-mei & Gao Xiao-lan, *Er Xue Zhi Bai Bing* (*The Treatment of Hundreds of Diseases with Ear Acupuncture*), People's Army Medical Press, Beijing, 1995

Cheng Shi-de, *Nei Jing Jiang Yi* (*Inner Classic Teaching Materials*), Shanghai Science & Technology Publishing Co., Shanghai, 1985

Cui Shu-gui et al., *Shi Yong Zhen Jiu Nei Ke Xue* (*A Study of Practical Acupuncture-moxibustion in Internal Medicine*), White Mountain Press, Chenyang, 1991

Dan Shu-jian & Chen Zi-hua, *Xiao Ke Juan* (*The Wasting & Thirsting Book*), Chinese National Chinese Medicine & Medicinals Publishing Co., Beijing, 1999

Dong Zhen-hua et al., *Zhu Chen Zi Jing An Ji* (*A Collection of Zhu Chen-zi's Experiences*), People's Health & Hygiene Publishing Co., Beijing, 2000

Gan Rui-feng & Lü Ren-he, *Tang Niao Bing* (*Diabetes*), People's Health & Hygiene Publishing Co., Beijing, 1985

Gao Yan-bin, *Zhong Guo Tang Niao Bing Fang Zhi Tie Se* (*The Characteristics of the Chinese National Prevention & Treatment of Diabetes*), Heilongjiang Science & Technology Publishing Co., Harbin, 1995

Gao Ying-sen et al., *Zhong Yi Nei Ke Lin Chuang Shou Ce* (*A Clinical Handbook of Chinese Medicine Internal Medicine*), People's Health & Hygiene Publishing Co., Beijing, 1996

Guo Zhen-qiu, *Zhong Yi Er Ke Xue* (*A Study of Chinese Medical Pediatrics*), Changchun Publishing Co., Beijing, 2000

Han Guang-mei, *Zhong Yi Nei Ke Zhi Yan* (*Chinese Internal Medicine Treatments*), Guizhou Science & Technology Press, Guizhou, 1992

Hu Zhao-ming, *Zhong Guo Zhong Yi Mi Fang Da Quan* (*A Great Compendium of Chinese National Chinese Medical Secret Formulas*), Literary Propagation Publishing Co., Shanghai, 1992

Huang Wen-dong, *Shi Yong Zhong Yi Nei Ke Xue* (*A Study of Practical Chinese Medicine Internal Medicine*), Shanghai Science & Technology Publishing Co., Shanghai, 1985

Huang Yong-yuan, *Qi Nan Za Zheng Jing Xuan* (*A*

Carefully Chosen [Collection of] Strange, Difficult Miscellaneous Conditions), Guangdong Science & Technology Publishing Co., Guangzhou, 1996

Huang Xiao-kai, Han Ying Chang Yong Yi Xue Ci Hui (Chinese-English Glossary of Commonly Used Medical Terms), People's Health & Hygiene Publishing Co., Beijing, 1982

Ji Qing-shan & Li Jie, Zu Liao Zhi Bai Bing (The Foot Therapy Treatment of Hundreds of Diseases), Jilin Science & Technology Publishing Co., Hua Dian, 1993

Jiang Ming, Yi Nan Bing Zhong Yi Lin Zheng Zhi Nan (A Clinical Guide to the Treatment of Difficult Diseases in Chinese Medicine), China Medical Publishing Co., Beijing, 1993

Jiang Qing-yun, Shi Zhi Ben Cao (A Food Treatment Materia Medica), Earthen Repository of Ancient Books, Beijing, 1990

Jiangsu College of New Medicine, Zhong Yao Da Ci Dian (Great Dictionary of Chinese Medicinals), Shanghai Science & Technology Publishing Co., Shanghai, 1991

Li Cong-fu & Liu Bing-fan, Jin Yuan Si Da Yi Xue Zhu Si Xiang Zhi Yan Jiu (A Study of the Thinking of the Four Great Schools of Medicine of the Jin-Yuan [Dynasties]), People's Health & Hygiene Publishing Co., Beijing, 1983

Li, Guo-qing et al., Pian Fang Da Quan (A Great Collection of Folk Formulas), Beijing Science & Technology Press, Beijing, 1987

Li Wen-liang & Qi Qiang, Qian Jia Miao Fang (Ten Thousand Families' Wondrous Formulas), People's Liberation Army Publishing Co., Beijing, 1985

Li Yi, Zhi Zhen Zhi Bai Bing (The Finger-needling Treatment of Hundreds of Diseases), New Era Publishing Co., Beijing, 1997

Li Yong-zhi & Meng Fan-yi, Xiao Ke (Wasting & Thirsting), Chinese National Chinese Medicine & Medicinal Publishing Co., Beijing, 1995

Liu Bin, Lin Chuang Bian Zheng Shi Zhi Xue (A Study of the Clinical Basing of Treatment on Pattern Discrimination), Science, Technology & Literature Publishing Co., Beijing, 1992

Liu Dong-liang, Nei Ke Nan Zhi Bing De Zhong Yi Zhi Liao

(Chinese Medical Treatment of Difficult to Treat Diseases in Internal Medicine), People's Army Medical Publishing Co., Beijing, 1994

Lu Ren-he, Tang Niao Bing Ji Qi Bing Fa Zheng Zhong Xi Yi Zhen Zhi Xue (The Onset of Diabetes and Its Diagnosis & Treatment by Chinese & Western Medicine), People'sHealth & Hygiene Publishing Co., Beijing, 1997

Lun Xin et al., Yi Nan Zha Zheng Zhen Jiu Yan Fang Jing (A Selection of Proven Acupuncture & Moxibustion Formulas for Strange & Difficult Diseases), Guangdong Science & Technology Publishing Co., Guangzhou, 2000

Qiu Chang-hua & Sun Ying-jie, Tang Niao Bing Shi Yong Fang (Practical Formulas for Diabetes), People's Health & Hygiene Publishing Co., Beijing, 2000

Research Institute, Guangzhou College of Chinese Medicine, Jian Ming Zhong Yi Da Ci Dian (A Plain & Clear Dictionary of Chinese Medicine), People's Health & Hygiene Publishing Co., Beijing, 1986

Shanghai College of Chinese Medicine, Zhong Yi Tui Na Xue (A Study of Chinese Medical Tuina), People's Health & Hygiene Publishing Co., Beijing, 1985

Shanghai Municipal Department of Health, Shang Hai Lao Zhong Yi Jiang Yan Xuan Bian (A Selected Compilation of Shanghai Old Chinese Doctors Experiences), Shanghai Science & Technology Publishing Co., Shanghai, 1984

Shi Yu-guang & Dan Shu-jian, Xiao Ke Zhuan Zhi (Wasting & Thirsting Expertise), Chinese Medicine Ancient Books Publishing, Co., Beijing, 1997

Sun Guo-jie & Tu Jin-wen, Zhong Yi Zhi Liao Xue (A Study of Chinese Medical Treatments), Chinese Medicine & Medicinal Science & Technology Publishing Co., Beijing, 1990

Tang Rong-chuan, Xue Zheng Lun (Treatise on Bleeding Disorders), Chinese National Chinese Medicine & Medicinals Publishing Co., Beijing, 1996

Tian Cong-huo, Zhen Jiu Yi Xue Yan Ji (An Examination & Assembly of Acupuncture & Moxibustion Medical Studies), Science, Technology & Literature Publishing Co., Beijing, 1985

Wang Xue-tai & Liu Guan-jun, Zhong Guo Dang Dai Zhen Jiu Ming Jia Yi An (Contemporary Chinese National

Acupuncture & Moxibustion Famous Masters Case Histories), Jilin Science & Technology Publishing Co., Changchun, 1991

Wang Zhan-xi, et al., Nei Ke Zhen Jiu Pei Xue Xin Bian (A New Compilation of Acupuncture & Moxibustion for Internal Medicine), Science, Technology & Literature Publishing Co., Beijing, 1988

Wu Da-zhou & Ge Xiu-ke, Nan Zhi Bing De Liang Fang Miao Fa (Fine Formulas & Miraculous Methods for Difficult to Treat Diseases), Chinese National Chinese Medicine & Medicinal Publishing Co., Beijing, 1992

Wu Dun-xu, Zhong Yi Bing Yin Bing Ji Xue (A Study of Chinese Medical Disease Causes & Disease Mechanisms), Shanghai College of Chinese Medicine Publishing Co., Shanghai, 1989

Wu Jun-xi, Lao Nian Chang Xian Bing Zheng Fang Zhi Fa (The Prevention & Treatment of Commonly Seen Diseases in the Elderly), Chinese National Chinese Medicine & Medicinal Publishing Co., Beijing, 1998

Wu Jun-yu & Bai Yong-ke, Xian Zai Nan Zhi Bing Zhong Yi Zhen Liao Xue (A Study of the Diagnosis & Treatment of Modern, Difficult to Treat Diseases), Chinese Medicine Ancient Books Publishing, Co., Beijing, 1993

Xia De-xin, Zhong Yi Nei Ke Lin Chuang Shou Ce (A Clinical Handbook of Chinese Medicine Internal Medicine), Shanghai Science & Technology Publishing Co., Shanghai, 1989

Xia Zhi-ping, Shi Yong Zhen Jiu Tui Na Zhi Liao Xue (A Study of Practical Acupuncture-moxibustion & Tuina Treatments), Shanghai College of Chinese Medicine Publishing Co., Shanghai, 1990

Xiao Shao-qing, Zhong Guo Zhen Jiu Chu Fang Xue (A Study of Chinese Acupuncture & Moxibustion Prescription-writing), Ningxia People's Publishing Co., Yinchuan, 1986

Xu Ji-qun et al., Fang Ji Xue (A Study of Formulas & Prescriptions), Shanghai Science & Technology Publishing Co., Shanghai, 1986

Xu Xiao-ting, Zhong Yi Nei Ke Tang Zheng Jue (Chinese Medicine Internal Medicine Prescription Protocols), People's Army Medical Press, Beijing, 1995

Yan De-xin, Yan De Xin Zhen Zhi Ning Nan Bing Mi Chi (A Secret Satchel of Yan De-xin's Diagnosis & Treatment of Knotty, Difficult to Treat Diseases), Literary Press Publishing Co., Shanghai, 1997

Yang Fei et al., Da Zhong Yao Shan (Medicinal Meals of the Masses), Sichuan Science & Technology Publishing Co., Chengdu, 1985

Ye Chuan & Jian Yi, Jin Yuan Si Da Yi Xue Jia Ming Zhu Ji Cheng (An Anthology of Famous Jin-Yuan Four Great Schools Medical Studies), Chinese National Chinese Medicine & Medicinal Publishing Co., Beijing, 1997

Ye Ku-quan, Shi Wu Zhong Yao Yu Pian Fang (Food Stuffs, Chinese Medicinals & Folk Formulas), Jiangsu Science & Technology Press, Nanjing, 1980

Zhang Bo-yu, Zhong Yi Nei Ke Xue (A Study of Chinese Medicine Internal Medicine), People's Health & Hygiene Publishing Co., Beijing, 1988

Zhang Geng-yang et al., Lin Chuang Zhong Yi Zheng Zhi Shou Ce (A Handbook of Clinical Chinese Medicine Confirmed Treatments), Tianjin Science & Technology Publishing Co., Tianjin, 1999

Zhang Ren et al., Zhong Yi Zhi Liao Xian Dai Nan Bing Ji Cheng (A Collection of Chinese Medicine Treatments for the Difficult Diseases of Modern Times), Wen Hui Press, Beijing, 1998

Zhang Wen-long, Tang Niao Bing Zhong Yi Zhi Liao Yu Pao Jian (The Chinese Medical Treatment & Health Care of Diabetes), Inner Mongolia Science & Technology Publishing Co., Chifeng, 1999

JOURNAL ARTICLES

Bai Jing, "The Treatment of 38 Cases of Diabetic Nephropathy with Bu Yang Huan Wu Tang Jia Wei (Supplement Yang & Restore Five [Tenths] Decoction with Added Flavors)," Si Chuan Zhong Yi (Sichuan Chinese Medicine), #9, 2001, p. 33

Bi Ya-an, "The Treatment of Diabetic Ketosis with Cooked Radix Rehmanniae (Shu Di)," Jiang Su Zhong Yi (Jiangsu Journal of Chinese Medicine), #1, 2000, p. 33

Bu Lu-nuo & Bu Lu-ke, "Overeating Sugar & Sweets [Causes] Detriment & Damage to the Five Viscera," Jiang Xi Zhong Yi Yao (Jiangxi Chinese Medicine & Medicinals), #1, 1995, p. 31-32

Bu Xian-chun & Zhou Shen, "A Survey of the Efficacy of

Treating 107 Cases of Diabetic Peripheral Neuropathy by the Method of Foot Baths," *Hu Nan Zhong Yi Za Zhi* (*Hunan Journal of Chinese Medicine*), #9, 2000, p. 15-16

Cai Chang-long et al., "The Integrated Chinese-Western Medical Treatment of 48 Cases of Diabetic Upper Back Welling Abscesses," *Hu Nan Zhong Yi Za Zhi* (*Hunan Journal of Chinese Medicine*), #9, 2001, p. 42

Cai Xiao-ping, "A Survey of the Treatment Efficacy of Master Li's *Qing Shu Qi Qi Tang* (Clear Summerheat & Boost the Qi Decoction) in the Treatment of 40 Cases of Diabetes Accompanied by Summer-Fall Diarrhea," *Xin Zhong Yi* (*New Chinese Medicine*), #6, 2001, p. 33-34

Cao He-xin, "The Influence of *Tang Shen Ning* (Sugar Kidney Calmer) on the High Filtration of Rats in Early Diabetic Nephropathy," *Shang Hai Zhong Yi Yao Za Zhi* (*Shanghai Journal of Chinese Medicine & Medicinals*), #5, 2001, p. 19-21

Cao Hui-fen, "Diabetic Dietary Therapy," *Yun Nan Zhong Yi Zhong Yao Za Zhi* (*Yunnan Journal of Chinese Medicine & Medicinals*), #4, 1996, p. 66-67

Cao Su-lan et al., "The Treatment of Diabetic Retinopathy with *Zeng Shi Jiao Nang* (Improve the Vision Gelatin Capsules)," *Shan Dong Zhong Yi Za Zhi* (*Shandong Journal of Chinese Medicine*), #5, 2000, p. 281-282

Chang Zong-fan & Wang Xiu-zhen, "The Treatment of 58 Cases of Diabetic Peripheral Neuropathy Using *Yi Qi Huo Xue Tong Luo Tang* (Boost the Qi, Quicken the Blood & Free the Flow of the Network Vessels Decoction)," *Shi Yong Zhong Yi Nei Ke Za Zhi* (*Journal of Practical Chinese Medicine Internal Medicine*), #2, 2001, p. 17-18

Chen Bao-sheng et al., "Analysis of the Treatment of Diabetic Coronary Heart Disease Using *Xiao Ke An Jiao Nang* (Wasting & Thirsting Calming Capsules)," *Guo Yi Lun Tan* (*Chinese Medicine Forum*), #3, 1997, p. 33

Chen Fu-bin, "The Treatment of 98 Cases of Eye Ground Bleeding with Self-composed *Pu Huang Tang* (Pollen Typhae Decoction)," *Bei Jing Zhong Yi* (*Beijing Chinese Medicine*), #5, 1999, p. 27

Chen Gang, "The Treatment of 48 Cases of Decreased Glucose Tolerance with *Jian Pi Yun Dan Tang* (Fortify the Spleen & Counter Pure Heat Decoction)," *Si Chuan Zhong Yi* (*Sichuan Chinese Medicine*), #11, 2001, p. 43

Chen Gang & Dan Wei-li, "The Treatment of 64 Cases of

Type II Diabetes with *Shu Gan Zi Yin Jian* (Course the Liver & Enrich Yin Decoction)," *Si Chuan Zhong Yi* (*Sichuan Chinese Medicine*), #3, 1999, p. 16-17

Chen Hun-fang, "The Treatment of Diabetes with the Bio-spectrum Physiatrics Apparatus," *Hei Long Jiang Zhong Yi Yao* (*Heilongjiang Chinese Medicine & Medicinals*), #2, 1999, p. 49-50

Chen Jian-fei et al., "The Treatment of 10 Cases of Diabetes Treated by Transplanting Pancreatic Islets to Acupoints," *Zhong Yi Za Zhi* (*Journal of Chinese Medicine*), #8, 1999, p. 484-486

Chen Jin, "The Treatment of 46 Cases of Type II Diabetes with *Qing Gan Xie Huo Tang* (Clear the Liver & Drain Fire Decoction)," *Jiang Xi Zhong Yi Yao* (*Jiangxi Chinese Medicine & Medicinals*), #2, 2000, p. 21

Chen Peng, "The Influence of *Fu Mai Pian* (Recover the Vessels Tablets) on Insulin Resistance in SMI [Symptomless Myocardial Infarction] Patients," *He Nan Zhong Yi* (*Henan Chinese Medicine*), # 1, 2001, p. 39-40

Chen Rong-sheng, "The Treatment of 43 Cases of Diabetic Peripheral Neuritis Using *Tong Mai Huo Xue Tang* (Free the Flow of the Vessels & Quicken the Blood Decoction)," *Jiang Xi Zhong Yi Yao* (*Jiangxi Chinese Medicine & Medicinals*), #5, 1999, p. 23

Chen Shao-lian, "A Survey of the Efficacy of Treating 63 Cases of Type II Diabetes with Integrated Chinese-Western Medicine," *Hu Nan Zhong Yi Za Zhi* (*Hunan Journal of Chinese Medicine*), #2, 2000, p. 24

Chen Xi et al., "The Treatment of 39 Cases of Diabetes Mellitus (NIDDM) by the Methods of Nourishing Yin & Quickening the Blood," *Zhe Jiang Zhong Yi Za Zhi* (*Zhejiang Journal of Chinese Medicine*), #10, 1999, p. 427

Chen Xia-bo, "An Analysis of the Patterns of 54 Cases of Type II Diabetes For Whom Orally Administered Hypoglycemic Medicines Are Ineffective – With a Comparison to 67 Cases For Whom They Are Effective," *Zhe Jiang Zhong Yi Za Zhi* (*Zhejiang Journal of Chinese Medicine*), #5, 2000, p. 188-189

Chen Xiao, "A Clinical Audit on the Treatment of Diabetic Secondary Hypertriglyceridemia by the Methods of Supplementing the Liver & Boosting the Kidneys, Flushing Phlegm & Transforming Stasis," *Zhe Jiang Zhong Yi Za Zhi* (*Zhejiang Journal of Chinese Medicine*), #1, 2000, p. 34-35

Chen Xu & Shan Wei-li, "The Treatment of 64 Cases of Type II Diabetes with *Shu Gan Zi Yin Jian* (Course the Liver & Enrich Yin Decoction)," *Si Chuan Zhong Yi (Sichuan Chinese Medicine)*, #3, 1999, p. 16-17

Chen Xu-ling & Yao Wei, "A Clinical Audit of 100 Cases of Diabetes Treated with Self-composed *Xiao Ke Yin* (Wasting & Thirsting Drink) plus a Comparison to 82 Cases Treated with Western Medicinals," *Zhe Jiang Zhong Yi Za Zhi (Zhejiang Journal of Chinese Medicine)*, #7, 2001, p. 290

Chen Yun-wang, "The Treatment of 69 Cases of Diabetic Gastric Paresis by the Methods of Fortifying the Spleen & Harmonizing the Stomach – Plus a Comparison with 35 Cases Treated with Ma Ding Lin," *Zhe Jiang Zhong Yi Za Zhi (Zhejiang Journal of Chinese Medicine)*, #4, 2001, p. 144

Cheng Han-qiao, "An Analysis of Wasting & Thirsting Disease as Described in the *Nei Jing (Inner Classic)*," *Shan Dong Zhong Yi Za Zhi (Shandong Journal of Chinese Medicine)*, #3, 2000, p. 134-135

Cheng Xin-lu *et al.*, "The Treatment of 72 Cases of Diabetic Foot with Self-composed *Tang Zu Yin* (Diabetic Foot Drink)," *Si Chuan Zhong Yi (Sichuan Chinese Medicine)*, #12, 1999, p. 30

Chinese National Chinese Medical Association Nephropathy Commission, "Experiences in the Use of Chinese Medicinals & the Chinese Medical Treatment of Diabetic Nephropathy," *Shang Hai Zhong Yi Yao Za Zhi (Shanghai Journal of Chinese Medicine & Medicinals)*, #5, 2001, p. 15-18

Cui Xian, "The Chinese Medical Pattern Discrimination & Treatment of Type II Diabetes," *He Nan Zhong Yi (Henan Chinese Medicine)*, #6, 2000, p. 51-52

Dai Fang-fang & Zhu Guang-hua, "A Discussion of the Disease Causes & Disease Mechanisms of Glucose Tolerance Reduction," *Jiang Su Zhong Yi (Jiangsu Chinese Medicine)*, #5, 2000, p. 17

Dai Xiao-man, "The Treatment of 33 Cases of Type II Diabetes Using Self-composed *Qi Xiong Xiao Ke Fang* (Astragalus & Ligusticum Wasting & Thirsting Formula)," *Hu Nan Zhong Yi Za Zhi (Hunan Journal of Chinese Medicine)*, #2, 1998, p. 42-43

Deng Yi-hui *et al.*, "The Influence of *Zuo Gui Jiang Tang Ling* (Restore the Left [Kidney] & Lower Sugar Efficacious

[Remedy]) on Peroxide Injury of Lipids in Experimental Diabetes in Rats," *Zhong Yi Za Zhi (Journal of Chinese Medicine)*, #5, 1999, p. 305-306

Ding Xue-ping *et al.*, "A Study of the Relationship Between Chinese Medical Pattern Discrimination and Non-insulin-dependent Diabetes with Glucagon & Insulin Sensitivity," *Shang Hai Zhong Yi Yao Za Zhi (Shanghai Journal of Chinese Medicine & Medicinals)*, # 9, 1999, p. 18-20

Ding Yi *et al.*, "A Clinical Audit of the Treatment of Foot Infection Stage Diabetes with *Si Miao Yong An Tang Jia Wei* (Four Wonders Brave & Quiet Decoction with Added Flavors)," *Bei Jing Zhong Yi (Beijing Chinese Medicine)*, #3, 2001, p. 30-31

Dong Ying *et al.*, The Treatment of 32 Cases of Diabetic Nephropathy with Integrated Chinese-Western Medicine," *Hu Nan Zhong Yi Za Zhi (Hunan Journal of Chinese Medicine)*, #2, 2001, p. 45

Dong Zhen-hua & Li Yuan, "The Treatment of 50 Cases of Diabetes Using Dr. Zhu's *Jiang Tang Sheng Mai Fang* (Lower Sugar Engender the Pulse Formula)," *Shan Xi Zhong Yi (Shanxi Chinese Medicine)*, #2, 1997, p. 9-10

Du Ji-hui & Sun Zhi-sheng, "The Treatment of 30 Cases of Diabetic Acromelic Gangrene with External Application of *Xiao Chung Ye* (Disperse Sore Liquid)," *Shan Dong Zhong Yi Za Zhi (Shandong Journal of Chinese Medicine)*, #2, 2000, p. 88

Du Ji-hui *et al.*, "The Treatment of 52 Cases of Type II Diabetes Early Stage Nephropathy with *Tang Shen Xiao* (Sugar Kidney Wasting)," *Shan Dong Zhong Yi Za Zhi (Shandong Journal of Chinese Medicine)*, #6, 2000, p. 335-336

Du Ting-hai & Lu Xiao-hong, "Prof. Lu Jing-zhong's Experiences in the Pattern Discrimination & Treatment of Asymptomatic Diabetes," *Xin Zhong Yi (New Chinese Medicine)*, #7, 2001, p. 11-12

Duan Shang-qin, "The Treatment of 50 Cases of Diabetic Light Paralysis of the Stomach with *Zi Sheng Wan* (Endow Life Pills)," *Zhong Yi Za Zhi (Journal of Chinese Medicine)*, #4, 1999, p. 248-249

Fan Jian-kai & Wang Yao-ping, "A Survey of the Internal and External Treatment of Diabetic Acromelic Gangrene in 33 Cases," *Zhong Yi Za Zhi (Journal of Chinese Medicine)*, #2, 1999, p. 95-97

Fan Shi-ping et al., "An Experimental Study of the Treatment of Diabetic Coronary Heart Disease with Tang Xin Ning Jiao Nong (Sugar Heart Calming Gelatin Capsules)," Xin Zhong Yi (New Chinese Medicine), #7, 2001, p. 75-76

Fan Yi-shan, "The Clinical Application of Shu Gan Huo Xue Jiang Tang Yin (Course the Liver, Quicken the Blood & Lower Sugar Drink) in the Treatment of Diabetes," Shi Yong Zhong Yi Nei Ke Za Zhi (Journal of Practical Chinese Internal Medicine), #1, 2001, p. 23-24

Fang Lian-shun, "The Treatment of 30 Cases of Diabetic Nephropathy with Zhen Wu Tang (True Warrior Decoction)," Fu Jian Zhong Yi Yao (Fujian Chinese Medicine & Medicinals), #3, 2000, p. 34

Feng Ming-xiu et al., "The Treatment of 309 Cases of Diabetes Using a Combination of Acupuncture & Xiao Ke Gao (Wasting & Thirsting Ointment) Applied to Acupoints," Zhong Yi Za Zhi (Journal of Chinese Medicine), #1, 1994, p. 25-26

Fu Dai-yu, "Advances in Chinese Medicinal & Specific Formulas for the Treatment of Diabetes," Si Chuan Zhong Yi (Sichuan Chinese Medicine), #7, 2001, p. 17-19

Fu Deng-yun, "The Nei Jing's Understanding of Diabetes," Zhong Yi Za Zhi (Journal of Chinese Medicine), #10, 1999, p. 636

Fu Qi-wu, "Understanding Based on Experience Treating Chronic Nephritis by Quickening the Blood & Transforming Stasis," Jiang Su Zhong Yi (Jiangsu Chinese Medicine), #7, 1998, p. 17

Gan Li, "The Treatment of 58 Cases of Diabetic Constipation Using Jia Wei Si Mo Tang (Added Flavors Four Milled Ingredients Decoction)," Zhe Jiang Zhong Yi Za Zhi (Zhejiang Journal of Traditional Chinese Medicine), #6, 1999, p. 384

Gao Ai-ai, "The Treatment of 52 Cases of Diabetic Peripheral Neuropathy with Xiao Ke Tong Luo Yin (Wasting & Thirsting Free the Flow of the Network Vessels Drink)," Bei Jing Zhong Yi (Beijing Chinese Medicine), #3, 2000, p. 19-20

Gao Hong-mei et al., "The Acupuncture-moxibustion Treatment of 34 Cases of Uremic Pruritus," Zhong Yi Za Zhi (Journal of Chinese Medicine), #5, 2001, p. 312

Gao Lu-wen, "Wen Dan Tang (Warm the Gallbladder

Decoction) & Diabetic Retinopathy," Zhong Yi Za Zhi (Journal of Chinese Medicine), #2, 2000, p. 20-22

Gao Ming-song & Xu Jie, "The Treatment of 68 Cases of Type II Diabetic Microalbuminuria with Integrated Chinese-Western Medicine," He Nan Zhong Yi (Henan Chinese Medicine), #3, 2001, p. 39

Gao Ya & Li Geng-sheng, "A Clinical Audit of the Treatment of 61 Cases of Diabetic Sexual Function Disturbance with Le Er Jiao Nong (So Happy Gelatin Capsules)," Zhong Yi Za Zhi (Journal of Chinese Medicine), #11, 2001, p. 673-674

Gong Wen-jun, "Recent Developments in Using Chinese Medicinals to Treat Diabetic Nephropathy," Shan Dong Zhong Yi Za Zhi (Shandong Journal of Chinese Medicine), #3, 2000, p. 187-189

Gu Li, "Lifting the Borders of the Treatment of Diabetes by Boosting the Qi, Enriching Yin & Clearing Heat," Si Chuan Zhong Yi (Sichuan Chinese Medicine), #11, 1999, p. 26

Guo Rui-lin, "Gao Hui-yuan's Experiences in the Treatment of Diabetes," Zhong Yi Za Zhi (Journal of Chinese Medicine), #4, 2001, p. 203

Guo Yan-bao & Shan Zhi-dan, "The Effect of Injectible Astragalus on Reducing Albuminuria in Early Stage Diabetic Nephropathy," Shan Dong Zhong Yi Za Zhi (Shandong Journal of Chinese Medicine), #6, 2000, p. 351

Han Mei-ying, "Discussion on the Treatment of Hepatogenic Diabetes," Guo Yi Lun Tan (National Medicine Forum), #4, 1997, p. 41-42

Han Zhen-chong et al., "The Treatment of Diabetic Peripheral Neuropathy by the Methods of Nourishing Yin, Boosting the Qi & Quickening the Blood," Si Chuan Zhong Yi (Sichuan Chinese Medicine), #11, 1999, p. 20-21

Hao Ming-qiang, "The Treatment of 40 Cases of Diabetic Nephropathy with Jiang Tang Li Shen Fang (Lower Sugar & Rectify the Kidneys Formula)," Si Chuan Zhong Yi (Sichuan Chinese Medicine), #10, 2000, p. 21

Hao Pei-shun & Hou Rong-hui, "Observations on the Treatment Efficacy of the Treatment of 118 Cases of Type II Diabetes Complicated by Peripheral Neuritis with Integrated Chinese-Western Medicine," Shan Xi Zhong Yi (Shanxi Chinese Medicine), #3, 2001, p. 28-29

He Gang, "The Treatment of 21 Cases of Painful Diabetic

Neuropathy Using *Huo Luo Xiao Ling Dan Jia Wei* (Quicken the Network Vessels Efficacious Elixir with Added Flavors)," *Jiang Xi Zhong Yi Yao (Jiangxi Chinese Medicine & Medicinals)*," 5, 1999, p. 23

He Gang, "The Treatment of 36 Cases of Diabetic Restless Leg with *San Ren Tang Jia Jian* (Three Seeds Decoction with Additions & Subtractions)," *Jiang Su Zhong Yi (Jiangsu Chinese Medicine)*, #5, 1999, p. 17

He Gang, "The Treatment of 42 Cases of Diabetic Constipation Using *Yi Yu Tang* (Benefit & Foster Decoction)," *Ji Lin Zhong Yi Yao (Jilin Chinese Medicine & Medicinals)*, #3, 1999, p. 29

He Jian, "The Treatment of Diabetic Nephropathy Using *Yi Qi Huo Xue Tang* (Boost the Qi & Quicken the Blood Decoction)," *Shan Dong Zhong Yi Za Zhi (Shandong Journal of Chinese Medicine)*, #11, 1999, p. 495-496

He Qing-hua, "The Treatment of 30 Cases of Diabetic Oral Thrush Using *Shen Ling Bai Zhu San* (Ginseng, Poria & Atractylodes Powder)," *Si Chuan Zhong Yi (Sichuan Chinese Medicine)*, #9, 1999, p. 19-20

He Xuan-min, "The Treatment of 30 Cases of Type II Diabetes with Self-composed *Yu Ye Tang* (Jade Humor Decoction)," *Hu Nan Zhong Yi Za Zhi (Hunan Journal of Chinese Medicine)*, #1, 2001, p. 36

He Ya-lu, "The Treatment of 36 Cases of Diabetic Diarrhea with Chinese Medicinals Applied to the Navel," *Zhe Jiang Zhong Yi Za Zhi (Zhejiang Journal of Chinese Medicine)*, #8, 2000, p. 332

Heng Xian-pei, "A Discussion on the Complicated Relationship Between Liver Depression & Blood Sugar in Diabetics," *Guang Ming Zhong Yi (Guangming Chinese Medicine)*, #2, 2000, p. 15-17

Hu Jian-ping, "A Survey of the Treatment Efficacy of *Dan Qi Yi Shen Tang* (Salvia & Astragalus Boost the Kidneys Decoction) in the Treatment of Diabetic Nephropathy," *Bei Jing Zhong Yi (Beijing Chinese Medicine)*, #5, 2001, p. 16-17

Hu Jian-ping, "The Treatment of 21 Cases of Asymptomatic Diabetes with *Liu Wei Di Huang Wan Jia Wei* (Six Flavors Rehmannia Pills with Added Flavors)," *Si Chuan Zhong Yi (Sichuan Chinese Medicine)*, #11, 1999, p. 35

Hu Jian-ping, "The Treatment of 48 Cases of Diabetic Nephropathy Proteinuria Treated with *Dan Qi Yi Shen*

Tang (Salvia & Astragalus Boost the Kidneys Decoction)," *Shang Hai Zhong Yi Yao Za Zhi (Shanghai Journal of Chinese Medicine & Medicinals)*, #8, 2001, p. 24-25

Hua Shi-zuo & Chen Wei-ping, "The Treatment of 24 Cases of Recurrent Transient Ischemic Attacks with *Ling Dan Tang* (Campsis & Salvia Decoction)," *Si Chuan Zhong Yi (Sichuan Chinese Medicine)*, #9, 2000, p. 28

Hua Zhuan-jin & Quan Xiao-lin, "Advances in the Chinese Medical Treatment of Diabetic Foot," *Bei Jing Zhong Yi (Beijing Chinese Medicine)*, #3, 2000, p. 54-56

Huang Fei-xiang *et al.*, "The Relationship Between Left Ventricular Hypertrophy and Chinese Medical Patterns Among Patients with Hypertension & Diabetes," *Zhong Yi Za Zhi (Journal of Chinese Medicine)*, #7, 2001, p. 432-433

Huang Jian-liang & Yu Gan-long, "The Treatment of 38 Cases of Diabetic Retinopathy by the Methods of Quickening the Blood & Transforming Stasis," *Hu Nan Zhong Yi Za Zhi (Hunan Journal of Chinese Medicine)*, #1, 2000, p. 29

Huang Xiao-zhi, "The Treatment of 38 Cases of Diabetic Urinary Tract Infection with *Yi Qi Yu Yin Tong Lin Tang* (Boost the Qi, Foster Yin & Free the Flow of Strangury Decoction)," *Xin Zhong Yi (New Chinese Medicine)*, #12, 1998, p. 16-18

Huang Yong-yan, "The Treatment of 32 Cases of Type II Diabetic Constipation Based on Stasis Heat," *Jiang Su Zhong Yi (Jiangsu Chinese Medicine)*, #11, 1999, p. 18

Huang Zhen-peng, "The Treatment of 26 Cases of Diabetes & Accompanying Peripheral Neuropathy with *Xiao Ke Bi Tong Tang* (Wasting & Thirsting Painful Impediment Decoction)," *Xin Zhong Yi (New Chinese Medicine)*, #12, 1996, p. 21-22

Ji Yun-hai, "The Treatment of 50 Cases of Type II Diabetes with *Jiang Tang Dan* (Lower Sugar Elixir)," *Si Chuan Zhong Yi (Sichuan Chinese Medicine)*, #3, 1999, p. 25

Jiang Hua, "The Use of *Shen Mai Zhu She Ye* (Ginseng & Ophiopogon Injectible Liquid) in the Treatment of Non-insulin-dependent Diabetic Nephropathy," *Jiang Su Zhong Yi (Jiangsu Chinese Medicine)*, #2, 1999, p. 27-28

Jiang Xi-lin, "The Treatment of 40 Cases of Diabetic Foot with Integrated Chinese-Western Medicine," *Zhe Jiang Zhong Yi Za Zhi (Zhejiang Journal of Chinese Medicine)*, #9, 2000, p. 388

Jiang Ying-hong, "An Inquiry into the Chinese Medical Conceptualization of the Diagnosis & Treatment of Diabetes," *Bei Jing Zhong Yi (Beijing Chinese Medicine)*, #2, 2000, p. 12-13

Jiang Zhi-cheng *et al.*, "A Small Discussion of the Treatment of 42 Cases of Diabetic Peripheral Neuropathy with Integrated Chinese-Western Medicine," *Hu Nan Zhong Yi Za Zhi (Hunan Journal of Chinese Medicine)*, #1, 2000, p. 8-9

Jiao Peng, "The Treatment of 40 Cases of Early Stage Diabetic Nephropathy by the Methods of Boosting the Qi, Quickening the Blood & Transforming Stasis," *Xin Zhong Yi (New Chinese Medicine)*, #9, 2001, p. 34

Jin Jie *et al.*, "Professor Zhang Fa-rong's Experiences in the Treatment of Diabetic Peripheral Neuropathy," *Si Chuan Zhong Yi (Sichuan Chinese Medicine)*, #6, 2000, p. 1-2

Jin Lan, "A Clinical Audit of the Treatment of 42 Cases of Type II Diabetes with *Yi Qi Yang Yin Huo Xue Tang* (Boost the Qi, Nourish Yin & Quicken the Blood Decoction)," *Hu Nan Zhong Yi Za Zhi (Hunan Journal of Chinese Medicine)*, #9, 2001, p. 19-20

Jin Ling-jiao, "The Treatment of 25 Cases of Diabetic Peripheral Neuropathy with Integrated Chinese-Western Medicine," *Hu Nan Zhong Yi Za Zhi (Hunan Journal of Chinese Medicine)*, #5, 2000, p. 39

Jun Cui-mei & Li Zhen-zhong, "An Investigation of the Pathological Changes of Diabetic Vascular Disease," *Shan Xi Zhong Yi (Shanxi Chinese Medicine)*, #3, 2001, p. 60

Kang Lu-wa, "An Inquiry into the Treatment of Diabetic Ketosis," *Si Chuan Zhong Yi (Sichuan Chinese Medicine)*, #8, 1999, p. 12-13

Kang Lu-wa, "The Treatment of Diabetes by Pattern Discrimination of the Tongue," *Zhong Yi Za Zhi (Journal of Chinese Medicine)*, 1999, #9, p. 530-531

Lai Xiao-yang, "The Treatment of 48 Cases of TypeII Diabetes Using *Jiang Tang Jia Pian* (Lower Sugar Grade A Tablets)," *Jiang Xi Zhong Yi Yao (Jiangxi Chinese Medicine & Medicinals)*, #4, 1999, p. 50

Li Chuang-peng & Chen Jian-fei, "The Treatment of Qi Vacuity & Blood Stasis in 30 Cases of Diabetes Using *Jiang Tang Er Hao* (Lower Sugar No. 2)," *Xin Zhong Yi (New Chinese Medicine)*, #12, 1998, p. 24-25

Li De-zhen, "An Exploration & Analysis of Shi Jin-mo's Treatment of Diabetes," *Zhong Yi Za Zhi (Journal of Chinese Medicine)*, #5, 2001, p. 261-262

Li Hong *et al.*, "The Treatment of Early Stage Diabetic Nephropathy with *Zhi Tang Bao Shen Chong Ji* (Treat Sugar & Protect the Kidneys Soluble Granules)," *Shang Hai Zhong Yi Yao Za Zhi (Shanghai Journal of Chinese Medicine & Medicinals)*, #10, 2001, p. 30-31

Li Hong & Fan Shi-ping, "A Clinical Audit of the Treatment of 42 Cases of Diabetic Nephropathy with Integrated Chinese-Western Medicine," *Fu Jian Zhong Yi Yao (Fujian Chinese Medicine & Medicinals)*, #4, 2000, p. 17-18

Li Hong & Hou Feng-ying, "A Clinical Audit of the Integrated Chinese-Western Medical Treatment of Diabetic Gastric Paresis," *Xin Zhong Yi (New Chinese Medicine)*, #5, 2001, p. 34

Li Hong & Xia Jian-sheng, "A Clinical Study of the Pattern Discrimination of Diabetic Retinopathy," *He Nan Zhong Yi (Henan Chinese Medicine)*, #5, 2000, p. 33

Li Hong-wei, "A Survey of the Treatment Efficacy of the Integrated Chinese-Western Medical Treatment of Diabetic Nephropathy in 34 Cases," *Xin Zhong Yi (New Chinese Medicine)*, #10, 2001, p. 35-36

Li Guang-ping, "The Treatment of 30 Cases of Sulfonylurea-type Hypoglycemic Medicine Subsequent Loss of Effectiveness with Integrated Chinese-Western Medicine," *Fu Jian Zhong Yi Yao (Fujian Chinese Medicine & Medicinals)*, #6, 2000, p. 13-14

Li Ming-rui, "A Discussion of Diabetic Yin Vacuity Complicated by Dampness," *Zhong Yi Za Zhi (Journal of Chinese Medicine)*, #4, 1999, p. 251-252

Li She-li & Cheng Yong, "The Treatment of 36 Cases of Diabetic Neurogenic Bladder with Integrated Chinese-Western Medicine," *Zhong Yi Za Zhi (Journal of Chinese Medicine)*, #2, 1999, p. 93-94

Li Wen-hong, "The Treatment of Diabetic Bullosis with Integrated Chinese-Western Medicine," *Si Chuan Zhong Yi (Sichuan Chinese Medicine)*, #7, 1999, p. 44

Li Xiang-hong, "Knowledge Based on Experience in the Integrated Chinese-Western Medical Nursing of Diabetic Vesicular Disease," *Si Chuan Zhong Yi (Sichuan Chinese Medicine)*, #7, 1999, p. 44

Li Xin-song, "The Treatment of 32 Cases of Yin Vacuity Dry Heat Type II Diabetes Using *Zi Yin Xie Re Yin* (Enrich Yin & Drain Heat Drink)," *Yun Nan Zhong Yi Yao Za Zhi (Yunnan Journal of Chinese Medicine & Medicinals)*, #1, 1997, p. 15-16

Li Xiu-juan, "The Treatment of Diabetic Gangrene with *Huai Ju Xun Xi Fang* (Gangrene Steaming & Washing Formula)," *Zhe Jiang Zhong Yi Za Zhi (Zhejiang Journal of Chinese Medicine)*, #3, 2000, p. 103

Li Yi, "The Treatment of 26 Cases of Diabetes Using the Methods of Boosting the Qi, Nourishing Yin & Quickening the Blood," *Yun Nan Zhong Yi Yao Za Zhi (Yunnan Journal of Chinese Medicine & Medicinals)*, #1, 1997, p. 12

Li Yi, "The Treatment of 156 Cases of Type II Diabetes with Self-composed *Xiao Ke Wu Chong Fang* (Wasting & Thirsting Five Worms Formula)," *Shang Hai Zhong Yo Yao Za Zhi (Shanghai Journal of Chinese Medicine & Medicinals)* #8, 1999, p. 18-19

Li Ying, "A Clinical Audit of the Treatment of Type II Diabetes with *Tang Zhi Xiao Wan* (Sugar & Fat Wasting Pills)," *He Nan Zhong Yi (Henan Chinese Medicine)*, #3, 2000, p. 31-32

Li Yu-zhong, "The Treatment of 30 Cases of Geriatric Diabetes Using *San Huang Xiao Ke Kang Nian* (Three Yellows Wasting & Thirsting Capsules)," *Guang Ming Zhong Yi (Guangming Chinese Medicine)*, #4, 2001, p. 45-48

Li Ze-yi, "The Treatment of 60 Cases of Diabetes by the Methods of Transforming Stasis & Dispelling Phlegm," *Si Chuan Zhong Yi (Sichuan Chinese Medicine)*, #6, 1999, p. 33

Li Zhen-zhong *et al.*, "The Disease Causes and Mechanisms of Diabetic Proliferative Retinopathy," *Jiang Su Zhong Yi (Jiangsu Chinese Medicine)*, #3, 2000, p. 12-13

Li Zhi-jie, "An Inquiry into the Relationship Between Obesity & Metabolism as Differentiated by Chinese Medical Pattern Discrimination for Type II Diabetes," *Shan Xi Zhong Yi (Shanxi Chinese Medicine)*, #5, 1999, p. 20-21

Liang Guang-yu, "A Brief Introduction to Professor Feng Ming-qing's Theory & Understanding of the Treatment of Diabetes," *He Nan Zhong Yi (Henan Chinese Medicine)*, #1, 2000, p. 15

Liang Guo-gang, "The Chinese & Western Medical

Approaches to the Treatment of Diabetes Mellitus," *Guang Ming Zhong Yi (Guangming Chinese Medicine)*, #4, 2001, p. 33-34

Liang Kai-fa, "The Treatment of 31 Cases of Diabetic Impotence by the Combined Methods of Boosting the Kidneys, Quickening the Blood & Standing Up the Wilted," *Si Chuan Zhong Yi (Sichuan Chinese Medicine)*, #3, 2001, p. 35

Liang Ping-mao, "The Treatment of 31 Cases of Diabetic Orthostatic Hypotension with Integrated Chinese-Western Medicine," *Hu Nan Zhong Yi Za Zhi (Hunan Journal of Chinese Medicine)*, #3, 1998, p. 47-48

Liang Shao-yong, "The Treatment of 58 Cases of Lower Limb Chronic Ulcers by the Methods of Boosting the Qi & Dispelling Stasis," *Hu Nan Zhong Yi Za Zhi (Hunan Journal of Chinese Medicine)*, #3, 2001, p. 28

Liang Xiao-chun & Guo Sai-shan, "A Way of Thinking About & Methodology for the Treatment of Diabetic Neuropathy," *Zhong Yi Za Zhi (Journal of Chinese Medicine)*, #1, 1999, p. 52-53

Liao Wei-ku & Lin Chun-yang, "Knowledge Gained from Experience in the Chinese Medical Pattern Discrimination Treatment of Diabetes Complicated by Upper Back Welling Abscesses," *Xin Zhong Yi (New Chinese Medicine)*, #3, 2001, p. 36-37

Lin Chen, "Knowledge Based on Experience of Treating Senile Diabetes by Fortifying & Moving the Spleen & Stomach," *Fu Jian Zhong Yi Yao (Fujian Chinese Medicine & Medicinals)*, #1, 2000, p. 28

Lin Hai-fei, "The Treatment of 26 Cases of Mild Diabetic Gastric Paresis with *Fu Ling Ze Xie Tang* (Poria & Alisma Decoction)," *Zhe Jiang Zhong Yi Za Zhi (Zhejiang Journal of Chinese Medicine)*, #9, 2001, p. 381

Lin Shao-zhi *et al.*, "Treating Diabetes Based on Phlegm Dampness—Plus An Analysis of 35 Cases of Type II Diabetes," *Shang Hai Zhong Yi Yao Za Zhi (Shanghai Journal of Chinese Medicine & Medicinals)*, #2, 1999, p. 8-9

Lin Xiao-hong, "The Treatment of 164 Cases of Diabetes with *Yi Qi Zi Yin Yin* (Boost the Qi & Enrich Yin Drink)," *Si Chuan Zhong Yi (Sichuan Chinese Medicine)*, #10, 1999, p. 31

Lin Zhi-gang, "A Study of the Efficacy of Treating Type II

Diabetes with Integrated Acupuncture & Medicinals," *Fu Jian Zhong Yi Yao (Fujian Chinese Medicine & Medicinals)*, #2, 2000, p. 19-20

Ling Bi-da, "The Treatment of Diabetic Eye Ground Bleeding with Integrated Chinese-Western Medicine," *Bei Jing Zhong Yi (Beijing Chinese Medicine)*, #3, 1999, p. 17-18

Liu Chang-zheng, "The Treatment of 25 Cases of Diabetic Gastric Paresis with Acupuncture & Western Medicine," *Hu Nan Zhong Yi Za Zhi (Hunan Journal of Chinese Medicine)*, #3, 2001, p. 33

Liu De-hua, "Lifting the Borders on the Treatment of Diabetic Impotence with *Si Teng Yi Xian Tang Jia Wei* (Four Vines & One Immortal Decoction with Added Flavors)," *Xin Zhong Yi (New Chinese Medicine)*, #8, 2001, p. 61

Liu Deng-xiang, "The Treatment of 27 Cases of Diabetes with *Gua Lou Qu Mai Wan Jia Wei* (Trichosanthes & Dianthus Pills with Added Flavors)," *Si Chuan Zhong Yi (Sichuan Chinese Medicine)*, #1, 1999, p. 24

Liu Gui-bin, "Four Methods Based on the Spleen for Treating Senile Diabetes," *Si Chuan Zhong Yi (Sichuan Chinese Medicine)*, #10, 2000, p. 7-8

Li Guo-sheng *et al.*, "The Treatment of 86 Cases of Type II Diabetes Using the Method of Supplementing the Kidneys," *Shi Yong Zhong Yi Nei Ke Za Zhi (Journal of Practical Chinese Medicine Internal Medicine)*, #2, 2001, p. 38

Liu Hong-hua & Tong Xiao-lin, "The Application of Standard Chinese Prescriptions in the Treatment of Diabetic Nephropathy," *Shi Yong Zhong Yi Nei Ke Za Zhi (Journal of Practical Chinese Medicine Internal Medicine)*, #2, 2001, p. 1-2, 4

Liu Hong-lu, "Herba Epimedii (*Yin Yang Huo*) in the Treatment of Type II Diabetes," *Zhong Yi Za Zhi (Journal of Chinese Medicine)*, #11, 1999, p. 645

Liu Ji-lin, "A Survey of Materia Medica Theory on Rhizoma Coptidis Chinesis (*Huang Lian*), Its Treatment of Wasting & Thirsting, and Its Functions," *Si Chuan Zhong Yi (Sichuan Chinese Medicine)*, #11, 1999, p. 17-19

Liu Jin-ping, "The Treatment of 47 Cases of Diabetic Peripheral Neuropathy with *Da Bu Yin Wan Jia Jian* (Greatly Supplementing Yin Pills with Additions & Subtractions)," *Hu Nan Zhong Yi Za Zhi (Hunan Journal of Chinese Medicine)*, #5, 2000, p. 40

Liu Ling, "The Treatment of Diabetic Retinopathy Via the Blood," *Si Chuan Zhong Yi (Sichuan Chinese Medicine)*, #2, 1999, p. 7

Liu Ling & Guo Xia, "The Treatment of Diabetic Retinopathy with *Tang Niao Bing Mu Qing Tang* (Diabetic Eye-clearing Decoction)," *Shan Dong Zhong Yi Za Zhi (Shandong Journal of Chinese Medicine)*, #3, 2000, p. 145-146

Liu Min-xing, "The Treatment of 60 Cases of Type II Diabetes with *Yu Xiao Jiang Tang Yin* (Cure Wasting & Lower Sugar Drink)," *Si Chuan Zhong Yi (Sichuan Chinese Medicine)*, #8, 2001, p. 42

Liu Wen, "The Treatment of 30 Cases of Diabetes Using Gao Hui-yun's Method of Boosting the Qi & Nourishing Yin," *Hu Bei Zhong Yi Za Zhi (Hubei Journal of Chinese Medicine)*, #1, 1994, p. 20

Liu Wu-jing *et al.*, "The Treatment of 48 Cases of Diabetic Peripheral Neuropathy with Ligustrazine & Anisodamine," *Xin Zhong Yi (New Chinese Medicine)*, #6, 2001, p. 35-36

Liu Ya-li, "The Treatment of 32 Cases of Diabetic Peripheral Neuropathy with *Huang Qi Mai Luo Ning Zhu She Ye* (Astragalus Vessel & Network Vessel Calming Injectible Fluid)," *Shan Xi Zhong Yi (Shanxi Chinese Medicine)*, #4, 2001, p. 12-13

Lu Jie-yun & Xu Hong-lan, "The Treatment of 42 Cases of Diabetic Peripheral Neuritis Using *Huang Qi Gui Zhi Wu Wu Tang Jia Wei* (Astragalus & Cinnamon Twig Five Materials Decoction with Added Flavors)," *Hei Long Jiang Zhong Yi Yao (Heilongjiang Chinese Medicine & Medicinals)*, #4, 1998, p. 17-18

Lu Ren-he, Zhao Jin-xi & Wang Shi-dong, "A Clincal Study on Diabetes & Its Complications," *Xin Zhong Yi (New Chinese Medicine)*, #3, 2001, p. 3-5

Lu Yan-ping *et al.*, "The Treatment of 41 Cases of Diabetic Cholecystitis by the Methods of Coursing the Liver & Disinhibiting the Gallbladder," *Si Chuan Zhong Yi (Sichuan Chinese Medicine)*, # 5 , 2000, p. 22-23

Lu Yu-zheng, "The Treatment of 32 Cases of Diabetic Peripheral Neuropathy with Self-composed *Ma Tong Tang* (Numbness & Pain Decoction)," *Si Chuan Zhong Yi (Sichuan Chinese Medicine)*, #9, 2000, p. 16

Lu Yuan-zhong & Wu Yu-ning, "Clinical Observations on

the Treatment of 50 Cases of Menopausal Diabetes with *Bu Shen Fang* (Supplement the Kidneys Formula)," *Shan Xi Zhong Yi (Shanxi Chinese Medicine)*, #3, 2001, p. 16-18

Luo Shan, "The Treatment of Diabetes Using the Methods of Boosting the Qi, Enriching Yin & Draining Fire," *Hu Bei Zhong Yi Za Zhi (Hubei Journal of Chinese Medicine)*, #3, 1998, p. 41-42

Mao Gao-feng & Zhang Bin, "An Experimental Study on the Effect of *Er Huang Tang* (Two Yellows Decoction) on Blood Sugar & Serum Insulin on an Empty Stomach in Mice Modeled with Alloxan Tetraoxypyrimidine," *He Nan Zhong Yi (Henan Chinese Medicine)*, #1, 2001, p. 37-38

Ni Yan-xia, "The Treatment of 30 Cases of Diabetic Uroschesis Using Chinese Medicinals," *Ji Lin Zhong Yi Yao (Jilin Chinese Medicine & Medicinals)*, #1, 1999, p. 32

Pan Zhao-xi, "The Disease Causes, Disease Mechanisms & Treatment Methods for Diabetes," *Jiang Su Zhong Yi (Jiangsu Chinese Medicine)*, #1, 2000, p. 1-3

Pang Shu-zhen, "The Treatment of 27 Cases of Diabetic Neurogenic Bladder with *Bu Zhong Yi Qi Tang* (Supplement the Center & Boost the Qi Decoction)," *Si Chuan Zhong Yi (Sichuan Chinese Medicine)*, #3, 2001, p. 42

Peng Bo, "A Survey of the Chinese Medical Medicinal Treatment of Diabetic Retinopathy," *Hu Nan Zhong Yi Za Zhi (Hunan Journal of Chinese Medicine)*, #9, 2001, p. 58-59

Peng Geng-ru & Zhao Lin, "A Clincial Audit of the Treatment of 92 Cases of Type II Diabetes with *Xiao Ke Tang* (Wasting & Thirsting Decoction) & Glyburide," *Hu Nan Zhong Yi Za Zhi (Hunan Journal of Chinese Medicine)*, #2, 2002, p. 17-18

Peng Wan-nian, "A Discussion of Damp Heat Patterns in Wasting & Thirsting Disease," *Xin Zhong Yi (New Chinese Medicine)*, #12, 1998, p. 3-4

Peng Zhen-sheng, "The Treatment of 102 Cases of Non-insulin-dependent Diabetes with *Ping Xiao Jiang Tang Tang* (Calm Wasting & Lower Sugar Decoction)," *Zhe Jiang Zhong Yi Za Zhi (Zhejiang Journal of Chinese Medicine)*, #8, 2000, p. 331

Pu Xian-chun *et al.*, "A Summary of 94 Cases of Mild Cerebral Ischemia Caused by Diabetic Hyperviscosity Syndrome Treated by *Zi Cui Tong Mai Jiao Nang* (Burst Fat & Free the Flow of the Vessels Gelatin Capsules)," *Hu*

Nan Zhong Yi Za Zhi (Hunan Journal of Chinese Medicine), #4, 2001, p. 17-18

Qi Fang *et al.*, "Clinical Observations on the Treatment of 331 Cases of Diabetes Using *Xiao Ke Jiang Tang Dan Nang Bao* (Wasting & Thirsting Lower Sugar Elixir Gelatin Capsules)," *Bei Jing Zhong Yi Za Zhi (Beijing Journal of Chinese Medicine)*, #1, 1994, p. 50-52

Qi Fang *et al.*, "Clinical Research on the Treatment of Diabetes Mellitus (NIDDM) Using *Xiao Ke Chong Ji* (Wasting & Thirsting Soluble Granules)," *Bei Jing Zhong Yi (Beijing Chinese Medicine)*, #4, 1998, p. 42-44

Qi Xiao-yan, "Experiences in the Integrated Chinese-Western Medical Approach to Diabetes," *Shi Yong Zhong Yi Nei Ke Za Zhi (Journal of Practical Chinese Medicine Internal Medicine)*, #31, 2001, p. 47

Qiao Yu-qiu & Xie Mao-ling, "The Treatment of 26 Cases of Diabetic Ketoacidosis with *Huang Lian Wen Dan Tang* (Coptis Warm the Gallbladder Decoction) Combined with Western Medicinals," *Zhe Jiang Zhong Yi Za Zhi (Zhejiang Journal of Chinese Medicine)*, #3, 2000, p. 112

Qing Zhao-qian, "A Survey of the Treatment of 60 Cases of Type II Diabetes with *Shen Qi Yu Xiao Tang* (Ginseng & Astragalus Cure Wasting Decoction – Plus a Comparison with 30 Cases Treated with *Glyburide*," *Zhe Jiang Zhong Yi Za Zhi (Zhejiang Journal of Chinese Medicine)*, #5, 2001, p. 190-191

Qiu Feng-wu & Zhao Shu-zhe, "The Treatment of 56 Cases of Diabetes Using the Methods of Fortifying the Spleen & Disinhibiting Dampness," *Ji Lin Zhong Yi Yao (Jilin Chinese Medicine & Medicinals)*, #2, 1999, p. 14

Qiu Yin-xiang, "Experiences in the Treatment of Diabetic Peripheral Neuropathy," *Bei Jing Zhong Yi (Beijing Chinese Medicine)*, #4, 2000, p. 54

Qu Li-qing, "A Discussion of Pattern Discrimination in the Treatment of Diabetic Psychological Disturbance," *Shan Dong Zhong Yi Za Zhi (Shandong Journal of Chinese Medicine)*, #11, 1999, p. 496-497

Quan Xiao-lin, "Six Treatises on Wasting & Thirsting," *Zhong Yi Za Zhi (Journal of Chinese Medicine)*, #4, 2001, p. 252-253
Ren Ai-hua & Kan Fang-xu, "The Triple Burner Pattern Discrimination & Treatment of Diabetic Nephropathy," *Shan Dong Zhong Yi Za Zhi (Shandong Journal of Chinese Medicine)*, #6, 2000, p. 328-329

Shang Wen-bin & Cheng Hai-bo, "Advances in the Study of Chinese Medicine & Medicinals in Insulin-resistant Diabetes," *Zhong Yi Za Zhi (Journal of Chinese Medicine)*, #11, 1999, p. 692-695

Shen Zhao-xiong, "Raising the Borders of [Zhang] Zhong-jing's Formulas for the Treatment of Wasting & Thirsting," *Jiang Su Zhong Yi (Jiangsu Chinese Medicine)*, #5, 1999, p. 30

Shi Su-yu, "The Treatment of 30 Cases of Diabetes by the Methods of Fortifying the Spleen & Upbearing the Clear—With a Comparison to 30 Cases Treated with *Yu Quan Wan* (Jade Spring Pills)," *Zhe Jiang Zhong Yi Za Zhi (Zhejiang Journal of Chinese Medicine)*," #2, 2000, p. 52-53

Shi Xi-zhi *et al.*, "The Chinese Medical Treatment of Diabetic Pruritus Vulvae," *Ji Lin Zhong Yi Yao (Jilin Chinese Medicine & Medicinals)*, #2, 1999, p. 31-32

Shi Ya-hong, "The Treatment of 32 Cases of Diabetic Nephropathy with Integrated Chinese-Western Medicine," *Si Chuan Zhong Yi (Sichuan Chinese Medicine)*, #4, 1999, p. 27

Shi Zhi-yun *et al.*, "The Clinical Significance of Thrombo-molecular Markers in Blood Stasis Pattern in Diabetes," *Zhong Yi Za Zhi (Journal of Chinese Medicine)*, #9, 1999, p. 554-555

Shui Rui-ying & Teng Shu-wen, "The Treatment of 30 Cases of Diabetic Peripheral Neuritis Using *Huo Xue Bu Shen Tang* (Quicken the Blood & Supplement the Kidneys Decoction)," *Zhe Jiang Zhong Yi Za Zhi (Zhejiang Journal of Chinese Medicine)*," 8, 1999, p. 329

Si Fu-quan, "The Treatment of 25 Cases of Diabetic Nephropathy with Integrated Chinese-Western Medicine," *Ji Lin Zhong Yi Yao (Jilin Chinese Medicine & Medicinals)*, #3, 1999, p. 37-38

Song Ju-min *et al.*, "The Influence of *Tang Niao Ning* (Diabetes Calmer) on Blood Glucose, Insulin & Sciatic Nerve Conduction in Rats with Diabetic Neuropathy," *Shang Hai Zhong Yi Yao Za Zhi (Shanghai Journal of Chinese Medicine & Medicinals)*, #7, 2001, p. 42-43

Su Ping-mao & Zhang Guo-xia, "A Summary of the Treatment of 57 Cases of Diabetic Dawn Phenomenon with Master Lei's *Su Xiang Hua Zuo Fang* (Penetratingly Aromatic Transforming Turbidity Formula)," *Hu Nan Zhong Yi Za Zhi (Hunan Journal of Chinese Medicine)*, #2, 2001, p. 16-17

Su You-min *et al.*, "The Treatment of 35 Cases of Retinal Vascular Obstruction with Integrated Chinese-Western Medicine," *Hu Nan Zhong Yi Za Zhi (Hunan Journal of Chinese Medicine)*, #1, 2001, p. 46

Su Yu-dian & Niu Tong-zhou, "Experiences in the Treatment of Diabetes with Rhizoma Atractylodis (*Cang Zhu*)," *Zhong Yi Za Zhi (Journal of Chinese Medicine)*, #9, 1998, p. 573

Sun Jun, "A Review of the State of Research on the Chinese Medicine & Medicinal Treatment of Diabetic Nephropathy," *Bei Jing Zhong Yi (Beijing Chinese Medicine)*, #6, 1999, p. 44-46

Sun Jun, "Clinical Research on the Treatment of Early Stage Diabetic Nephropathy with *Zhi Xiao Tong Mai Ning* (Stop Wasting & Free the Flow of the Vessels Calmer)," *Bei Jing Zhong Yi (Beijing Chinese Medicine)*, #4, 1999, p. 50-52

Sun Xue-dong, "The Treatment of 82 Cases of Diabetes-induced Skin Itching with Self-composed *Zhi Yang Tang* (Stop Itching Decoction)," *Bei Jing Zhong Yi (Beijing Chinese Medicine)*, #3, 2000, p. 22

Sun Yuan-bo & Sun Yuan-ping, "The Treatment of 52 Cases of Type II Diabetes with *Li Qi Huo Xue Bu Shen Fang* (Rectify the Qi, Quicken the Blood & Supplement the Kidneys Formula)," *Bei Jing Zhong Yi (Beijing Chinese Medicine)*, #2, 1999, p. 41

Tai Shu-xian, "The Treatment of Diabetes," *Yun Nan Zhong Yi Yao Za Zhi (Yunnan Journal of Chinese Medicine & Medicinals)*, #4, 1996, p. 6-8

Tan Xian-fang & Yang Yun-jun, "The Treatment of 32 Cases of Diabetic Bladder Pathology with Integrated Chinese-Western Medicine," *Hu Nan Zhong Yi Za Zhi (Hunan Journal of Chinese Medicine)*, #5, 2000, p. 40-41

Tan Yong-dong, "Herba Pycnostelmae (*Xu Chang Jing*) in the Treatment of Diabetic Nephropathy & Peripheral Neuropathy," *Zhong Yi Za Zhi (Journal of Chinese Medicine)*, #10, 2001, p. 584

Tang Dai-yi, "The Chinese Medical Pattern Discrimination of Diabetes & Advances in the Study of Related Experimental Criteria," *Si Chuan Zhong Yi (Sichuan Chinese Medicine)*, #6, 1999, p. 16-18

Tang Dai-yi & Pan Ming-zheng, "Research into the Relationship Between Obesity & the Chinese Medical Pattern Discrimination of the Diabetic Patient," *Si Chuan Zhong Yi (Sichuan Chinese Medicine)*, #2, 1999, p. 15-17

Tang Hong *et al.*, "The Influence of the Qi-boosting, Blood-quickening & Kidney-supplementing Method on Vaso-active Substances in Early Stage Diabetic Nephropathy," *Shang Hai Zhong Yi Yao Za Zhi (Shanghai Journal of Chinese Medicine & Medicinals)*, #12, 2001, p. 19-20

Tang Ju-rong, "A Survey of Chinese Medicinals in the Treatment of Diabetes," *Hu Bei Zhong Yi Za Zhi (Hubei Journal of Chinese Medicine)*, #5, 1998, p. 57-58

Tang Ting-han, "The Treatment of 50 Cases of Mild Diabetic Stomach Paresis with *Ban Xia Xie Xin Tang* (Pinellia Drain the Heart Decoction)," *Si Chuan Zhong Yi (Sichuan Chinese Medicine)*, #9, 2001, p. 35

Tang Yuan-shan, "The Pattern Discrimination Treatment of Diabetic Foot," *Si Chuan Zhong Yi (Sichuan Chinese Medicine)*, #10, 2001, p. 11-12

Tong Jia-luo, "The Treatment of Blood Stasis in 60 Cases of Type II Diabetes," *Shan Dong Zhong Yi Za Zhi (Shandong Journal of Chinese Medicine)*, #8, 1999, p. 350-351

Tong Jie *et al.*, "The Treatment of 122 Cases of Diabetic Hypertension with *Ping Gan Huo Xue Jiao Nang* (Level the Liver & Quicken the Blood Capsules)," *Shan Dong Zhong Yi Za Zhi (Shandong Journal of Chinese Medicine)*, #2, 2000, p. 78-79

Tong Xiao-lin *et al.*, "Clinical Research in the Treatment of Diabetic Insulin Resistance Using *Kai Yu Qing Wei He Ji* (Open Depression & Clear the Stomach Granules)," *Shi Yong Zhong Yi Nei Ke Za Zhi (Journal of Practical Chinese Medicine Internal Medicine)*, #2, 2001, p. 10-11

Tong Yan-ling, "The Treatment of Non-insulin-dependent Diabetes with *Yang Yin Jiang Tang Tang* (Nourish Yin & Lower Sugar Decoction) – With a Comparison to 36 Cases Treated with *Xiao Ke Wan* (Wasting & Thirsting Pills)," *Zhe Jiang Zhong Yi Za Zhi (Zhejiang Journal of Chinese Medicine)*, #7, 2000, p. 289

Wang Da-qian, "A Clinical Audit of the Treatment of 161 Cases of Diabetic Retinal Hemorrhage with *Dan Qi Di Huang Tang* (Salvia & Pseudoginseng Rehmannia Decoction)," *Bei Jing Zhong Yi (Beijing Chinese Medicine)*, #5, 1999, p. 25-26

Wang Fan, "The Treatment of 28 Cases of Diabetic Foot with the Methods of Boosting the Qi & Quickening the Blood Combined with the Use of Agkistrodon Antithrombotic Enzyme," *Zhong Yi Za Zhi (Journal of Chinese Medicine)*, #3, 2001, p. 170

Wang Hui-lan, "A Clinical Analysis of the Treatment of 62 Cases of Type II Diabetes with Integrated Chinese-Western Medicine," *Bei Jing Zhong Yi (Beijing Chinese Medicine)*, #4, 2000, p. 35-36

Wang Jia-zhan & Qu Wei-yi, "A Discussion of Toxins in the Treatment of Diabetes," *Shan Dong Zhong Yi Za Zhi (Shandong Journal of Chinese Medicine)*, #8, 1999, p. 339-341

Wang Jian, "A New Exploration of the Disease Mechanisms, Patterns & Treatments of Wasting & Thirsting," *Si Chuan Zhong Yi (Sichuan Chinese Medicine)*, #4, 2001, p. 14-15

Wang Jian & Xu Qing, "A Clinical Audit of the Treatment of 32 Cases of Diabetic Peripheral Neuropathy with Specific Electromagnetic Waves & *Gui Long Er Chuan Tang* (Dang Gui, Lumbricus & Two Chuans Decoction)," *Xin Zhong Yi (New Chinese Medicine)*, #8, 2001, p. 27-28

Wang Jin-tao, "The Treatment of 18 Cases of Diabetes with *Song Zhen* Method of *Tui Na*," *Shan Dong Zhong Yi Za Zhi (Shandong Journal of Chinese Medicine)*, #11, 1999, p. 502

Wang Jing-fang, "An Analysis of the Chinese Medical Patterns in 96 Cases of Senile Diabetes," *Shang Hai Zhong Yi Yao Za Zhi (Shanghai Journal of Chinese Medicine & Medicinals)*, #7, 1999, p. 21-22

Wang Jun-hua & Wang Cheng-cui, "The Treatment of 30 Cases of Type II Diabetes with Integrated Chinese-Western Medicine," *Shan Xi Zhong Yi (Shanxi Chinese Medicine)*, #2, 2001, p. 25-26

Wang Ling *et al.*, "The Effectiveness of *Shen Di Jiang Tang Ke Li* (Ginseng & Rehmannia Lower Sugar Granules) on Insulin Resistance in High Fructose Rats," *Zhong Yi Za Zhi (Journal of Chinese Medicine)*, #11, 2001, p. 686-688

Wang Ling-lu, "The Chinese Medicinal Treatment of Diabetic Peripheral Neuropathy," *Bei Jing Zhong Yi (Beijing Chinese Medicine)*, #4, 1999, p. 35-36

Wang Ling-xia, "The Treatment of Diabetic Peripheral Neuropathy Using Chinese Medicinals," *Bei Jing Zhong Yi (Beijing Chinese Medicine)*, #4, 1999, p. 35-36

Wang Min-han, "The Treatment of 80 Cases of Type II Diabetes Stomach Function Disturbance with *Jian Zhong Jiang Ni Tang* (Fortify the Center & Downbear Counterflow Decoction)," *Si Chuan Zhong Yi (Sichuan Chinese Medicine)*, #4, 2001, p. 46-47

Wang Shu-ling, "Clinical Observations on the Treatment of Blood Stasis in 27 Cases of Diabetes," *Bei Jing Zhong Yi (Beijing Chinese Medicine)*, #3, 1998, p. 26

Wang Wei, "The Pattern Discrimination Treatment of Diabetic Eye Ground Bleeding," *Si Chuan Zhong Yi (Sichuan Chinese Medicine)*, #4, 2001, p. 73-74

Wang Xiao-hong, "The Treatment of Diabetic Complications Using *Bu Yang Huan Wu Tang* (Supplement Yang & Restore Five [Tenths] Decoction)," *Zhe Jiang Zhong Yi Za Zhi (Zhejiang Journal of Chinese Medicine)*, #11, 1999, p. 494

Wang Xin-ling *et al.*, "The Treatment of 84 Cases of Diabetic Nephropathy Using Integrated Chinese-Western Medicine," *Shi Yong Zhong Yi Nei Ke Za Zhi (Journal of Practical Chinese Medicine Internal Medicine)*, #2, 2001, p. 36-37

Wang Yan-bin, "The Treatment of 34 Cases of Diabetic Nephropathy by the Methods of Boosting the Qi & Transforming Stasis," *Si Chuan Zhong Yi (Sichuan Chinese Medicine)*, #6, 2001, p. 26-27

Wang Yong, "Knowledge Based on Experience of the Discrimination & Treatment of Yang Vacuity Pattern Diabetes," *Si Chuan Zhong Yi (Sichuan Chinese Medicine)*, #7, 2001, p. 4-5

Wang You-gan, "Distinguishing What Are Called Diabetes and Wasting & Thirsting Disease," *Jiang Su Zhong Yi (Jiangsu Chinese Medicine)*, #5, 1999, p. 48

Wang Zhao-yu *et al.*, "Comparisons of Glycometabolism & Lipometabolism in Hypertension Patients with Different Chinese Medical Patterns," *Zhong Yi Za Zhi (Journal of Chinese Medicine)*, #7, 2001, p. 428-431

Wang Zhen-qing, "A Clinical Study of the Treatment of Diabetes by the Methods of Quickening the Blood & Boosting the Qi," *Hu Nan Zhong Yi (Hunan Chinese Medicine)*, #5, 2001, p. 33-34

Wei Ling-ling *et al.*, "A Clinical Audit of the Treatment of 40 Cases of Diabetic Peripheral Neuropathy by the Methods of Supplementing the Qi & Quickening the Blood," *Zhong Yi Za Zhi (Journal of Chinese Medicine)*, #7, 2001, p. 421-422

Wei Su-xia, "The Treatment of 40 Cases of Hepatogenic Diabetes Via the Liver," *Si Chuan Zhong Yi (Sichuan Chinese Medicine)*, #10, 1999, p. 16-17

Wei Zhan-chun, "A Clinical Audit of the Treatment of 42 Cases of Diabetes with *Shen Mai Zhu She Ye* (Ginseng & Ophiopogon Injectible Fluid) & *Yun Nan Deng Zhan Hua Zhu She Ye* (Yunnan Hibiscus Flower Injectible Fluid)," *Xin Zhong Yi (New Chinese Medicine)*, #8, 2001, p. 29

Wen Xiao-min & Yang Shou, "A Survey of the Chinese Medical Diagnosis & Treatment of Diabetes," *Si Chuan Zhong Yi (Sichuan Chinese Medicine)*, #3, 2000, p. 14-16

Wen Zi-long, "Deng Tie-tao's Experiences in the Treatment of Middle-aged & Geriatric Diabetes," *Zhe Jiang Zhong Yi Za Zhi (Zhejiang Journal of Chinese Medicine)*, #9, 2001, p. 369

Wu Chen *et al.*, "A Clinical Analysis of the Influence of Acupuncture on Blood Glucose & Blood Lipids in Patients with Diabetes," *He Nan Zhong Yi (Henan Chinese Medicine)*, #1, 2001, p. 42-43

Wu De-yin, "The Treatment of 32 Cases of Diabetic Retinopathy Mainly by Quickening the Blood & Transforming Stasis," *Zhe Jiang Zhong Yi Za Zhi (Zhejiang Journal of Chinese Medicine)*, #4, 2000, p. 158

Wu De-yong, "A Simple [*i.e.*, Short] Treatise on the Disease Causes & Disease Mechanisms of Wasting & Thirsting," *Hu Nan Zhong Yi Za Zhi (Hunan Journal of Chinese Medicine)*, #9, 2000, p. 7

Wu Ji-hai *et al.*, "An Inquiry into Zhang Zhong-jing's Treatment of Wasting & Thirsting Disease Formulas & Patterns," *He Nan Zhong Yi (Henan Chinese Medicine)*, #4, 2000, p. 5-6

Wu Jian-mei, "The Treatment of 27 Cases of Retinal Vascular Obstruction with Integrated Chinese-Western Medicine," *He Nan Zhong Yi (Henan Chinese Medicine)*, #5, 2000, p. 42-43

Wu Shen-tao, "Insulin Resistance Should be Treated by the Methods of Boosting the Kidneys, Transforming Stasis

& Coursing and Disinhibiting the *Shao Yang*," *Zhong Yi Za Zhi (Journal of Chinese Medicine)*, #6, 2001, p. 332-333

Wu Song-shou, "The Treatment of 58 Cases of Diabetes with *Jia Wei Shen Qi Wan* (Added Flavors Kidney Qi Pills) Plus Western Medicines—With a Comparison to 52 Patients Treated with Glyburide," *Zhe Jiang Zhong Yi Za Zhi (Zhejiang Journal of Chinese Medicine)*, #5, 2000, p. 194

Xia Cheng-dong, "An Exploration of the *Nei Jing*'s Treatise on Wasting & Thirsting," *Si Chuan Zhong Yi (Sichuan Chinese Medicine)*, #8, 2001, p. 15-16

Xia Cheng-dong, "Plucking the Essentials of Professor Ding Xue-bing's Experiences in Treating Diabetes," *Xin Zhong Yi (New Chinese Medicine)*, #2, 2001, p. 16-17

Xian Hui, "Clinical Observations on the Treatment of 30 Cases of Diabetes Using *Huo Xue Zhi Xiao Tang* (Quicken the Blood & Stop Wasting Decoction)," *Jiang Su Zhong Yi (Jiangsu Chinese Medicine)*, #5, 2000, p. 19-20

Xiao Yan-qian, "Important Examples in the Discrimination & Treatment of Diabetes," *Shang Hai Zhong Yi Yao Za Zhi (Shanghai Journal of Chinese Medicine & Medicinals)*, #9, 1997, p. 14-15

Xie Xi-sheng, "Feng Zhi-rong's Understanding & Experiences in the Treatment of Type II Diabetes," *Si Chuan Zhong Yi (Sichuan Chinese Medicine)*, #1, 1999, p. 1-2

Xin Jun *et al.*, "The Treatment of 52 Cases of Diabetic Nephropathy with Integrated Chinese-Western Medicine," *Shan Xi Zhong Yi (Shanxi Chinese Medicine)*, #6, 1999, p. 23

Xing Hai-yan, "An Experimental Study of the Treatment of Type II Diabetes & Its Chronic Complications with *Tang Yu Ping* (Sugar & Stasis Leveler)," *He Nan Zhong Yi (Henan Chinese Medicine)*, #5, 2000, p. 29-30

Xiong Man-qi *et al.*, "Clinical Observations on Changes of the Bones in Different Chinese Medical Patterns of Diabetes," *Zhong Yi Za Zhi (Journal of Chinese Medicine)*, #10, 1998, p. 597-598

Xu De-yi, "The Treatment of 36 Cases of Diabetic Peripheral Neuropathy Using *Juan Bi Tong Luo* (Alleviate Impediment & Free the Flow of the Network Vessels [Decoction])," *Hei Long Jiang Zhong Yi Yao (Heilongjiang Chinese Medicine & Medicinals)*, #5, 1998, p. 26

Xu Pei-ying *et al.*, "A Clinical Audit of the Treatment of Type II Diabetes (Qi & Yin Dual Vacuity Pattern) with *Yi Qi Yang Yin Fang* (Boost the Qi & Nourish Yin Formula)," *Shang Hai Zhong Yi Yao Za Zhi (Shanghai Journal of Chinese Medicine & Medicinals)*, #11, 2001, p. 20-21

Xu Sheng-sheng, "The Treatment of 32 Cases of Diabetic Neurogenic Bladder Using *Tong Quan Tang* (Free the Flow of the Spring Decoction)," *Si Chuan Zhong Yi (Sichuan Chinese Medicine)*, #11, 1998, p. 23

Xu Sheng-sheng, "The Use of *Yi Qi Zhu Yu Tong Mai Tang* (Boost the Qi, Dispel Stasis & Free the Flow of the Vessels Decoction) in the Treatment of Diabetic Peripheral Neuropathy," *Jiang Su Zhong Yi (Jiangsu Chinese Medicine)*, #3, 1999, p. 23

Xu Yuan, "Yin Hui's Important Issues in Understanding How to Treat Diabetes," *Shan Dong Zhong Yi Za Zhi (Shandong Journal of Chinese Medicine)*, #1, 2000, p. 40-41

Xu Yun-sheng & Cheng Yi-chun, "Experiences in the Treatment of Two Cases of Diabetes & Amenorrhea," *Zhong Yi Za Zhi (Journal of Chinese Medicine)*, #6, 1997, p. 338

Xu Zhao-shan, "The Treatment of 42 Cases of Diabetic Gastric Paresis with Pattern Discrimination—Plus a Comparison with 40 Cases Treated with Western Medicine," *Zhe Jiang Zhong Yi Za Zhi (Zhejiang Journal of Chinese Medicine)*, #4, 2001, p. 145-146

Xu Zhu-ting, "The Treatment of 76 Cases of Diabetes Accompanied by Hyperlipidemia with Self-composed *Jiu Wei Jiang Zhi Tang* (Nine Flavors Lower Fat Decoction)," *Shang Hai Zhong Yi Yao Za Zhi (Shanghai Journal of Chinese Medicine & Medicinals)*, #12, 1999, p. 30-31

Xue Fu-yu, "A Clinical Audit of the Treatment of 63 Cases of Type II Diabetes with *Jiang Tang Huo Xue Fang* (Lower Sugar & Quicken the Blood Formula)," *Bei Jing Zhong Yi (Beijing Chinese Medicine)*, #2, 1999, p. 19-20

Xue Wen-sen, "Observations on the Effectiveness of Self-composed *Jiang Tang Yin* (Lower Sugar Drink) on the Treatment of 42 Cases of Diabetes," *Ji Lin Zhong Yi Yao (Jilin Chinese Medicine & Medicinals)*, #2, 1994, p. 11-12

Ya Dao-zheng, "A Clinical Audit on the Treatment of 66 Cases of Type II Diabetes with *Tang Xiao Ping Tang* (Sugar Wasting Leveling Decoction)," *Zhe Jiang Zhong Yi Za Zhi (Zhejiang Journal of Chinese Medicine)*, #9, 1999, p. 407

Yan Juan, "Examination & Analysis of the *Nei Jing*'s Treatment of Wasting & Thirsting Disease," *Si Chuan Zhong Yi* (*Sichuan Chinese Medicine*), #11, 1998, p. 5

Yang Hai-yan & Yang Jian-hua, "Clinical & TCD Observations on Frequency Spectrum of Ophthalmic Arterial Blood Flow in 61 Eyes with Diabetic Retinopathy Treated with *Yi Shen Huo Xue Fang* (Boost the Kidneys & Quicken the Blood Formula)," *Zhe Jiang Zhong Yi Za Zhi* (*Zhejiang Journal of Chinese Medicine*), #1, 2001, p. 30-31

Yang Jun, "A Discussion of the Treatment of Diabetes Caused by Middle Burner Dampness & Turbidity," *Zhong Yi Za Zhi* (*Journal of Chinese Medicine*), #3, 1999, p. 187

Yang Shou, "The Use of the Methods of Clearing Heat & Disinhibiting Dampness in Diabetes," *Si Chuan Zhong Yi* (*Sichuan Chinese Medicine*), #8, 1999, p. 17-18

Yang Yong-hua *et al.*, "The Treatment of 30 Cases of Type II Diabetes Using the Methods of Boosting the Qi & Nourishing Yin," *Shan Xi Zhong Yi* (*Shanxi Chinese Medicine*), #6, 1997, p. 18

Yang You-xin *et al.*, "The Treatment of 35 Cases of Type II Diabetes by the Methods of Boosting the Qi, Nourishing Yin & Quickening the Blood," *Si Chuan Zhong Yi* (*Sichuan Chinese Medicine*), #8, 1999, p. 40-41

Yang Yu-lian, "New Methods for the Treatment of Diabetic Foot Using Combined Internal & External Applications," *Shan Xi Zhong Yi* (*Shanxi Chinese Medicine*), #4, 1999, p. 22

Yang Yun-jun & Tan Xian-fang, "The Treatment of 49 Cases of Type II Diabetes with Integrated Chinese-Western Medicine," *Hu Nan Zhong Yi Za Zhi* (*Hunan Journal of Chinese Medicine*), #1, 2001, p. 35

Yang Zao, "The Pattern Discrimination of 60 Cases of Type II Diabetes," *Shi Yong Zhong Yi Nei Ke Za Zhi* (*Journal of Practical Chinese Medicine Internal Medicine*), #1, 2001, p. 28

Yin Cui-mei & Li Zhen-zhong, "An Inquiry into the Treatment of Diabetic Angiopathy," *Shan Xi Zhong Yi* (*Shanxi Chinese Medicine*), #3, 2001, p. 60

Yu Hong *et al.*, "A Survey of the Efficacy of Treating 30 Cases of Diabetes with the Method of Acridly Moistening Combined with *You Jiang Tang* (Outstanding Lowering

Sugar [Tablets])," *Hu Nan Zhong Yi Za Zhi* (*Hunan Journal of Chinese Medicine*), #1, 2000, p. 9-10

Yu Jun-sheng & Wang Yan-lin, "A Discussion of the Mutual Engenderment of Phlegm, Stasis & Toxins," *Shan Dong Zhong Yi Za Zhi* (*Shandong Journal of Chinese Medicine*), #6, 2000, 323-325

Yu Shao-qing, "The Treatment of 39 Cases of Diabetic Neuropathy with *Yang Yin Huo Luo Tang* (Nourish Yin & Quicken the Network Vessels Decoction)," *Hu Nan Zhong Yi Za Zhi* (*Hunan Journal of Chinese Medicine*), #1, 2000, p. 28-29

Yu Wen-ping & Qin Ai-lin, "A Discussion of the Disease Causes & Disease Mechanisms of Diabetic Nephropathy," *Ji Lin Zhong Yi Yao* (*Jilin Chinese Medicine & Medicinals*), #5, 1999, p. 4-5

Yuan Guang-ping, "*Fu Fang Dan Shen Di Wan* (Compound Salvia Drip Pills) & Disturbances in Nail Microcirculation in Those with Geriatric Diabetes," *Hu Nan Zhong Yi* (*Hunan Chinese Medicine*), #5, 2001, p. 35

Yuan Jin-hong *et al.*, "The Influence of Acupuncture on the Nulceus Supra-opticus Hypothalmi in Experimental Non-insulin Dependent Diabetic Rats," *Zhe Jiang Zhong Yi Za Zhi* (*Zhejiang Journal of Chinese Medicine*), #11, 2000, p. 498-500

Yuan Ling *et al.*, "The Treatment of Nine Cases of Diabetic Nephropathy Using Chinese Medicinals," *Guo Yi Lun Tan* (*National Medical Forum*), #5, 1996, p. 28

Yuan Shun-xing *et al.*, "The Influence of Kidney-supplementing & Body-strengthening [Qi]gong on Insulin-resistant Type II Diabetes," *Shang Hai Zhong Yi Yao Za Zhi* (*Shanghai Journal of Chinese Medicine & Medicinals*), #11, 1999, p. 37-38

Zeng Zhi-yong, "The Influence of Acupuncture on Diabetic Rabbit Blood Sugar & Pancreatic Glucagon," *Si Chuan Zhong Yi* (*Sichuan Chinese Medicine*), #11, 2000, p. 8-9

Zhang Cheng-lu & Tan Jin-ling, "The Integrated Chinese-Western Medical Treatment of 16 Cases of Diabetic Foot," *Hu Nan Zhong Yi Za Zhi* (*Hunan Journal of Chinese Medicine*), #1, 2000, p. 28

Zhang Fu-nan, "The Treatment of Chronic Diabetic Diarrhea," *Guang Ming Zhong Yi* (*Guangming Chinese Medicine*), #4, 2001, p. 31-33

Zhang Guang-hui, "The Discrimination & Treatment of Diabetic Peripheral Neuropathy Via the Methods of Cooling the Blood & Scattering Stasis and Warming & Freeing the Flow of the Channels & Vessels," *Bei Jing Zhong Yi (Beijing Chinese Medicine)*, #4, 2001, p. 54

Zhang Hong & Cui De-zhi, "Concepts for Increasing the Vitality of the Spleen & Stomach in the Treatment of Diabetic Diarrhea," *Jiang Su Zhong Yi (Jiangsu Chinese Medicine)*, #3, 2000, p. 7

Zhang Hong-ming, "The Treatment of 50 Cases of Diabetic Retinopathy with *Jiang Tang Yin* (Lower Sugar Drink)," *Si Chuan Zhong Yi (Sichuan Chinese Medicine)*, #3, 1999, p. 45

Zhang Hong-ying, "Characteristic Analysis of Medicinals Used in Ancient Formulas to Treat Wasting & Thirsting Disease," *Bei Jing Zhong Yi (Beijing Chinese Medicine)*, #3, 1998, p. 49-51

Zhang Hui-zhen & Guo Shi-lin, "The Treatment of 56 Cases of Diabetes Using an Insulin Umbilical Plaster," *Shan Xi Zhong Yi (Shanxi Chinese Medicine)*, #5, 1999, p. 36

Zhang Jun-rong & Wan Yun-li, "A Survey of the Efficacy of Treating Diabetic Multiple Onset Peripheral Neuropathy with *Xue Fu Zhu Yu Jiao Nong* (Blood Mansion Dispel Stasis Gelatin Capsules)," *Bei Jing Zhong Yi (Beijing Chinese Medicine)*, #1, 2000, p. 61

Zhang Ming, "The Treatment of 40 Cases of Diabetic Neurogenic Bladder with *Gui Qi Tang* (Cinnamon & Astragalus Decoction)," *Si Chuan Zhong Yi (Sichuan Chinese Medicine)*, #1, 2001, p. 31

Zhang Min, "A Survey of Treatment Efficacy in the Treatment of 35 Cases of Diabetic Constipation by the Methods of Boosting the Qi & Nourishing Yin, Transforming Stasis & Freeing the Flow of the Network Vessels," *Xin Zhong Yi (New Chinese Medicine)*, #7, 2001, p. 29-30

Zhang Ming *et al.*, "The Treatment of 30 Cases of Diabetes & Cerebral Infarction with Internally Administered Chinese Medicinals & Blood Clot Freeing Flow Intravenous Drip," *Zhe Jiang Zhong Yi Za Zhi (Zhejiang Journal of Chinese Medicine)*, #4, 2001, p. 143

Zhang Wen-qu, "A Discussion of the Integrated Chinese-Medical Treatment of the Common Complications of Diabetes," *Hu Bei Zhong Yi Za Zhi (Hubei Journal of Chinese Medicine)*, #5, 1998, p. 5-7

Zhang Xue-hong, "The Treatment of 32 Cases of Type II Diabetes Using *Jia Wei Er Chen Tang* (Added Flavors Two Aged [Ingredients] Decoction)," *Zhe Jiang Zhong Yi Za Zhi (Zhejiang Journal of Chinese Medicine)*, #1, 1994, p. 9

Zhang Xue-jan & Hu Ke-jie, "A Discussion of the Treatment of Diabetic Hypertension with Chinese Medicinals," *Hei Long Jiang Zhong Yi Yao (Heilongjiang Chinese Medicine & Medicinals)*, #5, 1998, p. 21-22

Zhang Yan, "Pattern Discrimination in Wasting & Thirsting Disease," *Hei Long Jiang Zhong Yi Yao (Heilongjiang Chinese Medicine & Medicinals)*, #2, 1999, p. 42-43

Zhang Ying-qiang, "Professor Zhang Fa-rong's Experiences in the Treatment of Diabetic Encephalopathy," *Si Chuan Zhong Yi (Sichuan Chinese Medicine)*, #11, 2000, p. 1-2

Zhang Ying-wen, "The Treatment of 52 Cases of Diabetic Nephropathy Using Self-composed *Jiang Tang Shen Ning* (Lower Sugar Kidney Calmer)," *Hei Long Jiang Zhong Yi Yao (Heilongjiang Chinese Medicine & Medicinals)*, #4, 1998, p. 23

Zhang Yong-tao, "A Treatise on the Relationship between the Spleen & Type II Diabetic Insulin Resistance," *Xia Zhong Yi (New Chinese Medicine)* #6, 2001, p. 3-5

Zhang Yu-jin & Zhang Wen-zhi, "An Exploration of the Pattern Discrimination of Hypertension & Insulin Resistance," *He Nan Zhong Yi (Henan Chinese Medicine)*, #1, 2001, p. 35-36

Zhang Ze-sheng *et al.*, "A Clinical Audit of the Treatment of 64 Cases of Diabetic Nephropathy by the Methods of Boosting the Kidneys, Supporting the Spleen, Transforming Stasis & Downbearing Turbidity," *Xin Zhong Yi (New Chinese Medicine)*, #11, 2001, p. 36-37

Zhang Zhe & Niu Xi-wei, "The Treatment of 36 Cases of Diabetic Peripheral Neuritis with *Liao Bi Tong Luo Tang* (Treat Impediment & Free the Flow of the Network Vessels Decoction)," *Si Chuan Zhong Yi (Sichuan Chinese Medicine)*, #10, 2000, p. 24

Zhang Zhen-che & Zhang Wen-jian, "The Treatment of 45 Cases of Diabetes & Recalcitrant Oral Thrush by Enriching Yin & Clearing Heat," *Zhe Jiang Zhong Yi Za Zhi (Zhejiang Journal of Chinese Medicine)*, #1, 1994, p. 8

Zhao Hong, "The Treatment of Diabetic Retinopathy

Based on Pattern Discrimination," *He Nan Zhong Yi* (*Henan Chinese Medicine*), #3, 2001, p. 54

Zhao Huo-xiang, "The Treatment of 79 Cases of Diabetic Gastric Paresis by the Methods of Arousing the Spleen & Moving the Spleen," *Bei Jing Zhong Yi* (*Beijing Chinese Medicine*), #4, 2000, p. 18-19

Zhao Jie, "Understanding Based on Experience of the Pattern Discrimination Treatment of Diabetes à la Spleen Yin Vacuity," *Si Chuan Zhong Yi* (*Sichuan Chinese Medicine*), #6, 2001, p. 10-11

Zhao Kun *et al.*, "Professor Zhang Su-qing's Experience of the Diagnosis & Treatment of Diabetes," *Xin Zhong Yi* (*New Chinese Medicine*), #5, 2001, p. 14-15

Zhao Yuan-ying *et al.*, "The Treatment of Diabetic Peripheral Angioneuropathy Using *Bu Qi Huo Xue Tang* (Supplement the Qi & Quicken the Blood Decoction)," *Ji Lin Zhong Yi Yao* (*Jilin Chinese Medicine & Medicinals*), #2, 1999, p. 28

Zheng Bi-fang & Zhang Yi, "The Treatment of 21 Cases of Diabetic Nephropathy with Integrated Chinese- Western Medicine," *Shan Xi Zhong Yi* (*Shanxi Chinese Medicine*), #1, 2001, p. 33

Zheng Qiang, "The Treatment of 60 Cases of Geriatric Diabetic Profuse Sweating with *Bu Yang Huan Wu Tang* (Supplement Yang & Restore Five [Tenths] Decoction) plus *Sheng Mai Yin* (Engender the Pulse Drink)," *Zhe Jiang Zhong Yi Za Zhi* (*Zhejiang Journal of Chinese Medicine*), #11, 2001, p. 472

Zheng Xiao-jun *et al.*, "The Treatment of 48 Cases of Mild Diabetic Gastric Paresis with *Sheng Yang Yi Wei Tang* (Upbear Yang & Boost the Stomach Decoction)," *Si Chuan Zhong Yi* (*Sichuan Chinese Medicine*), #7, 2001, p. 29-30

Zhong Song-cai, "A Clinical Audit of the Treatment of 64 Cases of Type II Diabetes by Simultaneously Treating the Spleen & Kidneys," *Hu Nan Zhong Yi Za Zhi* (*Hunan Journal of Chinese Medicine*), #6, 2000, p. 13-14

Zhou Guo-ying *et al.*, "A Study of the Relationship Between the Pattern of Qi & Yin Vacuity Type II Diabetes and Insulin Resistance," *Fu Jian Zhong Yi Yao* (*Fujian Chinese Medicine & Medicinals*), #2, 2000, p. 7-8

Zhou Jian, "The Treatment of 93 Cases of Diabetic Peripheral Neuropathy Using *Yi Qi Yang Yin Huo Xue*

Tang (Boost the Qi, Nourish Yin & Quicken the Blood Decoction)," *Shi Yong Zhong Yi Nei Ke Za Zhi* (*Journal of Practical Chinese Medicine Internal Medicine*), #1, 2001, p. 25

Zhou Jian-yang, "Sublingual Vessels & Network Vessels Static Blood & Diabetes," *Zhe Jiang Zhong Yi Za Zhi* (*Zhejiang Journal of Chinese Medicine*), #2, 2000, p. 88-89

Zhou Jun-huai, "The Integrated Chinese-Western Medical Treatment of 50 Cases of Type II Diabetes," *Hu Nan Zhong Yi Za Zhi* (*Hunan Journal of Chinese Medicine*), #2, 2001, p. 44

Zhou Miao-ying, "The Treatment of Blood Stasis in 38 Cases of Type II Diabetes Using *Fu Yuan Huo Xue Tang Jia Wei* (Restore the Source & Quicken the Blood Decoction with Added Flavors)," *Ji Lin Zhong Yi Yao* (*Jilin Chinese Medicine & Medicinals*), #2, 1999, p. 13

Zhou Qi-xuan, "A Clinical Audit of the Treatment of 61 Cases of Diabetes with *Qi Ling Tang* (Astragalus & Clematis Decoction)," *Bei Jing Zhong Yi* (*Beijing Chinese Medicine*), #6, 2000, p. 32-33

Zhou Xin, "Recent Developments in Using Chinese Medicinals in the Treatment of Diabetic Nephropathy," *Si Chuan Zhong Yi* (*Sichuan Chinese Medicine*), #11, 1998, p. 14-16

Zhou Xun-ru & Wu Geng-yu, "The Treatment of 60 Cases of Type II Diabetes with *Zi Yin Jiang Tang Tang* (Enrich Yin & Lower Sugar Decoction)," *Zhe Jiang Zhong Yi Za Zhi* (*Zhejiang Journal of Chinese Medicine*), #8, 1999, p. 328

Zhu Fang-shi *et al.*, "A Study of the Chinese Medical Patterns of Diabetic Gastroparesis," *Jiang Su Zhong Yi* (*Jiangsu Chinese Medicine*), #6, 2000, p. 13-15

Zhu Yong-juan, "A Clinical Audit of the Treatment of 100 Cases of Type II Diabetes Via the Liver," *Shang Hai Zhong Yi Za Zhi* (*Shanghai Journal of Chinese Medicine & Medicinals*), #7, 1999, p. 19-20

Zhuang Xiao-ming, "A Discussion on the Pattern Discrimination & Treatment of 56 Cases of Diabetes," *Gan Su Zhong Yi* (*Gansu Chinese Medicine*), #2, 1998, p. 9

Zou Shi-chang, "A Clinical Audit of the Treatment of 42 Cases of Slight Diabetic Gastroparesis with *Wu Mei Wan* (Mume Pills)," *Xin Zhong Yi* (*New Chinese Medicine*), #12, 2001, p. 34-35

Zou Yuan *et al.*, "The Treatment of 64 Cases of Diabetes with *Shen Li Jiang Tang Kou Fu Ye* (Ginseng Lower Sugar Orally Administered Liquid)," *Si Chuan Zhong Yi (Sichuan Chinese Medicine)*, #9, 1999, p. 28

ENGLISH LANGUAGE BIBLIOGRAPHY

BOOKS

Adams, R. & Victor, M., *Principles of Neurology*, 6th edition, McGraw-Hill Co., NY, 1997

American Association of Clinical Endocrinologists, *Medical Guidelines for the Management of Diabetes Mellitus: The AACE System of Intensive Diabetes Self-management*, AACE, Jacksonville, FL, 2000

American Diabetes Association, *Complete Guide to Diabetes*, Bantam Books, NY, 1999

Becker, Simon, *A Handbook of Chinese Hematology*, Blue Poppy Press, Boulder, CO, 2000

Beers, Mark H. & Berkow, Robert, *The Merck Manual*, 17th edition, Merck Research Laboratories, Whitehouse Station, NJ, 1999

Bensky, Dan & Barolet, Randall, *Chinese Herbal Medicine: Formulas & Strategies*, Eastland Press, Seattle, 1990

Bensky, Dan & Gamble, Andrew, *Chinese Herbal Medicine: Materia Medica*, Eastland Press, Seattle, 1993

Bliss, Michael, *The Discovery of Insulin*, University of Chicago Press, Chicago, 1982

Braunwald, Isselbacher, Petersdorf *et al.*, *Harrison's Principles of Internal Medicine*, 14th edition, McGraw-Hill Co., NY, 1997

Brooks, G.A., *Exercise Physiology*, Macmillan Publishing Co., NY, 1985

Chen Ji-rui & Wang, Nissi, *Acupuncture Case Histories from China*, Eastland Press, Seattle, 1988

Chen Jin-ding, *The Treatment of Diabetes with Traditional Chinese Medicine*, trans. by Sun Ying-kui & Zhou Shu-hui, revised by Lu Yu-bin, Shandong Science & Technology Press, Jinan, 1994

Chen Ke-ji, *Traditional Chinese Medicine: Clinical Case Studies*, Foreign Languages Press, Beijing, 1994

Chen You-bang & Deng Liang-yue, *Essentials of Contemporary Chinese Acupuncturists' Clinical Experiences*, Foreign Languages Press, Beijing, 1989

Cheng Yi-chun, *Nonpharmacotherapies for Diabetes*, Shandong Science & Technology Press, Jinan, 1997

Cohen, Kenneth S., *The Way of Qigong: The Art and Science of Chinese Energy Healing*, Balantine Books, NY, 1997

Ellis, Andrew, Wiseman, Nigel & Boss, Ken, *Fundamentals of Chinese Acupuncture*, Paradigm Publications, Brookline, MA, 1988

Fallon, Sally & Enig Mary, Ph.D., *Nourishing Traditions*, New Trends Publishing, Inc., Washington DC, 1999

Flaws, Bob, *A Handbook of TCM Pediatrics*, Blue Poppy Press, Boulder, CO, 1997

Flaws, Bob, *The Book of Jook*, Blue Poppy Press, Boulder, CO, 2001

Flaws, Bob, *The Tao of Healthy Eating*, Blue Poppy Press, Boulder, CO, 1998

Franz, M.J. & Norstrom, J., *Diabetes Actively Staying Healthy (DASH): Your Game Plan for Diabetes and Exercise*, International Diabetes Center, Minneapolis, 1990

Gates, J.L., *Diabetes and Diabetic Foot: Etiology, Prevention, and Management*, Johnson & Johnson Medical, Arlington, TX, 1999

Gates, Judy, *Diabetes: Etiology, Management Advances, and Early Interventions*, Primedia Healthcare, Carrollton, TX, 2001

Hollander, P. *et al.*, *Intensified Insulin Management and You*, International Diabetes Center, Minneapolis, 1990

Hou Jing-lun *et al.*, *Traditional Chinese Treatment for Hypertension*, Academy Press, Beijing, 1995

Huang-fu Mi, *The Systematic Classic of Acupuncture & Moxibustion*, trans. by Yang Shou-zhong & Charles Chace, Blue Poppy Press, Boulder, CO, 1994

Kahn, R. & Weir, G.C., *Joslin's Diabetes Mellitus*, 13th edition, Lea & Febiger, Macern, PA, 1994

Kahn, R., *Medical Management of Non-insulin Dependent (Type II) Diabetes*, American Diabetes Association, Alexandria, VA, 1994

Kuchinski, Lynn M., *Controlling Diabetes Naturally with Chinese Medicine*, Blue Poppy Press, Boulder, CO, 1999

Kushi, Michio, *Diabetes and Hypoglycemia*, Japan Publications, Inc., NY, 1985

Lee, Miriam, *Insights of a Senior Acupuncturist*, Blue Poppy Press, Boulder, CO, 1992

Lee, Miriam, *Master Tong's Acupuncture: An Ancient Alternative Style in Modern Clinical Practice*, 2nd edition, Blue Poppy Press, Boulder, CO, 1998

Leovitz, H.E., *Therapy for Diabetes Mellitus and Related Disorders*, American Diabetes Association, Alexandria, VA, 1994

Li Dong-yuan, *The Treatise on the Spleen & Stomach*, trans. by Yang Shou-zhong, Blue Poppy Press, Boulder, CO, 1993

Lu, Henry C., *Chinese System of Food Cures*, Sterling Publishing Company, Inc., NY, 1986

National Diabetes Data Group, *Diabetes in America*, 2nd edition, National Institutes of Health, Bethesda, MD, 1995

Pastors, J.G., *Nutritional Care of Diabetes*, Nutrition Dimensions, San Marcos, CA, 1992

Peragalla-Dittko, V. *et al.*, *A Core Curriculum for Diabetes Education*, 2nd edition, American Association for Diabetes Education, Chicago, 1993

Ruderman, N. & Devlin, J.T., *The Health Professional's Guide to Diabetes and Exercise*, American Diabetes Association, Alexandria, VA, 1995

Shang Xian-min *et al.*, *Practical Traditional Chinese Medicine & Pharmacology: Clinical Experiences*, New World Press, Beijing, 1990

Shao Nian-fang, *The Treatment of Knotty Diseases with Chinese Acupuncture and Chinese Herbal Medicine*, trans. by Xiao Gong & Zuo Lian-jun, Shandong Science & Technology Press, Jinan, 1990

Sionneau, Philippe & Lü Gang, *The Treatment of Disease in TCM, Vol. 1-7*, Blue Poppy Press, Boulder, CO, 2000

Temple, Robert, *The Genius of China: 3,000 Years of Science, Discovery and Invention*, Simon & Schuster, Inc., NY, 1986

Tsay, Kuei-shi, *Acupuncturist's Handbook: A Practical Encyclopedia*, CPM Whole Health, Chestnut Hill, MA, 1995

Wexu, Mario, *The Ear: Gateway to Balancing the Body*, Aurora Press, Santa Fe, NM, 1985

Wiseman, Nigel & Feng Ye, *A Practical Dictionary of Chinese Medicine*, Paradigm Publications, Brookline, MA, 1998

Wolfe, Honora Lee & Crescenz, Rose, *Highlights of Ancient Acupuncture Prescriptions*, Blue Poppy Press, Boulder, CO, 1991

Yan De-xin, *Aging & Blood Stasis: A New TCM Approach to Geriatrics*, trans. by Tang Guo-shun & Bob Flaws, Blue Poppy Press, Boulder, CO, 2000

Yu Hui-chan & Han Fu-ru, *Golden Needle Wang Le-ting*, trans. by Shuai Xue-zhong, Blue Poppy Press, Boulder, CO, 1997

Yu Jin, *Obstetrics and Gynecology in Chinese Medicine*, Eastland Press, Seattle, 1998

Zheng Mei-quan, *The Chinese Plum Blossom Needle Therapy*, People's Medical Publishing Co., Beijing, 1984

Zhu Dan-xi, *The Heart & Essence of Dan-xi's Methods of Treatment*, trans. by Yang Shou-zhong, Blue Poppy Press, Boulder, CO, 1993

JOURNAL ARTICLES

American Diabetes Association, "Economic Consequences of Diabetes Mellitus in the U.S. in 1997," *Diabetes Care*, #2, 1998, p. 296-309

Chen Jian-fei, "A Hemorrheological Study on the Effect of Acupuncture in Treating Diabetes Mellitus," *Journal of Traditional Chinese Medicine*, #2, 1987, p. 95-100

Choate, Clinton J., "Diabetes Mellitus: Modern Medicine and Traditional Chinese Medicine (Part One)," *Journal of Chinese Medicine*, UK, #58, 1998, p. 5-14 http://www.acupuncture.com

Choate, Clinton J., "Diabetes Mellitus: Modern Medicine and Traditional Chinese Medicine (Part Two)," *Journal of Chinese Medicine*, UK, #59, 1999, p. 5-12

Choate, Clinton J., "Diabetes Mellitus: Modern Medicine and Traditional Chinese Medicine (Part Three)," *Journal of Chinese Medicine*, UK, #60, 1999, p. 27-36

Darlington, Joy, "Beat the Sugar Blues," *Vegetarian Times*, Apr. 2000, p. 66-77

Davis, Ted, "Diabetes Mellitus, Part 1," *Australian Journal of Acupuncture*, Apr. 1991, p. 23-31

Davis, Ted, "Diabetes Mellitus, Part 2," *Australian Journal of Acupuncture*, Sept. 1991, p. 17-23

Davis, Ted, "Diabetes Mellitus: West Meets East, Some Reflections Upon TCM Theory," *Australian Journal of Acupuncture*, Spring, 1992, p. 9-19

Dharmanada, Subhuti, "Treatment of Diabetes with Acupuncture and Chinese Herbs," *Institute for Traditional Medicine*, Portland, OR, 1996

Dufty, William, *Sugar Blues*, Warner Books, Padnor, PA, 1975

Fan Guan-jie *et al.*, "Treatment of Diabetic Gangrene by Stage Differentiation," *Journal of Chinese Medicine*, UK, #65, 2001, p. 50-51

Fischman, Josh, "Facing Down a Killer Disease," *U.S. News and World Report*, Jun. 25, 2001, p. 59-69

Fruehauf, Heiner, "The Treatment of Kidney Failure and Uraemia with Chinese Herbs," *Journal of Chinese Medicine*, UK, #60, 1999, 13-17

Gao Lu-wen, "Regulating Qi and Resolving Phlegm to Treat the Complications of Diabetes," *Journal of Chinese Medicine*, UK, #64, 2000, p. 20-21

Gavin, James *et al.*, "Oral Antidiabetic Drugs: One Size Does Not Fit All," *Patient Care Nurse Practitioner*, Mar. 1998, p. 18-32

Genouth, Saul *et al.*, "Diabetes Treatment Moves Forward: New Criteria for Diagnosis, Screening, and Classification," *Patient Care Nurse Practitioner*, Mar. 1998, p. 12-17

Hsu Chou-xin & Chen Ze-lin, "Prevention and

Treatment of Diabetic Foot," *The International Journal of Oriental Medicine*, #1, 1995, p. 13-16

Ikeda, Masakazu, "Diabetes," trans. by Edward Obaidey, *Pacific Journal of Oriental Medicine*, #7, p. 18-19

Jiang Jing, "Diabetes & Hypoglycemia," *Oriental Medicine*, #4, 1993, p. 50-53

Krieger, Diane *et al.*, "Insulin: Recent Developments and Common Quandaries," *Patient Care Nurse Practitioner*, Mar. 1998, p. 33-39

Lade, Heiko, "Diabetes," *Pacific Journal of Oriental Medicine*, #12, p. 34-42

Leslie, C.A., "New Insulin Replacement Technologies: Overcoming Barriers to Tight Glycemic Control," *Cleveland Journal of Medicine*, #66, 1999, p. 293-302

Li Rui-yi *et al.*, "The TCM Treatment of Diabetic Hearing Loss," *Journal of Chinese Medicine*, UK, #65, 2001, p. 52

Lin Yun-gui *et al.*, "Treatment of Diabetes with Moxibustion," *Journal of Traditional Chinese Medicine*, #1, 1987, p. 12-14

Lu Xian & Rodriguez, "The Application of Tonifying Yang for the Treatment of Diabetes," *Journal of Chinese Medicine*, UK, #67, 2001, p. 32-34

Luger, Todd, "Treatment of Diabetes Mellitus with Chinese Medicinal Substances," *International Journal of Oriental Medicine*, #1, 1995, p. 1-12

Ren Hui-ya, "A Clinical Study of the Treatment of Diabetic Peripheral Neuropathy with *Tang Zhi Min* Capsules," *Journal of Chinese Medicine*, UK, #65, 2001, p. 50

Saudek, Christopher D. & Daly, Anne E., "Diabetes Update," *Newsweek*, Aug. 27, 2001, special advertising section, p. 1-8

Schwartz, R.S., "Exercise Training in the Treatment of Diabetes Mellitus in Elderly Patients," *Diabetes Care*, #2, 1990, p. 77-84

Sun Pei-lun, "The Treatment of Polyneuritis by TCM," *Journal of Chinese Medicine*, UK, #46, 1994, p. 33-35

Wang Jia-xiu, "Classics on Dietotherapy," *Journal of Traditional Chinese Medicine*, #7, 1987, p.233-234

Wei Zhi-hua *et al.*, "Fructus Schisandrae Protects Vascular Endothelial Cells from Oxidative Injury," *Journal of Oriental Medicine in America*, #1, 1997, p. 31-37

Wu Shen-tao *et al.*, "The Treatment of Early Stage Diabetic Neuropathy by Clearing Stomach Heat, Purging Heart Fire, Strengthening the Spleen, and Supplementing the Kidneys," *Journal of Chinese Medicine*, UK, #65, 2001, p. 51-52

Xiao Fei & Liu Wei, "Observation on the Treatment of Dysphasia Due to Cerebrovascular Accident with Electroacupuncture at *She Gen* Point," *Journal of Chinese Medicine*, UK, #50, 1996, p. 27-29

Yin Guang-yao & Yin Yu-fen, "Clinical Research into Zhuchun Capsule Effect [*sic*] on Immune and Endocrine Function in Geriatric Patients with Kidney Yang Vacuity," *International Journal of Oriental Medicine*, #2, 1993, p. 100-102

Zhang Han-jun, "Efficacy of Acupuncture in the Treatment of Post-stroke Aphasia," "*Journal of Traditional Chinese Medicine*, #9, 1989, p.87-89

FORMULA INDEX

GENERAL INDEX

ACUPOINT POCKET REFERENCE
by Bob Flaws
ISBN 0-936185-93-7

ACUPUNCTURE AND MOXIBUSTION
FORMULAS & TREATMENTS
by Cheng Dan-an, trans. by Wu Ming
ISBN 0-936185-68-6

ACUPUNCTURE PHYSICAL
MEDICINE: An Acupuncture Touchpoint
Approach to the Treatment of Chronic Pain,
Fatigue, and Stress Disorders
by Mark Seem
ISBN 1-891845-13-6

AGING & BLOOD STASIS: A New Approach
to TCM Geriatrics
by Yan De-xin
ISBN 0-936185-63-5

BETTER BREAST HEALTH NATURALLY
WITH CHINESE MEDICINE
by Honora Lee Wolfe & Bob Flaws
ISBN 0-936185-90-2

THE BOOK OF JOOK:
Chinese Medicinal Porridges
by Bob Flaws
ISBN 0-936185-60-0

CHANNEL DIVERGENCES:
Deeper Pathways of the Web
by Miki Shima & Charles Chase
ISBN 1-891845-15-2

CHINESE MEDICAL PALMISTRY:
Your Health in Your Hand
by Zong Xiao-fan & Gary Liscum
ISBN 0-936185-64-3

CHINESE MEDICAL PSYCHIATRY:
A Textbook and Clinical Manual
by Bob Flaws & James Lake, MD
ISBN 1-845891-17-9

CHINESE MEDICINAL TEAS: Simple, Proven,
Folk Formulas for Common Diseases &
Promoting Health
by Zong Xiao-fan & Gary Liscum
ISBN 0-936185-76-7

CHINESE MEDICINAL
WINES & ELIXIRS
by Bob Flaws
ISBN 0-936185-58-9

CHINESE PEDIATRIC MASSAGE
THERAPY: A Parent's & Practitioner's Guide
to the Prevention & Treatment
of Childhood Illness
by Fan Ya-li
ISBN 0-936185-54-6

CHINESE SELF-MASSAGE THERAPY:
The Easy Way to Health
by Fan Ya-li
ISBN 0-936185-74-0

THE CLASSIC OF DIFFICULTIES:
A Translation of the Nan Jing
translation by Bob Flaws
ISBN 1-891845-07-1

CONTROLLING DIABETES NATURALLY
WITH CHINESE MEDICINE
by Lynn Kuchinski
ISBN 0-936185-06-3

CURING ARTHRITIS NATURALLY
WITH CHINESE MEDICINE
by Douglas Frank & Bob Flaws
ISBN 0-936185-87-2

CURING DEPRESSION NATURALLY
WITH CHINESE MEDICINE
by Rosa Schnyer & Bob Flaws
ISBN 0-936185-94-5

CURING FIBROMYALGIA NATURALLY
WITH CHINESE MEDICINE
by Bob Flaws
ISBN 1-891845-08-9

CURING HAY FEVER NATURALLY
WITH CHINESE MEDICINE
by Bob Flaws
ISBN 0-936185-91-0

CURING HEADACHES NATURALLY
WITH CHINESE MEDICINE
by Bob Flaws
ISBN 0-936185-95-3-X

CURING IBS NATURALLY WITH
CHINESE MEDICINE
by Jane Bean Oberski
ISBN 1-891845-11-X

CURING INSOMNIA NATURALLY
WITH CHINESE MEDICINE
by Bob Flaws
ISBN 0-936185-85-6

CURING PMS NATURALLY
WITH CHINESE MEDICINE
by Bob Flaws
ISBN 0-936185-85-6

THE DIVINE FARMER'S MATERIA
MEDICA: A Translation of the
Shen Nong Ben Cao
translation by Yang Shouz-zhong
ISBN 0-936185-96-1

THE DIVINELY RESPONDING CLASSIC:
A Translation of the Shen Ying Jing from Zhen
Jiu Da Cheng
trans. by Yang Shou-zhong & Liu Feng-ting
ISBN 0-936185-55-4

DUI YAO: The Art of Combining Chinese
Herbal Medicinals
by Philippe Sionneau
ISBN 0-936185-81-3

ENDOMETRIOSIS, INFERTILITY AND
TRADITIONAL CHINESE MEDICINE:
A Laywoman's Guide
by Bob Flaws
ISBN 0-936185-14-7

THE ESSENCE OF LIU FENG-WU'S
GYNECOLOGY
by Liu Feng-wu, translated by Yang Shou-zhong
ISBN 0-936185-88-0

EXTRA TREATISES BASED ON INVESTIGA-
TION & INQUIRY: A Translation of Zhu Dan-
xi's Ge Zhi Yu Lun
translation by Yang Shou-zhong
ISBN 0-936185-53-8

FIRE IN THE VALLEY: TCM Diagnosis &
Treatment of Vaginal Diseases
by Bob Flaws
ISBN 0-936185-25-2

FU QING-ZHU'S GYNECOLOGY
trans. by Yang Shou-zhong & Liu Da-wei
ISBN 0-936185-35-X

FULFILLING THE ESSENCE: A Handbook of
Traditional & Contemporary Treatments for
Female Infertility
by Bob Flaws
ISBN 0-936185-48-1

GOLDEN NEEDLE WANG LE-TING:
A 20th Century Master's Approach
to Acupuncture
by Yu Hui-chan & Han Fu-ru,
trans. by Shuai Xue-zhong
ISBN 0-936185-78-3

A GUIDE TO GYNECOLOGY
by Ye Heng-yin,
trans. by Bob Flaws & Shuai Xue-zhong
ISBN 1-891845-19-5

A HANDBOOK OF CHINESE
HEMATOLOGY
by Simon Becker
ISBN 1-891845-16-0

A HANDBOOK OF MENSTRUAL
DISEASES IN CHINESE MEDICINE
by Bob Flaws
ISBN 0-936185-82-1

A HANDBOOK OF TCM PATTERNS
& TREATMENTS
by Bob Flaws & Daniel Finney
ISBN 0-936185-70-8

A HANDBOOK OF TCM PEDIATRICS
by Bob Flaws
ISBN 0-936185-72-4

A HANDBOOK OF TCM UROLOGY & MALE
SEXUAL DYSFUNCTION
by Anna Lin, OMD
ISBN 0-936185-36-8

A HANDBOOK OF TRADITIONAL
CHINESE DERMATOLOGY
by Liang Jian-hui,
trans. by Zhang Ting-liang & Bob Flaws
ISBN 0-926185-07-4

STATEMENTS OF FACT IN
TRADITIONAL CHINESE MEDICINE
by Bob Flaws
ISBN 0-936185-52-X

STICKING TO THE POINT 1: A Rational
Methodology for the Step by Step Formulation
& Administration of an Acupuncture Treatment
by Bob Flaws
ISBN 0-936185-17-1

STICKING TO THE POINT 2: A Study of
Acupuncture & Moxibustion Formulas
and Strategies
by Bob Flaws
ISBN 0-936185-97-X

A STUDY OF DAOIST ACUPUNCTURE
& MOXIBUSTION
by Liu Zheng-cai
ISBN 1-891845-08-X

THE SYSTEMATIC CLASSIC OF
ACUPUNCTURE & MOXIBUSTION:
A Translation of the Jia Yi Jing
by Huang-fu Mi,
trans. by Yang Shou-zhong & Charles Chace
ISBN 0-936185-29-5

THE TAO OF HEALTHY EATING
ACCORDING TO CHINESE MEDICINE
by Bob Flaws
ISBN 0-936185-92-9

TEACH YOURSELF TO READ
MODERN MEDICAL CHINESE
by Bob Flaws
ISBN 0-936185-99-6

THE TREATMENT OF DIABETES
MELLITUS WITH CHINESE MEDICINE
by Bob Flaws, Lynn Kuchinski &
Robert Casañas, MD
ISBN 1-891845-21-7

THE TREATMENT OF DISEASE Vol. I:
Diseases of the Head & Face
Including Mental/Emotional Disorders
by Philippe Sionneau & Lü Gang
ISBN 0-936185-69-4

THE TREATMENT OF DISEASE, Vol. II:
Diseases of the Eyes, Ears, Nose, & Throat
by Sionneau & Lü
ISBN 0-936185-73-2

THE TREATMENT OF DISEASE, Vol. III:
Diseases of the Mouth, Lips, Tongue,
Teeth & Gums
by Sionneau & Lü
ISBN 0-936185-79-1

THE TREATMENT OF DISEASE, Vol. IV:
Diseases of the Neck, Shoulders, Back,
& Limbs
by Sionneau & Lü
ISBN 0-936185-89-9

THE TREATMENT OF DISEASE, Vol. V:
Diseases of the Chest & Abdomen
by Sionneau & Lü
ISBN 1-891845-02-0

THE TREATMENT OF DISEASE, Vol. VI:
Diseases of the Urogential System & Proctology
by Sionneau & Lü
ISBN 1-891845-05-5

THE TREATMENT OF DISEASE, Vol. VII:
General Symptoms
by Sionneau & Lü
ISBN 1-891845-14-4

THE TREATMENT OF EXTERNAL
DISEASES WITH ACUPUNCTURE
& MOXIBUSTION
by Yan Cui-lan & Zhu Yun-long,
trans. by Yang Shou-zhong
ISBN 0-936185-80-5

THE TREATMENT OF MODERN WESTERN
MEDICAL DISEASES WITH
CHINESE MEDICINE:
A Textbook and Clinical Manual
by Bob Flaws & Philippe Sionneau
ISBN 1-891845-20-9

160 ESSENTIAL CHINESE HERBAL
PATENT MEDICINES
by Bob Flaws
ISBN 1-891945-12-8

230 ESSENTIAL CHINESE
MEDICINALS
by Bob Flaws
ISBN 1-891845-03-9

630 QUESTIONS & ANSWERS ABOUT
CHINESE HERBAL MEDICINE:
A Workbook & Study Guide
by Bob Flaws
ISBN 1-891845-04-7

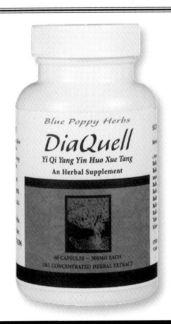

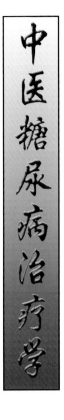

Don't forget to visit
The companion website for this book at

www.chinesemedicaldiabetes.com

This website is meant as a companion to Bob Flaws, Lynn Kuchinski & Robert Casañas's book, *The Treatment of Diabetes Mellitus with Chinese Medicine* available from Blue Poppy Press in Summer 2002. This site is intended for students and practitioners of Chinese medicine as well as practitioners of other health care systems interested in Chinese medicine and diabetes and its complications to do further research in this area. Hopefully, the resources it contains will be of use to all those interested in further researching Chinese medicine and diabetes. This site also serves as a repository of newly found, developed, and/or translated materials that did not make it into the book at the time the text was frozen. It is our intention to continually add new materials on Chinese medicine, acupuncture, and diabetes to this site.

Here's some of what you will find at www.chinesemedicaldiabetes.com:

Many new articles, research reports, and clinical audits recently translated from Chinese medical journals with new articles being added regularly. Find out about:

❖ Insulin Resistance Syndrome & Treatment Based on
     Pattern Discrimination
❖ Diabetes & Acupuncture
❖ Diabetic Constipation
❖ The Integrated Chinese-Western Medical Treatment of
     Diabetic Retinopathy
❖ Chinese Medicine & Impaired Glucose Tolerance
❖ Diabetic Peripheral Neuropathy & Integrated
     Chinese-Western Medicine
❖ And many more free articles

Scores of hyperlinks to other sites on the Web for doing research into all aspects of Diabetes Mellitus

❖ An online glossary of Western medical terms
❖ An online listing of the side effects of common diabetic drugs
❖ A bibliography of Chinese medical sources on diabetes
❖ Biographies of Bob Flaws, Lynn Kuchinski & Robert Casañas, MD

This is the premier site on the web for the research and discussion of all topics and issues related to Chinese medicine & Diabetes. It can also be accessed via **www.bluepoppy.com**.